Clinical Decision-Making in Fluency Disorders

Second Edition

Walter H. Manning, Ph.D.
The University of Memphis

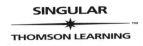

SINGULAR

™

THOMSON LEARNING

Vancouver, Canada   Auckland, New Zealand   Calgary, Canada

SINGULAR

✳ ™

THOMSON LEARNING

Clinical Decision-Making in Fluency Disorders , Second Edition

by Walter H. Manning, Ph.D.

Business Unit Director:
William Brottmiller

Acquisitions Editor:
Marie Linvill

Editorial Assistant:
Cara Jenkins

Executive Marketing Manager:
Dawn Gerrain

Channel Manager:
Kathryn Bamberger

Executive Production Editor:
Barb Bullock

Production Editor:
Brad Bielawski

Library of Congress Cataloging-in-Publication Data Available upon request

NOTICE TO THE READER

Dedication

The second edition of this book, as was the first, is dedicated to Sallie Starr Hillard. Sallie was a friend, a colleague, and a counselor to many people. She was a grand clinician because she was a person with marvelous wisdom and grace. We had intended to write the first edition together. Many of her thoughts continue to flow through this edition, and I believe, as with the first edition, that she is able to know of its completion.

Contents

Preface

The writing of the book proved one of its central points: that we write to find out what we know and what we want to say. I thought of how often as a writer I had made clear to myself some subject I had previously known nothing about by just putting one sentence after another—by reasoning my way in sequential steps to its meaning. I thought of how often the act of writing even the simplest document—a letter, for instance—had clarified my half-formed ideas. Writing and thinking and learning were the same process. (p. ix)

William Zinsser (1988). *Learning to Write.*

A primary goal of this book is to convey the enthusiasm and excitement of working, experimenting, and learning with people who stutter. I also want to provide the reader with overall strategies as well as a variety of specific techniques for conducting effective assessment and intervention for people who stutter or who have related fluency disorders. The readers who I have in mind as I write are graduate students who are beginning their first in-depth experience in the area of fluency disorders, as well as those experienced professionals who want to learn more about this specialty area. In some cases, the information and ideas discussed in these pages may also be helpful for individuals who stutter, for the intent of the book is to make stuttering less of a mystery and to provide a sense of direction for the (self-) treatment process.

This second edition includes information that has become available in the last few years. There are two new chapters. Chapter 3 describes the characteristics of onset and development apart from theories of etiology and sets the stage for subsequent chapters describing assessment procedures. Chapter 6 (Facilitating the Change Process) describes some basic aspects of human behavioral change and provides a context for many of the treatment suggestions found in subsequent chapters. There has also been a reordering of selected chapters so that information about the diagnosis and treatment of adults and adolescents is presented before information about younger children is discussed. At first, this may seem a bit awkward for some readers, since it is more common to discuss our clients in chronological order, describing children before adolescents and adults. However, we begin with the older speakers in order to present the many features of stuttering as they are manifested in its fully developed adult form, before describing issues more specific to younger speakers.

Although it is uncommon, I have again chosen to begin the text with a discussion of the characteristics of an ideal clinician. This is because I continue to believe that the clinician is at the center of a successful therapy experience. Although there are many similarities to be found in those who have chosen a career of helping people with communication disorders, there are some unique qualities that are desirable for those who are likely to be successful with individuals who stutter. Furthermore, many favorable comments about the first edition were in response to the information about clinicians, including humor as a variable in treatment (Chapter 1) and counseling (Chapter 7), and accordingly I have included additional information in these chapters. Finally, two features have been included to assist new clinicians in the process of clinical decision-making. First, there are several examples of clinical decisions that clinicians frequently make during assessment and treatment activities. Also in this edition we have included several study questions at the end of each chapter that readers may use for self-assessment.

The fundamental objectives that have guided the preparation of this text are the following:

1. to generate an enthusiasm in clinicians, especially graduate students, for working with children, adolescents, and adults who stutter;
2. to discuss clinical decision-making from the perspective of individual client needs;
3. to provide the clinician with choices of treatment strategies and associated techniques;
4. to discuss aspects of diagnosis and treatment that have been discussed very little or not at all in the literature; and
5. to suggest questions for clinical investigation in the general area of fluency disorders.

During the formulation and development of the profession of speech pathology in this country, particularly during the decades from the late 1920s through the 1960s, the area of fluency disorders was a major area of interest in our professional journals and texts. A review of the early issues of the *Journal of Speech Disorders* (published from 1936 through 1946) or the initial volumes of the *Journal of Speech and Hearing Disorders* confirms that a large proportion of the articles addressed the nature and treatment of stuttering. As the scope of practice continues to expand in the field of communication disorders, fluency disorders has become only one of many areas that students are presented with during their academic and clinical program. Today, students and professionals are exposed to areas of study that were not even acknowledged in the field only a few years ago. As the scope of practice for the field has expanded dramatically during the past two decades, graduate students in speech-language pathology are asked to become generalists across the wide range of human communication disorders. Perhaps, as Henri (1994) has suggested, "our clinical areas have simply become too substantial" (p. 45).

The depth of the field is also changing. Because clinicians are asked to become knowledgeable about so many different communication disorders and related areas, there is concern that the qualifications of professionals for serving any one disorder are being compromised. As a result, at the outset of the 21st century, professional clinicians will have the opportunity to become recognized as specialists in specific disorder areas. Specialty recognition is being driven both by the obvious need to enhance professional qualifications as well as the consumer demand for better services. In March of 1998, the Special Interest Division 4 (Fluency and Fluency Disorders) became the first specialty area within The American Speech-Language-Hearing Association to receive approval for establishing a Specialty Commission to oversee a specialty recognition program. A brief description of the current requirements for achieving and maintaining specialty recognition are described in Chapter 1. As the field of communication disorders continues to evolve, the critical mass of information will rapidly expand. Even within a single area of study such as fluency disorders, the literature is extensive and additional material is continually becoming available, recently including information available via computer and electronic networks (Appendix B).

Reading the volumes of literature can be intimidating, even for someone who has been a clinician and researcher in the field for many years. As Conture (1990) pointed out, it is easy to feel as though you are drowning in a sea of information, especially when some of it is conflicting. One wonders, as other authors have, what there is to say that is new. So much about stuttering and people who stutter has been said before—in some cases, probably more times than it needs to be (the many investigations of adaptation and consistency effects come to mind, as well as the discussions about the terms disfluent and dysfluent). In any case, one of the reasons for writing this book is to find out what I know and what I need to know about fluency disorders. This work is based on knowledge gained from a variety of texts, an extensive review of representative descriptive and experimental research, and 30 years of research and clinical work with individuals who have fluency disorders. It is also based on a successful experience of managing my own stuttered speech.

The intervention philosophy in this text is comprehensive. That is, I believe that successful treatment involves many levels of change. Fluency problems are multidimensional, involving—at the very least—attitudinal, behavioral, and cognitive features (the ABCs of stuttering, as Gene Cooper has referred to them). The process of human change involves many levels, and for most people counseling is often an important component of long-term success. Indeed, counseling and treatment are often one and the same. For a successful treatment outcome, especially for long-term success, each of these levels usually needs to be addressed. We need to change speech behavior, to be sure, but we also need to change ways of interpreting what is occurring during our attempts to communicate with another person. Our goal is change, not only in the nature of the speaker's fluency, but—more importantly—in the nature of the *person* who comes to us in order to live a better life.

No clinician who has recently completed a graduate program should expect to be perfect in her work, including speech-language pathologists. One or more classes, a text, and the initial years of experience with clients provide only a beginning to a lifelong career of learning about how to help people who stutter. If we continue to learn and do our job well, we can expect that many of our clients will be able to independently assess the situation, make decisions that are informed and truthful, use appropriate techniques for conceptualizing the situation, self-manage their speech, and create a new interpretation of their internal control as it relates to their speech. That last sentence represented many aspects of change. If our clients are able to do most of those things most of the time, they will be in a much better position to cope with their speech and their lives. Moreover, they will be less handicapped and have more options, which, after all, is the true measure of successful intervention.

One of the most difficult choices in preparing a text is not so much what to include but what information to omit. There have been and continue to be many diligent authors who have contributed to our knowledge about the age-old problem of stuttering. There is a desire to pay homage to those who have gone before and to acknowledge the colleagues you feel privileged to be working alongside in—as Charles Van Riper so often said—the vineyard of stuttering.

It is fitting at the outset to comment on some of the terms used in this book. Throughout the chapters, the clinician or speech-language pathologist is referred to by using feminine pronouns and clients are referred to by using masculine pronouns. Obviously, there are both male and female clients and clinicians, but since this reflects the most common clinical situation, this description will be used to enhance the consistency and ease of reading.

A somewhat more complicated issue is what to call the person who is doing the stuttering. In various contexts, he is referred to as the speaker, client, patient, subject, participant, or even consumer. For several years, there has been discussion concerning the appropriateness of using the term *stutterer*. Some have argued that the term is insensitive, too all-encompassing, and serves as a label that can negatively stereotype and limit how we define the problem as well as the person. Clearly a person who happens to stutter also takes on many other roles. Some have suggested using the person-first terms such as "person who stutters" (PWS) or "child who stutters" (CWS). While such terms may be seen by some as being somewhat more objective, they also tend to become ambiguous and result in an awkward writing style that is difficult to read. A few years ago, a friend with a background in psycholinguistics pointed out that the suffix *-er* means someone or something that performs the action of the root verb: someone who *does*, not someone who *is*. As we shall see, the variability of stuttering behavior also contributes to the problem of what to call our clients. That is, unlike someone who is blind or deaf or has lost a limb, the person who stutters is often fluent. Indeed, many people who stutter have no difficulty calling themselves stutterers even when they become highly fluent and even show pride in using the term, particularly if they are actively involved with a self-help association.

The approach I have chosen for this book is to use *person who stutters*, *speaker*, or *client* whenever possible. However, I will also use the term *stutterer* when it facilitates the clarity of the writing. To my knowledge there is no research that supports the notion that person-first terminology, however well-intentioned, promotes better attitudes by professionals or the public about people who have various problems or handicaps. The research that has been conducted indicates that person-first nomenclature has minimal value in reducing negative impressions about the situation (St. Louis, 1996). In any case, I want to state at the outset the earnest belief that, indeed, terms and categories do not define a person. Clearly, each client is vastly more than someone who stutters. This view is at the heart of any comprehensive and humanistic approach to the problem of stuttering. Just as the clinician makes decisions based on the needs of the client and the timing of treatment activities throughout the intervention process, a choice can be made about what terms are best in each case. If the clinician determines that the client attaches a stigma to the term *stutterer* and would feel more comfortable being called *a person who stutters* or *PWS*, then—for the time being—these are likely to be the best terms. In any case, the terminology should not become part of the problem.

Finally, a few comments concerning the scientific nature of our field are in order. These thoughts have been stimulated by recent opinions concerning the current direction of research in our field and the degree to which our clinical decisions should be guided by the outcomes of empirical data gathering (Cordes, 1998; Ingham & Cordes, 1999; Onslow, 1999). This issue might be described (or overly simplified) as a "science versus art" continuum. One obvious and easy response to the argument that experimental findings should guide all of our clinical decisions is to state firmly, "Well yes, of course that should be the case!" Any well-trained researcher or clinician would support the view that the efficacy of a clinical field moves forward on the shoulders of researchers who conduct scientifically rigorous basic and applied investigations in order to understand the etiology, development, and nature of stuttering. How could one oppose the position that our intervention strategies and techniques should be empirically demonstrated as having a positive influence on the desired treatment outcomes? A scientific approach to many aspects of life is often the most logical, objective, and reasonable.

On the other hand, as necessary and valuable as these scientific principles may be, treatment involves a great deal more than the concepts of validity and reliability that are at the core of scientific inquiry. The cause-and-effect relationships of stuttering phenomena are often extreme-ly complex and, at the present time, are a long way from being under-stood. Humans are "notoriously nonsensical and unfit subjects for scien-tific scrutiny" (Bannister, 1966). Waiting to make clinical or even scientific decisions until we can base all of our choices on satisfactory empirical evidence would result in, at the most, clinical gridlock and, at the least, a lack of spontaneity and creativity during the process of treatment. It can easily be argued that behavioral sciences in general, and our field in par-ticular, are a good distance from true experimental inquiry—depending, of course, on one's perspective of how much control is required in order to infer cause-and-effect relationships. There is a tendency for social sci-entists to rely on investigative models used in the "hard" sciences, a strat-egy that often works well. It can also result in investigative strategies that study a phenomenon one variable at a time and a gross oversimplifica-tion of human behavior. Effective clinicians must do more than that as they attend to many variables and help a person change within the con-text of their world. Furthermore, clinical decisions are made in real-time, often without all of the information we would like to have. When we do have information about the nature of the person who stutters, some of it is likely to be incomplete or inaccurate. Plainly, there is no excuse for fail-ing to base clinical decisions on good data or documenting the efficacy of our intervention. On the other hand, much of what experienced, wise, and effective clinicians do has a great deal to do with artistry. What takes place during treatment is considerably more complex than what can be accepted in the laboratory. Taking the pompous stance that to be of any clinical value, all clinical decisions must be theory-based or fall within the framework of empirically-based scientific inquiry has the effect of nar-rowing both clinical and research options, as well as inhibiting creativity. It makes our field much less than what it actually is.* That being said, I believe that a reasonable view is that there are equal amounts of "sci-ence" and "art" that combine to produce effective treatment for stutter-ing. To discount one at the expense of the other is a disservice to our field and the people we are attempting to help.

The treatment of fluency disorders should be challenging and fun. It should also be exciting, for to the degree that we as clinicians enter the process, model the behavior we want to change, take risks with our clients, and even experience setbacks with them, we grow as well. Thus much of the process of fluency treatment is a shared psychotherapeutic experience and typically a good one. Welcome to the vineyard! If you stay awhile, it won't be long before you find that there is a wealth of knowledge, goodwill, and support to be found among your colleagues.

* Readers may enjoy reading some delightful comments on this issue in the field of psychology (Bannister, D. [1966]. Psychology as an exercise in paradox. *Bulletin of the British Psychological Society, 19,* 21–26.)

Acknowledgments

A sincere "thank you" to Anthony DiLollo and Julie Sable at the School of Audiology and Speech-Language Pathology at the University of Memphis, who provided thoughtful evaluations and suggestions for the many drafts of this manuscript. The encouragement of my wife Cheryl was essential for the completion of this project. Her love and support make all the difference. Finally, I want to express my deep appreciation to my friends and colleagues in the field, as well as the clients who continue to show me the many facets of fluency disorders, especially the courage and persistence essential for change.

CHAPTER

CLINICIAN CHARACTERISTICS

> *Perhaps the hardest of all the things a clinician must learn is how to live well. You cannot heal a person's wound if you are a dirty bandage. Unless you are a healthy, strong person, your impact will be minimal, no matter what methods you use. There have been times when I resented my clients' expectations of what I should be, but I have noticed that over the years I have become a much better man than I hoped (or desired) to be. I have found that therapy is a two-edged chisel; it shapes the therapist as well as the client. (p. 140)*
>
> Charles Van Riper (1979).
> A career in speech pathology.
> *Englewood Cliffs, NJ: Prentice-Hall.*

INTRODUCTION

To begin a book on fluency disorders by discussing the characteristics of the clinician is unusual. Typically, the first chapter describes the onset of stuttering, presents definitions of the disorder, or provides the reader with historical views of the problem. In this text these things are done in Chapter 2. However, because this book emphasizes the ability of the clinician to make clinical decisions and the choices that must be made during diagnosis and treatment, it seems an ideal place to begin. More than any other component, the clinician is central to the success of the treatment process. Not all clinicians—not even clinically certified or experienced clinicians—are equally effective when trying to assist children and adults with fluency disorders.

Having stated in the Preface that the primary goal of this book is to convey the enthusiasm and excitement of working with people who stutter, we will now step back a bit and place the learning process into a larger perspective. Following the intense years of formal education as a clinician, you will be on your own. Your role will no longer be that of a graduate student who is continually prodded by your instructors to demonstrate your knowledge and ability. You will be a professional who is likely to be considered the resident expert on the topic of communication disorders in general and stuttering in particular. This is likely to be a difficult role change, because during the years of graduate school, many clinicians have relatively little exposure to the field of fluency disorders. Most students have the opportunity to take, at most, one course in stuttering and obtain clinical experience with relatively few clients. Even those clinicians who are able to observe clients make progress do so for only a short time. When clinical change does occur, it is often difficult for the student clinician to know how much of a role she played in promoting the change. Furthermore, even if the student is fortunate enough to take a course on stuttering that is an especially good one and the clinical experience is instructive, it is only the beginning of learning about the complex communication disorder called stuttering.

You may be a little worn out as you successfully complete the rigors of a good graduate program. However, in order to become an experienced and wise professional, the learning can't slow down following your graduation. The clinical decisions you will be making one or two decades from now may have little to do with some of the information you are currently being taught. As the field continues to develop, you will find that some of the theories that you now believe to be true will not hold up. When people of my generation were students, many things we were taught—including the influence of parents on the onset and development of stuttering, the gradual development of stuttering through primary and secondary symptoms, the likelihood of spontaneous recovery, the possibility of relapse following treatment, and the role of the vocal folds in the etiology of stuttering—have since been shown to be partially or completely inaccurate. Inaccuracies, of course, also occur in other areas of communication disorders and other areas of behavioral science. Of course, your instructors are not intentionally providing you with information that is not correct. It's just that the profession has yet to climb the hills necessary to allow us a more accurate view of the phenomena we are investigating and the people we are attempting to help.

Carl Sagan's (1996) caution that "one of the great commandments of science is, Mistrust arguments from authority" (p. 28) is probably good advice for many aspects of life. It is good advice for consumers of all information, including the ideas discussed in this text. As you expand your knowledge and wisdom through continuing educational activities, you will begin to adopt your own style and way of doing things. You will choose new ideas and approaches that will spring from new research findings yet to be discovered. Moreover, as you continue to be a student of your field, you will be more likely to enjoy your work and less inclined to experience burnout.

The purpose of this chapter is twofold. First, we will examine some characteristics of the clinicians who have been identified as being especially effective in working with children and adults who stutter. We will discuss the attitudes as well as the personal and professional attributes that are most desirable for the clinician who effectively guides a client through the treatment process. In the second half of the chapter, we will introduce an attribute of the client-clinician relationship that reflects the essential properties of the therapeutic process: humor.

THE IMPORTANCE OF THE CLINICIAN

Experienced clinicians and even some clients have suggested that certain clinician characteristics are more desirable than others. If this is the reader's first exposure to the field of fluency disorders, this initial chapter may help you to determine whether or not helping people with such problems is likely to be satisfying, for both you and your clients.

There is no exclusive set of attributes that define the ideal clinician. Even if this were the case, no clinician could be expected to possess all or even most of the desirable characteristics described in this chapter. Each client comes to us with different needs and requires, at various points during the treatment process, different attributes and different roles of the clinician. Furthermore, the professional and personal attributes of the clinician will interact with the characteristics of the client, resulting in a unique and dynamic combination during each therapeutic relationship. After many years of observing both student and professional clinicians as well as asking clients about their perceptions of their clinicians, it is clear that some clinicians are considerably better than others at motivating their clients and guiding them through the treatment process. The attitudes and abilities these clinicians possess distinguish them from the clinicians who are less effective. It is the effective clinicians who are able to discover appropriate therapeutic strategies and use or design related techniques. Perhaps more than any other qualities, the best clinicians are uncommonly effective in understanding, encouraging, supporting, and guiding their clients along the sometimes long and arduous path of treatment.

In contrast to the numerous investigations of children and adults who stutter, relatively few questions have been asked about the attributes of the clinicians who provide the treatment. Those authors who have considered this side of the therapeutic process, specifically in the area of fluency disorders (Cooper & Cooper, 1985c; Emerick, 1974; Hood, 1974; Shaprio, 1999; Van Riper, 1975), provide convincing arguments that the clinician is *the* critical part of the process. For example, regardless of the treatment strategy and the associated techniques, Cooper and Cooper maintain that the person who is administering the treatment is the most important variable in creating the process of change.

The importance of the clinician is perhaps more apparent when a counseling-based treatment is used. Murphy and Fitzsimons (1960) contend that during counseling, the "most important single variable affecting the success in the treatment of stutterers is—the clinician" (p. 27). Even if treatment takes the form of an archetypal program of behavioral modification, Cooper and Cooper (1985b) argue that "it does matter who is doing the conditioning" (p. 21). Regardless of the treatment strategy, many authors agree that the clinician plays a critical role in orchestrating a successful treatment program (Emerick, 1974; Hood, 1974; Shapiro, 1999; Van Riper, 1975). For that matter, the clinician often is a major factor in determining whether the client even stays in treatment long enough for meaningful change to take place. Just as in parenting, teaching, and coaching, when treating fluency disorders, it makes a real difference who is serving as a guide and mentor.

Finally, the importance of the clinician in the process of therapeutic change is highlighted within the American Speech-Language-Hearing Association's (ASHA) "Guidelines for Practice in Stuttering Treatment" (Starkweather et al., 1995) developed by the Special Interest Division on Fluency and Fluency Disorders. This publication provides both general and specific guidelines for clinical practice, such as the timing, duration, and cost of treatment as well as goals or assessment, management, transfer and maintenance. This document also emphasizes the personal and learned attributes of competent clinicians by including descriptors as commitment, problem-solving ability, knowledge base, and communication skills. Anyone who specializes in helping individuals with fluency disorders should be aware of these inclusive guidelines. The complete set of these guidelines is found in Appendix D.

Clinician Attitudes About Stuttering and People Who Stutter

Our attitude about those who come to us for help and our understanding of their communication problems have a fundamental influence on how we approach them as people during both assessment and treatment. What the clinician has been told and what she has been able to observe about stuttering and the people who stutter will determine whether she will even have the desire to work with such clients.

There are many people who stutter (or have stuttered) who have gone on to become professional clinicians, often specializing in stuttering.

Assuming that a clinician with a history of stuttering has also acquired the necessary academic and clinical knowledge, life experience as a person who stutters may be an advantage for someone at the outset of a clinical career. Having traveled within the culture of stuttering and survived the many tribulations along the way tends to promote the understanding and empathy necessary for guiding others through treatment. There are many examples of this understanding in the helping professions. For example, ex-addicts often are extremely good therapists in alcohol and drug addiction programs. They understand from experience the nature of the problem and the many tricks that can be used to avoid change.

This does not mean that people who stutter or who have stuttered in the past will be more effective as clinicians or will necessarily have a greater understanding of the stuttering experience. With good training, nonstuttering clinicians can have equal understanding, so much so that I have often admonished nonstuttering clinicians not to acquiesce to stuttering clients who may attempt to tell them "You don't understand because you don't stutter." Speaking as a person with a history of stuttering, I do not believe this to be the case. Throughout this book it is implied that one does not have to stutter in order to understand the nature of the stuttering experience.

Although it may sound somewhat discouraging to a student new to the topic of fluency disorders, it is clear that there are many professional clinicians who feel unqualified and uncomfortable when working with children and adults who stutter. For many years, research has consistently supported this observation (Ainsworth, 1974; Brisk, Healey, & Hux, 1997; Cooper, 1975b, 1985; Kelly, Martin, Baker, Rivera, Bishop, Kriziske, Settlery, & Stealy, 1997; Mallard, Gardner, & Downey, 1988; Matkin, Rigel, & Snope, 1983; St. Louis & Durrenberger, 1992; Thompson, 1984; Van Riper, 1992a; Wingate, 1971). Clinicians who do not find it enjoyable and rewarding to work with people who stutter should not do so, as their lack of enjoyment will show.

Obviously, at the outset of training, it is natural for anyone to be anxious. Until the clinician has seen change occurring and until she has taken an active part in facilitating change, it is difficult to believe that she can truly be of any help to a person who is struggling to say even the simplest of utterances. However, if a clinician has received a quality education and continues to be apprehensive about working with people who stutter, such uncertainty is one indication that she is not yet qualified. People who stutter will not get the best possible treatment unless they can find a clinician who is not merely competent, but also enthusiastic about the process of change.

The disturbing results of several investigations indicate that some professional clinicians have opinions of stuttering, and particularly of the people who stutter, that are not accurate. The findings of these investigations are consistent and have included large numbers of both student and professional clinicians from many areas throughout the country (Cooper & Cooper, 1985a; Curlee, 1985; Lass, Ruscello, Pannbaker, Schmitt, & Everly-Myers, 1989; Mallard, Gardner, & Downey, 1988; Matkin, Ringle, & Snope, 1983; St. Louis & Lass, 1981). A survey of 597 certified professional clinicians completed by Matkin, Ringle, and Snope indicated that these clinicians rated themselves as being much less competent with fluency disorders than with other communication disorders (48% of those surveyed felt highly competent in treating persons who stuttered). Curlee found that 40% of the respondents from accredited programs did not believe that their students were being adequately prepared to serve clients with fluency disorders. Mallard et al. found that only 50% of school clinicians had taken a course in stuttering and that only 6% reported that the coursework emphasized methods of treatment.

A comprehensive review of clinician attitudes toward stuttering done by Cooper and Cooper (1992) provides an indication of some improvement in the opinions of clinicians. These authors determined the attitudes of 1,872 speech-language pathologists from 21 states. Seventy-five percent of the subjects held a graduate degree in education. The subjects completed the Clinician Attitudes Toward Stuttering Inventory (CATS) (Cooper, 1975a). Clinicians responded to 50 attitudinal statements by circling words on a five-point strength-of-agreement scale. The results of the 1991 survey were contrasted to an identical survey of 674 clinicians conducted between 1973 and 1983.

The results of the 1991 survey indicated that as a group, the clinicians showed attitude changes over the years that indicated the development of a more enlightened view of stuttering and people who stutter. For example, in comparison to the earlier results, the 1991 data indicated that a smaller percentage of the professional clinicians held the view that most people who stutter have psychological problems (35.7% versus 41.9%). The view that parents are the primary factor causing stuttering in their children became less frequently expressed (10.6% versus 17.9%). Moreover, a larger proportion of clinicians now held the view that early intervention with young children is likely to yield success (63.4% versus 49.5%).

However, the results from the 1991 survey also indicated that there continued to be large percentages of clinicians who held the following views:

➤ 12.6 percent of the subjects agreed that most speech clinicians are adept in treating stuttering (75.5% disagreed).
➤ 2.1 percent of the clinicians agreed that they felt more comfortable in working with individuals who stutter than working with articulatory defective individuals (93.2% disagreed).
➤ 57.8 percent of the clinicians agreed that there are some personality traits that are characteristic of stutterers (18.4% disagreed).

More recent investigations continue to yield similar results. Sommers and Caruso (1995) noted that directors of university training programs and public school supervisors found both graduate clinical experience and postgraduate in-service training to be lacking in the area of fluency disorders. University program directors reported that clinical clock hours for master's degree students in the area of fluency disorders were considerably less (average, 20.2 hours, standard deviation, 18.7) than for language disorders (average, 104.2 hours, standard deviation, 52.8) or articulation-phonology disorders (average, 77.4 hours, standard deviation, 56.3).

Finally, recent surveys indicate only somewhat more positive findings concerning student training and clinician competence for treating those who stutter. In 1997 Brisk, Healey, and Hux reported improvements in clinicians' training, confidence, and attitudes about assessment and intervention for school-age children who stutter. Of the 278 school-based clinicians surveyed across 20 states, 97% had taken at least one undergraduate or graduate course where fluency disorders was the major topic. These results suggested a slight improvement over the findings of St. Louis and Lass (1981) and Lass et al. (1989), who reported percentages of 57% and 91%, respectively. In addition, 90% of those surveyed by Brisk et al. indicated that they had the opportunity to treat clients who stuttered during their training, whereas St. Louis and Lass found that 43% of their subjects had this opportunity.

When asked about evaluating clients, Brisk et al. found that 57%, 77%, and 71% of their participants felt confident about evaluating preschool, elementary, and junior/senior high school students, respectively. This outcome is in contrast to the findings of Matkin et al. (1983) indicating that only 48% of clinicians felt confident evaluating persons who stutter. With respect to treatment, Brisk et al. also found that the majority of clinicians they surveyed agreed that they were confident about treating elementary or middle school children (64% and 54%, respectively). Brisk et al. also found that regardless of the age of the client or how recently they had received their degrees, clinicians felt that they were better prepared to evaluate than to treat children and adolescents who stutter. Finally, Brisk et al. noted a continual need for improved training and attributed the positive changes they found to the greater number of participants in their study who received their training at accredited institutions and who had received master's degrees (98%, in contrast to 43% of the respondents in the St. Louis and Lass study in 1980).

Also in 1997, Kelly, Martin, Baker, Rivera, Bishop, Kriziske, Stettler, and Stealy surveyed 150 clinicians in the Indiana schools. They found that 54% of bachelor's and 65% of master's students had taken a course that was "entirely or partially" devoted to stuttering (somewhat greater than the 43% reported by St. Louis and Lass, 1981). A total of 19% of these students had never had a course in stuttering. The largest percentage of the respondents (39%) indicated that theory was emphasized over the clinical aspects of intervention for both undergraduate and graduate courses. Kelly et al. points out that this could be a particular problem if Henri's assertion that "today's graduates have considerable difficulty moving from theory into practice" (1984, p. 45) is true. Whereas Brisk et al. (1997) found clinicians expressing little interest in continuing education, the clinicians surveyed by Kelly et al. indicated that there were too few opportunities to obtain continuing education in fluency disorders, particularly in the form of practical information regarding intervention techniques. Kelly et al. also found that approximately half of those surveyed failed to obtain any clinical hours in either the diagnosis or treatment of stuttering during either the undergraduate or graduate level. Approximately half of those surveyed indicated that they felt inadequate for helping people who stutter, most indicating that they wanted information and experience with techniques for managing stuttering, a consistent finding in the research cited in this chapter. Respondents felt most knowledgeable about managing articulation/phonological disorders, followed by language disorders, and considerably less competent or even incompetent when working with fluency, voice, and neurogenic disorders. When considering only clients who stutter, clinicians perceived themselves as being most competent in helping children who stutter and had no other communication problems. Clinicians noted greater feelings of inadequacy when dealing with emotional or motivational aspects of treatment.

Finally, Yaruss (1999) surveyed 239 master's-level programs accredited by the American Speech-Language-Hearing Association. A total of 134 questionnaires were returned for an overall response rate of 56%. Although not all programs completed all questions, the results indicated the following:

➤ Of 134 programs responding, 101 programs (75%) offered at least one full *required* course devoted specifically to fluency disorders.
➤ Of 134 programs responding, 39 programs (29%) offered at least one full *elective* course devoted specifically to fluency disorders.
➤ Of 129 programs responding, 23 (17.8%) programs indicated that it was possible to graduate without taking any class specifically devoted to fluency disorders. Of these programs, 19 (97%) reported that fluency disorders are covered as part of some other class.
➤ Of 128 programs responding, 72 (56%) indicated that diagnostic experience in fluency disorders is not required during clinical practicum.
➤ Of 128 programs responding, 65 (51%) indicated that treatment experience in fluency disorders is not required.
➤ Of 128 programs responding, 76 (59%) indicated that it is possible for a student to graduate without any clinical experience in fluency disorders.

The survey also found no significant relationships between program size and students' academic or clinical training in fluency disorders. As Yaruss concludes, these recent findings indicate that a significant percentage of students graduating from master's-level programs do not have even the most basic academic or clinical background necessary for working with individuals who stutter. Finally, there is some indication that these results may represent a more positive view than is actually the case. That is, although 40% of all accredited programs have a faculty member with enough interest in fluency disorders to join ASHA's Special Interest Division for Fluency and Fluency Disorders (Division 4), 61% of the programs responding to the survey had a faculty member belonging to this Special Interest Division. This suggests that the responses to the survey were more likely to have been completed by programs that had required courses on fluency disorders, greater clinical populations and clinical practicum requirements, and a greater degree of expertise among the faculty.

As the above series of studies demonstrates, the issue of questionable graduate preparation in the area of fluency disorders is not a new one. However, this ongoing problem may have been worsened in 1993 following a decision of the American Speech-Language-Hearing Association to alter the certification requirements and delete a required 25 hours of clinical contact with individuals who stutter. Although no specific coursework in fluency disorders was required at that time by ASHA, the Council on Academic Accreditation (CAA) requirement (standard 3.5) specifies that coursework in a disorder area should precede clinical experience. This requirement undoubtedly contributed to a decrease in university programs *requiring* graduate-level courses in fluency disorders. The recent survey by Yaruss (1999) indicated that one-half of the programs responding reported reductions in their own academic or clinical requirements. At the very least, such a lack of standards for graduate preparation in fluency disorders has contributed to greater variability for academic and clinical preparation in programs throughout the country.

Specialty Recognition in Fluency Disorders

It is hoped that the recent efforts toward specialty recognition through ASHA's Special Interest Division 4 will help to elevate the level of training received by many clinicians. Division 4 was the first of many special interest divisions to receive approval from ASHA to form a commission and begin processing applicants for specialty recognition. In order to receive the Certificate of Specialty Recognition in Fluency Disorders, the candidate completes the following steps:

1. Submission of a *Fluency Specialist Interest Form* alerting the Specialty Commission of the candidate's interest.

2. Identification of a Commission-approved mentor who will advise, guide, and support the candidate throughout the recognition process.

3. Submission of an *application* and *program plan form* describing how the candidate's proposed (a) educational experience and (b) guided practice activities will occur. Prior to submitting these forms, the candidate must present evidence of successful completion of a graduate-level course devoted to fluency and fluency disorders with a minimum grade of B from an accredited program.

Educational Activities

In addition to a graduate level course, the candidate's educational plan must include 100 clock hours (10 continuing education units) of educational activities. In the case of graduate coursework, each semester hour is equivalent to 12 clock hours or 1.2 CEUs. At least 50 of the 100 hours should directly relate to assessment and treatment of children and adults. At least 75 of the 100 hours must be completed subsequent to receiving the master's degree in SLP. Clock hours must be obtained no more than 10 years prior to the candidate's program submission date.

Guided Practice

The guided practice includes four phases of assessment and treatment activities, totaling 100 clock hours. *Phase one* involves observation of the mentor or another experienced (approved) clinician as the mentor models essential aspects of a variety of treatment approaches (maximum of 20 hours). *Phase two* involves the candidate's practicing role-playing with the mentor (or another approved clinician) for various clinical skills relating to affective, behavioral, cognitive, and linguistics features of fluency and stuttering (minimum of 10 hours). *Phase three* requires the demonstration to the mentor of the candidate's ability to carry out clinical skills during direct contact with clients and families (minimum of 10 hours). In *Phase four*, the candidate practices clinical skills under continued supervision of the mentor (minimum of 40 hours). At the completion of the education and guided practice activities, the candidate submits a report to the Commission describing these experiences. Finally, the candidate will complete a written examination covering the nature, assessment, and treatment of fluency disorders in children and adults.

The candidate has three opportunities to pass this examination. During the time the requirements are being met, the candidate submits an annual report to the Commission describing progress toward recognition. Finally, the candidate must complete the program within five years of the date of the Commission's approval of the candidate's program. The current address for submitting the information is included in Appendix B.

In order to promote currency of knowledge, every three years specialists submit a *Fluency Specialists Renewal Form* verifying that they continue to remain active in the management of clients by providing a minimum of 100 clock hours per year and have completed a minimum of 4.5 ASHA-approved continuing education units in fluency disorders or related areas. Clearly, the preparation of professional clinicians in fluency disorders needs improvement, and consumers of our services need the very best understanding and clinical skills that can be provided.

How Clinicians Interpret the Disorder

If stuttering is presented as a mysterious disorder—an enigma—clinicians will naturally be wary about treating these clients. Stuttering may indeed be an enigma, for the syndrome is complex and much of the problem lies under the surface. Van Riper (1982), responding to the suggestion that stuttering is like a riddle, stated that "[it] is more than a riddle. It is at least a complicated, multidimensional jigsaw puzzle, with many pieces still missing" (p. 1). Sheehan frequently argued the case that stuttering is like an iceberg, with only small portions of the problem visible to those who were unwilling to look below the surface (Sheehan, 1970). Years later, Sheehan (1980) offered the pointed comment that "defining stuttering as [only] a fluency problem borders on professional irresponsibility. It ignores the person. It ignores his feelings about himself" (p. 392).

On the other hand, Ham (1993) argues that stuttering is not significantly more complex than many other human behavioral problems. Much of stuttering behavior is rule governed with cause-and-effect relationships that are well known. Many of the factors that precipitate and maintain stuttering are understood, and many children and adults achieve extraordinary success in modifying both their speech and their handicap as a result of treatment. As students have the opportunity to observe clinicians who are unafraid of stuttering and have had success with several people, they will be more likely to be enthusiastic about the assessment and treatment of people with fluency disorders. Experienced clinicians know what success looks and sounds like, and these changes can be shown to the new clinician. As with most things in life, there is no simple substitute for experience. Only continual practice of your craft will enable you to learn by your successes as well as your failures. Fortunately, for those who are excited by learning, the process is never really complete.

One of the substantial problems faced by students taking part in any clinical experience is that they are not likely to see a long view of progress. They are not able to follow clients throughout the continuum of change (see Chapters 10 and 11). For many practical reasons it is rare, even for a professional clinician, to follow a client for more than a few months or years following dismissal from treatment. Most students lack the chance to observe and work with a client for a substantial portion of their formal treatment, the time during which the client pays a professional for services, let alone informal treatment, the much longer period when the client gradually assumes the role of clinician and develops the "response-ability" required for self-treatment. The window available to student clinicians in graduate programs is a small one. When the overall picture of behavioral, affective, and cognitive change is unavailable, it is understandable that the treatment process will appear enigmatic. Then again, if student clinicians know what to look for and can be shown progress during treatment (both for behavioral changes and cognitive/ attitudinal changes), then helping these speakers will be more likely to be viewed as a positive rather than an aversive experience. A central principle is indicated in the comments of Daly (1988), who noted that the better clinicians tend to be those who hold a belief that their clients have the capacity for success as a result of treatment. Such conviction by the clinician is essential according to Van Riper (1973), who stated the belief that "out of the therapist's faith can come the stutterer's hope" (p. 230).

CLINICIAN PERSONALITY ATTRIBUTES

The therapeutic relationship has been studied extensively in the fields of counseling and clinical psychology. The results of these investigations began finding their way into the literature in speech-language pathology during the 1960s. Although the clinician-client relationship is clearly important in all aspects of clinical intervention in communication disorders, it is especially critical in the area of fluency disorders because of the strong interactive therapeutic component. Research in the fields of counseling and psychology has provided consistent evidence that therapeutic exchanges are more likely to facilitate optimum change or gain if the clinician is able to communicate messages of empathy, positive regard, genuineness, and concreteness (Berenson & Carkhuff, 1967; Carkhuff & Berenson, 1967; Truax & Carkhuff, 1966). Crowe (1997a) cites The American Psychological Association (1947) as recommending the following personal attributes for counselors and psychotherapists: resourcefulness, versatility, curiosity, respect for the integrity of others, awareness of one's own personality traits, humor, tolerance, ability to relate warmly to others, industry, responsibility, integrity, stability, and ethics. As we will discuss in Chapter 7, and as Crowe and others describe in his 1997 text *Applications of Counseling in Speech-Language Pathology and Audiology*, counseling activities are at the core of the assessment and treatment process of all communication disorders.

Van Riper (1975) provided the first comprehensive description of the desirable attributes of clinicians who help children and adults who stutter. He described personality characteristics such as *empathy*, an authentic sensitivity for the client; *warmth*, a respect or positive regard for the client; *genuineness*, an openness and the ability to disclose oneself as a real person; and *charisma*, an ability to arouse hope, appearing confident yet humble, frank yet tactful. As Van Riper (1973) stated: "Like fishermen, good therapists are optimists. Most of them have come to have profound respect for the latent potential for self-healing that exists in all troubled souls" (p. 230).

A slightly different view of clinician characteristics was proposed by Zinker (1977), who considers therapy as a creative process of changing awareness and behavior. Although Zinker was not discussing therapy for stuttering or describing clinicians in this field, he views therapy as a creative process and feels that a common malady among therapists is that they fail to see themselves as artists involved in a creative process. As the clinician becomes involved in the dynamic and shared process of change, the opportunity for creativity becomes more apparent. As we will discuss in succeeding chapters, the experienced clinician is a guide who has a map of the territory. The clinician has a sense of direction about where the client may benefit from traveling and a notion of when it might be appropriate to initiate a secondary trip. As Zinker states and as we will also discuss in Chapter 7 under the topic of counseling, the challenge for the clinician is to "establish an adequate cognitive map which includes the client's experience of himself and then to point to action steps to make the solution possible for the client" (p. 11). In order to do these things, Zinker suggests that it is useful if the clinician possesses several characteristics that nurture the creative process. Some of the characteristics of a creative clinician suggested by Zinker include a childlike wonderment and excitement; patience for change without forcing; a love of play; a sense of humor; a positive attitude about risk taking; a willingness to experiment with different approaches and techniques; the ability to distinguish the boundaries between themselves and a client; a willingness to push, confront, persuade, and energize another person in order to accomplish the work that needs to be done; and a lifestyle that promotes a rich background with a range of life experiences.

Zinker further suggests that blocks to the clinician's creativity lead to becoming stuck in a particular theoretical or professional stance or stuck with the view that science and art do not mix: a science-versus-art dichotomy. Some examples of blocks to creativity include a fear of failure (playing it safe and not taking risks), a reluctance to play (fear of experimenting with ideas and techniques and looking silly), over-certainty concerning a particular school of thought (a rigidity concerning the nature of the problem-solving approach), giving up too soon when an approach or a technique does not appear to be "working," a reluctance to push hard enough to help others, or an inability to accept contrasting ways of interpreting things and events (believing that there is only one way or one best way to define success during therapy).

Cooper and Cooper (1985b) also provide a description of several desirable attributes of the effective clinician. Many of the attributes described by these authors coincide with their view of fluency treatment as an interpersonal communication experience. The effective clinician brings to this interpersonal experience certain desirable attitudes and personality attributes. The Coopers suggested that, especially during the early stages of treatment, the client-clinician relationship should be a major focus of discussion. They stated that the clinician should be able to *openly express* both negative and positive feelings to the client. However, as the clinician is expressing these feelings, it is important that the clinician also *indicate a belief in the worth and potential* of the client. As treatment becomes challenging and the client is asked to make behavioral, attitudinal, and cognitive changes, the clinician should be *continually honest* in reinforcing the client's feelings of self-worth. Such honesty, the Coopers prudently note, is much easier to do when the clinician enjoys working with the client, which may not always be the case. They warn that clinicians need to resist the urge to tell clients how they should feel. Instead, they should foster an expression of client feelings. The clinician may, however, indicate that although she understands a client's feelings, she does not share them or at least does not necessarily agree that they are warranted by the situation. Importantly, experienced clinicians are able to indicate the difference between disapproval of feelings expressed by the client and the client's worth.

Cooper and Cooper (1985b) state that the clinician should be *"devoid of dogma"* and have the ability to adapt the therapeutic approach to the client's uniqueness and needs. This is another way of saying that good clinicians are client directed rather than treatment directed. The clinician must be able to recognize subtle client responses that provide cues for direction and indicate progress. Experienced clinicians are not slowed down by a client's negative response to the demands and challenges. They are, in short, able to be a constant ally and to persevere along with the client when the process of change becomes difficult. Experienced clinicians *inform the client* by providing information about the latter's status and progress in treatment. Cooper and Cooper submit that clients, at any point in treatment and regardless of age or mental abilities, should be able to describe just where they are in treatment in both behavioral and attitudinal terms. Finally, effective clinicians are able to attend to the details of record keeping and report writing.

Undoubtedly, the characteristics we have discussed would be desirable for any clinician working with a person for any reason. They would be valuable characteristics to have in a friend or colleague. Moreover, just as it is possible to be successful as a friend or colleague without all of these attributes, it is possible to be a successful clinician without possessing enormous amounts of each. Clinicians who possess such characteristics not only make the treatment process more effective, they also make it more enjoyable.

Most people come to the professional field of speech-language pathology with many of these basic personality attributes, attitudes, and abilities. It is not clear whether some or all of these basic characteristics can be created or enhanced as a function of academic and clinical experience. What is clear, however, is that given these basic personality characteristics, clinicians can achieve proficiency in several intervention skills that increase their effectiveness.

CLINICIAN INTERVENTION SKILLS

This section will discuss, given the aforementioned attitudes and personality attributes, some of the intervention abilities that can be acquired and developed during the student's education. There is, of course, considerable overlap across each of these abilities.

Becoming Less Inhibited as a Clinician

Becoming desensitized to stuttering is an important first step in understanding the behavior and the person we are treating. Only after the clinician is able to become uninhibited about stuttering in general, and about herself in particular, will treatment proceed (Van Riper, 1982).

The clinician needs to become less inhibited about many aspects of stuttering. First of all, clinicians often need to overcome a concern about doing something "wrong" in therapy that will hurt the speaker and somehow make things worse. This common perspective is most likely related to the notion that there is something psychologically amiss or unstable about the person who stutters and that such clients are especially susceptible to emotional trauma. In part, this attitude may be a result of the diagnosogenic view of stuttering etiology advocated during the period from the early 1950s through the late 1960s, which stated that stuttering was created by inappropriate listener reactions to the fluency breaks of young children (See Chapter 2). Alternately, such a cautious approach may be related to the idea that any increase in the frequency of stuttering is necessarily bad. As we will discuss in later chapters, an increase in the frequency of stuttering may be a sign of progress. In addition, stuttering is highly variable, and changes in the frequency of the overt behaviors can be attributable to many factors, only one of which is the clinician.

In extreme instances it may be possible to make the stuttering, or even the person who is stuttering, in some sense worse. If, for example, the clinician is truly an unqualified, uncaring, and insensitive person, the client and, conceivably, the stuttering could become worse. However, a qualified clinician who is inhibited about saying or doing something during treatment for fear of somehow injuring a client most likely possesses a naive view of the person doing the stuttering. On the contrary, most people who stutter are stable and highly durable, especially those who have the courage to ask for help and initiate treatment. Clinicians, if they have enough training and experience, should have no more fear about doing the "wrong" thing during the treatment of a child or adult who stutters than they would have with a client with any other communication disorder.

The relationship between clinician and client is an important aspect of the process of change during treatment. There is no question, especially with adults who stutter, that there is a strong counseling or psychotherapeutic component at the center. As suggested by the opening quote of this chapter, there are aspects of this process change and growth that impact on the clinician as well as the client. It is rare that only one person grows during good, interactive treatment. Indeed, such growth is often experienced most clearly during the mixture of personalities and perceptions that take place in group treatment activities. Students have often commented after completing their clinical experiences in fluency disorders that they miss the exciting and challenging experiences of group treatment.

Nevertheless, because the process of change and growth is a dynamic one, it is not necessarily something that all clinicians are initially comfortable about entering. One alluring aspect of the early behavior modification programs with fluency disorders in the late 1950s, 1960s, and 1970s was the belief that the role of the clinician could be limited to the identification and modification of overt stuttering behaviors. The behaviors that were audible and visible on the surface were the major focus of treatment. Certainly clinicians were making decisions. Frequency counts were made, contingencies were agreed upon or at least implied, and rewards and punishments were dispensed based on the client's performance. The treatment process was clear, goals were explicit, and fluency was charted and changed. The approach was relatively easy to teach to students as well as to clients. Some clients did well, as some clients will do in nearly all treatment approaches. Some even stayed well. However, the point is not whether behavior modification approaches are effective. A particular treatment strategy can only be evaluated based on the needs and response of the client. The point is that when using any treatment, including current behavioral modification programs (which tend to include a more broad-based approach that focuses on more than the speaker's surface behaviors), the clinician needs to be unafraid. She needs to be uninhibited about stuttering and the people doing the stuttering if she expects the client, parents, teacher, or spouse to also adopt this attitude.

Obtaining experience with clients in any clinical area is difficult: It can be frightening. Although the clinician may have a sense of the overall direction of treatment and know a variety of treatment techniques, at best she has seen only a portion of the total treatment sequence and sees only the tip of the iceberg regarding the client's characteristics. Although there may have been the opportunity to observe clients on videotape in the clinic, *she* has not been the one who has made the process happen.

One of the best aspects about the series of treatment videotapes produced by the Stuttering Foundation of America is that the clinician, Charles Van Riper, demonstrates an uninhibited and assertive interactive style with the young adult, male client. He models attributes of empathy, genuineness, warmth, charisma, and particularly frankness, as he works through the treatment process with his young adult client. Because of changes in dress, Van Riper's interpersonal style, and current aspects of "political correctness," it is usually necessary for new clinicians to view the tapes several times before they begin to appreciate these characteristics of Dr. Van Riper's personality. Before long, however, it becomes clear that Van Riper is obviously unafraid of stuttering. He moves forward in treatment with an uninhibited attitude and a distinct sense of direction.

Another beneficial aspect of this video series is that the student has the opportunity to see an enlarged window of change as the client progresses through treatment. There is some indication that students can increase their level of self-efficacy about clinical performance with fluency clients as a function of (only) academic training (Rudolf, Manning, & Sewell, 1983). There is, of course, no substitute for a successful clinical experience.

Avoiding Dogmatic Decisions

Being able to see beyond the dogma of one treatment strategy is a sign of clinical wisdom. Egan (1990) cautions that we should "beware the person of one book" (p. 26). The message of a single book or single author can too easily become a calling. It is true that the discovery of *the method* can be empowering and give a sense of direction to the clinician and, therefore, the client. However, as Egan points out, such devotion to a single treatment path can also lead to a closing down of new ideas and new growth. The foundation for choosing a strategy or technique for a professional should not be the method, but the nature and needs of the client.

Several years ago, at a professional meeting of a state association of speech-language pathologists, I was a member of a panel that was asked, along with the audience, to view a series of videotapes of children and adults with fluency disorders. The panel's task was to react to these hypothetical clients and discuss the strategies and techniques that we speculated might be appropriate for them. As we took our turns offering suggestions about each tape segment, it became apparent that one member of the panel was giving the identical response each time. Regardless of the client's age, severity, or nature of stuttering, this clinician would take the microphone and say something similar to: "I believe strongly in the _____ _____ method and feel that this approach would be ideal for this client. I have seen this method work for many clients and would prefer to use this approach with this person."

Beyond the demonstrated efficacy of this particular method (note: in this case there was a frightful lack of such data), we were all witnessing a clear example of a "one book" approach to helping clients. Clinical decisions should be driven primarily by the needs of the client rather than the dogma from a book. If you want to be a technician, make all of your clinical decisions according to a treatment manual. If you want to be a professional, however, make your decisions primarily according to the needs of the client.

Opening Your Treatment Focus

One of the characteristics of someone who is learning a new activity is the amount of attention given to the techniques. When first learning a sport such as soccer, for example, it is necessary to learn such techniques as passing, receiving, and shooting the ball. Later, with more experience, one moves beyond the techniques. The accomplished player has a broader, less technical view of the game. With experience, the view includes the strategies of the event, and particularly an analysis of the other team's strengths and weaknesses. The player's focus begins to open up. Although the techniques remain essential to the accomplishment of the overall strategy, the most important aspect of the process is not so much what to do or how, but when to do it and why. Similar to inexperienced players or coaches, new clinicians tend to focus on techniques of the moment rather than the overall, long-term strategies. Even more to the point, new clinicians are more likely to focus on the techniques rather than the person they are trying to help. They are apt to think to themselves, "What do I *do* in therapy today?" rather than, "What does my client need from me now, and how does that fit with the long-term goal of treatment?"

We are not suggesting that specific treatment techniques are unimportant. They are, of course, every bit as essential as knowing how to pass and control the ball is to playing soccer. You cannot play the game if you are not good at the techniques and you cannot treat people who stutter if you fail to develop skill at identifying specific accessory behaviors, tabulating the percentage of syllables stuttered, and modeling specific stuttering- or fluency-modification techniques. Techniques are unquestionably important: The professional clinician must know many of them and know them well. However, they are not the most important aspect of the process. The ability to look beyond the techniques—even beyond the treatment program—and see the client is something that distinguishes the experienced clinician from the novice, the technician from the professional.

Just as the new instructor is less likely to vary from prepared notes or stray more than a few steps away from the podium, the less experienced player is more likely to have a rigid, preplanned attack. A preplanned strategy may work for awhile, particularly if the opponent is easy. However, the plan may not work indefinitely, especially if the opponent is challenging. The accomplished participant is flexible; he or she can see what is occurring on the field in a broader sense. The accomplished athlete (or coach) is more likely to be aware of, and willing to change, strategy, based on the circumstances and the competition. The clinician's decisions and actions are primarily dictated by the other players. They most certainly are not dictated by a textbook or by dogma. Table 1.1 suggests several continuums that serve to distinguish the technician from the professional.

For decades, Van Riper stated that "the client is the guide," not the clinician, and certainly not the text or the treatment techniques. There is no one path up the mountain. Rather, the path is likely to be different for each client because people are beginning the journey from different places. This seems rather complicated—and sometimes it is. However, before we throw up our hands at the challenge facing us with each new client, it is important to realize that most clients have common needs and we can expect to see certain patterns of thinking and behavior. Moreover, there are basic clinician as well as client skills that will contribute to the process of change.

Calibrating to the Client

At the outset of the first several treatment sessions, we clinicians find ourselves overloaded with information presented by the client. Not only are we introduced to expected surface behaviors that we have seen before, but we will also be presented with some new behaviors that are unique to this speaker. Some of these behaviors may be obvious and explicit. Other behaviors may occur rarely or not at all during the initial sessions. Some of the behaviors that were learned long ago and have become part of this person's response to stuttering may only surface during more stressful speaking situations. These behaviors may be observed only rarely, if at all, during treatment sessions. We may see these surface behaviors only if we accompany the person into the speaking situations

Table 1-1. Two continuums that distinguish clinical decision-making by a technician and by an experienced clinician.

Technician	Professional
Technique directed	Client directed
Preplanned procedures	Flexile procedures
Dogmatic treatment	Treatment alternatives
Narrow focus on problem	Open focus on person

they enter daily, at school or at work. Alternately, we may note these behaviors if we call clients unexpectedly at home or by chance meet them in some location outside of the formal clinical setting. In any case, there are apt to be many surface behaviors, several of them unique to this one person, and it will take some time to become calibrated to them.

In addition to tuning in to the stuttering behaviors, it will also take awhile to become calibrated to the way the new client speaks when not stuttering. In order to specify the nature of the client's stuttered speech, it is essential to specify the quality of the person's nonstuttered speech. What is it about the surface behaviors of this speaker that indicates to us that they are not stuttering? Is the client able to produce truly fluent speech that, as Starkweather (1987) indicates, is characterized by an easy, smooth, relatively effortless flow? On the other hand, is their speech characterized by something less than a smooth, effortless quality? Is the client achieving fluency or just "not stuttering"? Is the speech fluent in a technical sense but characterized by a degree of instability? An essential step in calibrating yourself to the client is being able to differentiate and contrast at least three levels of fluency: stuttered speech, unstable speech, and fluent speech.

One procedure that aids in the calibration process, especially during the first several meetings, is to pantomime the client's speech (Van Riper, 1973). That is, the clinician follows the client's speech by shadowing what he is saying. In this way the clinician is able to get a feel (literally) for how the client may, for example, slightly slow his speech before a feared word. The clinician can begin to sense how the client scans ahead and "pretastes" words while considering whether to try moving through them. Using audio- or videotapes early in treatment can assist clinicians in tuning in to their new client. The clinician can become calibrated to the client's speech patterns by pantomiming the tapes at the office, at home, or while driving in the car. Although on the surface, the client may appear to be fluent, with time the clinician will be able to detect instances when the client is speaking carefully and making a concerted effort not to stutter. The speech is unstable and the clinician will get the sensation that the client is "talking on thin ice"; the client is not stuttering in a technical sense yet seems as though he may fall through the surface of the fluency at any moment.

There is some interesting preliminary support for this notion of vocal tract instability found in the results of a recent study by Robb, Blomgren, and Chen (1998). Steady-state portions of the vowel from *fluently produced* consonant + vowel + /t/ utterances were analyzed (5 to 10 pitch periods) for second formant (F_2) frequency fluctuation (FFF). The fluent productions ($N = 145$) of five untreated adult males were compared to fluent productions ($N = 147$) by five treated clients and fluent productions ($N = 143$) of five nonstuttering speakers. The untreated speakers showed significantly ($p < 0.05$) larger formant frequency fluctuation compared to the control group of nonstuttering speakers (approximately 30 Hz larger) and to the treated clients. No significant difference was found between the control group and the treated speakers. That is, the untreated speakers demonstrated the greatest amount of vocal tract instability during the production of what were perceptually evaluated as *fluent* C-V-*t* utterances.

As we become calibrated to the new client, we will begin to notice how the client's speech looks as well as how it sounds. We can begin to tune in not only to the surface structure, but perhaps even more importantly, to the deep structure of the person. What are the cues signaling that this speaker may feel some loss of control, some helplessness, as he approaches, and even goes through, a feared word? Although the speaker may not have overtly stuttered on a word, he may not have felt completely in control of his speech. It is as though the stuttering were just under the surface. Until we become calibrated to that person, we are not likely to detect such occurrences. Detecting this loss of control, a key feature of the stuttering experience, is discussed in greater detail in Chapter 4.

Using Silence

In observing the surface and deep structure of the client's speech, experienced clinicians are apt to minimize talk and maximize observation. One way to tune in to someone is to stop talking. More experienced clinicians use silence rather than being intimidated by it. They use the silence as a time for reflecting on what the client has said. Interpersonal communication is not stopped during silence. Body language, eye contact, and facial expressions tell much about the status of what has been said—and left unsaid. Silence on the part of the clinician may even be thought of as providing the client with a degree of independence. Van Riper (1975) suggested that when the clinician finds herself uttering more than four or five sentences in a row, "warning lights should go off." This is especially true, he suggested, if the sentences contain many *I*'s and *We*'s.

Modeling Risk Taking

Clinicians must be prepared to lead the way in treatment. We must be able to demonstrate our willingness to take risks if we are asking our client to do so. Sheehan (1970) made the insightful comment that "the Achilles heel of most normal speaking therapists who try to work with stutterers is simply that they are not willing to do what they ask their stutterers to do" (p. 283). If we are afraid of stuttering and the tasks that await our client on the road to change, how can we expect him to follow our recommendations and to move forward? We do not have to do so often, but we will occasionally be called upon to demonstrate our willingness to take risks and to lead the way into speaking situations. Each situation is an opportunity to demonstrate that it is possible to be reasonably calm in the midst of stuttering; it is possible to openly stutter and not completely lose control. Alternately, depending on how difficult this experience is for you as a clinician, it is a chance to demonstrate that, despite your obvious anxiety, you are committed to helping the client. You will, for example, voluntarily stutter to a stranger on the street as your client observes. You will openly stutter on the question, "Pardon me, do you have the ta . . . ta . . . ta . . ." until the listener gives you the time of day. It is fine to tell the client that you are committed to helping him, but showing him is far better.

It is easy to talk about the tasks, what needs to be done to change the behaviors and attitudes associated with the problem. However, it is quite another thing to enter into the hard, often grueling, tasks that must be done. As Peck (1978) suggested, the cornerstone of any clinical relationship is the commitment on the part of the clinician, who must be willing to join in the struggle rather than sitting back and playing a professional role. There will be times during successful treatment when the clinician will be asked to take the field and join in the struggle, not to talk about commitment, but to demonstrate it (see Manning, 1991a). If the clinician is able to do so and to show that she is a stable and understanding ally, the client will be much more likely to go beyond his previously established boundaries.

There are times during treatment—especially if it is conducted outside of the safe environment of the clinic room or building—that you as the clinician will need to "step up to the plate" and lead the way. If clients know that you are willing, they will come to know that you understand the dynamics of stuttering and what it is to be a person who stutters. Moreover, they will know that you are committed to the treatment process. Take your turn at stuttering with a stranger on the street, in a store, on the telephone. Don't talk about it—just do it! Do not tell, but rather *show* the client that it is possible to change both stuttering itself and ways of thinking about it.

The clinician may model risk-taking behavior in speech as well as non-speech activities. Just as the client is asked to venture outside his previously established speech boundaries, the clinician can model behavior that includes presentations to colleagues or social groups. Alternately, the clinician can take on athletic challenges (such as walking, running, or swimming) or professional challenges (such as coordinating a social event or writing an article, pamphlet, or book). By taking risks yourself, it is possible to model new limits for the client; to extend a little beyond previous boundaries.

Challenging the Client

Assuming that we are able to provide the security of a committed clinical relationship and a strategy for change with the client, we then must begin

✓ **CLINICAL DECISION-MAKING**

Several years ago when I was a doctoral student conducting therapy with a young man in his 20s, we left the safety of the clinic room in order to obtain some realistic examples of his stuttering behavior as well as typical listener reactions. As we walked around a large midwestern campus, his task was to stop people and inquire about the location of various buildings. We were early in the treatment process and he was stuttering severely at this point. Nevertheless, he was willing to take part in the activity. Finally, following a particularly difficult speaking situation where he became completely stuck and unable to say anything, his listener, not knowing what else to do, apologized and walked away. My client was devastated and unable to continue. Perhaps I had asked too much of this man. Perhaps I should have done what I was asking him to do. So I took my turn. I asked my client what I should say and how I should stutter. His task was to verify that I stuttered in the preplanned way and to discover specific listener responses. After we had successfully done this with several strangers he was more than willing to enter again into the battle and we continued gathering the information we had set out to find.

pushing the person forward. However, change is difficult even when the motivation exists. Changing the surface structure and, especially, the deep structure of stuttering is difficult. If it were easy, anyone could do it and there would be far fewer people handicapped by the problem of stuttering. However, it is difficult to alter the equilibrium that has been established in one's psyche and in the roles that the stutterer and his listeners have developed over many years. Change involves work; it is time-consuming, and it can be expensive. At the very least, it is an inconvenience.

Because of the difficulties involved, change is not apt to occur without some applied force. The current ways of speaking and thinking about speaking must be moved off-center. There will be times during treatment when the clinician will have to push hard, and demand that specific, concrete tasks be accomplished. Moreover, on more than a few of those occasions, even the most motivated of our clients will not comply. They may not comply because they do not understand the task, because we ask them to move too fast, because the task is too difficult, or simply because they do not want to do what needs to be done. Nonetheless, pushing the client—just as in parenting, teaching, or coaching—beyond his previous levels of performance also shows respect for his potential.

If clinicians, including myself, are to be faulted for any one thing, we are most likely guilty of not pushing our adult clients hard enough. Most adult clients come to us knowing that the task is difficult. They often want us to push them harder, but we are fearful of eliciting a negative reaction. There is some evidence that greater progress in fluency treatment is made when the client is pushed to the point of eliciting negative feelings toward the clinician (Cooper & Cooper, 1965; Manning & Cooper, 1969). As Cooper and his associates have suggested, the dynamic process of change is not likely to yield a consistently positive client-clinician relationship. Just as change is a function of a teacher-student, parent-child, or coach-player relationship, there will be times when progress is especially hard and the mentor must do what is necessary, not what the client would prefer to do. Thus there will be times during treatment when the effective clinician will say and demand things that the client does not want to hear or do. Moreover, there will be periods when, based on our clinical experience and our long-range view of the treatment process, we will have to stand firm in our clinical decisions. However, temporarily being the "bad guy" can sometimes be good, especially when it promotes the long-term progress of our clients.

HUMOR AND THE CLINICIAN

We turn now to a final but potentially sensitive indicator of successful clinicians, the ability to use humor during the clinical process. The reader may have recognized that some authors already cited have suggested humor as a valuable characteristic of clinicians. The focus of our discussion on humor in this chapter concerns clinician attributes. However, our discussion of these attributes and the rationale behind the use of humor will also provide the basis for information found in subsequent chapters on assessment and intervention. Furthermore, a sense of humor is essential for coping with life on a daily basis, particularly if you are working hard to help people with serious communication problems.

A Historical Perspective

Kuhlman (1984) reported that during the first two decades of behavior therapy (1950–1970) there was not a single reference to humor in the literature. This lack of interest in the therapeutic value of humor was clearly the case in the area of fluency disorders. Van Riper (1973) commented briefly about the significance of humor for the person who stutters, describing it in terms of an antiexpectancy device used to lessen the severity of stuttering. He also referred to Bryngelson (1935), as well as Luper and Mulder (1964), who recommended that people who stutter learn to joke about their stuttering in order to help others feel more at ease and to themselves develop more optimistic attitudes about their problem. More recently, Guitar (1997) suggested using humor during the transfer stage of treatment with children as a way of showing them how to become open about their stuttering.

Since the early 1970s there has been a substantial and progressive increase in the therapeutic use of humor, particularly in the professional fields of clinical psychology, counseling, and allied health. During the last twenty-five years, the value of humor began to be recognized as a legitimate part of the human healing process, a way to maintain both physical and psychological health (McGhee & Goldstein, 1977).

The interest in humor in the clinical setting during the 1970s may have occurred, at least in part, because of an increased interest in the humanistic tradition and a renewed appreciation of the cognitive aspects of behavioral intervention in psychology, counseling, and related fields. The research on humor in general, and especially as applied to various forms of treatment for human physical and behavioral problems, began to blossom in the mid-1970s. Perhaps more than any single event, the publishing of Norman Cousins' book, *Anatomy of an Illness,* in 1979 (describing his recovery from the life-threatening disease of ankylosing spondylitis) provided a major impetus for the appreciation of the therapeutic potential of humor by the general public as well as researchers in many areas of human development. Writing and research on humor increased dramatically. Formal and informal networks of professionals interested in the potential of humor in human growth and adjustment were formed (Robinson, 1991). The need to understand the uses and benefits of humor was becoming obvious to researchers throughout the world. Subsequent years have seen the formation of many groups with associated newsletters and meetings, all with an interest in promoting the benefits of humor in various aspects of personal and professional life. Although it is evident that empirical support is needed for much of what is discussed in the literature, the benefits are often striking and the therapeutic potential is obvious.

Beginning in the 1970s, the field of psychotherapy saw an increased call for clinicians who were empathic, spontaneous, flexible, and creative (Kuhlman, 1984). It was reasoned that selecting such a person was the best way to increase the likelihood of creating an effective professional through the academic and clinical training processes. Most of us would choose as a colleague someone who possessed these characteristics—and most clients would be likely to choose such a clinician.

The characteristics proposed by Kuhlman are closely related to another personality characteristic: the ability to appreciate and use humor with yourself and with others. Morreall (1982) noted that a person with a sense of humor is more likely to interact well with others than a person lacking humor. Individuals with a sense of humor tend to be more imaginative and flexible and correspondingly less likely to become obsessed with a particular issue or approach to a problem. In addition, a person with a sense of humor is more likely to be open to suggestions from others and more approachable (Morreall).

Alport (1937, 1961), Maslow (1968), Rogers (1951, 1961), and Combs and Snygg (1959) all identified humor as an essential attribute of a healthy and fully functioning person. It is only recently, however, that this attribute has been acknowledged as a vital characteristic of clinicians. Burton (1972) stated the issue clearly: "One thing every therapist must have is a feeling for the comic. This balances his feeling for the tragic. I am suspicious of any therapist who never laughs" (p. 93). Zinker (1977), in describing the creative nature of (gestalt) therapy, argues that a love of play is a fundamental aspect of the creative life and essential for change. In a similar vein, Rosenheim (1974) commented on the therapeutic potential of humor by saying:

> The unique value and potency of humor in psychotherapy derives mainly from its intrinsic attributes of intimacy, directness and humaneness. Thus, it draws patient and therapist into a closer alliance than is often possible through a more formal, purely rational modality. Laughing with a patient . . . puts to the test and strengthens the accurate perception of both internal and interpersonal realities. (p. 591)

As indicated earlier in this chapter, Zinker (1977) viewed a sense of humor as an important characteristic of an effective clinician. Humor enables us to "turn the world upside down, to make the familiar strange" (p. 45). He indicates that humor has allowed him to view the action of the treatment session with a broader view or from a different angle than would have otherwise been possible. It also enabled him to laugh at his own self-importance. Humor can open a gate for taking a behavior or event and turning it just enough to see the humorous colors. Sometimes it can help loosen what is stuck.

What's So Funny?

Kuhlman (1984) suggested that trying to define and understand humor is like trying to do so for the concept of "learning." When theories of humor are contrasted, there is little agreement on many of the fundamental points (Davis & Farina, 1970). However, a review of even a portion of the literature on humor, especially in the area of "therapeutic humor," clearly indicates that there are some valuable concepts for the speech-language pathologist. The fact that humor has been positively correlated with such personality characteristics as enthusiasm, playfulness, hopefulness, excitement, and vigorousness and negatively correlated with fear, depression, anger, indifference, and aloofness (McGhee & Goldstein, 1977) should alert the clinician to the importance of humor during both the assessment and intervention aspects of treatment.

Attempts to understand the essence of humor and its therapeutic potential have evolved through at least three stages of research. The initial stage of research on humor has been defined by Goldstein (1976) as the *pretheoretical* stage. This stage began during the early part of the 20th century and continued until about 1940. Published manuscripts during this period consisted largely of correlational and observational studies of laughter and smiling: when and how people responded to humor-producing stimuli. There were relatively few attempts to develop or test a particular theory. Goldstein termed the next stage of humor research the *psychoanalytic* phase. Beginning in the 1940s and continuing until the 1970s, this phase was concerned almost exclusively with Freudian theory of wit and humor. Sigmund Freud viewed humor as a potential reducer of stress and placed it alongside the neurotic and psychotic disorders as a basic mechanism of adaptation to human suffering. The essential difference was that humor was thought of as a nonpathological adaptation. In addition, Freud (1928, 1961) asserted that perceived humorousness is related to the degree with which one is able to empathize and assume the role of the person who is the focus of humor.

The third and current stage of research on humor began during the 1970s and stressed the *cognitive* foundations of humor: what it is that causes a person to interpret a particular event as humorous. The change from a Freudian view of humor to a cognitive approach corresponded to the loss of interest in the psychoanalytic view of human behavior and a corresponding increase in Jean Piaget's cognitive-structural view of humor development and behavior.

Two similar views of humor provide a good beginning for appreciating the possibilities for intervention with individuals who stutter. Morreall (1982) suggested that laughter is the natural expression of the feeling of amusement in response to a *sudden conceptual shift*. He suggested that the essence of humor is found in the enjoyment of incongruity. Associated with incongruity is a conceptual shift (not necessarily an emotional one) in the way we consider an event. This conceptual shift must be *immediate,* and the change in the conceptual states be relatively large. When the shift is predictable or anticipated, the degree of humor decreases accordingly. Davis and Farina (1970) advance a similar explanation for a humorous event. They include as basic features of humor *contradiction* or *incongruity*, as well as the *integration* of contradictory ideas or concepts, which takes place *suddenly*. These authors also emphasize a sudden shift that results in new *insight* about the relationship of ideas or concepts. Furthermore, this new insight results in an objective—in contrast to an emotional—experience of the concepts. "We may say that on the cognitive side, laughter results from the sudden insightful integration of contradictory or incongruous ideas, attitudes, or sentiments which are experienced objectively" (Davis & Farina, 1970, p. 307).

Humor in Psychotherapy

Psychotherapists and counselors have differing views on the efficacy and worth of humor during the treatment process. To some clinicians, treatment is "serious business" and not a place where humorous things are likely to take place. On the other hand, there are clinicians who argue that a humorous view of the circumstances presented to us by life could be considered an appropriate issue for the process of treatment (Schimel, 1978). Because of the inherent difficulty of persuading clinicians to consider the possibilities of humor during treatment, some authors have attempted to relate humor to prevailing theoretical approaches. This, of course, is one way of assigning some importance to an aspect of treatment that is likely to have little credibility for some clinicians. One can imagine this group reacting to the suggestion of using humor in the treatment of a handicapping problem by saying "Be serious! Change is difficult, even painful. How can you possibly imply that there is something humorous about such an overwhelming problem." Not surprisingly, clients also may have this initial response to the appropriateness of humor during treatment.

USING HUMOR IN TREATMENT

It is important to consider the way we think about humor in a treatment sense. The semantics of the phrase "using humor" suggests that humor is a device that the clinician brings to the treatment session in the same way that one might bring a questionnaire or treatment technique. To think in terms of *using* humor gives the impression that a clinician will arrive at the treatment session with a well-rehearsed series of jokes (Kuhlman, 1984) or wearing a red clown nose.

Rather than thinking of using humor in this sense, Kuhlman (1984) proposed that humor is more appropriately viewed as an integral part of the *interactional* aspects of treatment. Rather than a device or tool, humor is related to the client-clinician relationship and to the sense of timing therein. He suggested that spontaneity is the essence of all effective humor, and certainly of humor occurring during treatment. Accordingly, until the clinician is calibrated to the client and until some level of intimacy has been established in the therapeutic relationship, humor is not likely to serve a beneficial purpose.

The fact is, humor and laughter frequently take place during successful treatment, including treatment for fluency disorders. Until recently though, it has not been discussed in the literature (Manning & Beachy, 1995). There is, during effective treatment, the enthusiasm and excitement of exploration. The resulting change in insight often leads to an expression of humor, and conversely, humor can lead to insight. E. B. White (1954/1960) wrote that "humor at its best is a kind of heightened truth—a super truth." Most behavioral strategies seek to expand the client's awareness of the problem that brought him to treatment. Alport (1961) demonstrated the close relationship between insight and humor, finding a positive correlation of .88 between the two. He further noted that insight and humor were related to an individual's capacity for self-objectification and the ability to construe oneself as both subject and object (Kuhlman, 1984). That is, humor reflects a person's ability to step away and *distance* himself from his situation in order to gain a degree of insight. The distance provides for a degree of objectivity that allows us to see ourselves from a new angle or with a "God's eye" view. The new view that we are able to provide through humor is the first of three basic qualities (conceptual shift, distancing, and mastery) that make humor an effective force for the clinician.

The Conceptual Shift

The conceptual shift that is an integral part of humor and permits a more objective view is not likely to be part of the treatment process early in the therapeutic relationship. The initial treatment sessions often are spent gathering information such as acquiring baseline performance, obtaining demographic data, developing procedural guidelines, and becoming calibrated to the client. During and following these initial stages, the clinician begins to become attuned to the client. Once the therapeutic relationship becomes stable, humor is more likely to become part of the relationship. As the sessions continue, an interactional environment will begin to be established in which spontaneity and the expression of something other than the preliminary aspects of the relationship can occur.

As more intimacy is established in the clinician-client relationship, the limits of appropriate humor can expand, as can the number and severity of the taboos that may be violated in safety (Kuhlman, 1984). Humor creates a relaxed atmosphere and encourages communication, particularly on sensitive matters (McGhee & Goldstein, 1977). Although humor is not the only force in the process of promoting a client's conceptual shift about himself and his problem, it can play an important role in the process of change during treatment (Kuhlman).

As humor facilitates a new insight about an old problem, the client may respond with pleasure or laughter. A kind of catharsis may take place, and for the first time, a new way of looking at the problem may result. According to Kuhlman (1984), the client's laughter, if spontaneous and genuine, can be taken as a sign of validation of a change in insight. On occasion, a client's initial reaction to a new view of the problem or the situation may be one of anger. He may not like the view that the new insight provides, especially if the old view is comforting. Consequently, the appropriateness of a humorous interpretation of an event must be judged within the context of the therapeutic relationship *at that particular moment*. To be appropriate as well as effective, the timing must be both accurate and spontaneous.

It has often been suggested that an integral part of a comprehensive behavioral treatment strategy involves the client's development of a new belief system—a paradigm shift—about himself and the problem (Cooper, 1993; Covey, 1989; Kuhlman, 1984; Hayhow & Levy, 1989, Peck, 1978; Van Riper, 1973). During that process, the client tends to, more or less effectively, ward off the clinician's views and perspective on the problem. As Kuhlman (1984) suggested, although people seek treatment in order to feel better, they are often less than enthusiastic about the behavioral and cognitive changes necessary to achieve the goals of treatment. The client is apt to cling to established perspectives and belief patterns because they are familiar, comfortable, and self-protective (Hayhow & Levy, 1989). The client is often too close to the situation, especially a threatening or emotionally laden one, to see it any other way. Alternately, he has viewed the situation for so long from a particular angle that no other view seems possible. Humor can assist both the clinician and the client in viewing the situation from other angles, other perspectives. As Kuhlman (1984) stated, before a client is able to adopt a new belief system, he must acknowledge and dismiss the old one as being in error in some way. Although humor does not have to be a part of the process, it is often an effective and pleasurable way to facilitate and share the changes that are occurring.

Distancing With Humor

In order to facilitate the development of a new cognitive perspective and begin to form a new belief system about both oneself and the problem, it is necessary to step away from the situation somewhat (Kuhlman, 1984). It is not necessary to step back a great distance, but only far enough to see its paradoxical aspects. Until the person is able to move back somewhat, especially from a threatening experience or a problem that creates anxiety, the paradoxical aspects of the situation will not be readily appar-

---

⌕ CLINICAL INSIGHT

On the afternoon of one of our first therapy sessions, I was helping Joyce, a woman in her 50s, to identify some of the characteristic behaviors that accompanied her moments of stuttering. As we worked together to replicate the various behaviors we were seeing and hearing, I commented on a particularly severe example. With a good deal of enthusiasm I told her that what she had just done was "a really fascinating and wonderful way of stuttering." My interest and positive attitude about a behavior that had represented only embarrassment, shame, and misery for more than 50 years elicited abrupt laughter from her that we both enjoyed.

ent. However, as the client, with the clinician's assistance, is able to achieve greater distance, it will be possible to gradually gain objectivity by viewing the problem with the third eye of humor. Rather than endlessly reliving earlier experiences with the old view, new interpretations will become possible. Humor promotes the possibility that the client will begin to play with the possibilities and have fun considering a variety of new interpretations of the experience.

Morreall (1982) also discussed the role of distancing in humor. He suggested that humor has a liberating effect. Often something is funny because it violates what is supposed to be sacrosanct, or it goes against the rational or, certainly, the accepted order of things. Morreall made the astute observation that humor enables us to achieve some distance and perspective, not only in situations where we are failing, but also in situations where we are succeeding; humor can prevent us from overrating our achievements. The more developed a person's sense of humor, the wider the range of situations in which the clinician can achieve the distance required to laugh. For the clinician, and certainly for the client, it is important to appreciate that to the extent that we can achieve this distance from the practical aspects of a situation, we will be free from being dominated by it. Moreover, to the degree that a person can appreciate the humor in his or her own personal situation, that person will be liberated from the dominance of emotions and more likely to develop an objective view.

🔍 CLINICAL INSIGHT

One afternoon during our group therapy session, Marcy was reporting to the others that she had finally, after many failures, willed herself to order something at a drive-through restaurant. Since we were at the early stages of treatment, the goal of this activity was simply to do the task regardless of any stuttering that might occur. In vivid detail, Marcy described her fear as she approached the enclosed microphone-speaker and her attempt to place her order. The typical unintelligible voice asked her what she wanted and she promptly responded by saying "I would like an order of fries, a coke, and a hambur- hambur- hambur- hambur- hamburger. The group responded with applause at her courage for taking such a risk and carry out an action that she had rigorously avoided for many years. She thanked us all but added that the only real problem she had was when she pulled around to receive her lunch. The cashier handed her an order of fries, a coke, and five hamburgers. The laughter of Marcy and the group members suggested that she had achieved some distance from an event that had always been thought of as an absolutely dreadful experience.

Mastery and Humor

Lefcourt and Martin (1989) found that the expression of humor is also related to a feeling of mastery of a task or situation. Their interpretation of this relationship relates to the view of humor as a reducer of stress. As Kuhlman (1984) pointed out, the relationship between mastery and humor is readily observed in children as they face problem-solving situations. Laughter is often a by-product of children's shift from one cognitive stage to another as they master a new problem. Problem solving, especially when the experience is a new one, is exhilarating (Levine, 1977). The client's subsequent behavior change suggests that some reorganization of internal reality (insight) has been achieved, which allowed the problem to be solved.

This perspective of humor and mastery also coincides with the view of humor suggested by Freud (1928). That is, the humor process includes a cognitive reorientation in the face of stress (Martin & Lefcourt, 1983; Nezu, Nezu, & Blissett, 1988). The ability to appreciate as well as use humor has been shown to be related to a person's internal locus of control, which provides an indication of how much the individual perceives events as a consequence of his or her own behavior (Craig, Franklin, & Andrews, 1984). Subjects who hold an internal locus of control were found to smile and laugh more in the face of stress (Lefcourt, Sordoni, & Sordoni, 1974). Martin and Lefcourt (1984) found that people with better internal locus of control scores demonstrate greater ability to take multiple perspectives when problem solving as well as to resist the effects of persuasion. Persons whose locus of control is more internally based are more able to consider alternative constructions for their experiences. Though having multiple perspectives regarding an issue does not necessarily lead to humor, the experience of humor is believed to require a person's ability to view a situation or event from multiple perspectives (Lefcourt & Martin, 1989).

Lefcourt and Martin (1989) suggested that in order to have a greater ability to entertain alternative interpretations for experiences, one must perceive oneself as an actor, a determiner of one's fate, and an active maker of choices. Only by making choices among available options can one be free. In the absence of choice, one is more likely to feel controlled and constrained. Thus, in the exercise of choice and the ability to consider alternative interpretations, there is a connection between a sense of mastery and the potential for humor (Lefcourt & Martin, 1989).

Everyone has experienced relief following the successful completion of a particularly daunting activity and, as with children, laughter often accompanies the retelling of the experience. As people who stutter achieve the ability to vary and change their behavior, there are likely to be reports of humorous reactions and experiences that could not have been regarded as humorous only a few weeks or months earlier. This relief is also the case for nonstuttering clinicians who are asked to take the role of a person who is stuttering in order to understand the fear and avoidance that is part of the experience.

CONCLUSION

We have addressed in this chapter the most important component of the treatment process for people who stutter: the clinician. We have considered the impact of the clinician's attitudes and intervention skills on the treatment process and described many of the characteristics of the experienced and wise clinician. We have also introduced the variable of humor, as both a clinician characteristic as well as an indication of client change and progress during treatment. Humor seems to be a factor worthy of consideration in the treatment process, for many features of change are indicated by humor as people achieve mastery, distance, and a conceptual shift concerning their situation. Effective clinicians are able to lead the way in viewing the situation from different angles, often with the help of humorous interpretations. As we will see in the chapters to follow, many variables influence the likelihood of success, both during and after treatment.

However, one important constant is the person guiding the process. It takes energy and optimism on the part of the clinician, for the work is sometimes demanding. Each client provides a challenge that tests us repeatedly, and it is necessary and appropriate that we ask ourselves if we are up to the task. It can be hard to prevent burnout. However, if being a clinician is thought of as a continual process of learning and growth, we can renew ourselves with continuing educational opportunities and other avenues of personal enrichment. Much of our growth

---

🔍 CLINICAL INSIGHT

In order to complete their assignment of posing as a moderately severe stutterer, two graduate students were going around a local mall and engaging in conversations with people at several stores. As they entered a bookstore, one of the students realistically stuttered as she asked for a book on the topic of physical therapy. The clerk checked her computer and indicated that no books on that topic were available. The student, still obviously stuttering, asked for something on the topic of occupational therapy. The clerk was unsuccessful yet again. After a brief pause, the clerk cautiously asked "Would you consider something on speech therapy?"

comes from the people we are trying so hard to help. The best clinicians know that clients have much to teach us and that we often benefit nearly as much from the treatment process as they do. Although we have been down this path before, the territory and timing of the steps will be new for our companion, to whom we must attend closely with both determination and esteem.

STUDY QUESTIONS

➤ What attitudes and stereotypes do you have about people who stutter? What stereotypes do you feel have changed as a result of reading this chapter?

➤ What reasons can you give to explain why many clinicians are anxious about providing treatment for people who stutter?

➤ Provide examples of how people who stutter are portrayed in movies and television. (See the Stuttering Home Page, Appendix B)

➤ Which of the personality characteristics of clinicians described in this chapter do you believe are characteristic of you?

➤ Which of the clinician intervention skills described do you feel will be the most difficult for you to demonstrate in a clinical situation?

➤ Write a humorous interpretation of your attempts to learn a new athletic skill.

➤ Provide at least two examples of past experiences or situations that were embarrassing or frightening at the time that with some distance, mastery, and paradigm shift, have since become humorous.

RECOMMENDED READINGS

Cousins, N. (1979). *Anatomy of an illness*. New York: Norton.

Robinson, V. M. (1991). *Humor and the health professions*. Throrfare, NJ: Slack, Inc. (See the chapters in the section titled, "Humor in Health and Illness".)

Van Riper, C. (1975). The stutterer's clinician. In Jon Eisenson (Ed.), *Stuttering, a second symposium* (pp. 453–492).

Van Riper, C. (1979). *A career in speech pathology*. Englewood Cliffs, NJ: Prentice Hall Inc. (See chapters titled, "The Clinician's Skill," pp. 103–114; "The Rewards of Therapy," pp. 115–138.)

CHAPTER

2

THEORIES OF ETIOLOGY

> *"Again, the reason science works so well is partly that built-in error-correcting machinery. There are no forbidden questions in science, no matters too sensitive or delicate to be probed, no sacred truths. That openness to new ideas, combined with the most rigorous, skeptical scrutiny of all ideas, sifts the wheat from the chaff. It makes no difference how smart, august, or believed you are. You must prove your case in the face of determined, expert criticism. Diversity and debate are valued. (p. 31)*
>
> Carl Sagan (1996).
> The Demon-Haunted World: Science as a
> Candle in the Dark. *New York: Random House*

INTRODUCTION

Perhaps no other disorder of human communication has been described in so many different ways. Stuttering has been called, among other things, a mystery, an enigma, a puzzle, and a riddle (Bluemel, 1957). Because stuttering can look and feel very different depending on how one experiences it (particularly whether or not one is a person who stutters), Wendell Johnson (1958) used the analogy of a group of blind men examining an elephant, each arriving at a very different conclusion because they were examining a different aspect of the animal and because they were unable to see the entire structure. Similarly, because the large majority of the syndrome of stuttering lies beneath the surface, stuttering also has been equated to an iceberg (Sheehan, 1970). These characterizations suggest that stuttering is a complex disorder composed of many levels or factors. However, they also indicate the confusion that the syndrome holds for even the most experienced researcher and clinician in the field. While there appears to be gradually increasing agreement about the most appropriate possibilities for intervention, the etiology of the disorder continues to be an appealing mystery that many dedicated researchers are attempting to answer.

This uncertainty is such that it could be argued that one sign of the competent clinician is that she does not effortlessly provide an answer to the question of etiology. As we shall see, glib answers about such a complex syndrome may be one sign of a less than knowledgeable (or ethical) professional. However, even though clinicians and researchers may not yet have a complete answer about the etiology of the problem, it is important for the clinician to have an opinion. The clinician should have, if not a complete answer, at least a reasonable response to the question of causation, and she should be able to demonstrate her awareness of the etiological possibilities for the clients (and the parents of clients) whom she will see.

One of the first and most frequent questions the clinician will be asked by clients, parents, and other professionals is, "What causes stuttering?" The clinician's response to this question will frequently be her first opportunity to demonstrate her competence and understanding concerning the syndrome. The response will also set the stage for the client's interpretation of himself and his speech. Telling someone that the stuttering is a symptom of a psychological conflict resulting from a pregenital conversion neurosis is likely to have a considerably different effect than saying that his stuttering may be the result of a combination of physiological predisposing factors and learned (mal)adaptive behaviors. In addition, as many current authors suggest , the clinician's understanding about the possible etiologies of the problem will have an influence on the clinician's treatment decisions (Bloodstein, 1995; Conture, 1990; Culatta & Goldberg, 1995; Ham, 1990; Peters & Guitar, 1991; Riley & Riley, 2000; Silverman, 1996; Starkweather, Gottwald, & Halfond, 1990). If the clinician believes that fluency failure can result from communication demands that exceed a child's limited capacity for speech and language production, some treatment decisions will undoubtedly be more appropriate than others. The clinician's explanation of etiology will influence the parents' response to their situation, including how they deal with any guilt or shame they may have about their child's speech and how they react when their child produces fluent or stuttered speech.

Although stuttering can be a highly aversive phenomenon, it nevertheless holds a fascination for most people. Characters who stutter appear with some regularity in movies and books. No doubt much of this appeal centers on the mystery of the etiology and the unique, sometimes humorous, situations that stuttering sometimes creates. Students of the field only have to mention to one or more people that they are taking a course in stuttering in order to elicit a flood of queries about the disorder. The initial questions will usually center on etiology, the psychological components of the problem, and the possibilities of treatment.

Undoubtedly, the problem of stuttering is complex. In a few select cases we are able to identify, with reasonable certainty, a likely cause. For example, there are instances of sudden onset, such as in neurogenic or psychogenic stuttering, where it is possible to identify specific events that appear to have precipitated the problem (see Chapter 4). As we will see, however, these are exceptional cases. Given our current understanding, the precise reasons for the large majority of *developmental* stuttering are unknown. This is because there is no single reason. At least in most cases, the syndrome appears to arise from a combination of several factors that come together within a requisite time interval. In addition, combination of forces that result in stuttering may well be novel for different individuals. Fish (1995) suggested that efforts to determine the past causes of many current human problems may be unnecessary, misguided, or even counterproductive. Fortunately, in most cases, it is not necessary for the clinician to know the precise cause of the problem in order to provide the speaker with substantial help.

Throughout history, there has been no shortage of writers proposing simplistic solutions concerning the etiology of stuttering. Today, a student of the field who is exploring the many worthwhile sources of information about stuttering on the Internet does not have to travel far before coming face-to-face with such claims. These are typically accompanied by testimonials of former clients who now profess to be as fluent as an anchor person on the national news. To be sure, there have always been beguiling leads that result in a wave of furious investigations. Although there are some etiological models that appear to explain much of what is known about the onset and development of the problem, there are many speakers who are exceptions to each model: people who fail to follow the prescribed developmental path.

Silverman (1996) makes the barbed—but accurate—comment that should any so-called authority propose to understand the cause, let alone a cure for this disorder, all but the most naive clinicians will tend to be highly suspicious of anything else the person may say. Conture (1990) reflects the understanding of those who have worked for years in the field when he says that no one has developed a program that provides an answer to all people who stutter. He provides a forthright opinion when he says:

> I don't know what causes stuttering. I also don't know the best way to treat it. I don't even know if there is *one* way. I'm not sure if anyone else does either. Of one thing I am sure, however: The history of stuttering reflects a multidimensional problem that has repeatedly and successfully defied unidimensional solutions. (p. 1)

So, despite claims to the contrary, it is good to suspect *anyone* who appears to have all the answers and to claim consistently high levels of success with those who stutter. The problem, especially for adolescents and adults, is plainly not a simple one. If there were a single or obvious reason why people stutter, the answer would have been found long ago. Many intelligent and dedicated people have spent lifetimes (see Van Riper, 1979, 1990) searching for a cause. Moreover, though explanations about etiology vary across researchers and clinicians, there are probably seeds of truth in many.

ATTEMPTS TO DEFINE STUTTERING AND RELATED TERMS

Before discussing etiological models of stuttering, we will define some related terms. The term *stammering* can be found in some early literature in this country, where it tended to be used interchangeably with stuttering. While currently the term *stuttering* is used in the United States, *stammering* is often used to mean essentially the same thing in Europe. The major self-help group in Great Britain, for example, is called the British Stammering Association.

The term *disfluent* is often used in the literature to indicate the fluency breaks of normal speakers, while the term *dysfluent* is used to describe the abnormal fluency breaks of people who stutter. According to a variety of medical dictionaries, the prefix *dis* means reversal, separation, or duplication. The prefix *dys*, on the other hand, means difficult, impaired, painful, bad, or disordered. However, because there is considerable overlap in the nature of the fluency breaks of normal and stuttering speakers, there have been ambiguous findings. The speech of people who stutter contains many "normal" fluency breaks, and it is not always clear which surface behaviors differentiate disfluent and dysfluent speech. Often, of course, it is a matter of degree. The fact that the two words are pronounced the same can lead to additional confusion. As we will see later, normal speakers have many fluency breaks, with some of them characterized by tension and struggle behavior, features that are associated with stuttered speech. In part because of this overlap along the continuum of normal and abnormal fluency, several authors use the term *disfluent* speech when referring to normal as well as abnormal fluency breaks. As we have stated, fluent speech is characterized by both ease of production and flow of information. Fluency allows the listener to attend to the content of the speech rather than the way it is being produced. When production is effortful and information does not easily flow from the speaker to the listener, speech is apt to be considered disfluent.

It is important to point out that the following discussion concerns the development of stuttering in young children. Although the onset of developmental stuttering may begin (or at least is diagnosed) as late as the early years of adolescence (ages 8 through 11), the vast majority of people who stutter begin doing so during the early childhood years, ages 2 through 6 (Andrews & Harris, 1964).

A term that has appeared in the literature on stuttering for many years is *primary stuttering*. Bluemel (1932) described primary stuttering as a transient phenomenon in which a child's fluency breaks are easy and he is generally unaware of his problem. The child displays no special effort or tension during speaking. The motoric behaviors taking place in the speech production mechanism at the outset of the behavior are sometimes referred to as *core* (Van Riper, 1982) or *Alpha* (Conture, Rothenberg, & Molitor, 1986) behaviors. These primary—or initial—behaviors are differentiated from the *secondary* or *accessory* behaviors that gradually develop around the core of the small breaks and pauses in speech. It is generally agreed that secondary behaviors are learned responses or attempts to cope with the initial breaks in speech flow. The initial breaks in the timing of speech sometimes indicate the incipient stages of stuttering in young children. These breaks, at their most basic level, take the form of easy repetitions and prolongations. However, as awareness increases and struggle behavior develops, there may be blockages or disruptions in airflow, phonation, or even respiration. The essential question that theories of etiology attempt to explain is why these core behaviors take place and why they occur in some children and not in others.

Writers have often conceptualized the development of stuttering as progressing in a more or less linear fashion from primary to secondary stuttering. More recent findings indicate that many children who stutter do not go through a period of primary stuttering, but rather present with complex and severe behaviors at the time stuttering is first observed (Yairi & Ambrose, 1992a,b, 1999; Yairi, Ambrose, & Niermann, 1993). As we shall see, this will have important implications for the clinician when making decisions about whether or not to initiate treatment.

Some Definitions of Stuttering

The variety of definitions that have been offered over the years gives the reader an indication of the many ways of viewing this problem. Many definitions reflect the author's view of etiology rather than actually defining the problem. Johnson's 1946 definition, for example, reflected his view of etiology when he argued that stuttering was what the person who stutters does to avoid stuttering. During the 1940s and 1950s Johnson came to define stuttering as an anticipatory, apprehensive, hypertonic avoidance reaction. His view was that stuttering was a learned response to environmental events and something that the person (a) does, not something that happens to him; (b) expects to (anticipates will) occur; (c) is fearful (apprehensive) about doing; (d) is tense (hypertonic) about; and (e) tries to keep from happening (avoidance). Most agree that this was a somewhat restrictive definition and that stuttering can occur in the absence of some or even many of these attributes.

Another definition of stuttering is offered by the World Health Organization (1977). This definition points out that, in contrast to the view of many nonprofessionals, people who stutter know what they want to say. Although people who stutter certainly can experience word finding problems, for someone to tell a person who stutters to stop and think what he wants to say indicates a lack of understanding about the nature of the problem. The person who stutters generally knows precisely what he wants to say. He is unable, however, to move through the sounds or make the transitions from one sound to another so that it can be said. The World Health Organization states that stuttering includes "disorders in the rhythm of speech in which the individual knows precisely what he wishes to say, but at the time is unable to say it because of an involuntary, repetitive prolongation or cessation of a sound" (p. 202). There are aspects of this definition that will reoccur throughout this text. That is, the word "disorders" implies that the symptoms of stuttering can take many forms and have more than one etiology (hence the title of this text). Furthermore, the core behaviors of the problem are involuntary.

Taking a similar approach, Van Riper (1982) and Perkins (1983) suggest that a fluency break is more likely to be *normal* if it is the result of "linguistic uncertainty." That is, the speaker is hesitating because he has not yet formulated how to express himself. Stuttering is more likely to be occurring if formulation is not the major issue and if there is a physical constriction or closure of the vocal tract.

Views of stuttering as a classical and operant conditioned behavior are reflected in Brutten & Shoemaker's 1967 definition that "stuttering is that form of fluency failure that results from conditioned negative emotion" (p. 61). For those who view stuttering as a type of primary neurosis, a symptom of a basic emotional or psychological conflict, there is the trend to define stuttering by citing the presumed source of the conflict rather than describing the stuttering behavior (symptoms). Coriat (1943), for example, describes stuttering as a psychoneurosis characterized by the persistence of early, pregenital oral nursing, oral sadistic, and anal sadistic elements. Taking a similar approach, Glauber (1958) described stuttering as "a symptom in a psychopathological condition classified as a pregenital conversion neurosis" (p. 78). Perhaps the most memorable explanation of this type was offered by Fenichel in 1945 who stated, "Stuttering is a pregenital conversion neurosis in that the early problems of dealing with retention and expulsion of feces have been displaced upwards into the sphincters of the mouth" (as cited in Van Riper, 1982, p. 264).

One of the most frequently cited is that of Wingate (1964). For many years this definition has been used to describe subjects in clinical studies since it provides a comprehensive list of both behaviors and attitudes that the clinician can expect to see across a variety of clients.

> The term "stuttering" means: 1. (a) Disruption in the fluency of verbal expression, which is (b) characterized by involuntary, audible, or silent repetitions or prolongations in the utterance of short speech elements, namely: sounds, syllables, and words of one syllable. These disruptions (c) usually occur frequently or are marked in character and (d) are not readily controllable. 2. Sometimes the disruptions are (e) accompanied by accessory activities involving the speech apparatus, related or unrelated body structures, or stereotyped speech utterances. These activities give the appearance of being speech-related struggle. 3. Also, there not infrequently are (f) indications or reports of the presence of an emotional state, ranging from a general condition of "excitement" or "tension" to more specific emotions of a negative nature such as fear, embarrassment, irritation, or the like. The immediate source of stuttering is some incoordination expressed in the peripheral speech mechanism; the ultimate cause is presently unknown and may be complex or compound. (p. 488)

Following years of study concerning the psycholinguistic features of stuttering and his conclusion that the language skills (word fluency, word association, storytelling) of people who stutter are atypical, Wingate (1988) proposed that "stuttering is a deficit in the language production system, a defect that extends beyond the level of motor execution . . . [and that] the defect is not simply one of motor control or coordination, but . . . involves more central functions of the language production system" (p. 239).

It is common for definitions of stuttering to include the perceptual effect of the stuttering on a *listener* but fail to consider the reaction of the *speaker* that occurs before, during, and following the most obvious aspect of the stuttering moment. This is an important shortcoming in some definitions because, as much and possibly more than anything else, it is the *speaker's* response to the breaks in fluency that differentiates people who stutter from those who experience normal and usual disruptions of fluency. Perkins (1983) discusses this idea when he points out the shortcomings of definitions that depend exclusively on listener perception. Although the listener is able to identify the acoustic features of the fluency break, he or she may not distinguish the cognitive and affective experience of the event. Thus definitions that deal only with the surface (audible and visible) features of the problem fail to thoroughly describe the stuttering experience. A comprehensive definition of stuttering must also take into account the effect of the experience on the speaker. Van Riper acknowledged this when, in 1982, he stated that "stuttering occurs when the forward flow of speech is interrupted by a motorically disrupted sound, syllable, or word, or *by the speaker's reactions thereto* [italics added]" (p. 15).

How the speaker reacts—what he tells himself about his stuttering experience (or even the possibility of stuttering)—helps to define himself and his speech. In a related issue, Silverman (1996) takes a pragmatic approach when discussing the *handicapping* effect of stuttering. He maintains that the number of choices and activities that stuttering prevents the person from doing defines the degree of handicap. Citing several personal accounts (Attanasio, 1987; Carlisle, 1985; Johnson, 1930; Murray & Edwards, 1980; Shields, 1989; Sugarman, 1980; Van Riper, 1984), he points out that the actual handicap that can result from being a person who stutters can be considerably different (often greater) than the surface features of the stuttering would indicate. It is not uncommon for the handicapping effects associated with stuttering to result from the speaker's reaction to his situation and his attempts to alter or adapt to the problem, often in less than effectual ways.

The issue of handicap has been addressed within the classification scheme proposed by the World Health Organization (WHO, 1980). The International Classification of Impairments, Disabilities, and Handicaps (ICIDH), developed by the WHO, describes separate but related levels of a disease or disorder: impairment, disability, and handicap. Yaruss (1998) provides a comprehensive review of how the these three levels have been applied to the disorder of stuttering and suggests a model for describing the experience of stuttering and for bringing consistency to how the terms impairment, disability, and handicap are used. Yaruss (p. 253) suggests the following suggestions for defining the three basic levels of the model:

Impairment: Disruption of speech-language production typically characterized by certain interruptions in the forward flow of speech (e.g., unusually long or physically tense hesitations; repetitions of sounds, syllables, or words; or prolongations of sounds or articulatory postures beyond their usual duration), and including any associated audible or visible characteristics of those interruptions, if present (e.g., physical tension, nonspeech behaviors, and struggle in the speech musculature or periphery).

Disability: Limitations in an individual's ability to communicate with others or to engage in social or work-related activities, resulting directly from the individual's stuttering impairment, or form the individual's affective, behavioral, or cognitive reactions to the stuttering impairment.

Handicap: Disadvantages experienced by an individual, resulting from the stuttering impairment and associated disabilities, or from reactions to them (exhibited either by the individual or by those with whom the individual interacts), that *limit* the individual's ability to fulfill social, occupational, or economic roles that would otherwise be considered normal and attainable for that individual.

Yaruss expands the WHO model to include an additional level of (presumed) etiology which was not part of the impairment level of the WHO model (Figure 2-1). The model also includes three levels of reactions (affective, behavioral, and cognitive) which influence the interplay between the impairments and disabilities. Finally, the model is a dynamic one with bidirectional interactions between levels. That is, there is the possibility of developing other impairments in reaction to certain disabilities and handicaps, and there is an interplay between environmental influences, such as the speaker's unique reaction to environmental influences in the development of handicaps.

Finally, the involuntary nature of the problem and the associated loss of control and helplessness are a crucial feature that defines the experience of being a person who stutters. The many clinical implications of such a loss of control over one's ability to speak are discussed again in the following chapters. At this point, however, we want to emphasize that the experience of losing control is an important part of a definition of stuttering.

Several authors agree that a fundamental and distinguishing characteristic of the stuttering moment is the *loss of control* by the speaker (Bloodstein, 1987; Cooper, 1968; Manning, 1977; Manning & Shrum, 1973; Perkins, 1983; Van Riper, 1937). Van Riper stated that "the stutterer feels he has no control over his stuttering performance." (p. 151). Bloodstein felt that for the person who stutters, the fundamental difference between real and fake stuttering is the awareness of tension and being out of control associated with real stuttering. It is also noteworthy that the involuntary aspect of the syndrome is included in the previously discussed World Health Organization (1977) definition.

While the concept of "involuntary" can be difficult for the clinician or researcher to identify and quantify, Manning and Shrum state that such a loss of control

> can be extremely identifiable and specific to the stuttering client. The client is able to "know" whether he is completely "in charge" of his speech or whether "the block has assumed command." Certainly the stutterer could indicate to the clinician when such control has been achieved. In many instances, though, the experienced clinician is able to identify such control or the lack of it. (1973, p. 33)

Perkins (1983) argues that the involuntary nature of stuttering should form the core of any definition. In 1990 he suggested that although listeners can demonstrate reasonably good reliability in identifying the surface features of stuttering, a more valid and authentic indicator of stuttering is provided by the person who is producing (or attempting to produce) the speech. Precisely because it is possible for the speaker to distinguish

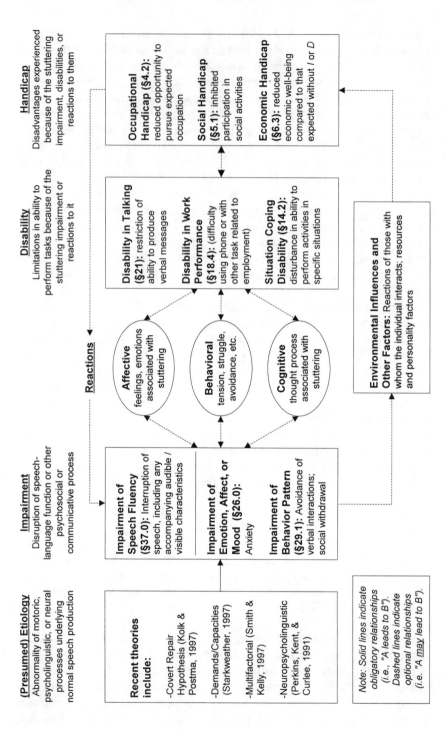

Figure 2-1. A model for viewing the experience of stuttering based on the International Classification of Impairments, Disabilities, and Handicaps (ICIDH) by the World Health Organization (WHO, 1980).

whether he is in control of his speech, Perkins describes stuttering as being categorically different from nonstuttered speech.

> The essence of stuttering, in my view, is not what is perceived by listeners as stuttering in the acoustical signal, but rather what occurs in the production of stuttered speech. . . . Stuttering is the involuntary disruption of a continuing attempt to produce a spoken utterance. . . . From the stutterer's vantage point, however, the judgement is categorical: Either involuntary blockage has or has not occurred to some degree. If it has not occurred, then what sounds like stuttering to the observer would not feel like stuttering to the speaker. The reason that this distinction is categorical is because the proposed definition posits that loss of control of the ability to voluntarily continue a disrupted utterance is the essence of stuttering. If the disruption is not involuntary to some degree, then it is not a stuttered disfluency. Moreover, the stutterer would not react to it with apprehension, struggle, or avoidance if it were stuttered. (p. 376)

Thus, Perkins sees stuttering as being *qualitatively* unique because the speaker, during a moment of stuttering, is not in control (see Chapters 3 and 9 for examples). While this view may seem intuitively appealing and a feature of stuttering that has important clinical implications, it has proven to be difficult to identify empirically (Martin & Haroldson, 1986; Moore & Perkins, 1990).

In summary, although the surface features of stuttering are sometimes obvious and distinguishable, it would appear that some of the most telling features lie under the surface and reside in the more subtle cognitive and affective layers of the syndrome. As Conture (1990, pp. 17–20) suggests, there are many nonverbal features such as body movement, tension, and psychosocial discomfort that help to more precisely distinguish and define stuttering.

A comprehensive definition of stuttering by Peters and Guitar (1991) incorporates both the physiological capacities of the speaker as well as the adaptive learning that takes place. These authors define stuttering as "a disorder of the neuromotor control of speech, influenced by the interactive process of language production, and intensified by complex learning processes" (p. 18).

Although another definition is probably unnecessary, the following sentences indicate the view of the present author. Stuttering behavior is indicated by an involuntary break in the sequence of motor movements necessary for verbal communication. The speaker typically knows what he or she wants to say. Breaks in fluency are often accompanied by physical tension that restricts the efficient and coordinated functioning of the vocal tract and the entire speech production system. Many of the overt features are learned, often maladaptive behaviors that the speaker uses to avoid, postpone, or escape from the stuttering experience. Breaks in fluency are generally accompanied by a sense of helplessness and loss of control. The etiology of (developmental) stuttering is due to a combination of factors rather than a unitary cause. Current research on the etiology of the disorder suggests a combination of subtle neurological factors, some of which may be genetically influenced, combining with responses to environmental stimuli at critical stages in the early (preschool) acquisition of language and speech.

THEORIES OF ETIOLOGY— A HISTORICAL PERSPECTIVE

Students may not always appreciate the value of learning about past views of stuttering etiology. Silverman provides a fine justification for such reflection when he says:

> Our present views on both the etiology and management of stuttering are built upon the experience of the past. Clinicians who are unaware of how stuttering has been treated in the past are more likely to use intervention strategies that have been shown again and again to be of little or no long-term value than are those who have this knowledge. These strategies may produce a rapid reduction in stuttering severity, but the vast majority of clients on whom they are used are likely to relapse within five years following termination of therapy. (Silverman, 1996, p. 10)

There is some measure of support as well as conflicting evidence for nearly all reasonable theories of stuttering onset. In addition, there are exceptions to all attempts to explain stuttering behavior even in small subgroups of individuals (Daly, 1981; Schwartz & Conture, 1988), let alone across the variety of different people who stutter. Since the conclusions about theories are tentative and subject to change with the availability of fresh data, Silverman (1996) suggests that the clinician must continuously evaluate each theory in the light of new evidence.

Wingate (1968) pointed out that the questions that are asked in a field are influenced by the *zeitgeist* (the spirit of the times). What is published is driven, to some degree, by what is fashionable as much as it is by the decisions of reviewers and editors. Those issues that are considered important enough to be supported by available funds are influenced by the zeitgeist. Questions are researched and the results of investigations generate further considerations along a line of inquiry. The zeitgeist gradually changes and the pendulum swings back and forth, often returning again to views that—at one time—were thought to have outlived their usefulness. Sometimes the published articles—particularly review articles—summarize research that has pursued a particular direction for a time. These review articles, in turn, have their own influence on the zeitgeist. On the other hand, review articles may simply reflect and document a change in the zeitgeist that has already occurred. For example, views of stuttering as a (neuro)physiological problem that were popular during the first third of the 20th century have again achieved favor, in large part due to new theories of normal speech and language acquisition, as well as a variety of technological advances.

Although there have been many attempts to formulate models that explain the onset of stuttering, one thing remains clear—stuttering is a multidimensional problem. Determining onset is complicated by the fact that there are no absolute definitions or criteria that enable the clinician to entirely differentiate stuttered speech from nonstuttered speech and to identify those who are and are not stuttering (Ingham, 1984; Onslow, 1992). Using an interesting analogy, Conture (1990) compares stuttering to the common cold. That is, despite years of trying, no one has come up with a cause or a solution to the problem. There are a variety of explanations and a variety of remedies. Sometimes, for some people, a remedy will work. In other instances, possibly because of the interaction of the remedy and the person—or the timing of this interaction—the remedy is less effective. Each treatment comes with its own cadre of supporters. Nevertheless, there appears to be no clear-cut cause and no consistent cure. There may be one difference, however, between the common cold and stuttering. The likelihood of successfully treating a cold is considerably better than altering the network of behaviors and attitudes that are united by the helplessness and fear found in stuttering.

Excellent descriptions of the long and fascinating history of proposed stuttering causation are provided by Van Riper (1982) and Silverman (1996). Perhaps the oldest view is that stuttering is a form of punishment for wrongdoing on the part of the child or the parent. Undoubtedly this view continues to be held today in some cultures and socio-economic groups throughout the world. Stuttering has been around for a long time throughout human history. There is, in fact, debate about the possibility that Moses was a person who stuttered (Attanasio, 1997; Bobrick, 1995; Fibiger, 1994).

The earliest recorded indication of stuttering is provided by the Egyptians, who used a sequence of hieroglyphics to represent the term *"nitnit"* or *"njtjt"* which meant "to talk hesitantly" (Faulkner, 1962). The verb *"to stutter"* appeared in a papyrus copy of a narrative dating from the Middle Kingdom of Egypt titled "The Tale of the Shipwrecked Sailor" (DeBuck, 1970, p. 100). Reading Figure 2-2 from right to left, the symbols represent the concept of *impediment* or *impede*, and the final portion, the *determinative*, indicates human speech. This reference to stuttering is the earliest known evidence of a human communication disorder.

The references to stuttering in this narrative tale of a high official returning to the royal court after a failed expedition include the sentences: "You must speak to the king with presence of mind. You must answer without stuttering! A man's mouth can save him. His speech

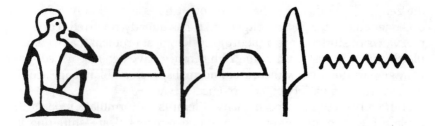

Figure 2-2. Reading from right to left are the Egyptian hieroglyphic symbols from the Middle Kingdom indicating "impediment," followed by the determinative designating human speech. From L. H. Corcoran and A. Webb, Institute of Egyptian Art and Archaeology, The University of Memphis. Reprinted with permission.

makes one forgive him" (p. 212). In addition, as a sailor in the story makes his way about the island on which he is shipwrecked, he encounters a large snake who repeats sentences: "Who brought you, who brought you, fellow, who brought you? Don't be afraid, don't be afraid" (Lichtheim, 1973).

At the most basic level, models of stuttering etiology can be separated into intrinsic (physiological or psychological) or extrinsic (environmental) models or some combination of these two. We will first discuss stuttering as a physical (structural or functional) problem, an idea that—in recent years—has gained renewed interest.

Stuttering From a Physiological Perspective

There is a long tradition in the literature of attributing stuttering to physiological processes not directly related to speech and language production. Nearly every structure of the body, whether associated with speech production or not, has been implicated in the search for a cause of stuttering. Examples include—but are not limited to—dryness of the tongue or problems in the hyoid bone, the hard palate, the uvula, the root of the tongue, the larynx, various aspects of the hearing mechanism including the higher auditory pathway, assorted bones of the head, the endocrine and autonomic nervous systems, and the central nervous system. Since the tongue is often involved during moments of stuttering, that structure has often been implicated as the culprit. According to Silverman (1996), the belief that stuttering results from an abnormality in the tongue's structure, function, or both, appears to have been the most widely held view between the time of Aristotle and the Renaissance, approximately 1500 A.D.

Since one or more anatomical structures were thought to be implicated, it was not uncommon to recommend various forms of surgery for those who stuttered. Believing a spasm of the glottis to be responsible for stuttering, Johann Dieffenbach, a German surgeon, performed more than 250 operations on the tongues of people who stuttered in France and Germany in 1841. Performed without anesthesia, the operation involved making a horizontal incision at the base of the tongue and the excising of a triangular wedge. As self-proclaimed experts in stuttering are fond of doing, Dieffenbach claimed that his technique was highly successful— except, of course, for those who died as a result of infection. As his claims failed to be confirmed by others, the technique was abandoned by the end of the same year (Hunt, 1861). (Interestingly, the common house-plant *Dieffenbachia,* known for its bitter-tasting leaves, is named after this somewhat infamous surgeon.)

Other "cures" for offending parts of the anatomy included severing the hypoglossal nerve, piercing the tongue with hot needles or blistering it with fluids, encouraging smoking as a sedative for the vocal folds, and both tonsil- and adenoidectomies. According to Blanton and Blanton (1936), such procedures continued in the United States during the first few decades of the 20th century.

There is also a long history of placing objects in the mouth or next to a variety of locations in the vocal tract (both externally and internally) in order to elicit fluency. The first reported example of such an approach may be that of Demosthenes, who was told to place pebbles under his tongue and practice speaking loudly to the sea. During the past several centuries there have been a multitude of devices (see Silverman, 1996; Van Riper, 1982) that facilitated fluency by both distracting the speaker from his habitual method of speech production and producing altered forms of phonation and articulatory proprioception and timing. With few exceptions, however, these devices provide, at best, only temporary fluency.

It was popular during the late 1960s and 1970s to attribute an ineffi-ciency or overadduction of the vocal folds as a core aspect of stuttering etiology. Wingate's (1969) publication titled "Sound and pattern in 'artifi-cial fluency' " and his proposal of a "modified vocalization hypothesis" led to many investigations of vocal fold function during both stuttered and fluent speech. More recently, Starkweather (1995), although not specifically implicating the vocal folds, stated that "elevated muscle activity is itself the proximal cause of stuttering behavior (p. 91). Subsequent findings by several investigators (Caruso, Gracco, & Abbs, 1987; Conture, McCall, & Brewer, 1977; Denny & Smith, 1992; McClean, Goldsmith, & Cerf, 1884; Smith, 1989; Smith, Denny, & Wood, 1991; Smith, Denny, Shaffer, Kelly, & Hirano, 1996) have failed to support the notion of a consistent pattern of adduction or abduction during stutter-ing or excessively high intrinsic muscle activity during either fluent and/or nonfluent speech of adults who stutter.

During the later part of the last century, attempts to explore possible differences or deficits in the physical makeup of individuals who stutter have focused on more subtle tasks of speech and nonspeech activities such as auditory and visual tracking, finger tapping, and reaction time. Although there are exceptions, several authors have used a variety of tasks on which subjects who stutter perform less accurately or slower than those who do not. For example, stuttering subjects have been found to be somewhat slower in starting and stopping a sound when they hear a buzzer (Adams & Hayden, 1976; Starkweather, Hirschman, & Tannenbaum, 1976). Stuttering subjects have been found to be somewhat slower when reacting to respiration (exhalation) and articulation (lip-closing) movements. The results of number of studies (see Silverman, 1996, pp. 60–61) indicate that people who stutter have slower phonatory reaction times (the time it takes to initiate or terminate phonation in response to a signal). In a related study, Cross and Luper (1983) found that stuttering subjects took longer than control subjects to perform non-speech movements, such as finger tapping.

There have also been many investigations suggesting that adults who stutter have a neuro-physiological deficit that results in an inability to achieve accurate articulatory targets or move their articulators as quickly as their nonstuttering counterparts (e.g., Alfonso, Watson, & Baer, 1987; Caruso, Abbs, & Gracco, 1988; De Nil & Abbs, 1990; Zimmerman, 1980, 1981). This seems especially to be the case for people who stutter more severely. Some of these studies are discussed in more detail in the next chapter.

Theories of Cerebral Dominance

In the 1920s a number of anecdotal reports suggested that individuals who stutter are more likely to be left-handed or ambidextrous than non-stutterers and that the onset of stuttering had occurred in conjunction with attempts to change their handedness in some way (Bloodstein, 1993). In response to this evidence, and within a scientific environment that had embraced the concept of a left-hemisphere dominance for speech and language, Samuel T. Orton proposed a theory of stuttering that would become known as "the Cerebral Dominance" theory (Orton, 1927). With the subsequent publication of a text by one of his students (Travis, 1931), Lee Edward Travis popularized Orton's theory.

Orton and Travis theorized that because the muscles of the speech mechanism receive nerve impulses from both the left and right hemi-spheres of the brain, one hemisphere needed to be dominant over the other in order for speech movements to be properly synchronized. They suggested that the nervous system of people who stutter had not matured sufficiently to achieve hemispheric dominance over speech movements, and that this maturational failure could have resulted from hereditary influences, disease, injury, or even emotional arousal and fatigue.

Initially, research on the theory focused on investigating the handedness of individuals who stutter, and the results were encouraging. However, later studies questioned these results, prompting researchers to develop new ways of studying the innate "sidedness"—rather than simply the handedness—of subjects. When by the 1940s investigations yielded inconsistent findings, interest in the cerebral dominance theory had subsided, as there was little consistent support for the idea that people who stutter as a group differed from nonstuttering speakers on measures of handedness or sidedness.

By the 1960s new interest in the cerebral dominance theory emerged with the development of procedures that could more specifically examine hemispheric dominance for language functions. For example, the Wada test involved injecting sodium amytol into the left and right carotid arteries of a conscious speaker, resulting in a temporary loss of the ability to produce speech. Wada and Rasmussen (1960) found that four patients who stuttered demonstrated transient aphasia regardless of either right or left side injection, suggesting a lack of cortical dominance for speech (see Bloodstein, 1987). Follow-up studies (e.g., Andrews, Quinn, & Sorby, 1972; Branch, Milner, & Rasmussen, 1964) failed to find significant differences between those who stuttered and those who did not with regard to hemispheric dominance for language. Little research has continued using the Wada test, in part because of the discouraging results, and in part because the procedure can have potentially harmful side effects for the patient.

Dichotic listening procedures have also been used to demonstrate cerebral dominance for language, with a moderate degree of success. Dichotic listening tasks involve the simultaneous (competing) presentation of two different speech signals to opposite ears, with subjects being required to repeat back what was heard in one or both ears (Mueller & Bright, 1994). As the auditory-cortical system is taxed by the simultaneous presentation, auditory processing via the primary (contralateral) pathways may indicate accuracy and response time advantages for right-ear–left-hemisphere or left-ear–right-hemisphere stimuli. Studies employing this technique with (nonstuttering) normal listeners have reported a significant right-ear advantage (REA) in the recognition of *linguistic stimuli* (e.g., Broadbent & Gregory, 1964; Kimura, 1961; Lowe-Bell, Cullen, Berlin, Thompson, & Willett, 1970) while other studies (e.g., Kimura, 1964) have reported a left-ear advantage (LEA) for the recognition of dichotically presented *melodic tones*. These findings have suggested hemispheric dominance for certain psychological phenomena such as speech and language, which have been associated with left-hemisphere processing (Kimura, 1961; Studdert-Kennedy & Shankweiler, 1970) for most right-handed individuals. Furthermore, numerous studies have found REAs for both right- and left-handed subjects (e.g., Berlin,

Lowe-Bell, Cullen, Thompson, & Loovis, 1973; Kimura, 1961; Studdard-Kennedy & Shankweiler, 1970) but results have not been as consistent or overwhelming as with other techniques (e.g., direct electrical stimulation and the Wada test). Despite these findings, the dichotic listening paradigm has been employed in the investigation of cerebral dominance differences between stutterers and nonstutterers.

The cerebral dominance theory of stuttering (Orton, 1927; Travis, 1931) suggests that due to the stutterer's lack of a dominant hemisphere for language, his or her performance on a dichotic listening task should demonstrate a reduced or nonexistent REA or perhaps even an LEA. Curry and Gregory (1969) were the first to use a dichotic listening approach with speakers who stuttered. They presented both verbal and non-verbal dichotic stimuli to adults who stuttered and a group of nonstutterers, and found that on a verbal task, 75% of the nonstutterers demonstrated an REA, whereas 55% of the participants who stuttered demonstrated an LEA. They reported that no differences were found between the two groups on the non-verbal tasks. Similar results have been found by other researchers (Brady & Berson, 1975; Moore, 1984; Moore & Haynes, 1980; Sommers, Brady, & Moore, 1975) using meaningful words as stimuli.

Hall and Jerger (1978) also found differences between the performance of stutterers and nonstutterers on some dichotic listening tasks given as part of a central auditory processing (CAP) test battery. They stated that their results indicated that participants who stuttered demonstrated a mild CAP dysfunction not associated with hemispheric specialization, but in the area of the brain-stem. This finding has received support from other researchers (Dietrich, 1997; Hageman & Greene, 1989; Liebetrau & Daly, 1981; Toscher & Rupp, 1978) who have found differences between stutterers and nonstutterers on selected central auditory processing subtests. Toscher and Rupp, for example, found a statistically significant difference between stutterers and nonstutterers on one of three subtests (the Ipsilateral Competing Message subtest) of the Synthetic Sentence Identification test. They concluded that this was the only subtest that was sufficiently difficult to activate the central integrative functions of the central auditory system.

Additional conflicting evidence regarding the performance of stutterers relative to nonstutterers on dichotic listening tasks was found by Sussman and MacNeilage (1975). Sussman and MacNeilage used a dichotic listening task and a pursuit auditory tracking task to assess the hemispheric specialization in a group of 28 stutterers and 31 nonstutterers. The pursuit auditory tracking task was similar to that used by Sussman (1971) and Sussman et al. (1974, 1975), where subjects are asked to match a control tone presented to one ear with a target tone presented to the other ear that was controlled by either movements of a speech articulator (tongue or jaw) or by the subject's dominant hand. In their initial studies Sussman et al. found that normal speakers demonstrated a significant REA on this task. Sussman and MacNeilage found that stutterers demonstrated an REA similar to nonstutterers on the dichotic listening task, but failed to demonstrate a significant REA on the pursuit auditory tracking task. These results led them to conclude that stutterers may differ from nonstutterers in terms of hemispheric specialization for speech production but not for speech perception. However, Berlin et al. (1973) and Berlin and McNeil (1976) proposed an interpretation of Sussman's original work with pursuit auditory tracking that suggested the existence of a left-hemisphere speech analyzer involved in analysis of acoustic events that contain rapid gliding motions of the vocal tract. This interpretation suggests that the stimuli used by Sussman and MacNeilage did not possess the appropriate characteristics to activate this speech analyzer.

Pinsky and McAdam (1980) also found conflicting evidence regarding the cerebral laterality of speakers who stutter. They performed a comprehensive study of five stutterers and five nonstutterers using four experimental paradigms: dichotic listening, alpha localization, contingent negative variation, and readiness potential. Results indicated a left-hemisphere dominance for language in 9 of the 10 subjects, prompting the authors to state that "no support was found for the Orton-Travis hypothesis of a contribution of bilaterality to dysfluent speech" (p. 418). This conclusion was also supported by the results of studies by Dorman and Porter (1975) and Liebetrau and Daly (1981), both of which failed to find differences in performance on dichotic listening tasks between speakers who stuttered and those who did not. The results of other studies indicate that for individuals who stutter, control of speech production, perception, or both may be shared by both hemispheres (Cerf & Prins, 1974; Curry & Gregory, 1969; Haefner, 1929; Oates, 1929; Ojemann, 1931).

One possible explanation for these discrepancies was presented by Moore (1976, 1984). Moore suggested that differences in the dichotic verbal stimuli (e.g., syllables, digits, words) between the various studies may have influenced the results. He stated that studies that employed meaningful linguistic stimuli rather than syllables in their dichotic listening tasks (e.g., Curry & Gregory, 1969; Sommers, Brady, & Moore, 1975) did indicate that stutterers as a group failed to demonstrate an REA.

Similarly, Molt and Brading (1994) questioned the accuracy of dichotic listening measures of hemispheric specialization that used CV-syllables. They compared the performance of a group of stutterers to a group of nonstutterers on a dichotic listening task that used CV-syllables, while also measuring hemispheric activity via recording of event-related potentials (ERP). They found no significant differences between the groups on the dichotic listening measure, but did find laterality differences between the groups based on the ERP recordings: a finding that they suggested was "especially notable in that the scalp-recorded electroencephalographic activity should reflect actual hemispheric patterns to a greater extent than dichotic ear advantage measures" (p. 149).

Evidence from Neuroimaging Techniques

In an effort to find evidence to support his theory, Lee Travis pioneered the area of neuroimaging (beginning with EEG studies) with stutterers (e.g., Travis & Knott, 1936, 1937; Travis & Malamud, 1937). As suggested by Molt and Brading (1994), neuroimaging approaches to the investigation of hemispheric laterality in those who stutter is a more direct and, potentially, more accurate approach than previous methods. Although both structural and functional neuroimaging techniques have been applied to the study of cerebral dominance in stuttering speakers, the number of studies is small and, due to the expense associated with these techniques, the number of participants in many studies is low. Despite these problems, new insights into the functioning of the brains of those who stutter have been achieved utilizing these techniques.

Neuroimaging is a general term that refers to radiologic and physiologic techniques that can provide a visual representation of intact, functioning neurological systems. Neuroimaging techniques can be divided into two broad categories:

1. Structural
2. Functional

Structural neuroimaging studies identify anatomical structures of the brain and include *Computerized Tomography* (CT) and *Magnetic Resonance Imaging* (MRI) techniques. CT uses a narrow x-ray beam to examine the head in a series of thin "slices." Data regarding the absorption of x-rays by the various structures in the cranium (e.g., bones of the skull, soft tissue of the brain, etc.) is fed into a computer which then produces absorption maps of the structures (Bhatnagar & Andy, 1995). CT scanning has become routine for any persons suspected of brain lesion (e.g., suspected CVA), and has been demonstrated to be an effective technique for accurately localizing such lesions. MRI creates brain images by using the magnetic properties of hydrogen atomic nuclei. The structure to be imaged is placed into a large magnetic field and shortwave radio-frequency pulses are directed toward it. Transmission of these pulses temporarily aligns the hydrogen atoms. When the pulses cease, the atoms return to their previous alignment, and in doing so discharge electromagnetic signals. These signals are converted by a computer into shades of black, gray, and white. Because of the varying water (and therefore hydrogen) content of brain structures, MRI provides greater resolution of brain tissue than does CT scanning (Bhatnagar & Andy, 1995; Kertesz, 1989).

With structural imaging techniques, an indication of hemispheric localization of language must be deduced by comparing site of lesion with behavioral characteristics. For example, Broca's aphasia has been associated with CT scans identifying lesions in Broca's area as well as lesions in inferior parietal and anterior temporal regions (Kertesz, 1989).

Functional brain imaging techniques can generally be divided into two categories. The first are radiographic techniques that investigate the physiological and biochemical properties of the brain and include *Functional Magnetic Resonance Imaging* (fMRI), *Regional Cerebral Blood Flow* (rCBF), *Positron Emission Tomography* (PET), and *Single Photon Emission Computed Tomography* (SPECT). Functional MRI combines the structural imaging technique described previously with real-time representation of physiological activity in the brain (Bhatnagar & Andy, 1995). Regional cerebral blood flow techniques utilize a radioactive "tracer" to measure the flow of blood to functionally active areas of the brain. This technique is based on the assumption that areas of the brain that are activated during the performance of activities will require increased blood flow (Bhatnagar & Andy). PET scanning, like rCBF, also uses a radioactive tracer to measure physiological events in the brain. However, the PET technique involves using a positron-emitting isotope "tagged" to a natural body substance (e.g., water or glucose) that will be metabolized by cells in the brain. When the tagged substance is metabolized, it releases radiation that is scanned and interpreted by the computer. According to Bhatnagar and Andy (1995) and Kertesz (1989), PET scans allow the study of physiological activity within the brain that directly reflects cognitive functioning. SPECT is generally a "refined blood flow measurement" (Bhatnagar & Andy; p. 317) and is functionally similar to PET but does not provide as much detail.

Radiographic functional imaging techniques have been used in the investigation of brain activation patterns during speech and language tasks with a wide range of results. For example, Lauter, Herscovitch, Formby, and Raichle (1985) used a PET technique to study activation of the auditory cortex by speech and non-speech stimuli. They found that different areas of the auditory cortex were activated in response to the speech stimuli than in response to the pure-tone non-speech stimuli. Alternately, Shaywitz, Pugh, Constable, Shaywitz, Bronen, Fulbright, Shankweiler, Katz, Fletcher, Skudlarski, and Gore (1994) reported fMRI results that indicated left anterior temporal lobe activation during a phonologic processing task, but *bilateral* activation of inferior frontal lobes and activation of left posterior frontal lobe during a semantic processing task. Wood, Flowers, and Naylor (1991) reported that although some studies using radiographic functional imaging techniques in the investigation of hemispheric laterality for language have found expected asymmetries, there have been many exceptions. They suggest that the small sample size in many of these studies makes it difficult to explain inter-subject variance and has restricted the statistical procedures available for assessing the patterns of activation.

The second category of functional imaging techniques are techniques that measure the brain's electrical activity and include *Electroencephalography* (EEG) and *Evoked Potentials* (EPs). EEG is a graphic representation of the potential differences between two separated points on the scalp surface that represent brain transmitted electrical potentials, or brain waves (Bhatnagar & Andy, 1995). EPs are measurements of changes in neural activity that occur after the presentation of a stimulus. EPs can be analyzed in terms of certain parameters such as amplitude or latency (Springer & Deutsch, 1989). One specific type of EP that is commonly used in the investigation of speech and language is the *Auditory Evoked Potential* (AEP). The AEP is a measure of changes in the auditory system in response to controlled presentation of auditory stimuli. Both EEG and EPs/AEPs are recorded via metal electrodes arranged in certain standard configurations, known as the international 10-20 system, on the scalp. These recordings can be topographically mapped, with different brain wave patterns representing different physiological functioning, and presented as different colors on the topographical map (Bhatnagar & Andy).

Very few studies have been reported that utilize structural neuroimaging techniques in the study of cerebral dominance in people who stutter. Watson and Freeman (1997) reported that they had obtained MRI data for 20 adults with developmental stuttering and found no significant differences in the scans of the stutterers compared to normal controls. Strub, Black, and Naeser (1987) reported a CT study of two adult subjects (a brother and sister) who had been diagnosed with developmental stuttering. Their findings indicated no focal lesions for either subject, but did reveal some structural anomalies in their scans. Both subjects showed enlargements of the anterior horns of the ventricles as well as a focal anatomical asymmetry (right wider than left) in the occipital lobe. For the brother, the asymmetry was noted in scans that covered both Wernicke's area and the supramarginal gyrus. For the sister, the asymmetry was noted only in scans that covered Wernicke's area.

Structural imaging techniques have, overall, provided little data regarding the cerebral dominance of speakers who stutter. Strub et al. (1987) suggested that their findings provided physical evidence to support the cerebral dominance theory of Orton (1927) and Travis (1931). However, it is difficult to confidently draw conclusions from a study with only two subjects, and Watson and Freeman (1997) also point out that the observed anatomical asymmetries reported by Strub et al. are "often difficult to interpret and may not be replicable with higher-resolution scans" (p. 145).

Functional neuroimaging techniques appear to provide a greater potential for identifying differences between speakers who stutter and those who do not. Pinsky and McAdam (1980) used four techniques (a dichotic listening task, alpha localization, contingent negative variation [CNV], and readiness potential [RP] measures) to assess hemispheric differences in speech and language processing between five adults who stuttered and a group of control speakers. Their findings provided indication that adults who stutter demonstrate either a lack of cerebral dominance or a right-hemisphere dominance for speech and language processing. In fact, a greater number of their control subjects demonstrated a right-hemisphere dominance, particularly on the CNV measure. Similarly, Fitch and Batson (1989) used alpha wave suppression measures to investigate the cerebral dominance for speech and language in stuttering speakers. They also found no evidence of hemispheric differences between experimental and control subjects in the processing of a linguistic task. On the other hand, several researchers have found between-group differences for stuttering and control speakers.

Finitzo, Pool, Freeman, Devous, and Watson (1991) used quantitative electroencephalographic (QEEG) techniques in a study of resting EEG and auditory evoked potential (AEP) for 20 adults with developmental stuttering. They placed electrodes at 20 sites over the scalp and had additional electrodes as extracerebral monitors and linked earlobe references. Subjects received binaural presentation of 103 dB SPL pure-tone bursts as the auditory stimuli. Results indicated a global reduction of EEG amplitude in the Beta frequency region when compared to a group of 12 adult nonstutterers. AEP data indicated differences for the participants who stuttered, implicating temporal cortex (P1 and N1) and cingulate cortex (P2) dysfunction.

In a related study, Pool, Devous, Freeman, Watson, and Finitzo (1991) collected SPECT regional cerebral blood flow (rCBF) data (also during a resting state) for the same 20 adult developmental stutterers studied by Finitzo et al. (1991). Their results indicated a global reduction in absolute blood flow for individuals who stuttered when compared to a control group. In addition, asymmetries in the cerebral blood flow in 20 of 20 regions of interest (ROIs) were noted for the stuttering participants. The rCBF asymmetries observed in the stutterers were consistent with cortical areas usually identified as being involved in speech motor control (inferior frontal), language processing (middle temporal), and motor initiation (anterior cingulate).

Watson, Pool, Devous, Freeman, and Finitzo (1992) performed SPECT rCBF scans on 16 adult males with developmental stuttering (a subgroup of the experimental subjects from their previous studies) and compared them to the subjects' performance on a laryngeal reaction time (LRT) task. Control data for this study were from two separate databases, one for SPECT rCBF and one for LRT. Findings indicated significant differences between the control data and the performance of a subgroup of the stuttering subjects who demonstrated low rCBF for left superior and middle temporal areas.

Watson, Freeman, Devous, Chapman, Finitzo, and Pool (1994) also reported SPECT rCBF data for 16 adult male developmental stutterers and 10 adult male nonstutterers. These groups represented subgroups of both stutterers and controls from the Pool et al. (1991) study. The SPECT rCBF data was compared to performance on a discourse (linguistic) task. Findings identified three ROIs related to language processing (superior temporal, middle temporal, and inferior frontal). No rCBF differences were found between nonstutterers and stutterers who performed normally on the linguistic task. However, significant rCBF differences were found between the linguistically impaired stutterers and the normal controls in the middle temporal and inferior frontal ROIs. Watson et al. (1994) suggested that these findings indicate a subgroup of stuttering speakers who have involvement of linguistic processing areas of the brain. The studies by the Watson et al. research group have been criticized on methodological grounds (e.g., Viswanath, Rosenfield, & Nudelman, 1992; Fox, Lancaster, & Ingham, 1993) regarding the appropriateness of control groups used, analytical techniques, and accuracy of scanning procedures.

In addition to the studies indicating that adults who stutter demonstrate greater involvement of right-hemisphere processing of linguistic data, a number of studies have compared cortical activation patterns for linguistic tasks prior to, and after, the application of a fluency enhancing intervention. Wood, Stump, McKeehan, Sheldon, and Proctor (1980) reported SPECT results for one male adult and one female adult who stuttered in both resting and reading aloud conditions both prior to, and following, a two-week trial of Haloperidol, a psychoactive drug used in the treatment of some neurogenic motor control and psychiatric disorders. They found severe stuttering and significant differences in cerebral blood flow (right greater than left) between specific regions of the hemispheres for both subjects in the unmedicated reading-aloud condition, and less severe stuttering and a reversal of comparative cerebral blood flow (left greater than right) for both subjects in the medicated reading-aloud condition. They suggested that these results supported the lack of cerebral dominance for speech production as a potential etiological factor of stuttering.

Ingham, Fox, and Ingham (1994) reported PET rCBF data for four adults with developmental stuttering and four normal speakers during resting, solo reading, and choral reading conditions. Their data indicated that the adults who stuttered showed increased blood flow to the supplementary motor area (left greater than right) and the superior lateral premotor cortex (right greater than left) during the solo reading condition, but that "activation" of these regions was significantly reduced during the fluency enhancing choral reading condition. However, Ingham et al. (1996) failed to find differences in brain blood flow between groups of stuttering and nonstuttering speakers.

Similarly, Wu et al. (1995) also studied PET scans of stuttering and nonstuttering adults in solo and choral reading conditions. Four adults who stuttered were compared to their performance during choral speech (a fluency-enhancing condition) and to normal-speaking controls. The speakers who stuttered showed decreased cerebral activation in several unilateral and bilateral regions, including Broca's and Wernicke's regions in the left hemisphere. These results coincided with Pool et al.'s observations for stuttering speakers during a resting state. They identified a left caudate hypometabolism that was observed during both stuttering and induced fluency and suggested that this was a "trait characteristic" of a "functional neuroanatomical circuit" that may be basic to stuttering. They also identified a hypoactivity in Broca's area, Werneke's area, the superior frontal cortex, and the right cerebellum, and hyperactivity in substantia nigra/ventral tegmental areas and the limbic system, which they described as "state-dependent" characteristics of the circuit, meaning that they occurred only during stuttering and not during induced fluency.

Three studies have found a "reversal" of location of hemispheric processing of linguistic tasks after short periods of behavioral treatment that increased fluency. Boberg, Yeudall, Schopflocher, and Bo-Lassen (1983) used an EEG technique to gather alpha wave suppression data for verbal tasks with a group of stuttering clients before and after fluency shaping treatment. Normal-speaking subjects usually demonstrate alpha suppression in the left hemisphere for linguistic tasks (Moore, 1990); however, prior to treatment, the clients in this study demonstrated decreased alpha over the right posterior frontal region. After a short period of fluency-shaping treatment, however, Boberg et al. reported normal EEG results (left posterior frontal alpha suppression) for the same (stuttering) subjects. McFarland and Moore (1982) also measured alpha wave suppression for a group of adults who stuttered and were treated using a biofeedback design. Pretreatment recordings indicated right-hemisphere alpha suppression. However, as fluency increased with the use of the biofeedback treatment, a gradual and consistent suppression of left-hemisphere alpha was noted. Similarly, DeNil, Kroll, Kapur and Houle (2000) used PET scanning procedures to investigate 10 right-handed male adults who stuttered and a control group of normally individuals. Participants were asked to read individually presented single words silently or aloud. Between- and within-group differences were obtained by subtracting the functional brain images obtained during the two reading tasks and a baseline non-linguistic task. During silent reading, stuttering speakers showed increased activation in the left anterior cingulate cortex (ACC) while nonstuttering speakers did not. The authors suggested that increased activation in the ACC reflected cognitive anticipatory reactions associated with stuttering. During oral reading, both stuttering and non-stuttering speakers showed bilateral cortical and subcortical activation. However, nonstuttering speakers showed greater left-hemisphere activation while stuttering speakers showed greater right-hemisphere activation.

Fox et al. (1996) performed a functional-activation study with 10 adult males with developmental stuttering and 10 adult male nonstutterers, matched for age and handedness. They took three 40s PET scans for each of three conditions; solo reading, chorus reading, and eyes-closed rest. Their results indicated significant differences between stuttering and nonstuttering subjects in both activations and deactivations for areas of both hemispheres of the brain. Fox et al. state that the findings suggest that the neural systems of stuttering include a diffuse overactivity of the cerebral and cerebellar motor systems, a right dominance of the cerebral motor system, a lack of normal self-monitoring activations of left anterior superior temporal phonological circuits, and a deactivation of a verbal fluency circuit between left frontal and left temporal cortex. This type of study, however, provides information only with regard to what was happening in the brain at the time of the stuttering event. As such, the findings could be interpreted as reflecting the systems *response* to breakdowns rather than what actually caused the system to breakdown.

Ingham et al. (1996) performed a systematic replication of the Pool et al. (1991) study but utilized a more modern imaging PET technique. Subjects for this study were 10 adult males who were diagnosed with chronic developmental stuttering and 19 adult males who did not stutter. The groups were rigorously matched for age and "body-dominance." All subjects underwent three 40s PET-acquisition scans and a full-brain MRI scan. MRI data was used to accurately identify regions of interest (ROIs) for each individual subject. Results indicated a lack of evidence for any functional or anatomical lesions in the brains of men who stutter. Therefore, Ingham et al. state that their findings "do not support theories or previous research findings using other methodologies indicating that developmental stuttering is associated with, or due to, focal functional lesions (e.g., Pool et al., 1991). Nor do the present findings support the conjecture that developmental stuttering is associated with an absence of normal asymmetry between the cerebral hemispheres" (p. 1222).

Although inconsistent results have been found, neuroimaging data regarding hemispheric specialization differences for speech and language processing in adults who stutter appear to have some support. Watson and Freeman (1997) state that neuroimaging techniques have demonstrated evidence of "multifocal anomalous brain functions" for speech and language processing in adult speakers, suggesting that there appears to be a significant amount of inter and intra-subject variability regarding the location of these anomalous brain functions, but that they generally appear to involve regions classically associated with speech motor (anterior cingulate and inferior frontal) and language (temporal) processing. However, the recent findings by Fox et al. (1996) and Ingham et al. (1996) dispute such a statement, and suggest that further study is necessary to be able to make even general statements regarding the hemispheric dominance of adults who stutter. There appears to be a need for additional systematic replications as accomplished by Ingham et al. in order to reconsider many of the established findings in this area of research using new technology and more rigorous methodologies. As De Nil (1997) states, "At the present time, one cannot exclude the possibility that this atypical lateralization develops as the result of some compensatory mechanism at some time following the onset of stuttering" (p 95). With advancing technology, investigators will continue to replicate and advance many of these designs that may help to answer that question.

Temporal-Processing Abilities

Another area where the results of many investigations are consistent indicates that people who stutter are unable to process information about the precise temporal features necessary to monitor and produce speech. The theme of these investigations is that people who stutter experience a subtle breakdown in speech or speech-related functioning. This breakdown, particularly when the speaker is experiencing internal or externally generated stress, may result in a reduced ability to achieve fluency. Or as Bannister (1966) whimsically explains, some models of information theory suggest that humans are "basically a digital computer constructed by someone who had run out of insulating tape" (p. 22).

Kent's (1983) description of stuttering as a reduced ability to generate temporal patterns is a good example of this view and is one example of the return, during the later decades of this century, to exploring stuttering from a physiologic perspective. Kent proposed that stuttering is a result of a central nervous system disturbance that results in a "reduced ability to generate temporal patterns, whether for sensory or motor purposes, but especially the latter" (p. 252). Speakers who stutter appear to lack the ability to smoothly sequence the movement or gestures of speech. There is some indication that people who stutter perform less well than nonstuttering controls on tasks requiring the discrimination of subtle temporal differences in signals (Hall & Jerger, 1978; Kramer, Green, & Guitar, 1987; Toscher & Rupp, 1978). The suggestion is that those who stutter may be demonstrating a lack of central nervous function that allows for the control of both incoming and outgoing signals.

Related to this general line of thinking is the fact that many more males than females are found to stutter, with ratios from three-to-one to five-to-one often cited (American Psychiatric Association, 1994; Andrews & Harris, 1964; Beech & Fransella, 1968; Bloodstein, 1987; Van Riper, 1982). The findings of Geschwind and Galaburda (1985) suggest the possibility that because of the secretion of testosterone during fetal development, males have more disorders involving less-than-ideal development in the left hemisphere. The result is less obvious hemispheric dominance for speech activities, and thus, a central nervous system that is more vulnerable to fluency disruptions.

Although researchers continue to find intriguing differences in speech-related performances of subjects who stutter, the perplexing result continues to be that many of these subjects *do not* show any difference in performance. As Peters and Guitar (1991) and Guitar (1998) point out, the differences, even when they can be noted, are not in and of themselves a direct cause of fluency breaks. Rather, these authors view such findings as conditions that provide fertile ground in which stuttering may grow. That is, such deficits may be neither necessary nor sufficient to *cause* stuttering (Bloodstein, 1995). It may also be, of course, that some of these differences are a *result* of stuttering, particularly for adults who have been stuttering for decades.

Genetic Influences

It has often been noted that stuttering tends to run in families, a fact that suggests a genetic link for the disorder. This supposition for stuttering onset has gained support during recent decades and seems to tie in nicely with the above-mentioned proposal of an inability to precisely process temporal patterns. Investigations of family genetics and the characteristics of twin pairs suggest that, as for many other human characteristics, there may be genetic influences that at least predispose a person to develop stuttering. Andrews and Harris (1964) traced the family history of 80 stuttering children. They found that more males than females were likely to stutter, that females were more likely to have relatives who stuttered than males, and that stutterers were more likely than nonstutterers to have stuttering relatives. Several experimenters indicate that the risk to first-degree male relatives of an individual who stutterers is about fivefold greater than in the general population (Kay, 1964; Ambrose, Yairi, & Cox, 1993; Kidd, 1984). Investigators who have considered the occurrence of stuttering in identical twins (monozygotic [MZ] pairs, with identical genetic makeup) and fraternal twins (dizygotic pairs [DZ], sharing only about half of their genes) have found stuttering to occur more often for both children in monozygotic pairs than in dizygotic twins (Andrews, Yates-Morris, Howie, & Martin, 1991; Howie, 1981). The genetic term *concordance* indicates the presence of a particular characteristic for both twin pairs, and thus stuttering is said to have a higher concordance in monozygotic than in dizygotic twin pairs. However, some identical twins are also discordant. Howie (1981) found, for example, that 6 out of 16 identical twin pairs did not result in stuttering in both subjects. Kidd and his associates (Kidd, 1977; Kidd, Kidd, & Records, 1978; Kidd, Reich & Kessler, 1973) also found convincing evidence that the occurrence of stuttering follows familial patterns. These authors indicated that the occurrence of stuttering can be explained by a combination of genetic and environmental factors. In an analysis of the familial distribution of stuttering in the relatives of 69 school-age children who stutter, Ambrose, Yairi and Cox (1993) found evidence suggesting a single major genetic locus for the familial transmission of stuttering (see also Ambrose, Cox, & Yairi, 1997). Adoption studies suggest that stuttering is more closely related to whether or not a child's biological parents stutter than whether the adoptive parents stutter (Felsenfeld, 1997). With continuing advances in human genetics and improved statistical tools, many complex diseases and problems are being identified.

An international project that that was recently completed will have far-reaching benefits for the understanding both normal and pathological human conditions. The Human Genome Project, sponsored by the United States Department of Energy and the National Institutes of Health (NIH), undertook the goals of mapping, sequencing, and identifying the human gene map. A genome is all the DNA in an organism, including its genes. Genes carry information for making all the proteins necessary for an organism. In turn, these proteins determine such things as how an organism looks, how well it both metabolizes food or fights infections, and how it behaves. Originally conceived in 1990 as a 15-year project, new technological advances resulted in an expected completion date of June, 2000. A primary goal of this project was to discover the 80,000 to 100,000 human genes, making available detailed DNA information for scientists to understand the structure, organization, and function of DNA in chromosomes. Genome maps of other organisms will provide comparative information for understanding more complex systems. Another goal of the project was to determine the sequence of the 3 billion DNA subunits or pairs of bases/chemical pairs present in human DNA. The resulting genetic map is already being applied by scientists to identify and isolate genes that either directly cause human ailments or increase our susceptibility to disease. The importance of this project cannot be overestimated, since it will likely result in a quantum leap in the understanding of the human body and its related disorders. In essence, the project will provide a "users manual for the human body."

One of the many research sections of this undertaking is called the Stuttering Family Research Project and is designed to identify regions of the human genome with linkages to stuttering. DNA is obtained from both affected and unaffected adults and children using a buccal swab. The DNA will then be genotyped using markers distributed across the human genome, and the genotypic information analyzed to determine which markers show linkage to stuttering. Some studies will also consider such factors as motor skills, language skills, neuropsychological abilities and psychological responses to stuttering in order to identify subgroups in which the phenotype expression of the gene may differ. There seems to be little doubt that genetics plays a part in stuttering but it is not yet understood if few or many genes are involved. Understanding of how inherited (genotypic) traits are manifested in behavioral (phenotypic) responses may help explain much about the nature-nurture continuum as it applies to the onset and development of stuttering. Current status of the project, including new discoveries, may be found on the world wide web at:

http://www.ornl.gov/hgmis/project/hgp.html.

The ratio of stuttering in males and females may also interact with genetic loading for factors of fluency as well as recovery (Yairi & Ambrose, 1999). The sex difference suggests that males are more susceptible to stuttering, females are more resistant to it, or both. It may be that females will stutter only with a higher degree of genetic loading and also be more likely to pass it on to their offspring. Similar findings have been noted in the familial history of cluttering, and there seems to be some interaction of these two disorders throughout the generations of families (Weiss, 1964). People who stutter are far from a homogeneous population, and it appears that some, particularly those with a strong familial history of stuttering, may possess a strong neurophysiological loading for the disruption of speech fluency. As we will discuss in subsequent chapters, these findings have strong implications for both treatment as well as long-term success and the possibility of relapse.

In summary, our current understanding indicates that whatever predisposing factors may be inherited, they do not appear to be, in most cases at least, sufficient to result in stuttering. It may be that such predisposing characteristics must combine with environmental factors for stuttering to not only begin but to also continue. As Conture (1990) suggests, in this way, stuttering may be similar to asthma or migraine headaches.

Auditory Feedback

The nature of auditory feedback in those who stutter is another feature that has been the subject of research. Cybernetic theory holds that in a closed-loop system, various lines of feedback are used to regulate the output of a system, as with a thermostat that controls the temperature of a building. The goal of a such a system, termed a *servosystem*, is to match what is intended as system output to the actual output and reduce any differences between the two (the error signal) to zero. If for some reason there is a distortion of the information arriving via the feedback loop, the error signal will be incorrect. When this occurs, the system tends to go into oscillation. Fairbanks (1954) and Mysak (1960) described the nature of such systems and interpreted many aspects of speech production in this manner. The basic idea was that for speakers who stutter, the distorted feedback creates the misconception that an error has occurred in the flow of speech. Stuttering occurs when the speaker attempts to correct an error that has, in fact, not occurred.

Subsequent studies (Black, 1951; Lee, 1951; Neeley, 1961; Yates, 1963) provided some indication that what was occurring for speakers who stuttered was a distorted auditory feedback signal. They noted that for normal speakers, altering the auditory feedback by delaying the signal tended to produce stuttering-like behavior. For example, it was generally agreed that nonstutterers speak under delayed auditory feedback (DAF) in much the same way people do when they stutter. That is, the effect of DAF on normal speakers is to produce repetitions and prolongations of sounds, slowing of speech, pitch increases, and greater vocal intensity. In order to "beat" the effect of the delayed feedback, the speaker must disregard that signal, slow his speech, and focus attention to the undistorted tactile and proprioceptive feedback that is available to him from his articulators. When speakers who stutter respond (with or without DAF) in this manner, there tends to be a reduction in the severity of stuttering. Depending on how these fluency breaks are considered, there may also be a reduction in the frequency of stuttering (Hayden, Scott & Addicott, 1977). Because of these effects of DAF, some treatment programs have employed it as a way to establish fluency in some speakers (Ryan & VanKirk, 1974; Shames & Florance, 1980). Once the speaker has gradually learned to maintain improved fluency under the distorted feedback, the delay intervals are varied in the direction of instantaneous or normal feedback, and the client learns to speak without using the device as he continues to use the slow speech along with an emphasis on proprioceptive feedback.

More recent considerations of this view have failed to support the idea of an error in the feedback loop of subjects who stutter. Postma and Kolk (1992) investigated the effects of error monitoring in eighteen adults who stuttered and a group of control subjects. The speakers were asked to detect self-produced phonemic errors under normal and masked auditory feedback conditions. The results failed to indicate that the experimental (stuttering) subjects performed less well than nonstuttering speakers in either the accuracy or speed of their error detection. They concluded that speakers who stutter possess a deficit in their ability to self-monitor the accuracy of their speech production. They further speculated that rather than a deficit in any speech-monitoring ability, speakers, and particularly those who stutter, may be experiencing prearticulatory errors, which they are attempting to covertly repair.

The Covert Repair Hypothesis

A relatively recent extension of the above-mentioned view is the development and elaboration of what is called the covert repair hypothesis (CRH) (Postma, Kolk, & Povel, 1990; Postma & Kolk, 1993). This hypothesis also makes use of a monitoring device that checks on the accuracy of speech. In this case, however, the monitoring takes place as a central or internal function rather than at the output level in the form of auditory or proprioceptive sensory feedback. In this model, monitoring takes place during the formulation of the phonetic plan (see Figure 2-3) and *prior* to the implementation of articulatory commands. The model proposes that all speakers are able to detect errors in their internal phonetic plan as they internally prepare what they want to say. When errors in the phonetic plan are detected, the speaker interrupts the planning of the phonological sequence in order to make a repair. As a result of this covert repair of errors prior to their production, fluency breaks occur. This is the case for any speaker. It is proposed, however, that speakers who stutter are impaired in their ability to encode phonological sequences, such that the activation of target phonemes is delayed and placed in competition with other phonemes. Furthermore, individuals who stutter tend to

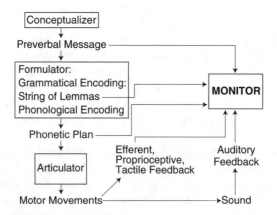

Figure 2-3. A neurophysiological model of stuttering as proposed by De Nil (1999).

begin speech rapidly, not allowing time for their slowed phonological encoding system to select phonological targets. The process of detection-and-repair in combination with a system that is not adept in selecting the correct phonological target before it is produced results in the overt manifestation of a speech disfluency.

Postma and Kolk suggest that this covert process may be thought of in much the same way as overt self-repairing. That is, the process involves an interruption of speech production and a revising of the necessary movements, followed by a new attempt with a revised plan. This hypothesis nicely explains many of the disfluencies of normal speakers and had been extended to explain the fluency breaks in stuttering speakers, for both loci and type of intrasyllabic disfluencies. It also coincides well with a number of reports of phonological-processing abilities of subjects who stutter (Bosshardt, 1990; Bosshardt & Nandyal, 1988; Postma, Kolk, & Povel, 1990; Wingate, 1988).

The Covert Repair Hypothesis appears to offer a number of testable ideas and has generated a good deal of research. However, as with other models, the reasoning is somewhat circular (Yaruss, 2000) in that the CRH assumes that individuals who stutter put demands on their phonological encoding mechanism that exceeds their (assumedly diminished) ability to rapidly and precisely select correct phonological units. Nevertheless, some studies and clinical observations have provided partial support for the CRH. Louko, Edwards, and Conture (1990) found that children who stutter also produce a greater number and variety of phonological processes (systematic or rule-governed sound changes). Authors have found that some children show an increase in speech disfluencies when undergoing treatment for articulation and phonological disorders (Hall, 1977; Ratner, 1995). An analysis by LaSalle and Conture (1995) of the disfluencies produced by preschool children who stuttered provided preliminary support for the notion that both overt and covert self-repairs may interact with a child's ability to perform phonological encoding in a timely manner. Yaruss and Conture (1996) studied nine boys who stuttered with normal phonology and nine boys who stuttered and exhibited disordered phonology. All the children were approximately five years old. They found that both groups were similar in their speech disfluencies, nonsystematic speech errors, and self-repair behaviors. Both groups of children exhibited similar speaking rates, and there was no association between faster speaking rates and more speech disfluencies. Neither group of children repaired their systematic speech errors during conversation, suggesting that these deviations from adult speech were not considered as errors by these children. Some support for the CRH was noted in that there were co-occurrences of disfluencies and speech errors for nonsystematic "slip-of-the-tongue" errors. That is, utterances containing nonsystematic speech errors were significantly more likely to contain within-word speech disfluencies for both groups of children, a finding similar to LaSalle and Conture (1995).

STUTTERING AS AN EMOTIONAL OR PSYCHOLOGICAL PROBLEM

Van Riper, after many decades of treating thousands of children and adults who stuttered, wrote an engaging article in what was then called the *Western Michigan University Journal of Speech Therapy*. Written in 1974, the article was titled "A Handful of Nuts" (see also Van Riper, 1979). From the many hundreds of clients he had seen up to that point in his career, Van Riper found only a very few who had severe emotional problems. These people, while they most certainly stuttered, also had emotional problems that were considerably more handicapping. His description of these clients makes for some exciting reading. As we shall see, however, there are relatively few people who have such deep-seated emotional problems that are directly related to their stuttering (see also Van Riper, 1979).

Through the first several decades of this century, many people who treated stuttering in this country were physicians, and some of these individuals held a psychoanalytic view of the disorder. Theories from the field of psychology have often been adapted to the field of communication disorders, and in this case psychoanalytic views held that stuttering was a psychopathology with the stuttering behaviors symptomatic of a deep-seated, psychological disorder. As Bannister cleverly describes it,

> Thus psychoanalytic theories seem to suggest that man is basically a battlefield. He is in a dark cellar in which a well-bred spinster lady and a sex-crazed monkey are forever engaged in mortal combat, the struggle being refereed by a rather nervous bank clerk. (p. 21)

With the development of university speech and hearing centers and the creation of the National Association of Teachers of Speech in 1925 (the precursor of the American Speech-Language-Hearing Association) (Paden, 1970), fewer physicians provided treatment. The new clinicians, who were trained in the behavioral sciences, were less likely to hold a psychoanalytic view of stuttering (Silverman, 1996).

The neurotic or psychoanalytic explanation of stuttering also has been termed the *repressed-need hypothesis* (Silverman, 1996). That is, stuttering is seen as a neurosis. Individuals who stutter do so as a result of a repressed, neurotic, unconscious conflict. Stuttering behavior is seen as a symptom, which is symbolic of this conflict. The origin of the conflict is a central question, and there has been no shortage of suggestions about the possible source. Some theorized that the source was psychosexual, a fixation of psychological development at an oral or anal stage of infant sexual development (Glauber, 1982). It was proposed, for example, that one who stuttered had not experienced oral erotic gratification as an infant, possibly due to a disturbance in the mother-child relationship. Others proposed a neo-Freudian view that the source of conflict was the result of inadequate interpersonal relationships (Barbara, 1965, 1982; Wyatt, 1969).

Many of these opinions sound strange and even preposterous to most current speech-language pathologists. The chapter by Travis, "The Unspeakable Feelings of People with Special Reference to Stuttering," in the two editions of his *Handbook of Speech Pathology* (1957, 1971) are lucid examples of this viewpoint. This chapter may represent the high-water mark of this psychoanalytical perspective. It is unlikely that a client or parent will have access to the opinions about stuttering etiology expressed in these chapters. However, the experienced clinician should be aware of these views and have an opinion about this view of fluency disorders.

Silverman (1996) indicates that an American physician Edward Scripture (1931) was one of the first to combine psychotherapy and speech treatment that focused on changing specific speech habits. This combined approach is similar to that of more recent clinicians who are psychoanalytically based (Barbara, 1982; Freund, 1966; Glauber, 1982). According to Silverman (1996) there has been relatively little success reported by those using a psychoanalytic approach for treating stuttering. Brill (1923) indicated that after eleven years of treating a total of sixty-nine individuals who stuttered through psychoanalysis, he was able to claim only five persons cured, one of whom was reported to have subsequently relapsed. There is the indication that Freud himself (Freund, 1966) did not believe that psychoanalytic techniques were particularly helpful in treating stuttering.

The psychological status of children who begin to stutter, and particularly the psychological characteristics of their parents, has received considerable discussion in the literature. In order to determine the possibility that the parents of children who stutter are emotionally or psychologically different from parents of nonstuttering children, Adams (1993) reviewed thirty-five articles that contrasted the attitudes, traits, emotions, psychological adjustment, and child-rearing practices and behaviors of parents of children who stutter. Adams found some limited support for the notion that the parents of young children who stuttered may possess some attributes that could have a negative effect on young children who stutter. For example, Zenner, Ritterman, Bowden, and Gronhovd (1978) found that parents of young stuttering children may exhibit higher than usual levels of both trait and state anxiety. Gildston (1967) noted that parents were perceived by some of the children who stuttered as being slightly less accepting. Quarrington, Seligman, and Kosower (1969) found that parents of young children who stutter set lower goals for their children than those of normally speaking children. However, Adams found that the vast majority of investigations indicated no differences between the experimental and control parents. In fact, some investigations identified characteristics in the parents of young children who stuttered that are generally viewed as psychologically healthy—for example, parents of stuttering children were found to be less possessive and less likely to exert hostile control (Yairi & Williams, 1971).

Adams summarized his findings by addressing three questions concerning the home environment of children who stutter:

1. Do children who stutter grow up in a home environment that can validly be described as blatantly pathologic or unhealthy emotionally? Adams's answer was a certain no.
2. Do children who stutter grow up in a home environment that can validly be described as "emotionally unsatisfactory or conducive to maladjustment"? Adams's answer to this question was that he found little support for this idea.
3. Do children who stutter grow up in a home environment that, although not obviously pathologic, is nonetheless unique or different from the home environment of youngsters who develop normal speech? Adams's answer to this final question was also a certain no.

In a recent review of studies that have investigated the influence of both home environment and parent-child interaction, Yairi (1997) also found that the evidence to date fails to support the view that parents of children who stutter have abnormal personalities or emotional or adjustment problems. Yairi concludes that "it is clearly time to declare that the belief that parents' personalities or attitudes are causally related to stuttering is null and void for purposes of counseling and treatment" (p. 44). Nonetheless, he suggests that clinicians should be aware of issues in the home environment that may impede progress.

STUTTERING AS LEARNED BEHAVIOR

This view of stuttering onset has been termed the *anticipatory-struggle model* (Silverman, 1992). The essence of this model is that stuttering is a learned behavior. Bannister (1966) provides this succinct, if basic view: "Learning theory seems to suggest that man is basically a ping-pong ball with a memory." This view, at least in an informal sense, also has a long history. Amman (1700/1965) was one of the first to state that stuttering was, in fact, a bad habit. In a precursor to the learning theories of the 20th century, in the 1800s, Erasmus Darwin (grandfather of Charles Darwin) attributed stuttering to emotionally conditioned interruptions of motoric speech. Arnott (1928) believed that stuttering resulted from a learned "spasm of the glottis." According to Van Riper (1982), this was the most popular view of stuttering onset and development in both the United States and Great Britain from the middle to the end of the nineteenth century. For example, during this time Alexander Melville Bell (grandfather of Alexander Graham Bell) wrote a number of books suggesting that stuttering was learned. One important implication of this view was to place this problem within the arena of the educator rather than a medical professional (Bell, 1853). Dunlap (1932) also considered much of stuttering to be learned and recommended weakening the behavior by having the speaker stutter on purpose, or voluntarily stutter. However, these views of stuttering as a learned behavior were the exception during the early part of the 20th century.

After several decades in which the zeitgeist favored physical and psychoanalytical views of stuttering etiology, there was a gradual change in viewing stuttering as learned behavior during the middle third of the 20th century, from approximately 1930 through 1950. Many people were entering the field at this time with backgrounds in psychology, and the majority had received their training at the University of Iowa. Many of these scholars had a profound influence on the general field of communication disorders. This concentration of researchers, clinicians, and authors led to what has been termed the "Iowa Development" (Bloodstein, 1995). A second generation of clinicians included such individuals as Hugo Gregory, Joseph Sheehan, David Williams, and Dean Williams.

A most influential result of the Iowa development was the diagnosogenic theory of stuttering onset as proposed by Johnson. This theory continues to be one of the most comprehensive theories of both stuttering onset and development. Having been influenced by the writings of Alfred Koszybski in his book *Science and Sanity* (1941) and his work in general semantics, Johnson developed a "semantic theory" of stuttering. General semantics is the study of the ways in which people use words to explain their lives and solve problems. Johnson's theory also became known as the semantogenic or interactional theory (Perkins, 1990), and it had both a profound and long-term impact in the area of fluency disorders. A key aspect of a general semantic approach to events and behavior is our interpretation of the events and our choice of labels for these occurrences. This theory held that stuttering evolves from normal fluency breaks that are overreacted to and mislabeled by the parents or other significant people in the child's environment. Two sentences contained in *An Open Letter to the Mother of a "Stuttering" Child* state the essence of this view.

> The diagnosis of stuttering—that is, the decision made by someone that a child is beginning to stutter—is one of the causes of the stuttering problem, and apparently one of the most potent causes. Having labeled the child's hesitations and repetitions as "stuttering," the listener—somewhat more often the mother than the father—reacts to them as if they were all that the label implies. (Johnson, 1962, p. 2)

The theory assumed that many children, including those who eventually stutter, experience a period of effortless fluency breaks. Furthermore, when children are penalized (typically by their parents) for producing these normal disfluencies, the result is both greater anticipation and increased struggle behavior. Stuttering, therefore, is created by the *listener* and normal breaks in fluency have been shaped into stuttering. Eventually, the speaker "learns" to stutter in his unique manner and the problem becomes self-reinforcing, eventually affecting many aspects of life.

Certainly much of the stuttering that we see on the surface, and some of what resides underneath the surface, is learned. That is, we are able to learn ways of escaping from experiences of fear and penalty. We can also learn ways of interpreting events and of thinking about ourselves. We can learn to play the role of a person who stutters (Sheehan, 1970). Perhaps most apparent are the assortment of escape and avoidance behaviors that become accessories to the experience of fluency breakdown. Escape behaviors are attempts to get away from the stuttering moment and include a multitude of activities, including eye blinks, head nods, interjections, and a wide variety of tension and struggle activities. As the speaker is able to move away from the moment of helplessness or through the sentence, the behavior that appeared to facilitate this escape is rewarded. A powerful link is formed between these behaviors and the escape from the stuttering: one that is extremely difficult to weaken, even with the assistance of an experienced clinician. Avoidance behaviors, on the other hand, are related to the anticipation of stuttering. Anticipating a difficult speaking situation, speaking partner, word, or sound, the speaker chooses to avoid or completely postpone the feared stimulus by using starter sounds or words ("ah, let me see") or timing and distraction devices (finger or head movement, audible or inaudible movements of the articulators). The point is that these behaviors gather around the initial fluency break, making it ever more complex, distracting, and handicapping.

As with other explanations of stuttering onset and development, there are several studies that provide support and several others that do not. That is, normally speaking preschool children do tend to repeat and hesitate (Johnson & Associates, 1959; Yairi, 1981, 1982). A central question, however, is whether these early fluency breaks are normal: whether they are a function of formulative processing or whether they are indicative of a motoric break in the system. There are data to support both arguments, with Johnson and Associates (1959) arguing that the initial fluency breaks are essentially normal. Other researchers (Bloodstein, 1958; McDearmon, 1968; Van Riper, 1982; Wingate, 1988; Yairi, 1997; Yairi & Lewis, 1984; Yairi and Ambrose, 1999; Yairi, Ambrose, & Niermann, 1993) suggest that the original fluency breaks are far from normal, both in terms of quantity and quality. In addition, an extensive review of the literature concerning the role of parents of young children who stutter by Nippold and Rudzinski (1995) found little evidence that parents of children who stutter differ in the way they respond to their children.

One of the more compelling studies indicating that stuttering can be created by misdiagnosing normal breaks in fluency is described by Silverman (1988b) in his accounting of an unpublished study conducted by Tudor in 1939 titled "An Experimental Study of the Effects of Evaluative Labeling on Speech Fluency." It is clear why Silverman (1988b, 1996) refers to this investigation as the "monster study" and why the research was never published. Although the investigation was conducted prior to the development of the diagnosogenic theory, it provided a direct test of this hypothesis. The goal of the study was to see if labeling someone as a stutterer would influence the speaker's fluency.

Children living in an orphanage in Davenport, Iowa, were subjects. From a total of 256 children, 12 were randomly selected. Ten children identified as stuttering during speech were also included. These children were divided into four groups. The first group of five children who apparently did stutter were designated by the experimenters as *not* being stutterers, and the attempt was made to remove the label of *stutterer* from these children. The second group of five children who did stutter were designated by the experimenters as true stutterers, a label they endorsed. The third group consisted of six normally speaking children with what was determined to be normal fluency. The ages of these children were 5, 9, 11, 12 (two children), and 15 years. As described below, the label of *stuttering* was endorsed for these children. The final group of six normally speaking children were not given the label of *stutterers* and were complimented on their speaking ability (e.g., "You speak very well. Your speech is of very good quality").

The study lasted for three months. During this time, both the normally speaking children in the third group as well as their teachers and the staff of the facility were told that these children were demonstrating classic signs of stuttering. For example, the children were told that they were found to be having

> a great deal of trouble with your speech. The types of interruptions which you have are very undesirable. These interruptions indicate stuttering. You have many of the symptoms of a child who is beginning to stutter. You must try to stop yourself immediately. . . . Do anything to keep from stuttering. . . . Don't ever speak unless you can do it right. . . . Whatever you do, speak fluently and avoid any interruptions whatsoever in your speech. (Tudor, 1939, pp. 10–11)

In addition, the childrens' teachers and staff were informed that

> these children show definite symptoms of stuttering. The types of interruptions they are having very frequently turn into stuttering. . . . Watch their speech all the time very carefully and stop them when they have interruptions; stop them and have them say it over. Don't allow them to speak unless they can say it right. (Tudor, 1939, pp. 12–13)

The children, the teachers, and the staff were consulted a minimum of once each month in order to reinforce the label of *stutterer*. Dictaphone recordings were made of all children for both reading and monologue speech at both the outset and conclusion of the study. Five judges rated the childrens' speech using a five-point, perceptual-fluency rating scale, and disfluencies were tabulated and placed into categories of syllable repetition, word repetition, phrase repetition, interjection, and pauses. Apparently no count was made of silent or audible prolongations.

Tudor provided a subjective analysis of the subjects from the third group by stating that by the end of the investigation, all six children showed varying degrees of speech disruptions and concern about their speech. According to Tudor:

> They were reluctant to speak and spoke only when they were urged to. . . . [T]heir rate of speaking was decreased. They spoke more slowly and with greater exactness. They had a tendency to weigh each word before they said it. . . . [T]he length of response was shortened. . . . [T]hey became more self-conscious. They appeared shy and embarrassed in many situations. . . . They accepted the fact that there was something definitely wrong with their speech. Some hung their heads, others gasped and covered their mouths with their hands. (pp. 147–148)

As Silverman (1996) points out, these results were especially striking since five of the six children were beyond the age at which stuttering usually begins. The investigation appears to provide reasonably strong support for the essence of the diagnosogenic theory of stuttering onset and development.

In the 1960s, stuttering as a learned behavior was formalized, in the form of both classical (instrumental) conditioning and operant (respondent) conditioning. Both approaches hold that the speaker gradually learns to stutter, but for slightly different reasons. With classical conditioning, the speaker learns to associate speaking with an emotional response. Just how this occurs is unclear, although some children—not necessarily those eventually diagnosed as stuttering—may have several characteristics that make it more difficult for them to achieve fluency. It may be that some children experience highly penalizing responses to natural fluency breaks that may become tied to the experience of speaking. In any case, the child learns that speaking is—or can be—difficult and begins to both anticipate and struggle during breaks in his fluency. Again, whether or not the initial fluency breaks are normal is a major issue of debate. If the initial breaks are normal, then the argument that stuttering is principally a learned behavior is strengthened. If the initial or core breaks in fluency are not normal, however, learning would assume somewhat less importance. That is, it would suggest that—at least at the outset—something is not functioning normally in the speaker's speech production system.

Models of operant or respondent conditioning do not explain the onset of stuttering as well as they do the evolution of the behavior. Operant models propose that the fluency breaks of young children are shaped by the response they elicit. These theories propose that listeners respond to the child's fluency breaks by reinforcing their occurrence. The breaks are then gradually shaped into greater abnormality, with associated struggle and secondary characteristics. Operant models do well in explaining the great variety of secondary behaviors that develop with each individual. The avoidance and escape behaviors, while somewhat similar across all people who stutter, tend to be uniquely shaped by listener responses so that individuals tend to develop distinctive behaviors. The fact that these secondary behaviors are not regularly reinforced makes them particularly resistant to change, since an intermittent schedule of reinforcement tends to strengthen behaviors, making them more difficult to extinguish.

Over time, the learned or secondary behaviors such as eye blinks, head movements, or gasping for air become part of an integrated and tightly bound pattern of behavior. In addition, it is suggested that negative reinforcement, or escape from punishment, is occurring. This may also be one explanation why the frequency of stuttering does not always decrease with what is perceived as punishment. That is, the "punishment" may help the speaker to escape from the stuttering moment by providing a highlighting affect (Cooper, Cady, & Robbins, 1970; Daly & Kimbarow, 1978).

Brutten and Shoemaker (1967) attempted to combine the best of the classical-conditioning and operant-conditioning models in a two-factor approach. They suggested that the initial fluency breaks occurred as a result of classically conditioned negative emotion being associated with the act of speaking. Via classical conditioning, learned, negative emotion disrupts the cognitive and motoric production of speech. The autonomic nervous system responds to this negative emotion. The development of secondary behaviors that follow are the result of respondent or operant conditioning.

The high-water mark for traditional learning theories was likely a review article by Gerald Siegel published in 1970. Siegel, one of the foremost researchers in the field of behavioral science, pointed out that operant-conditioning models fail to adequately explain stuttering behavior in the laboratory, let alone in the real world. Although research has shown that it was clearly possible to manipulate the secondary behaviors of stuttering, clinicians had much less success in explaining the development and modifying the core behavior of the disorder: that is, the cause of the fluency breaks in the first place.

A final account of stuttering as learned behavior is Bloodstein's (1961, 1993, 1995) *continuity hypothesis*. Like the diagnosogenic theory, this view also proposes that stuttering develops from the normal fluency breaks produced by young children. However, misdiagnosis and negative reactions by one or more significant listeners are *not* part of the problem. Bloodstein suggests that both the tension and the fragmentation of fluency breaks increase as a result of communicative pressure. The development of stuttering is not a consequence of the child's trying to avoid normal fluency breaks that have been mislabeled. As tension and fragmentation increase, especially for part-word repetitions, the pattern becomes chronic and the child is more likely to be identified as a someone who stutters.

MULTIFACTORIAL MODELS

As we said earlier in this chapter, for many reasons simplistic and unidimensional approaches to understanding stuttering onset and development are clearly far from adequate. As authors and researchers have increasingly appreciated the multidimensional nature of stuttering, there has been an increase of such models that describe the many intrinsic and extrinsic factors that influence one's ability to produce fluent speech (Andrews et al., 1983; Andrews & Neilson, 1981; Cooper & Cooper, 1985c; De Nil, 1999; Neilson & Neilson, 1987; Riley & Riley, 1979, 1984; Smith, 1990, 1999; Smith & Kelly, 1997; Wall & Myers, 1984). For example, Wall and Meyers (1994) identified psycholinguistic factors (phonology, prosody syntax, semantics/cognition, propositionality, and pragmatics), psychosocial factors (parents and other significant adults, peers, and social load of discourse), and physiological factors (voice onset and ter-mination time, laryngeal and supralaryngeal tension, sensorimotor coor-dination, autonomic nervous system, coarticulation, genetics, and respi-ration). These models by their nature involve many factors, are somewhat complex, and are therefore difficult to test. On the other hand, they have led to many empirical investigations as well as clinical tech-niques. We will continue this section by discussing examples of such models.

The Demands and Capacities Model

One of the more recent paradigms used to explain the onset of stuttering is called the demands and capacities model (DCM). The model is an appeal-ing one, particularly for clinicians, because it includes many of the factors that seem to influence fluent and nonfluent speech. It is a model that fits with current multifactoral and dynamic views of stuttering onset and development. From a clinical standpoint, it provides a straightforward and often much-appreciated explanation to parents of children who may be stuttering (see Curlee, 2000 [in press] and Gottwald & Starkweather, 1999).

This model considers both the capacities of the individual and the effects of both internal and environmental "demands" in the develop-ment of the disorder. The model proposes that children who stutter pos-sess genetically-influenced general tendencies for fluency breakdown that interact with environmental factors to both originate and maintain the problem. The model also addresses, in a preliminary way, the fact that human genotypes (the fundamental hereditary constitution of an individual) interact with their environment to create what we observe as the phenotype (the outward, visible expression of a specific human). Recent advances in the understanding of the nature-nurture interaction (epigenesis) have yielded fascinating explanations of the multiple inter-actions influencing this process (See Kelly, 2000; Smith, 1999; Smith & Kelly, 1997).

Variants of this model were first proposed by Andrews and colleagues (Andrews et al., 1983; Andrews & Neilson, 1981; Neilson & Neilson, 1987; Riley & Riley, 1979, 1984). For example, based on their accumulated diagnostic data, Riley and Riley proposed a component model that described factors that distinguished the ability of children to produce flu-ent speech. These components included attending, auditory processing, sentence formulation, and oral motor ability. Their treatment approaches concentrated on enhancing a child's ability to improve performance in one or more of these components rather than altering environmental demands. More recently, several authors (Adams, 1990; Gottwald, 1999; Gottwald & Starkweather, 1999; Starkweather, 1987; and Starkweather & Gottwald, 1990) have provided theoretical elaboration.

In the demands and capacities model the deterioration of fluency is viewed as reflecting an imbalance between the child's current capacities or abilities for producing fluent speech and the demands placed on the child. Capacities are viewed as inherited tendencies, strengths, weaknesses, and perceptions, which may influence a child's ability to speak fluently. They are dynamic and changing rather than static. According to this model, capacities include—but may not be limited to—the general categories of **motoric** (the ability to initiate and control coarticulatory movements smoothly, rapidly, and with minimal effort), **linguistic** (the ability to formulate sentences), **socio-emotional** (the ability to produce smooth movements when under communicative or emotional stress), and **cognitive** (the ability to use metalinguistic skills).

Demands may take the form of (external) environmental demands or (internal) self-imposed demands. Examples of demands are fast-speaking rates used by parents and other adults; time pressure to respond quickly; competition and lack of turn taking by other speakers; overstimulation of language and demand for language performance; including the need to formulate complex sentences; excitement and anxiety' and cognitive requirements for expressing complicated thoughts. It is important to point out that the child evidences no disorder or deficit. However, if the demands of the environment continue to exceed the capacities of that particular child, stuttering is more likely to occur. The model is dynamic in that internal or external demands interact with the speaker's skills at a given moment. The skills that are likely to enhance fluent speech production change as the child grows both physically and cognitively, just as internal and external demands change over time. As Starkweather and Gottwald (2000, in press) describe,

> When the positive forces (either environmental or organismic) outweigh negative ones, the person will be fluent, and when the negative forces outweigh the positive ones, the person will be dislfuent. Since these organismic and environmental variables have been identified in the literature as making it more or less likely that a person will speak fluently, it is certainly logical to suggest that a threshold may be present, different of course, for different individuals.

Conture (1990) states that neither the child's capacity alone nor his environment alone appear to be sufficient to cause stuttering. In most cases, both components seem to be necessary for the problem to develop. For example, Andrews, Yates-Morris, Howie, and Martin (1991) found that 71% of the variance contributing to the likelihood that one would stutter was accounted for by environmental factors, while 29% is accounted for by the individual's unique environment (factors affecting the fetus and following birth). Peters and Guitar (1991) and Guitar (1998) agree that predisposing physiological factors interact with developmental and environmental influences to enhance the problem.

The demands and capacities model, despite its intuitive appeal, has received criticism from those who suggest that for a variety of reasons it is not possible to test the model (Ingham & Cordes, 1997; Siegel, 2000). That is, the capacities that are suggested as being necessary for producing fluent speech are not directly measurable, and specific requirements for mismatches between demands and capacities are not defined. In addition, no thresholds are indicated for when mismatches may lead to the disruption of fluency. Finally, these authors suggest that the model invites circular reasoning: Stuttering occurs when demands exceed capacities indicating that demands are too great for the child (Ingham & Cordes, 1997).

Siegel (2000) suggests that reconfiguring the model as a "demands and performance model" would lead to empirical testing of the proposed relationships of a child's ability and behavior. However, others have questioned the necessity or value of such a change (Curlee, 2000; Kelly, 2000; Ratner, 2000; Starkwather & Gottwald, 2000; Yaruss, 2000). As Kelly (2000) indicates, performance (the execution of an action or reaction to stimuli) may be more measurable than capacities (faculties or potential), but the interaction of the two is clear and has been inferred in many areas of scientific study—including the behavioral sciences—for years. The demands and capacities model brings together many of the complexities that have been observed about stuttering and the people who speak in this fashion.

Ratner (1995, 1997; 2000) describes support for the model in the form of *trading relationship* between fluency and associated speech and language capacities in children. She notes that a proportion of children's fluency breaks evolve from linguistic pressures that exceed their productive capacities. That is, a fluent child sometimes begins to "stutter" following intervention to enhance expressive language or phonological skills (Hall, 1977; Meyers, Ghatak, & Woodford, 1990). Furthermore, Winslow and Guitar (1994) demonstrated a relationship between conversational turn-taking and fluency for a five-year-old child during family dinnertime interaction. Fluency increased when conversational demands were lessened with turn taking while stuttering increased when turn-taking rules were withdrawn. Yaruss et al. (1995) found that nine nonstuttering children exhibited a strong positive correlation between their articulatory speaking rate and their diadochokinetic (DDK) rate ($r = .81$), indicating that these children speak at rates in line with their abilities. On the other hand, the nine children who stuttered showed a mild negative correlation ($r = .24$) between speaking rate and DDK, suggesting that children who stutter may attempt to use speaking rates that exceed their ability to rapidly and precisely move their articulators. Yaruss (1997c) found a trade-off between production rate and DDK accuracy. Children exhibiting faster DDK rates also produced more errors than children with slower DDK rates, again suggesting that children who produced more errors were actually exceeding their ability to rapidly and precisely move their articulators in a speech-related task.

Additional study may help to specify the relationships between a child's capacity (such as diadochokinetic ability) for responding to demands of rapid speech. Of course, understanding the relationships between capacities and demands and determining thresholds for fluency disruption may be particularly difficult for socio-emotional and cognitive domains. Likewise, specifying and quantifying self-imposed demands will require some creative research designs. Defining and testing the model will likely lead to capacities as well as demands that are unique to particular children at different points in their development.

The Multifactorial-Dynamic Model

In an attempt to create a unified strategy for communicating about the disorder, Smith (1990; 1999) and Smith and Kelly (1997) provide a novel way of describing the multifactorial nature of the disorder within a dynamic framework. They suggest that viewing stuttering by tabulating the static units of disfluency form-types provides only a record of surface events. The problem with this approach is that stuttering is a dynamic disorder with many processes that underlie these surface behaviors. Using an analogy that fits nicely with stuttering, the scientific study of volcanoes, the authors explain that early volcanologists concentrated on surface events. They counted and classified volcanoes based on the shape of the landform and type of eruptive materials. After decades of this approach, researchers began to understand that classifying volcanoes by their surface features failed to explain the dynamic nature of the phenomena. Real understanding of volcano activity finally began once the theory of plate tectonics was applied to the problem. This explanation of what was occurring under the surface provided a unified framework for studying the many aspects of volcanic activity.

Smith and Kelly suggest that a major impediment to developing a global theory of stuttering is the belief in the "reality of the units of stuttering" (p. 29). These surface units of stuttering are akin to the smoke of the volcano and fail to provide insight to the true dynamic nature of the phenomenon. Moreover, concentrating on the surface behaviors of the disorder continues to obscure our understanding of the multifactoral nature of the disorder.

Perhaps the best argument in favor of this view is the fact that the stuttering experience is present even when a listener is unable to perceive the surface behaviors in the form of a traditional moment of stuttering. As we will discuss at several points in this book, it is possible for profound stuttering events to take place in the complete absence of any observable breaks in fluency. As we will see as we discuss treatment strategies, it is also possible to create highly realistic and disruptive stuttering behaviors in the absence of any underlying emotional or cognitive turmoil. As Smith and Kelly point out, even though stuttering events may appear to be highly specific on the surface of the speaker's behavior, the dynamic processes influencing the relative level of fluency-disfluency are distant in time and space from the "event" we perceive as stuttering. That is, there are many neurological and physiological events that occur long before the placement of some arbitrary timing mark suggesting the onset or termination of the stuttering event. Even though the "precise identification" of those stuttering events on the surface may be possible, they provide an artificial boundary for segmenting the dynamic process of speech production. The surface events of stuttering, as with volcanoes, provide only one window with which to view the disorder. Additionally, there is no one-to-one relationship between traditional classifications of fluency breaks and the many underlying events. Commenting on the use of traditional fluency form-types in analyzing stuttering, Smith (1999) states:

> Requiring researchers to use these units, to use "reliable means" of classification, and to interpret their data in relation to these units is analogous to asking the scientist who is recording seismic activity around volcanoes to interpret the data in relation to the pattern of smoke rising from the surface of the volcano. (p. 30)

Attempts to identify a single cause of stuttering, particularly based on surface features, are unlikely to be successful. In fact, after decades of hard work this approach has been remarkably unsuccessful. Attempting to discern the *cause* of stuttering by analyzing patterns of surface features seems to be an exercise in asking the wrong questions.

That stuttering is a multifactoral disorder is clear. Those who live with the problem of stuttering have compared it to the many layers of an onion, many of which must be peeled away in order to get at the core features of the problem during treatment. It is also clear that researchers and clinicians who work directly with those who stutter view the problem in this way. In spite of the attraction of a simplistic answer to the cause of stuttering, years of study have shown us that, at the very least, stuttering is not a simplistic problem. Smith (1999) suggests that creating a consensus on this point is the first step in formulating a global strategy for research and clinical practice.

Smith also provides other important insights that impact the way we look at theories of stuttering onset and development. She attempts to integrate the nature and nurture views of onset. All learning is organic.

While the genetic and physiological aspects of the CNS are currently being implicated in the etiology of stuttering, no single locus has been identified. Smith points out that the mammalian brain is constantly changing and responsive to environmental stimuli. Both the structure and the functioning of the brain are remodeled, not only during the early stages of development but during learning through all stages of life. That is, experience and learning influence the modeling of the adult brain. Rather than continuing to argue over the nature-nurture controversy for explaining the etiology of stuttering, Smith suggests that it would be useful to recognize that they are essentially, one in the same, an organic-learning combination.

Developmental stuttering likely results from the interaction of normal systems. That is, stuttering is not caused by a lesion in one or more sites but some form of multilayered interaction of the systems. Furthermore, this may be considerably different for each individual. When parents ask, "Is it organic (or inherited or neurological)?" we can say, "Yes, but it is also learned"; to say that a behavior is organic *or* neurobiological does not mean that the behavior cannot be modified by learning. Indeed, as the child learns to speak, he or she is making new connections between nerve cells and find-tuning neural networks in the brain. As Smith (1999) explains, "Successful behavioral therapy essentially helps the child to establish adaptive, stable patterns of operation and interaction among the widely distributed neural networks involved in language production" (p. 37). Fortunately, the mammalian brain is plastic and continually changing. Although the structure and cortical functioning of the brain are rapidly changing during early development, this remodeling also continues throughout life, resulting in an experience-determined plasticity in the adult brain.

The work of De Nil et al. (1998) and Kroll et al. (1997) using positron emission tomography (PET) indicate that such neural remodeling may be what occurs with the use of fluency-shaping techniques by adult subjects. These authors found that pretreatment adults who stuttered showed a preponderance of widely distributed right-hemisphere activation, which included primary and secondary cortical motor regions. Following intensive treatment emphasizing fluency-shaping techniques, these adults showed increased activation in the cortical motor regions of the left hemispheres. The authors interpreted this shift from right- to left-hemisphere activation as an indication of greater volitional control over their articulatory movements. These findings coincide with those of Boberg et al. (1983), who used electrophysiological measures of alpha-wave activity in the brain.

Smith also employs the concept of "attractor states" from dynamic systems theory to understand the development of both normal nonfluency and stuttering in children. Attractor states are observed when systems self-organize into models of behavior that are preferred (even though it may be very complex or even undesirable). Once the system is in a deep or stable attractor state, it takes more energy to move away from that state. Although the skills necessary for producing fluent speech are developing and are influenced by both nature and nurture, instability of speech is predictable. Children move between fluent and nonfluent attractors during development. Following years of development, the fluent young adult demonstrates a highly stable attractor for fluent speech and few unstable or disfluent attractors. For those who stutter, there is a combination of both fluent and disfluent attractors, resulting in instability and perpetuating breakdown in speech motor control. Furthermore, adults who stutter may have stable patterns of neuromuscular activity during stuttering (as in a tremor). The ultimate goal of this modeling is to study the factors that influence speech motor performance and "to understand the dynamic interplay of these factors as the developing brain seeks the stable, adaptive models of interaction among neural networks that generate . . . fluent speech" (p. 42).

A Neurophysiological Model

De Nil and his colleagues describe a model that also provides a comprehensive and unifying model of stuttering (De Nil, 1999). This model also includes capacities or skills similar to those noted in the demands and capacities model. In addition, De Nil also believes that just as nature and nurture are not separate phenomena, psychological and neurophysiological processes are not independent entities. This model also emphasizes the dynamic interplay among three levels of influence on human behavior—processing (central neurophysiological processes), output (motor, cognitive, language, social, and emotional), and contextual (environmental influences)—on all human behavior, and on stuttering in particular. Bidirectional-dynamic feedback takes place across all levels and continually influences output. That is, environmental stimuli and behavioral consequences are filtered through neurophysiological processes and vary both between individuals and within individuals over time. Long-term modification of behavior necessitates the modification of how information is processed centrally.

A SUMMARY OF MODELS

With so many ways of viewing the problem of stuttering, it can be difficult to explain the disorder to our clients and parents of clients. It can be extremely frustrating to students of the field who would like to have a clear, unequivocal answer to how and why stuttering is an aspect of human communication. On occasion, it is even difficult to agree about the nature of the problem when communicating with colleagues. Having many explanations about what seems on the surface to be essentially the same disorder would seem to detract from our credibility as a profession. The successful outcome of basic research such as the Human Genome Project, as it relates to stuttering, could go a long way toward building a consensus about the etiology of the problem.

Many researchers have found that people who stutter possess one or more predisposing characteristics that may, at the very least, set the stage for the onset of stuttering. None of these features, in and of itself, is likely to be sufficient to cause the problem. If the etiology of the syndrome were uncomplicated, the mystery would have been solved long ago. In more extreme cases—such as individuals undergoing injury to the central nervous system due to trauma, medication, or disease—traumatic emotional damage—including conversion neurosis, or extreme environmental or communicative pressure (as in the "monster" study described by Silverman [1988b])—one or relatively few factors may bring about a chronic disruption of fluency. However, in the vast majority of cases it takes a critical mass of factors that combine to tax the system over a critical time during the early development of speech and language.

CONCLUSION

The multifactorial and dynamic nature of stuttering has prevented the adoption of a single unifying theory that permits a comprehensive explanation concerning onset of this disorder. The many uncertainties about the skills or capacities that seem to be necessary for humans to produce fluent speech and the factors that make this so difficult for some people will continue to perplex and fascinate researchers in the field. The lack of a unified theory is often frustrating to clinicians. Despite this, the clinician should be familiar with the possibilities that have been proposed and have a reasonable response to questions such as, "Why is my child stuttering?"

Having considered the many possibilities for stuttering onset, it should be obvious that people who stutter are far from a homogeneous group. This may be one reason why there are so many divergent theories of stuttering onset throughout history. This also may help to explain why some speakers are more apt to recover than others, why treatment techniques that work well with one person do not work as well with another, and why relapse is an especially important issue with some clients. As a result of advanced technology as well as greater understanding of the human speech production system, there is increasing evidence of neuro-physiological factors that contribute to both the onset and maintenance of fluency problems. This is not to say that such factors indicate a deficit; they may indicate reduced capacities for producing fluent speech and language. Such intrinsic capacities, in combination with extrinsic demands (particularly during a critical developmental period of speech and language acquisition), may result in chronic stuttering—but some-times they do not. Current evidence indicates that although there are common surface characteristics, the development of stuttering often fol-lows a highly individual course and that people who stutter, just as flu-ent speakers, are far from unique.

STUDY QUESTIONS

➤ How will you respond when you are asked by the parents of a young stuttering child the inevitable question, "Why is my child stuttering?"
➤ Spend several hours on the Internet reviewing websites on stuttering. How would you describe the nature and quality of the theoretical views of stuttering etiology that are presented?
➤ Do you find the conflicting theories of stuttering etiology frustrating? Can you explain the reason(s) for your frustration?
➤ Of the various etiological theories discussed in this chapter, which one is most appealing to you?
➤ How would you respond if a friend commented that "Stuttering is mostly a psychological problem, isn't it?"
➤ Provide examples of impairment, disability, and handicap that are associated with stuttering.
➤ Give several of your own experiences when you experienced a "loss of control." Describe the emotional and cognitive characteristics of each experience.
➤ Which investigations described in this chapter do you feel provide the strongest support for the idea that stuttering has a neurophysiological basis?
➤ What are the basic similarities and differences in the three examples of multifactorial models presented in this chapter (capacities and demands, the multifactorial-dynamic model, and the neurophysiolog-ical model).

RECOMMENDED READINGS

Journal of Fluency Disorders (in press, 2000) Consideration of Multifactoral Models of Stuttering Onset and Development: The Demands and Capacities Model.

Smith A., & Kelly, E. (1997). Stuttering: A dynamic, multifactoral model. In R. F. Curlee & G. M. Siegel (Eds.), *The nature and treatment of stuttering: New directions* (2nd Ed.) (pp. 204–217). Needham Heights, MA: Allyn & Bacon.

Van Riper, C. (1974). A handful of nuts. *Western Michigan Journal of Speech Therapy, 11 (2).*

Van Riper, C. (1982). *The nature of stuttering* (2nd Ed.). Englewood Cliffs, NJ: Prentice-Hall. See Ch. 5, "The Development of Stuttering," pp. 88–110; Ch. 17, "The Nature of Stuttering: An Attempted Synthesis," pp. 415–453.

Van Riper, C. (1990). Final thoughts about stuttering. *Journal of Fluency Disorders, 15,* 317–318.

CHAPTER

3

CHARACTERISTICS OF STUTTERING ONSET AND DEVELOPMENT

> *When I asked my mother what she thought caused me to stutter, she told me about my Aunt Helen and about everything the psychologists and therapists she and my father consulted had told them, and then added, "You know, when you were very little, still a toddler, and were living on 178th Street in the Bronx, you were playing on the floor in the living room, and this mouse ran right past you. I had the superintendent come and plug up the hole, and it never happened again, but I always wondered." (p.32)*
>
> Marty Jezer (1997).
> Stuttering: A Life Bound Up in Words.
> *New York, NY: Basic Books.*

INTRODUCTION

In the previous chapter we described ways of considering the etiology of stuttering. In this chapter we will discuss some of the basic characteristics of normal and disordered fluency and elaborate on the characteristics of early stuttering development. The many characteristics of the speaker's fluency provide key features for the diagnostic decisions to be discussed in subsequent chapters. Beyond these surface features, we will continue to see that stuttering has many layers and is manifested in a variety of ways according to the individual's response to the problem.

STEREOTYPES OF STUTTERING AND PEOPLE WHO STUTTER

Nearly all the stereotypes pertaining to people who stutter tend to be negative (Bloodstein, 1995; Doopdy, Kalinowski, & Armonson, 1993; Lass et al., 1992). What clinicians and clients believe about the etiology of stuttering can have an influence on the various stereotypes held by the general public (Bloodstein, 1987; Silverman, 1992; Van Riper, 1982). The information the clinician is able to provide to other professionals as well as the general public should illuminate the problem rather than obscure it.

If the reader has doubts concerning the attitudes and reactions of listeners to someone who stutters, give yourself the following challenge. Pose as a person with a moderate-to-severe stuttering problem in a variety of social, educational, and vocational situations. This will be difficult so it is usually best to do it with a fellow student or colleague. With your partner to help you record your behavior as well as that of your listeners, make a series of telephone calls and enter into a series of face-to-face speaking situations. See if you can elicit "the look" that people who stutter are all too familiar with. We won't describe it now, but you will know it when you see it. And your clients will respond to you with a knowing understanding when you are able to describe it and relate your experience. As you accumulate several listener reactions, determine your level of anxiety in each situation. Keep a record of the verbal and nonverbal responses of your listeners. It is wise to enter at least ten to fifteen speaking situations during a single outing, for it will take a series of such encounters to begin to become desensitized to the experience.

There will be occasions during treatment sessions when it will be appropriate for you, the clinician, to take this role and do what you are asking your client to do. As you challenge yourself to this experience you will gradually become desensitized and appreciate the dynamics of the situation. You will also find that many listeners will react to you as though you are, at the very least, unintelligent. Listeners may respond minimally, for stuttering tends to act as a behavioral depressant (McDonald & Frick, 1954). Listeners may also respond by speaking slowly and carefully, using excessively simple vocabulary and syntax. Once they realize that you are stuttering, they may attempt to avoid you completely or try to exit from the conversation. Although many listeners also will demonstrate a surprising amount of empathy, the experience is apt to reveal the stereotypes that many people have about stuttering. As a clinician, you may notice that you would like to avoid certain people and situations, and you will rather quickly begin to make decisions based on your stuttering experience. What the clinician communicates to the general public about the etiology of the problem can help to shed light on the stereotypes people tend to have about stuttering and the people who are speaking that way. There is much to learn about fluency disorders, and it is the clinician's responsibility to enlighten all those who are interested enough to listen.

CHARACTERISTICS OF NORMAL FLUENCY

Another difficulty we face when assessing fluency is the lack of data describing the nature of fluency in normal speakers. For instance, we know relatively little about the fluency characteristics of normal children and their responses to fluency-disrupting stimuli. We know almost nothing about changes in fluency throughout the life cycle, particularly for older speakers (Manning, Dailey, & Wallace, 1984; Manning & Shirkey, 1981). Furthermore, few data have been accumulated about the fluency characteristics as a function of variables such as gender, race, culture, and socio-economic level. Given the changing demographics of the United States, there are many important questions that should be asked concerning these variables if we are to be in a position to help clients who stutter (Cole, 1986, 1989; Cooper & Cooper, 1991b; Satcher, 1986; Waldrop & Exter, 1990).

In order to appreciate the nature of nonfluent speech production, it is necessary to understand the dimensions of fluent speech. Even the best of speakers speaking under ideal conditions are apt to produce breaks in the flow of words. Language and speech production is a complex task; it takes many years of experience to do it well, especially under conditions of stress. As Van Riper (1982) and Starkweather (1987) have pointed out, it is fortunate that humans have the opportunity to practice speaking as much as they do.

Starkweather (1987) provides an elegant assessment of the research on the dimensions of fluent speech in both children and adults. The term *fluency*, derived from the Latin for *flowing*, describes what the listener perceives when listening to someone who is truly adept at producing speech. The speech flows easily and smoothly in terms of both sound *and* information. There are no disruptions of the stream, and the listener can attend to the message—the overall effect of the performance—rather than considering how it was produced. The effect is similar to observing any accomplished athletic performance that requires complicated sequential movements, such as gymnastics, ice skating, diving, or swimming. The impression when observing such athletes is one of smoothness and ease. The individual segments of the performance are blended together, with no obvious transition from one movement to the next. There is a consistency to the behavior, and little or no tension is evident.

As a matter of fact, it may look as though the performer is unencumbered by the force of gravity—almost floating—with relatively little effort being expended.

Most young adult speakers are able to achieve a level of speech production that results in a high level of fluency. Such fluency requires facility at a minimum of two levels of production: language and speech. Filmore (1979) described three types of language fluency, which are interpreted by Starkweather (1987) as syntactic, semantic, and pragmatic fluency. Starkweather adds a fourth component, which he describes as phonologic fluency. Speakers who are *syntactically* fluent are able to construct highly complex sentences. Speakers who are *semantically* fluent possess and are able to access large vocabularies. Speakers who are *pragmatically* fluent are adept at verbal response in a variety of speaking situations. Starkweather's term *phonologically* fluent describes those speakers who are able to pronounce long and complicated sequences of sounds and syllables, including nonsense and foreign words.

Although *language* fluency is a prerequisite for the production of fluent speech, it is not the case that individuals who stutter are deficient in these aspects of language competence or ability. People who stutter do, however, exhibit difficulties in *speech* fluency.

There are several dimensions of speech fluency. Starkweather (1987) defines speech fluency in terms of continuity, rate, duration, coarticulation, and effort. **Continuity** relates to the degree to which syllables and words are logically sequenced as well as the presence or absence of pauses. If the semantic units follow one another in a continual flow of information, the speech is interpreted as fluent. If, however, the units of speech fail to flow in a logical sequence, information does not flow. Despite a continual flow of sound and the absence of pauses, the speech is not thought of as fluent, as in the following paragraph offered by Starkweather:

> What I mean, what I mean is, that, uh, when you, you, go to the, uh, store because, uh, you, you want some, need some, uh food or supplies or something, and, and, uh, the storekee—the man, clerk, who, who waits, well not waits, but serves, you know, gets some—something for you is, well, if he, if he, well if he is sort of, well, stern, or you know angry or something, then, well, then, I find it, well, I find it difficult to talk. (p. 19)

Another aspect of continuity has to do with a disruption in the flow of sound in the form of pauses. The pauses in the sequence of speech can be viewed from several perspectives. Clark (1971) differentiates pauses as conventional and idiosyncratic. *Conventional pauses* are used by speakers to signal a linguistically important event. *Idiosyncratic pauses*, on the other hand, reflect hesitation or uncertainty on the part of the speaker. These pauses indicate a decision-making process concerning upcoming word choice, style, or syntax.

Pauses also have been considered as unfilled or filled. Unfilled pauses are characterized by a silence lasting *longer* than approximately 250 milliseconds (ms) (Goldman-Eisler, 1958). This duration is suggested as a convenient threshold for normal silent intervals during fluent speech, since normal word junctures rarely exceed this duration (e.g., the juncture necessary to distinguish *night rate* from *nitrate*). Filled pauses are characterized by essentially meaningless sounds such as "ah," "er," "uh," and "um." With filled pauses, the flow of sound continues, but again, the flow of information does not. Whether the speech is considered fluent depends on many other features, including the frequency of these pauses along with the occurrence of other aspects of fluency.

Rate of speech also signals the perception of fluency. Most people talk about as fast as they can, as indicated by Tiffany (1980), who noted that the maximum and ordinary rates of speech tend to be similar. Young adult speakers of English average approximately five syllables per second (Picket, 1980; Stetson, 1951; Walker & Black, 1950). Obviously, according to the speaking task, there is considerable variability in terms of such factors as formality of the speaking situation, time pressure, and interference from background noise or competing messages. There appears to be a reasonably wide range of acceptable rates in the judgment of fluency. It is well known that if communication failure is likely, such as when speaking in a noisy environment, speakers are likely to slow down (Longhurst & Siegel, 1973). Likewise, if a speaker is producing a lengthy utterance, the rate of speech is likely to be more rapid (Malecot, Johnston, & Kizziar, 1972). It is not surprising, then, that listeners provide speakers with a great deal of latitude in their judgments of nonfluency based on rate alone. That is, simply because the speaker is producing speech at a slow rate, everything else being equal, the speaker is not likely to be evaluated as being nonfluent. Conversely, simply because a speaker is producing speech at a very rapid rate, he or she is not likely to be evaluated as being fluent. Although the rate of speech production is obviously one aspect of fluency, it does not appear to be a primary dimension. The flow of speech and information is based not only on rate, but on a combination of many factors, particularly the ease of production.

Duration of speech segments relates closely to the *coarticulation* of the segments, so we will discuss them concurrently. The duration of the consonants and vowels of a language varies considerably with speech rate and phonetic and linguistic context. For example, stressed syllables are longer than unstressed ones (Umeda, 1975). Sound segments are longer at the initiation and termination of syllables, words, and phrases (Fowler, 1978). Segment durations are dramatically influenced by position in the syllable (initial consonants are longer than syllable-final consonants), length of the word (segments are shorter with longer words), and sentence length (segments and words are shorter during longer sentences) (Huggins, 1978). Much of what occurs in terms of the duration of individual sound segments and words appears to be related to the speaker's anticipated flow of information during an utterance (Stark-weather, 1987). That is, the speaker may not need to plan all aspects of the upcoming utterance in terms of the necessary respiratory, phonatory, and articulatory events. Rather, the speaker would only need to have some idea about the amount of information the utterance would contain. Once the intended information was anticipated, the relative length of the utterance and the corresponding duration of the units of the sentence would be consolidated into the planned production.

Closely related to the durational aspects of individual sound segments and words is the fact that during speech there is a considerable overlap of the movements associated with speech sounds. Each sequence of speech sounds is the result of several coordinated gestures, each with its own associated movements. The movements will result in differing productions for individual sounds, in terms of the velocity of movement as well as the location and degree of contact. Because adjoining sounds and their associated gestures overlap temporally to the degree that the movements are not conflicting, the sounds are coarticulated.

This overlap, or *coarticulation*, extends across many sound segments, both forward and backward in time (Kozhevnikov & Chistovich, 1965; Ohman, 1965). The effect extends forward in time because the speaker anticipates upcoming sounds and, to the degree possible and assuming there are no competing movements taking place, begins to move the articulators into position to produce upcoming sounds. That is, the anticipation of upcoming sounds will influence the current production of sounds. For example, in anticipation of the upcoming vowel in the word *see, s* is characterized by a higher tongue placement than during the production of the word *sue*. This is referred to as forward (in time) coarticulation.

Coarticulatory effects also extend backward in time when the inertial effects of sounds that have already been produced influence the location and degree of contact of sounds currently being produced. An example of this effect would be a slightly more posterior lingual-alveolar contact for the production of the *t* in the word *cat* than for the word *sat*. That is, the lingual-velar production of the already produced *k* results in the tongue having to move a greater distance to the front of the oral cavity to produce the *t*. The place of contact for the *t* in this case would be apt to be produced in a somewhat posterior position relative to the place of the *t* in the word *sat*. This type of coarticulation may thus be thought of as backward (in time) coarticulation. These coarticulatory effects are greater when the speech rate is increased (Gay, 1978; Gay & Hirose, 1973; Gay, Ushijima, Hirose, & Cooper, 1974). The point of this for our discussion of fluency is that these coarticulatory effects contribute to the timing and smoothness of speech. In fluent speech, articulatory movements between the sounds, syllables, and words are done with ease. The transitions are smooth, and there is a continuous flow of overlapping sounds.

The final dimension of fluency, and perhaps most important—particularly as it relates to stuttering—is *effort*. Starkweather (1987) distinguishes two types of effort: effort associated with linguistic planning and that associated with muscle movement. Clinically, it may be that the listener's perception of effort, in combination with the other dimensions of fluent speech production already discussed, is the most sensitive indicator of fluent speech. As Starkweather suggests, "Fluent speech is effortless in two distinct ways: It requires little thought, and it requires little muscular exertion" (p. 37). Fluent speech is characterized by little attention being paid to the process of production; speaking is "automatic." The focus is on what is being said, the information that is being communicated from one person to another. The thought process in fluent speech takes relatively little time, while the execution of the speech takes somewhat longer. To the degree that the focus of the speaker is on *how* speech is being produced, there is a good chance that attention will be taken away from *what* is being said.

Finally, in terms of effort, Starkweather (1987) suggests that the perception of effort and, thus, fluency is closely related to the force of contact between opposing articulators. Fluent speech is characterized by little sensation of opposition or constriction of airflow. The air, the movements, and the sounds are produced with evident ease and smoothness. On the other hand, people who stutter are at the opposite end of the continuum of effort. Greater effort is associated with all the following: greater contact between articulators; greater impedance between the flow of air and the structures of the vocal tract, beginning with the vocal folds; and greater subglottic air pressure. With the speaker producing speech in this fashion, it is likely that speech will be judged as nonfluent. The focus for these speakers, particularly during overt stuttering, is nearly completely centered on *how* the speech is produced.

WHEN IS IT STUTTERING?

We will take a moment to address the issue of whether the speech behavior of people who stutter and the speech of those who do not is essentially the same. That is, is it reasonable to consider the fluency breaks of people who stutter and those who do not on the same continuum? While there are some who argue that the fluency breaks of those who stutter and normal speakers are so distinctively different as to be mutually exclusive (Hamre, 1992), most investigators believe that the fluency breaks of all speakers fall on the same continuum (Bloodstein, 1992; Starkweather, 1992). Still others suggest that this discussion has gone on long enough and that it is time to move on to other more important issues (Conture & Zebrowski, 1992; Ham, 1992; Van Riper, 1992a).

Cooper (1993) provided a colorful commentary on such investigations when he stated:

> I am hopeful we have seen the last of studies concerned with differentiating a "dysfluency" from a "disfluency" on the basis of a series of sophisticated psychoacoustical measurements of vocalizations made without respect to the subjects' histories and their affective and cognitive states at the moment of the assessment. We have suffered, and I believe those we strive to serve have suffered, because too frequently we allow our energies to be dissipated in discussions over issues as relevant as how many angels can dance on the head of a pin. I think we can do better. (pp. 377–378)

People who stutter are making use of essentially the same speech production system as normal speakers. One would expect, even given some difficulties at one or more levels of their system, that there would be considerable overlap in the nature of the speech produced. Some people who stutter are clearly more distinguishable by both the amount and type of their fluency breaks. Some people who stutter do not do so in any easily observable way: at least they do not do so by producing the repetitions, prolongations, or blocking behavior of traditional stuttering. They may speak very carefully, avoiding sounds, words, people, or—in some instances—speaking altogether. The discussions concerning the continuity or discontinuity between the surface behavior of people who stutter and those who do not are interesting, if somewhat esoteric. If the focus of our decisions during assessment and intervention is on the *person* it is clear that we must go beneath the surface and consider the affective and cognitive features of the speaker's fluency breaks.

In this text we often use the terms *formulative* and *motoric fluency breaks*. We have chosen this nomenclature rather than terms such as *(normal) disfluencies, (abnormal) dysfluencies, stuttering moments*, and the like, primarily because they present a clearer picture of what appears to be happening for stuttering as well as nonstuttering speakers. Drawing from the writings of Starkweather (1987); Van Riper (1982); Bloodstein (1974); Yairi and Clifton (1972); and Gordon, Hutchinson, and Allen (1976), Manning and Shirkey (1981) suggested the use of these terms for describing the continuum of fluency breaks among speakers. Formulative fluency breaks are characterized by (1) breaks in fluency between words, phrases, and larger syntactic units (including whole-unit repetitions thereof), (2) lack of obvious tension during the breaks, and (3) interjections between whole-word or larger syntactic units. These breaks are typical of normal speakers and are often absent from the speech of people who stutter. However, they are also present in the speech of people who stutter. Motoric fluency breaks are characterized by (1) breaks between sounds or syllables (part-word breaks), (2) obvious tension in the vocal tract, (3) pauses with a possible cessation of airflow and voicing, and (4) an excessive prolongation of sounds or syllables.

These breaks are more typical of speakers who stutter but may also be present to a small degree in normal speakers.

With these terms in mind, we may begin to distinguish some differences in the fluency breaks of children and adults and in the patterns of breaks for stutterers as well as nonstutterers. The normally speaking young adult typically displays few motoric fluency breaks and only slightly more formulative fluency breaks (Manning & Shirkey, 1981). The relatively few studies conducted with older normal speakers provide preliminary evidence suggesting that formulative fluency breaks tend to increase somewhat during late adulthood, and that motoric fluency breaks continue to be infrequent (Gordon, Hutchinson, & Allen, 1976; Manning & Monte, 1981; Yairi & Clifton, 1972).

The fluency breaks of young adults who stutter are made up almost entirely of motoric fluency breaks. In fact, there appears to be a notable absence of formulative (or normal) fluency breaks, a fact that can also be used to distinguish stutterers from normal speakers (Manning & Shirkey, 1981). Although there is little research on how the *quality* of a speaker's fluency changes during and following treatment, it may be that progress in treatment is sometimes signaled by an *increase* in the frequency of formulative fluency breaks to levels typical of normal speakers. That is, as the person who stutters begins to consider the variety of ways of expressing a thought rather than dealing with the short-term problems inherent in avoiding or struggling through a motoric fluency break, formulative breaks may increase in frequency to normal or near-normal levels.

The fluency breaks of normally speaking children often contain a large number of formulative fluency breaks. Bloodstein (1974) suggested that such breaks may be a function of language learning. While motoric fluency breaks may occur, they are relatively infrequent. For the normally speaking child, the frequency of both formulative and motoric breaks decreases as the neurological system approaches maturity and psycholinguistic abilities develop. By early adolescence, the speaker will achieve the optimum level of fluency typical of the young adult (Manning & Shirkey, 1982).

THE FEATURES ON THE SURFACE

The nature of stuttering at onset has often been discussed in the literature and forms the basis for many diagnostic decisions when assessing young children who are suspected of stuttering (see Chapter 5). Rarely do the characteristics of stuttering begin after the early childhood years, although some instances of late onset will be discussed in Chapter 4. For this reason, stuttering has often been called a disorder of childhood (Bloodstein, 1995; Conture, 1990; Van Riper; 1982).

Because these features of stuttering onset in children sometimes develop slowly and are highly variable, determining their presence in young children can be difficult. Authors have noted that even during stuttering moments, young children who stutter produce relatively normal movement sequences (Caruso, Conture, & Colton, 1988). Furthermore, during perceptually fluent speech, children who stutter are nearly identical to normally speaking children in terms of temporal onsets, offsets, and durations of speech movements (Conture, Colton, & Gleason, 1988). The great overlap in the behaviors of young, normally speaking children and those who eventually emerge as young people who stutter can make it difficult for the clinician to make precise diagnostic choices, let alone predict future performance. There is no absolute standard for how often or how tense a fluency break must be before it will be called stuttering. As much as anything, the designation of stuttering may coincide with whether the child's manner of speaking takes away from the effective communication of the message. If the quality of the speaker's fluency begins to detract from the effective communication, it may be nearing the threshold of a problem.

If fluency can be described as the easy, automatic, and continuous flow of sound and information, then the essence of a fluency disorder is the difficult, broken sequence of sounds, information, or both. This is what occurs in one form or another for most children and adults who stutter. However, there are typically many other features of stuttering occurring on the surface that accompany the fragmented speech and may obscure this central facet of the problem. There are often highly individualized surface features that speakers develop to escape from, disguise, or minimize the handicapping effects of stuttering. These are often an important part of the stuttering behavior, and it is necessary to identify and map these features for each person. Throughout the assessment and treatment of both children and adults who stutter, we find ourselves returning repeatedly to the fact that the essence of what the speaker is doing is preventing the easy, open flow of smooth and continuous speech.

DISTINGUISHING NORMAL AND ABNORMAL SURFACE FEATURES

The fact that normal speakers also exhibit many breaks in their fluency forces us to distinguish between normal and abnormal types of breaks, a task that has been a historical point of contention in the field for decades. Even the semantics of what to call the fluency breaks of normal and stuttering speakers has always created some difficulty (Tables 3-1 and 3-2). At the center of the controversy is whether the fluency breaks of nonstuttering speakers are qualitatively different than those of stuttering speakers. This fundamental question has received as much research attention as any issue in the field.

Table 3-1. Guidelines for Differentiating Normal from Abnormal Disfluency. (From Van Riper, C. *The Nature of Stuttering* (2nd ed.). Copyright © 1982. All rights reserved. Adapted by permission of Allyn & Bacon).

Behavior	Stuttering	Normal Disfluency
Syllable Repetitions:		
a. Frequency per word	More than two	Less than two
b. Frequency for 100 words	More than two	Less than two
c. Tempo	Faster than normal	Normal Tempo
d. Regularity	Irregular	Regular
e. Schwa vowel	Often present	Absent or rare
f. Airflow	Often interrupted	Rarely interrupted
g. Vocal tension	Often apparent	Absent
Prolongations:		
h. Duration	Longer than one second	Less than one second
i. Frequency	More than 1 per 100 words	Less than 1 per 100 words
j. Regularity	Uneven or interrupted	Smooth
k. Tension	Important when present	Absent
l. When voiced	May show rise in pitch	No pitch rise
m. When unvoiced	Interrupted airflow	Airflow present
n. Termination	Sudden	Gradual
Gaps (silent pauses):		
o. Within the word boundary	May be present	Absent
p. Prior to speech attempt	Unusually long	Not marked
q. After the disfluency	May be present	Absent
Phonation:		
r. Inflections	Restricted; monotone	Normal
s. Phonatory arrest	May be present	Absent
t. Vocal fry	May be present	Usually absent
Articulatory Postures:		
u. Appropriateness	May be inappropriate	Appropriate
Reaction to Stress:		
v. Type	More broken words	Normal disfluencies
Evidence of awareness:		
w. Phonemic consistency	May be present	Absent
x. Frustration	May be present	Absent
y. Postponements	May be present	Absent
z. Eye contact	May waver	Normal

Table 3-2. Several ways of categorizing disfluencies. Fluencey breaks characteristic of individuals who *do* stutter are listed in the first column. Fluency breaks characteristic of individuals who *do not* stutter are listed in the second column. From Yaruss, 1997a.

Within-Word Disfluencies	*Between-Word Disfluencies*
Monosyllabic whole-word repetition	Phrase repetition
Sound/syllable repetition	Polysyllabic whole-word repetition
Audible prolongation	Interjection
Inaudible prolongation	Revision
Stuttering-Like Disfluencies (SLD)	*Other Disfluencies*
Part-word repetition	Interjection
Monosyllabic word repetition	Phrase repetition
Dysrhythmic phonation	Revision/Incomplete phrase
Stutter-Type Disfluencies	*Normal-Type Disfluencies*
Part-word repetition	Whole-word repetition
Prolongation	Phrase repetition
Broken word	Revision
Tense pause	Incomplete phrase
	Interjection
Less Typical Disfluencies	*More Typical Disfluencies*
Monosyllabic word repetition (3 or more repetitions)	Hesitation
Part-word syllable repetition (3 or more repetitions)	Interjection
Sound repetition	Revision
Prolongation	Phrase repetition
Block	Monosyllabic word repetition (2 or fewer repetitions: no tension)
	Part-word syllable repetition) (2 or fewer repetitions: no tension)

One of the first systems for differentiating the fluency breaks of young children, and one that was used for many years, was developed by Wendell Johnson and his associates (Johnson, 1961; Johnson & Associates, 1959) and modified by Williams, Silverman, and Kools (1968). This scheme placed some of the surface behaviors of stuttering into the following categories:

➤ part-word repetition
➤ single and multisyllabic word repetition

➤ phrase repetition
➤ interjections
➤ revision-incomplete phrase
➤ dysrhythmic phonation (sound prolongations within words, unusual stress or broken words)
➤ tense pause (barely audible heavy breathing and other tense sounds between words)

Although younger children who stutter tend to have a higher occurrence of nearly all form types (Yairi & Lewis, 1984; Yairi et al. 1996), the categories of part-word repetitions, word repetitions, dysrhythmic phonations, and tense pauses tend to occur most often (Silverman, 1974). Still, there is no fluency break that stuttering children produce and normal speakers do not. Yairi and his colleagues make use of what they call *stuttering-like disfluencies* (SLD) (e.g., Yairi, Ambrose, & Niermann, 1993), which include part-word repetition, monosyllabic word repetition, disrhythmic phonation, and tense pause. They contrast SLDs with what they call *other disfluencies*, which include polysyllable word repetition, phrase repetition, interjection, and revision-incomplete phrases. These authors have suggested that some combinations of fluency breaks, such as SLD, may provide more sensitive measures of early stuttering.

Van Riper (1982) also suggests criteria for differentiating normal from abnormal fluency breaks (Table 3-1). These often-cited guidelines distinguish stuttering and normal disfluency on the basis of speech characteristics and reaction of the speaker to forms of stress and awareness of the problem. It is apparent that more than speech attributes must be considered when differentiating between a normal speaker and someone who is stuttering. Because of the considerable overlap in the type of fluency breaks, it has been suggested that nonverbal behaviors also should be considered when describing the onset of stuttering. Conture (1990) suggests two types of nonspeech behavior that the clinician can look for: (a) body movement and tension and (b) psychosocial discomfort and concern. Conture and Kelly (1988) found that young children who stutter were more likely to move their eyeballs to the left or right or to partially or totally obscure their view of the listener by blinking. In addition, young children may indicate their frustration and anxiety about speaking. Although the young child may not be extremely concerned, he may be in the initial stages of thinking of himself as someone who has trouble talking (DeVore, Nandur, & Manning, 1984).

Yaruss (1997a) provides a summary of terms that are used to categorize the fluency breaks of individuals who do stutter and those who do not (Table 3-2). The four basic categories use somewhat different terminology in describing what are essentially formulative and motoric breaks, as described in the previous chapter. The fluency breaks of speakers who stutter are characterized by within-word breaks, and nonstuttered breaks tend to be between larger units of language production. The other basic characteristic is the duration and tension of the break, with both being noticeably greater during stuttered speech.

There has been considerable controversy over the differences, or lack thereof, in the fluency breaks of young stuttering and nonstuttering children. Much of the controversy stems from the fact that the very early stages of stuttering are difficult to investigate. As Yairi and Lewis (1984) pointed out, investigations of the fluency of young children have been beset by such problems as a reliance on parent accounts and the difficulty of obtaining speech samples in a natural environment. An even bigger problem, however, is the lag between the initial behaviors of stuttering and the referral for professional assistance. These problems have contributed to the conflict about whether the fluency breaks of young children who stutter are indistinguishable from those of normal speakers (Glasner & Rosenthal, 1957; Johnson & Associates, 1959; Johnson & Luetenegger, 1955) or are different in many clinical aspects from normal speakers (Bloodstein, 1974; McDearmon, 1968; Van Riper, 1982).

In an attempt to decrease the effect of the usual delay between the onset and diagnosis of stuttering, Yairi and Lewis (1984) conducted the first in a continuing studies of investigations by Yairi and his colleagues on the developing nature of stuttering in young children. They analyzed the fluency breaks of two- and three-year-old children within two months after the initial identification of stuttering behavior. Ten children identified as stuttering (five boys and five girls) were matched with a group of normally speaking children. A perceptual analysis was performed on audiotaped samples of spontaneous speech of all subjects, with intrajudge and interjudge agreements ranging from +.93 to +1.0. The results indicated considerable overlap in the type of fluency breaks of the two groups, especially for interjections and revision-incomplete phrases. The fluency breaks of the ten normally speaking children were characterized by a relatively even distribution across eight categories of fluency breaks. The most frequent fluency breaks for these normal speakers were, in order, interjection, part-word repetition, and revision-incomplete phrase.

Yairi and Lewis found that the most frequent fluency breaks for the stuttering children were, in order, part-word repetitions, dysrhythmic phonation, and single-syllable repetitions. The stuttering children had more than three times the number of fluency breaks of the normally speaking children (21.5 breaks and 6.2 breaks per 100 syllables, respectively). The stuttering children had significantly more fluency breaks for all categories of breaks, although significant differences ($p < .05$) were found only during part-word repetitions and dysrhythmic phonation. It has been suggested that whole-word repetitions may be a precursor to part-word repetitions (Bloodstein & Grossman, 1981). Finally, Yairi and Lewis found that the stuttering children distinguished themselves from the control subjects in the number of repetitions that occurred during the part-word repetitions. That is, while the normally speaking children rarely repeated a part-word repetition more than once (range of 1–2), the stuttering children typically repeated a portion of the word two or more times (range of 1–11).

In a subsequent study, Ambrose and Yairi (1995) analyzed 1,000 syllables of 29 experimental subjects recently diagnosed (mean of 2.14 months post-onset) as children who stuttered (average age, 34.76 months) and 29 control subjects (average age, 35.57 months). The young stuttering children demonstrated a significantly greater number of units per repetition ($p < .002$). The frequency per 100 syllables of disfluencies containing two or more repetition units for the experimental subjects was 3.70 ($SD = 3.77$), while for the control subjects it was 0.21 ($SD = .20$).

Continued investigation on one of these surface characteristics that may help to predict the course of stuttering, the rate of the repetitions, was investigated by Throneburg and Yairi (1994). Comparing the speech of 20 preschool children who stuttered and a control group of 20 nonstuttering children, they found that the stuttering children exhibited shorter silent intervals between the repeated units and thus a more rapid rate of repetitions than the nonstuttering children. These results supported the findings of Yairi and Hall (1993) that children in the early stages of stuttering tend to repeat at a faster rate than children who do not stutter.

Researchers have also noted the tendency for children who stutter to produce fluency breaks in clusters (Colburn, 1985; Hubbard & Yairi, 1988; LaSalle & Conture, 1995; Silverman, 1973). That is, children in the early stages of stuttering often produce a sequence of between- or within-word breaks in close proximity to one another. For example, when contrasting the conversational speech of 30 young (average age of four years, three months) children who stuttered (CWS) with a control group of children, LaSalle and Conture (1995) found that 32% of the clusters produced by the children who stuttered were within word groups of two stuttering sequences, while the children who did not stutter *never* produced such clusters in any of their 300-word speech samples. They also noted that the occurrence of clusters containing within-word disfluencies was positively correlated with greater severity of stuttering and, perhaps, chronic stuttering.

A thorough review of the literature on the disfluency characteristics of early childhood stuttering was developed by Yairi (1997). Normally disfluent children typically have two or fewer part-word and word repetitions. A sudden rise in short-element repetitions constitutes an unusual departure from the usual development course of normal disfluency. One of the more interesting findings was the fact that approximately one-third of children who stutter exhibit abrupt onsets, and even relatively gradual onsets of stuttering actually take place within two weeks. Compared with their nonstuttering counterparts, children who are beginning to stutter exhibit:

➤ two-and-a-half to three times as many total instances of disfluencies
➤ five to six times as many instances of stuttering-like disfluencies
➤ proportions of SLDs to total disfluency that are twice as large
➤ proportions of part-word and monosyllabic word repetitions having two or more extra repetition units that are three times larger
➤ six times as many disfluency clusters and proportionally at least twice as many clusters, with longer clusters
➤ repetitions in which intervals between iterations are shorter
➤ twice as many head and neck movements accompanying disfluencies.

Another important characteristic of the speech of children who stutter is the "co-effect," in that the combination of both a greater occurrence of repetitions and the larger number of repetitions results in an even greater differentiation between stuttering and nonstuttering children. When clustering and duration of fluency breaks are added in, the result is even more obvious, with concentrations of disfluencies that are longer and faster in rate than those produced by normally fluent children.

A SEQUENCE OF DEVELOPMENT?

The most traditional view of stuttering development is one of gradual increase in awareness and struggle, and thus severity. For example, Conture (1990) suggested a sequence that corresponds closely with Van Riper's (1982) tracks of stuttering development (see Van Riper, pp. 94–108). This model may describe the sequence of development for some children who stutter.

Alpha Behaviors are brief, subtle inefficiencies in speech production characterized by short within-word pauses, laryngeal catches, and articulatory arrests at the beginning of an utterance or at the transition between sounds and syllables. These subtle breaks appear to occur as a result of an interplay between the child's capacity for producing fluency and environmental stimuli or demands.

Beta Behaviors are oscillatory movements of the speech mechanism that are characterized by brief to lengthy repetitive productions. These are compensatory or coping reactions to the original Alpha factors and take the form of syllable repetitions, laryngeal adduction, and nostril flaring.

Gamma Behaviors are speech movements that are relatively tense, fixed, or both and are viewed as coping reactions to the Beta activities.

These behaviors take the form of fixed laryngeal adductory postures, labial contacts, and lingual posturing. They result in inaudible sound prolongations or a cessation of airflow or voicing. This stage is a significant step in the development of stuttering, marking a reduced likelihood that spontaneous recovery will take place.

Delta Behaviors are both nonverbal and verbal reactions to Beta, Gamma, and possibly Alpha behaviors and are seen as reactive speech and nonspeech behaviors. These coping reactions are in the form of such responses as pharyngeal muscle constriction, vocal fold lengthening (pitch rises), vocal fold shortening, blinking of eyelids, and eyeball movements.

In addition, Conture (1990) describes three possible patterns of development for young children who possess Alpha features. One possibility is the spontaneous resolution of the Alpha behavior. He suggests that this may occur for about 40 to 50% of children who begin demonstrating Alpha behaviors. Their fluency breaks are characterized as brief, often imperceptible. That is, they may have somewhat longer articulatory contacts and slightly slower trajectories to articulatory targets than controls. These children may exhibit cycles of Beta behavior, which eventually fade away. For whatever reasons, these children do not move to and stay at the next stage of stuttering development. They do not respond to the subtle motoric breaks with tense or fixed gestures. It may be important to note that for the most part, these children also have essentially normal articulation, language, and neuromotor development.

Another possible sequence has children reacting to the various Alpha features and progressing gradually through the Beta level. The difference for these children is that they will recover only with treatment. They also comprise about 40 to 50% of the total population of children who begin with Alpha behaviors. These children may demonstrate increased numbers of sound prolongations and associated nonspeech behaviors. It is likely consequential that they tend to also have some difficulty with articulation, deviant or delayed sound production, and phonological difficulties, as well as other language or voice problems (St. Louis & Hinzman, 1986). In an attempt to cope with the Alpha and Beta features, these children go on to develop Delta behaviors that make the problem even more apparent. Conture suggests that treatment intended to alter the Gamma behaviors will not solve the problem of the more central Alpha and Beta features.

Although this pattern of development assists in understanding how stuttering may sometimes evolve, there is a growing body of data that suggests that such development is not always the case. The longitudinal data accumulated by Yairi and his associates concerning onset and development (Yairi & Ambrose, 1992a, 1992b, 1999; Yairi, Ambrose, & Niermann, 1993; Yairi & Hall, 1993; Yairi & Lewis, 1984) suggest that stuttering in young children can reach an advanced form soon after onset (see also Chapter 5). This early stuttering can take complex forms that include head and facial movements and long, tense blocking behavior. Yairi, Ambrose, and Niermann conclude that for many children, the peak of stuttering is reached during the first two to three months post-onset. However, perhaps the most interesting finding is the observation that a substantial number of children show a dramatic decline in both the frequency and severity of stuttering within the first six months after onset (Yairi & Ambrose, 1992a; Yairi, Ambrose, & Niermann, 1993). Yairi and his colleagues have found that some stuttering form-types such as repetitions of sounds, syllables, monosyllabic whole-words, and sound prolongations tend to decrease for children who recover. Interestingly, other, more normal or formulative fluency breaks (revisions, interjections, phrase repetitions, and other between-word breaks) tend to remain stable or increase for this group of children.

CONDITIONS CONTRIBUTING TO ONSET

This section will consider two sets of conditions that have been related to the onset of stuttering. These are issues that clinicians are frequently questioned about by clients and parents. The first set of conditions are those that, while they have been considered in the literature, seem to have relatively little influence on stuttering causation. Although they may be prominent events in the child's life, these conditions are more likely to simply coincide with the initial observation that the child is beginning to stutter. We will then discuss conditions that may have a greater effect on onset. These are factors that relate more directly to the child's capacities for producing fluent speech. It is important to understand that many investigations of young stuttering children are descriptive studies that do not allow an assumption of cause-and-effect relationships between the speaker or environmental characteristics and the onset of stuttering behavior. While there may indeed be some relationship between these events, the fact that they covary in some manner may only signify that another unknown factor or factors are causing this relationship.

Less Influential Factors

These factors have not been shown, at least to date, to have a strong influence on precipitating the problem of stuttering. In many instances these factors are similar to the myths that tend to be associated with stuttering.

Physical Development

Children who stutter have the same general physical makeup as children who speak normally. There is no evidence that children who stutter are distinctive in terms of general developmental milestones such as ages of teething and weaning, as well as developing the ability to dress and feed themselves, acquire bowel and bladder control, sit, creep, stand, and walk (Andrews & Harris, 1964; Cox, Seider, & Kidd, 1984).

Illness

On occasion, parents will report that stuttering began following an illness. As Silverman (1996) points out, if the illness affects the central nervous system, a cause-and-effect relationship between the illness and the onset of stuttering may be possible. However, children who stutter do not appear to have more illnesses than those that do not (Andrews & Harris, 1964; Johnson & Associates, 1959). Illness is more likely to influence the nature of stuttering in those who already stutter. It is difficult for the child to maintain the energy to monitor speech production and use fluency-enhancing techniques when they are sick and resistance and energy are low (Luchsinger & Arnold, 1965; Van Riper, 1978).

Imitation

This consideration of stuttering onset may be influenced by the culture of the speaker. For example, Otsuki (1958, as cited by Silverman, 1992) reported that in Japan, imitation was viewed as a major causal factor in 70% of his cases. In his review of clinical cases, Van Riper (1982) indicated that although there were several instances where imitation appeared to be involved in the onset of stuttering, only one case appeared to be attributed to this cause. The strongest argument against imitation is that the early forms of stuttering are usually highly dissimilar from the more advanced forms.

Shock or Fright

Parents may report the onset of stuttering following a traumatic emotional event (Van Riper, 1982). However, as both Van Riper (1982) and Silverman (1996) point out, in many cases, the initial signs of stuttering often precede the suspected event. Rather than a cause of the stuttering, an event that happens to occur at approximately the same time as the stuttering was first observed may serve as a marker of that time period. Parents may report the onset of stuttering associated with an event without knowing that their child had been stuttering for some time in school and other locations outside the home. Moreover, as Silverman indicates, in almost all cases the "traumatic" events are not really very traumatic.

Emotional and Communicative Conflicts

Similar to shock or fright, some parents suspect that a variety of interpersonal and family stresses can bring about stuttering. There are, of course, many forms of emotional and communicative stress for children. The majority of authorities believe that although such forms of stress may well aggravate the fluency breaks of children who have already begun to stutter, there is little empirical support for this form of causation. There is no indication that children who stutter have a greater number of emotional conflicts than their normally speaking counterparts (Adams, 1993; Andrews & Harris, 1964; Bloch & Goodstein, 1971; Bloodstein, 1987; Johnson & Associates, 1959; Van Riper, 1982). Again, as with illness, shock, or fright, emotional or communicative stress undoubtedly enhances the possibility of breakdowns in the motor sequencing of speech (Van Riper, 1982).

Socioeconomic Status of the Family

The relatively few data that are available concerning this factor indicate that stuttering is present in all socioeconomic groups. Undoubtedly, factors of socio-economic level and race interact with—and cloud—this issue. A lack of diagnostic and treatment services are likely to underestimate the occurrence of stuttering for certain populations. Van Riper (1982) reviews several studies that report varying amounts of stuttering across both cultures and races. Gillespie and Cooper (1973) and Dyker and Pindzola (1995) report data showing a higher occurrence of stuttering in African-American populations. Bloodstein (1987) suggests that the occurrence of stuttering may be related to the imposition of high standards for the achievement of status and prestige, along with the intolerance of deviancy, values that may vary depending on the socioeconomic status of families.

Nationality

The occurrence of stuttering in technologically developed countries is typically reported at approximately 0.7–1.0% of the population. The occurrence is somewhat higher in several cultures throughout the world, possibly due to a combination of limited genetic pools and cultural responses to disfluency (Bullen, 1945; Lemert, 1953, 1962; Morgenstern, 1956; Snidecor, 1947).

More Influential Factors

Other factors do appear to have a somewhat greater influence on the likelihood of stuttering, although their precise impact remains unclear. Again, it is important to keep in mind that stuttering onset is most likely influenced by a combination of intrinsic and extrinsic factors, and no one aspect is likely to decrease a child's capacity or increase the environmental demands to the point where stuttering will occur. Rather, these conditions may be best thought of as predisposing factors that can place a child at greater risk for both *precipitating* and *maintaining* stuttering (Silverman, 1992).

Sex

Kent (1983) discussed the fact that the higher occurrence of stuttering in males is one of the few consistencies about the disorder. It appears, however, that stuttering behavior begins with approximately equal frequency with young boys and girls. However, females are much more likely to recover from stuttering during pre-school years than are males. The result is that by the early school years there are approximately three boys who stutter for every girl. The reasons why males consistently show a higher persistence of stuttering may relate to boys being less adept at language and speech activities or less able to adapt to communicative stress. The previously mentioned findings of Geschwind and Galaburda (1985) suggest that young male speakers may have greater difficulty in achieving or maintaining fluency. In addition, as discussed earlier, there may also be a sex-related genetic influence that, at the very least, precipitates stuttering (Kidd, Kidd, & Records, 1978). Based on the results of several studies, Yairi and Ambrose (1999) suggest that gender and genetics interact in such a way that young females who stutter are much less likely to persist in stuttering than young males.

Age

Children who are approximately two through seven years of age are much more likely to begin stuttering than older children, adolescents, or adults. There is a much greater chance of stuttering onset before age five than after age seven. Andrews (1984) suggests that the risk of developing stuttering drops by 50% after age four, 75% after age six, and is virtually nil by age twelve. The onset of stuttering during the middle or late adult years is extremely rare and is likely to occur only in cases of neurological or psychological origin. It is also important to appreciate that speaker age also appears to interact with speaker sex in a number of ways. Yairi and Ambrose (1992b) found that boys begin stuttering an average of five months later than girls. The later age of stuttering onset for boys may reflect a slower language/phonologic development. Furthermore, as we will discuss, chronic stuttering has been associated with somewhat poorer performance on linguistic and phonologic tasks.

Genetic Factors

As described in the previous chapter, there is a long history of documentation that stuttering occurs with much greater than usual frequency in some families. Bloodstein's (1995) review indicates that the percentage of persons who have relatives on the maternal or paternal side who stuttered ranges from 30 to 69%. Studies concerning the genetics of stuttering have focused on the occurrence of stuttering in families, particularly in instances where there is a high density of stuttering in the first and second degree relatives. Research during the past few decades has indicated a genetic component in selected groups of people who stutter (Cox, Seider, & Kidd, 1984; Falsenfeld, 1997; Johnson & Associates, 1959; Kidd, 1977; Kidd, 1884; Kidd, Heimbuch, Records, Oehlert, & Webster, 1980; Pauls, 1990; Poulos & Webster, 1991; Sheehan & Costley, 1977; Yairi, 1983). As suggested earlier, genetics and gender appear to interact in predictable patterns during stuttering development.

Twinning

The relationship of twinning to stuttering is, of course, closely connected to genetic factors. Approximately one third of all twin pairs are monozygotic (MZ) pairs and are genetically identical. The remaining twin pairs are dizygotic (DZ) or fraternal pairs and share about half of their polymorphic genes. A child is more likely to stutter if he is a member of a twin pair in which the other twin also stutters (Howie, 1981). This is especially true if the twins are monozygotic. It is less likely that both members of a fraternal twin pair will stutter (Howie, 1981). These findings seem to be explained by a genetic predisposition to stuttering (Howie, 1981; West & Ansberry, 1968) and to family and environmental factors.

Brain Injury

Van Riper (1982) summarizes findings that report considerably greater than a 1% occurrence of stuttering with brain injury, especially for speakers with cerebral palsy and epilepsy. However, it can sometimes be difficult to distinguish motor speech and language problems (particularly word finding) from fluency breaks. In addition, speakers who are developmentally delayed often have a higher than usual occurrence of stuttering, especially those with Down's syndrome. Van Riper (1982) summarized the results of seven independent studies indicating prevalence figures ranging from a low of 7% (Schaeffer & Shearer, 1968) to a high of 60% for clients with Down's syndrome (Preus, 1973). Averaging across all seven studies and the two reported categories of "general retardates" and "mongoloids" results in a prevalence figure of 24% (standard deviation [SD] = 18.1). Of course, with this population there is also a much higher occurrence of many speech and language problems, including cluttering. In addition, developmental delays and neuropathological influences can mask the identification of fluency disorders. Studies indicate that both verbal and nonverbal intelligence is slightly lower in speakers who stutter, in contrast to control subjects. For whatever reasons, individuals who possess less than normal cognitive abilities tend to have more fluency problems.

Speech and Language Development

There is an obvious interplay of factors such as intelligence, school performance, and language skills. Summarizing a series of studies by Andrews and Harris (1964), Berry (1938), Guitar (1998); Kline and Starkweather (1979), Murray and Reed (1977), and Wall (1980), Peters and Guitar (1991) concluded that children who stutter typically achieve lower scores than their peers on measures of receptive vocabulary, the age of speech and language onset, mean length of utterance, and expressive and receptive syntax. In addition, children who stutter frequently also exhibit other communicative problems. Especially for these children, speech and language production *is* likely to be more difficult, and there is a higher probability that they will find themselves exerting increased effort when they are speaking.

Recent investigations suggest that the relationship of stuttering and expressive language and phonological abilities is far from simple. Watkins, Yairi, and Ambrose (1999) studied 62 preschool children who recovered by stuttering and 22 who persisted in stuttering. Spontaneous language samples of 250–300 utterances were used to examine the children's expressive language skills (lexical, morphological, and syntactic measures). Both groups of children (those who recovered from and those who persisted in stuttering) displayed expressive language abilities near or above developmental expectations. For both groups of children, those who were the youngest when entering the investigation (two to three years old) had expressive language scores well above normative values. These results counter the frequently expressed opinion that young children who stutter demonstrate delays in expressive language.

Paden, Yairi, and Ambrose (1999) studied the phonological abilities of these same children. Those children who would eventually persist in stuttering were found at the outset of the investigation to have significantly poorer performance on all aspects of the Assessment of Phological Processes-Revised (APP-R) (Hodson, 1986). The authors concluded that there is mounting evidence that "preschool children who stutter and are slow to develop phonologically are usually in the group whose stuttering will be persistent" (p. 1122). Interestingly, both persistent and recovered children showed a pattern of relatively few errors on early-developing production patterns and much larger percentages of error on later-developing patterns. In addition, in comparison to the recovered group, twice the percentage of the children in the persistent group scored more than 40% error on Consonant Sequences, suggesting that such performance may indicate chronic stuttering.

Motor Coordination

There is some evidence that adults who stutter have somewhat greater difficulty in fine motor coordination (Riley & Riley, 1984, 2000; Starkweather, 1987; Van Riper, 1982). Interestingly, as mentioned earlier in this chapter, Conture et al. (1988) found no differences between the temporal coordination characteristics of the perceptually fluent speech of eight young children who stuttered and their normally fluent peers. Obviously, a significant part of the act of speaking is a motor skill, and any delay or deficit in this aspect could certainly adversely affect the development of normal fluency. There is, for example, some indication of a lack of appropriate interaction between laryngeal and supralaryngeal behaviors during fluent speech in young children who stutter (Zebrowski, Conture, & Cudahy, 1985), which was confirmed by Borden, Kim, and Spiegler (1987). Such oral-motor difficulties could be especially problematic for children who have above-average linguistic skill as well as a strong desire to communicate. Finally, Archibald and De Nil (1999) studied the oral kinesthetic ability of four adults with very mild and four adults with moderate-to-severe stuttering (as determined by the Stuttering Severity Instrument, Riley, 1980). Participants were instructed to make the smallest possible jaw movements from a defined starting position in response to a series of short tones. The participants performed the task with and without visual feedback. When only proprioceptive information was available to the speakers with moderate/severe stuttering, the subjects took significantly longer than either the subjects with mild stuttering or the non-stuttering controls. The findings provide additional support for the notion that some adults who stutter to a moderate or severe degree may have an oral kinesthetic deficit.

CONCLUSION

The features of stuttering that are on the surface, regardless of what they are called, are the primary characteristics of the person's speech that serve to differentiate speakers who are stuttering from those that are not. For many years a common sequence of development was thought to prevail for children who stuttered. Although it is somewhat difficult to differentiate the time of onset from subsequent development of the problem, recent studies have shown that some children begin stuttering abruptly and with obvious severity within a short time.

Many factors have been associated with both onset and development that appear to have little influence on the development of stuttering. Other factors, particularly those of speaker sex, age, family genetic factors, and phonological ability, appear to play a stronger role in influencing the nature of how the problem develops. As we will see in the following chapters, as stuttering continues to evolve, the individual's response to his situation can have an extensive and often negative impact on the speaker's interpretation of himself and his response to nearly all aspects of his life.

STUDY QUESTIONS

➤ Describe some common stereotypes that listeners often have about people who stutter. How do you think these views come about?
➤ Create a written description of the "the look" you receive from several listeners as you portray a speaker with moderate-to-severe stuttering behavior.
➤ What are the four basic characteristics of fluent speech?
➤ What are the most basic surface features that distinguish stuttering behavior in young children?
➤ For many years it has been suggested that children who stutter progress from primary to secondary stuttering. What are your thoughts about the likelihood of stuttering's developing in this way?
➤ If you were limited to only four or five verbal and nonverbal behaviors for distinguishing between normal and abnormal fluency of young children, which ones would you choose and why?
➤ What are examples of conditions or events that, although they have not been shown to be particularly influential in the etiology of stuttering, may be associated with stuttering onset by parents?
➤ What are the factors that seem to be related to the occurrence of stuttering?

RECOMMENDED READINGS

Paden, E. P, Yairi, E., & Ambrose, N. G. (1999). Early childhood stuttering II: Initial status of phonological abilities. *Journal of Speech, Language, and Hearing Research, 42,* 1113–1124.

Yairi, E. (1997). Home environment and parent-child interaction in childhood stuttering. In Curlee & G. Siegel (Eds.), *Nature and treatment of stuttering, New directions* (2nd ed., pp. 24-48). Needham Heights, MA: Allyn & Bacon.

Yaruss, J. S. (1977b). Clinical measurement of stuttering behaviors. *Contemporary Issues in Communication Science and Disorders, 24,* 33–44.

CHAPTER

4

ASSESSING ADOLESCENTS AND ADULTS

> *Talk is part of our very biological heritage by virtue of our membership in the human species. Talk is an imperative for us. It is an imperative for us to connect with others through talk, it is an imperative for us to explore our worlds through talk, and it is an imperative for us to express our self-hood through talk.*
> *J. W. Kindfors: Speaking creatures in the classroom. In S. Hynd and D. L. Rubin (Eds.),* Perspectives on Talk and Learning. *Urbana, IL: National Council of Teachers of English, 1992, p. 21)*

INTRODUCTION

Before discussing the assessment of adolescents and adults (in this chapter) and of preschool and school-age children (in Chapter 5), we will present several concepts that have a primary influence on our ability to characterize nonfluent speech and handicapped speakers, regardless of age. The differences between the assessment of younger speakers, who may or may not be starting (or continuing) on a road of stuttering, and those older speakers who have traveled the road for many years will become obvious. Of course, there also are many important similarities. As mentioned in the Preface, we describe both the diagnosis and treatment of older speakers (adolescents and adults) before presenting the corresponding chapters for younger speakers (preschool and school-age children). This sequence is selected because the disorder is most obviously manifested in adolescent and adult populations. The characteristics of somewhat older speakers provide the most comprehensive picture of the impairment, the reactions, the disability, and the handicapping effects of the disorder. Guitar (1998) also demonstrated the utility of this approach.

THE VARIABILITY OF FLUENCY

Our level of fluency varies widely across time and location. Most of the time we speak nearly automatically, with words flowing smoothly and effortlessly. We give no attention to our manner of communicating. On other occasions, particularly during communicative or emotional stress, the smoothness begins to disappear and breaks in our speech occur—or at least they become more obvious. Although fluency varies for all speakers, its variability is even more pronounced for the person who stutters. In most instances a person who stutters is more likely than the normally fluent speaker to react sooner and to a greater degree to fluency-disrupting stimuli such as time pressure and difficult communication situations. At the other extreme, people who stutter are sometimes able to "turn on their fluency." By avoiding feared sounds and words or—with heightened energy and emotion—momentarily "rising to the occasion," speakers who typically stutter are able to become uncharacteristically fluent.

The variability of stuttering behaviors is one of the facts about stuttering and something that contributes as much as anything else to the mystery of the disorder. It is difficult for listeners to understand how a speaker can be speaking fluently one moment and a word or two later struggle dramatically as they attempt to do something as common as say their name. The variability of stuttering behavior also makes it difficult for listeners to become accustomed to a speaker, for it is not always possible to predict whether or not a person will stutter. Such variability also presents a predicament for the person doing the stuttering. That is, the person who stutters can not always be certain of the amount and degree of difficulty he will have in any given speaking situation. It is difficult for the speaker to compensate for a problem that is so inconsistent. Of the many communication handicaps that people may suffer, perhaps none is more variable than stuttering.

The high degree of intra-speaker variability makes the assessment of fluency more formidable than it may first appear. As Bloodstein (1987) states, "The great variability of stuttering from time to time under different conditions is liable to result in assessments that are unrepresentative" (p. 386). Any single assessment protocol will provide only a glimpse of the complexity. Many aspects of the fluency disorder will go undetected unless the assessment is conducted in a variety of speaking situations, something that is especially true with younger speakers. Usually, the more these situations are similar to the daily activities of this person, the more likely we are to obtain a valid indication of the problem. The inconsistent nature of stuttering requires that the assessment of stuttering be an ongoing process that takes place over several assessment or treatment sessions.

SURFACE AND INTRINSIC FEATURES

Along with the great variability of both frequency and severity, the features of stuttering are often intricate and subtle. For these reasons it is not surprising that there have been many debates over what stuttering is and what it is not (Hamre, 1992; Perkins, 1990). This may also help to explain why we had to discuss (in Chapters 2 and 3) the many terms used to describe this phenomena.

Another more basic problem in assessing stuttering is that most of the events that we see and hear only indicate the surface features of the problem. Naïve listeners naturally tend to focus on these more obvious events such as the frequency, duration, and tension of stuttered moments, as well as the sometimes dramatic accessory features used by the speaker to postpone or escape from the moment of stuttering. Although it is not necessarily an uncomplicated perceptual task, these surface features of stuttering can be observed and recorded with good accuracy and reliability by an experienced clinician. Still, the variability of these features both within and across speakers complicates the task. Furthermore, the variability of a speaker's behavior can be further increased with the introduction of treatment techniques. Despite all these dilemmas, it is worthwhile to identify and follow both the quantity and quality of the surface features presented by the client. At the very least we want to determine the usual characteristics of frequency and the duration of formulative and motoric fluency breaks, as well as representative samples of the speaker's tension and fragmentation during moments of stuttering. These surface features provide one important view of the problem, as well as evidence of behavioral change during treatment.

On the other hand, even with younger speakers—and certainly with adolescents and adults—we must look below the surface in order to obtain a valid indication of the speaker's problem. Otherwise, as complex and interesting as these features may be, we are merely observing the smoke from the volcano and the superficial characteristics of the mountain. It is below the surface that we find the intrinsic features: the deep structure of the stuttering syndrome. They are the intrinsic aspects of the *person* who is doing the stuttering and require more from the clinician than a basic knowledge of the impairment. We will discuss these intrinsic features in many ways throughout these chapters, particularly in Chapters 6 and 7. It is important to appreciate that while these are less apparent aspects of the syndrome, they are, to varying degrees, normal and expected components of the stuttering experience.

To understand the intrinsic nature of stuttering is to appreciate the loss of control that occurs with stuttered speech. As discussed in Chapter 2, the loss of control is what makes the fluency breaks of people who stutter distinct from the fluency breaks produced by people who do not stutter. It is the critical difference between "real" and "fake" stuttering. This distinction, however, is usually only realized by the speaker and not by the listener. The surface features of stuttering often appear identical for fake and real stuttering. There can be part-word repetitions, prolongations, and even blocking of airflow. Still, the critical difference is the feeling by the speaker doing the real stuttering that they are not in control of their

---

◯ CLINICAL INSIGHT

My experience as a school-age child who stuttered illustrates the importance of appreciating the intrinsic aspects of stuttering. I think that all the clinicians who worked with me over the years knew about stuttering. They could identify stuttering moments and categorize the overt aspects of my surface behaviors. They helped me to understand, monitor, and—to some degree—modify these behaviors. On the other hand, most of the clinicians failed to indicate to me that they understood anything about what I was experiencing as the person who was struggling with my speech and my life. It seems to me, at least, that the fear and helplessness that were so strongly influencing my choices as they related to my speech were not apparent to them. Because the clinicians knew about the surface features of stuttering, these were what we focused on. At least I suspect that was the reason. Fortunately, later on I encountered clinicians who not only knew about the surface features of the problem but also showed me that they had insight about how this problem influenced my responses to my predicament. They understood something about the deep structure and the intrinsic nature of the problem. They knew that at the center of my daily decision-making was the fact that I often felt helpless. I had little or no sense of being able to control my speech. Sometimes I had what felt like "lucky fluency," which, at that time, I regarded as a good thing. But a moment later I would be unable to communicate even my most basic thoughts. Even when I wasn't overtly stuttering, I experienced the problem as I constantly altered my choices and constricted my options due to even the *possibility* of stuttering. In many instances, stuttering never reached the surface, but the choices I was making were examples of profound moments of stuttering even though they were not being tabulated as a repetition or prolongation.

speech and their speaking mechanism. They feel they are out of control and cannot stop the behavior when they want to. The essence of this difference between the two forms of stuttering is the sense of tension and being out of control that accompanies real moments of stuttering (Prins, 1997, p. 347). For years, authors have pointed to this cognitive-affective aspect of stuttering as a central feature of the stuttering experience (Bloodstein, 1987; Cooper, 1968, 1987, 1990; Manning, 1977; Manning & Shrum, 1973; Perkins, 1990). In describing this experience, Guitar (1997) cites the work of Mineka (1985), who suggested that anxiety increases the sense of losing control and leads to fear-based responses.

Although nonstuttering speakers do not typically experience a distinct loss of control while speaking, everyone has had a similar experience during an athletic or physical activity. There is an instant when you perceive that you are not in control of your body, a fleeting moment when you realize that you have lost your balance. It is at this moment that you recognize that you are not in charge and cannot determine the consequences of your helplessness. There is, at this moment, a level of anxiety and even fear. Such an experience is more likely to occur if you are taking part in activities that require some degree of precision, timing, and balance. Activities such as skiing, skating, paddling a kayak, and wind surfing are good examples. However, it is also possible to encounter similar situations during more common activities such as riding a bike, climbing stairs, walking, running, or even driving a car. For the nonstuttering clinician who is able to be genuine and open about herself, these experiences provide an opportunity to connect to the client and demonstrate her understanding about this primary aspect of the stuttering experience.

🔍 CLINICAL INSIGHT

As part of a class on stuttering, clinicians are often asked to take the part of a person who stutters in a series of daily speaking situations. On occasion, students completing this assignment report that they experience a distinct feeling of losing control as they are in the midst of stuttering. They describe having a feeling where, at least for a moment, they were not at all certain whether they were completely in control of their speech and were unsure if they would be able to stop voluntarily stuttering and continue on. Of course, this experience can be frightening. It can also provide the student with insight about why people who stutter, when they find themselves in such a condition, reflexively grasp for avoidance and escape behaviors that (as irrational as they may appear) have worked to get them unstuck in the past.

Another common example for adults is the feeling you have when sliding out of control in your car through an icy intersection. During these moments one can approach the level of fear and helplessness that occurs for a person who stutters during a moment of stuttering. This loss of control can be both profound and discrete. It has been suggested that it is measurable (Moore & Erkins, 1990), at least by the person doing the stuttering. Whether a clinician can identify such a loss of control in another speaker has yet to be demonstrated empirically. Nevertheless, over the years authors have suggested that it is possible for experienced clinicians to accurately identify such moments (Bloodstein & Shogan, 1972; Cooper, 1968; Manning & Shrum, 1973). In discussing the difficulty of identifying successful avoidance behavior by people who stutter, Starkweather (1987) makes an important point that is pertinent to this discussion. He argues that although we may not have the means to apply rigorously scientific study to what we consider to be the essential features of an event, it should not preclude our study of those features. "Our first duty as scientists is to be true to the validity of the phenomenon being observed. If we lack the means to examine it objectively, we cannot assume or pretend that it doesn't exist" (p. 122).

A recent qualitative study that investigated the experiences of eight adults provides additional insight about the central feature of helplessness for the person who stutters (Corcoran & Stewart, 1998). The goal of the study was to discover central themes that were consistent for adults with a history of stuttering. The authors attempted to include people who varied maximally in terms of age and sex. Participants included five men and three women and ranged in age from 25 to 50 years. The authors used a series of interviews with open-ended questions combined with probes to obtain narratives from the participants. The narratives were then analyzed using qualitative research procedures designed to provide understanding of meaningful categories and themes that would help to describe the core experiences of stuttering for the participants.

The primary theme that the authors noted was one of *suffering*. Four basic elements of suffering were a profound sense of *helplessness, shame, fear,* and *avoidance.* Participants felt *helpless* because of the involuntary nature of their stuttering and the general lack of control in their lives. They described being unable to perform even basic social activities (e.g., introducing oneself or asking questions). Participants described the fact that their stuttering seemed beyond their control as the core of their experience. In addition, participants consistently described *shame* and *stigma* that were experienced to a degree that other aspects of their self were obscured or discounted. Because of the lack of an accepted explanation for stuttering, they tended to assign blame to themselves for their stuttering and its continuation. Given the feelings of helplessness and shame, *fear* of the stuttering experience and of listener reactions was also a common theme. Lastly, *concealment* and *avoidance* of even the possibility of stuttering was a consistent pattern that often resulted in a dramatically constricted lifestyle. The authors propose that the clinician is the major agent for assisting clients to transform the meaning of their stuttering which, in turn, will provide both a reduction in suffering and facilitate the modification of overt behaviors. The processes of understanding the client's story and allowing the client to begin to consider alternate views about the experience of stuttering can begin during the initial diagnostic interview.

Suggesting that the clinician is capable of detecting affective components of stuttering such as moments of helplessness, loss of control, shame, and fear in another speaker may sound rather enigmatic. Assuming this is really possible, how might it be accomplished? For the nonstuttering clinician, the first step is to truly understand the nature of the stuttering experience and the significance of stuttering in the person's life. As we explain throughout these chapters, the nature of the fluent or nonfluent speech that we see on the surface is only one layer of the problem. Understanding the person who is doing the stuttering (or often trying terribly hard not to stutter or avoid communicating at all) is a good first step in helping to change the client's situation. The strategies and techniques of counseling that are discussed in Chapter 7 are particularly useful.

A useful procedure for becoming calibrated to the client's experience is to carefully observe the speaker's body language. As we will point out again in Chapter 7 when we discuss counseling issues, a person's body language has a way of "leaking" information (Egan, 1990). How do speakers stand or sit as they are producing fluent speech? Is the relaxed nature of their fluent speech reflected in their body position, or in the location and movement of their hands or their heads? In contrast, what are they doing with their bodies when they are producing overtly stuttered speech? Moreover, what do they do when they are producing speech that is not really stuttered, but also not entirely fluent? The cues provided by the speaker's body language are likely to be subtle and unique to each speaker. Some clients may reveal their status by subtle nostril flaring or by a slight alteration in the rate or tempo of their speech. Fluent speech sounds smooth and feels smooth to the clinician as it is being imitated. However, if the speech sounds flat or has the "sticky" quality associated with a constricted vocal tract, the speaker is apt to be experiencing something less than complete control. The client's speech may be "fluent" in a traditional sense, but it is really just "not stuttered." As the clinician pantomimes the client's speech characteristics, it should be apparent to the clinician that the client is "talking on thin ice." He is not stuttering in the usual sense, but as a clinician who is gradually becoming calibrated to the speaker, you will have the feeling that he is not completely in control of his speech. Moreover, when you ask the speaker if he is truly in charge of his speech, he will usually agree that he is not.

After the clinician has several sessions with a client, she will begin to understand how the person is apt to express himself during periods of fluent speech. Not only will she begin to anticipate the rate and tempo of the client's speech, but she will begin to predict what sentence structure and vocabulary the speaker is going to use. Moreover, when these usual patterns are not part of the client's speech, we may guess, often correctly, that he has avoided or substituted a word, or at the very least, that he has scanned ahead, is anticipating difficulty, and is speaking cautiously. The following interaction between a client and a clinician that took place after several treatment sessions is such an example.

> **Client:**   "We had a wonderful time. We drove to [the speaker slightly slows his speech and indicates minimal tension in the jaw] my hometown in Indiana for the weekend."
> **Clinician:** "Did you avoid the word of your hometown just now?"
> **Client:**   (smiling) "Yes. How did you know?"
> **Clinician:** "Because you slowed your speech, it sounded just a little sticky, and because I know that is one of your feared words."

Such exchanges take many forms but occur with regularity for most speakers who stutter. As the clinician gradually becomes attuned to the client's characteristics, these important events become more transparent.

TWO BASIC PRINCIPLES OF ASSESSMENT

Although the assessment of fluency can be intricate, it is useful to realize that much of what is done during both the assessment and the treatment of stuttering can be reduced to two basic principles. Often, during both assessment and treatment, we find ourselves returning to these principles, particularly when we are not certain of our next clinical decision. First, and perhaps most importantly, it is helpful to remember that the more an individual who stutters alters the choices and narrows the options that are available in life, the greater the handicap of stuttering is apt to be. Clinicians, as well as people who stutter, need to appreciate this. Assessment must focus on determining the degree of such altered decision-making in all its forms. In turn, many treatment goals will focus on increasing the person's ability to make choices based on information beyond the fact that stuttering is a possibility. In Chapter 8 we will describe the technique of asking the client to respond to the question "What do you do *because* you stutter?" His answers to this question provide a preliminary indication of the influence of how the even the *possibility* of stuttering impacts his decision-making. As the members of the National Stuttering Associaton proclaim in the title of their newsletter *Letting GO*, the person who stutters must learn to "let go" and live life as it can best be lived rather than basing so many decisions on the fact that, among other characteristics, he or she happens to be someone who stutters.

The second basic principle of assessment has to do with the various forms of struggle behavior. Everything else being equal, the more a speaker reacts to a situation by struggling, the greater the handicap. The clinician must determine how and to what degree a person is closing down or restricting the speech production system in general and the vocal tract in particular. What is the speaker doing with the source of energy in the respiratory system and the vocal tract resonator/filter that prevents these systems from being used efficiently? (See Baken, 1987; Kent, 1997; Zemlin, 1988). How is the speaker inhibiting normal voicing and articulation from occurring? What is the speaker doing to prohibit the transition from one sound or syllable to another? What is the speaker doing to keep from speaking (or stuttering) easily, openly, and smoothly? Much of what influences the clinician's assessment and treatment decisions can be based on these two principles:

➤ To what degree is the person using open decision-making about communicating with others?
➤ To what degree is the person attempting to speak with an open vocal tract?

ASSESSING OLDER SPEAKERS

The assessment or evaluation session provides our first opportunity to find out about the person who has come to us for help as well as others in his daily environment. It is also the client's first opportunity to find out about us. There is much for each person in this clinical relationship to learn about the other, and this learning will continue long after the initial diagnostic meeting. Although we will obtain background information and specific results by using our favorite assessment devices, continuing assessment of the client and the effectiveness of our intervention takes place during and following treatment. The foundation of an ongoing assessment is the interplay between the client and the clinician as they work together through the stages of treatment. The conversation, the behavior, and the learning that occur throughout treatment provide the information necessary for reasoned decision-making on the part of the clinician.

The most fundamental goal during the initial period of assessment is to understand the client's story. How a person tells his story reveals important characteristics of the person and his problem. The client may well have experienced previous treatment and know something about basic terminology concerning stuttering. He may have some insight about the therapeutic process. At the other extreme, a new client may know absolutely nothing about the true nature of stuttering and, depending on his cultural background and educational experience, bring with him a basket of myths often associated with the disorder. While some people have a degree of inquisitiveness and openness about their problem, others will indicate embarrassment and shame. Although they may not come to us often, there are those who are frustrated about former treatment experiences. On occasion, there are people who are angry because they feel (in some cases correctly) they have received less than competent help. Our task is to find out where they are on their journey of change, their understanding of their situation, and their willingness to enter into the hard work of making change happen. We know, of course, that the basic problem is stuttering, and we want to get some indication of their perception of their problem, the nature of their stuttered speech, the quality of their fluency, and the degree that the experience of stuttering is influencing their lives.

Generally, although not always, both the surface- and the deep-structure of stuttering are more severe and more obvious in adolescent and adult speakers. Even at the early stages of stuttering development, some young children will display well-developed tension (sound prolongations and body movements) and fragmentation (within-word fluency breaks), which are typically associated with advanced or established stuttering (Schwartz & Conture, 1988; Yairi, 1997). Usually, however, older speakers show much greater complexity of behavior and exhibit greater anxiety and fear. Adolescents and adults have coped and adjusted to the problem for years. Thus the features of their stuttering, especially those having to do with concealing the problem, tend to be more sophisticated and complex. Adolescent and adult speakers have had time to develop subtle patterns of avoidance that mask the surface features, and therefore the basic question to be answered during assessment is not so much whether formulative or motoric fluency breaks are occurring. The primary goal of assessment is focused on the nature of stuttering and the handicapping effects of the problem with *this* particular person.

SEVERITY VERSUS HANDICAP

It should be apparent from many of the comments in the previous chapters that the severity of stuttering is affected by the many levels of the disorder and goes far beyond the surface features. There will be cases where a person will come to us and it is not immediately apparent that the problem has anything to do with a fluency disorder. That is, in an attempt to lessen the impact of stuttering on their lives, adult speakers will sometimes shape their speech and overall behavior into a pattern of symptoms that resemble other problems such as motor-speech disorders, voice disorders, language disorders, or even emotional disturbances. For example, because of tension in a speaker's voice or the fact that he is speaking in a careful, slow, or labored manner, it may appear as though the person has a voice or word-finding problem. In order to protect themselves from the penalties associated with stuttering, the person may refuse to speak or choose to speak in a way that, although it is obvious that something is amiss, it is not clear that stuttering is the problem.

If a speaker is particularly adept at avoiding feared sounds and words, specific people, or speaking situations, he may rarely if ever be perceived as a person who stutters. He may, however, be thought of as someone who is introverted, shy, lazy, or at the very least, somewhat peculiar. He may be seen as a person who is a bit strange because, due to avoidance and word substitutions, he uses usual syntax, speech rates, or intonation patterns that are idiosyncratic or inappropriate. For example, one client answered his office telephone by saying "Hi" rather than saying "Hello" followed by his name and the name of the company. The person may not always respond in expected ways to simple questions, pretending he did not hear a question or does not know an answer when it is obvious that he does. He may avoid saying his own name or introducing friends or relatives when it is appropriate to do so. He may make excuses so that he will not have to participate in projects at work, school, or engage in social activities. In other words, this person will do the same things normal speakers do when they want to avoid aversive stimuli. As speakers develop such ways of adjusting to stuttering, they are sometimes able to mask the stuttering entirely or at least obscure the true nature of their situation and therefore the actual severity of their problem. In general, we have found that the more successful the speaker is at covering up the stuttering behavior, the more difficult it will be to change these choices during treatment.

When determining the nature and severity of the stuttering syndrome with older speakers, the clinician is faced with the natural variability of surface behaviors. Although this variability is not likely to be as great as when assessing children, obvious fluctuations do occur in both the quantity and quality of stuttering in most adults who stutter. Thus it is good to keep in mind that a formal evaluation can yield a relatively narrow view of these behaviors. The experienced clinician knows that she is unlikely to capture all the surface and intrinsic features of the problem in a single diagnostic interview. This variability is to be expected and, in fact, is an important diagnostic feature in distinguishing the more typical client with developmental stuttering from individuals who present with a sudden onset of stuttering following an emotional or physical trauma, as discussed in the final sections of this chapter.

Although it is not possible to obtain all the necessary information in a single attempt, it is usually possible to obtain a reasonable sample of the individual's surface behaviors and begin the process of understanding the deep structure of the person's response to his fluency problem. Nevertheless, assessment will continue for many days and weeks. As the clinician accompanies the client into a greater variety of more difficult speaking situations, the client is likely to exhibit stuttering behaviors not seen previously. In addition, behaviors that have been noted before may occur with greater frequency and intensity. As the clinician begins to calibrate herself to the new client—a process that will take several sessions even for an experienced clinician—additional subtle behavioral features will gradually become apparent.

Assessing the severity of stuttering is not as straightforward as determining the frequency or even the form of the stuttering events. Clearly, the frequency of the surface features may not correspond to a person's handicap. The person's response to the problem—what he tells himself about his situation—is a critical indicator of handicap (Emerick, 1988). The severity of the problem is much greater than the features that reside on the surface. The speaker reacts to his communication impairment as he experiences a diminished ability to perform daily functions (the disability) and a wide variety of disadvantages (the handicap). Any estimate of severity must include at least some appraisal of each level of the model as presented in Chapter 2, Figure 2-1. We have seen many people who would be judged as having a severe fluency problem based on the nature of the surface features of their speech production. They have frequent moments of stuttering accompanied by obvious tension and struggle behavior. However, it is as though they are not inclined to be handicapped. They make all or the majority of their decisions based on information apart from the possibility of stuttering. It is probable that most people who respond to their stuttering in this fashion never ask or seek our help. At the other extreme, we have seen adults who stutter only infrequently, with relatively little tension or obvious struggle. Their stuttering moments are exceedingly brief—hardly noticed by their listeners. Nevertheless, they are devastated by these moments. Even though by any objective standard the problem seems a minor one, the fact that they are a person who stutters is catastrophic. They have a difficult time tolerating the moments when they lose control of their speech, however infrequent or brief they may be. For these people and many others who stutter, stuttering is a problem that cuts across all aspects of their life: vocationally, academically, and socially. These two examples are end points of a continuum, and, of course, most speakers who stutter fall somewhere between these extremes of response. A primary task for the clinician is to help the client map both the surface behaviors of stuttering as well as the intrinsic features of the problem.

The field of counseling also faces a similar dilemma for assigning a severity level to a client's problem. Mehrabian and Reed (1969) suggest the following formula for determining severity:

Severity = Distress × Uncontrollability × Frequency.

This formula may be particularly appropriate for assessing the severity of stuttering, for this formula factors in the speaker's reaction in terms of affective and cognitive features of the problem. In addition, frequency of stuttering, while often a major contributor to severity, is not the only factor. It is important to note that the multiplication signs imply that even low levels of distress or lack of control can promptly contribute to the effective severity of the (stuttering) problem, preventing the client from fully taking part in life.

THE NONREPRESENTATIVE SAMPLE OF CLIENTS

Many people who stutter do not seek formal treatment and instead make it through life by compensating and adjusting to the problem (Manning, Dailey, & Wallace, 1984). These are certainly people who stutter but, for one reason or another, they do not seek professional help. They may not be aware that treatment is available. For some, the cost of treatment may be prohibitive. For others, it may be that the thought of treatment is so aversive that they would refuse treatment even if they are able to pay for it. For most of these people who stutter, however, it may be that although the disability is apparent, they do not seek assistance because the handicap is not sufficiently great.

Although there are no data to indicate how many never seek formal help, there is little doubt that the large majority of individuals who stutter never make contact with professional treatment centers. Consequently, these people never serve as subjects for the research on which we base our understanding of the problem and form the rationale for most of our clinical decisions. Perhaps it is good to keep in mind that our knowledge about stuttering and the people who stutter is based on a nonrepresentative sample of the total population of people who stutter. Furthermore, it is likely that this sample is skewed in the direction of people who, for whatever reasons, come to recognize not only that they need help, but that they are able to obtain assistance.

For those who are able to make changes on their own, some of the changes are good and some may not be so good, or at least not as good as they could be. An experienced guide can show the way or, at the very least, make the journey more efficient and often more pleasant. As people acquire new skills, there are many things that are counterintuitive. It is highly likely that people will do things wrong without the help of a good instructor. Swimmers will try to raise their head above the water rather than turn their head and breathe efficiently, soccer players will kick the ball with their toe rather than their instep, kayakers will pull away from a wave rather than leaning into it, and drivers will steer away from— rather than into—the direction of a slide. There are many examples. People who stutter usually try harder and harder not to stutter. When they do stutter, they tend to expend more and more effort to get through a sound or word and to "control" their stuttering. Because so many things are counterintuitive, without a good coach, teacher, or clinician, most people will not be aware of the best techniques.

This reasonably typical encounter reveals much about the characteristics of nonassisted recovery from stuttering. In my experience, this person is representative of many people who have stuttered into adulthood. Of course, there are many reasons why this particular person was able to

---

🔍 CLINICAL INSIGHT

A few months ago at a reception a woman introduced me to her husband. He was a young man in his early thirties who was a successful businessman and both extremely pleasant and outgoing. He also appeared to be spontaneously fluent. As we discussed my field and my interest in stuttering, he volunteered that he too had stuttered as a child and, on occasion, still had difficulty with certain words. His brother had also stuttered, and his description of the impact his stuttering had on his life as a young child and teenager left no doubt that he truly was a member of the clan of the tangled tongue. Although he had experienced some teasing about his speech, his close friends had been understanding and supportive. During his elementary school years he had been seen for a brief time by a clinician (the treatment emphasized speaking slower) but he felt that therapy provided little help. Now as a young adult, he explained that, for the most part, he had gotten over it. He mentioned that actually, rather than stuttering (repeating sounds and words), he stammered (blocking and "getting stuck" on words).

When I asked what he had done to "get over his stuttering," he informed me that he had several very specific techniques that he used. He had learned to adeptly change words or topics as he anticipated stuttering on a feared sound or word. He had adopted an assertive approach to life and "went for it" in many aspects of his life, including communication situations. It was clear that although stuttering had been a traumatic experience for him when was younger, he wasn't going to let something like that get in his way. He had been an outstanding athlete and had a broad circle of friends. By any standard he was successful. He explained that "everyone has their faults" and that he happened to stutter.

"overcome" the fact that he stuttered. As many—perhaps most—people who stutter are able to do, he had adjusted his approach to communication situations so that he could have success as a speaker. On the other hand, his stuttering continued to impact his life to some degree. It may be that he chose to describe his fluency breaks as stammering because that term, in this country at least, has less stigma associated with it than stuttering. His statement that "everyone has their faults," while an accurate and generally healthy comment, indicated that he viewed stuttering—to some degree at least—as his "fault." His strategy of changing words prevented him from being as spontaneous as he might have otherwise been and, at the very least, required that he scan ahead for feared stimuli that might result in stuttering. As I thought about this interaction with this young man, I couldn't help but think that the quality of his life might have been enhanced somewhat by learning more about stuttering. He may also have experienced some relief from his mission of hiding his stuttering by giving himself permission to easily stutter on some occasions. In any case, I suspect that some version of this reaction to stuttering is characteristic of a large number of "recovered stutterers."

ASSESSING INTRINSIC FEATURES

Because of their very nature, these covert features of the person are more difficult to identify and quantify. It takes several sessions before the clinician will become calibrated to a new client and be able to recognize such features. Because surface behaviors are more easily observable, there is a tendency to spend the majority of the assessment time on these features. However—and this is especially true with adults—the intrinsic features must also be identified and eventually modified if long-term success is to be a reality (Emerick, 1988; Guitar & Bass, 1978).

Identifying Loss of Control

As we become attuned to the client, we can begin to identify the three levels of fluency discussed in Chapter 1: stuttered, unstable, and fluent. These levels of fluency tend to reflect the degree of control by the speaker. By pantomiming—imitating his speech production with our own mouths—we can begin to distinguish when the speaker is at each level of control. We can begin to sense when he is experiencing some lack of control over his fluency and identify those moments when stuttering does not quite reach the surface.

At times, during what may initially appear to be seemingly fluent portions of speech, the person is, at best, on the edge of control. As discussed earlier, in order to prevent overt stuttering, the speaker may substitute and rearrange words. Although he may be producing "nonstuttered" speech, he is not in control and is far from producing the effortless, smooth, and continuous speech that characterizes authentic fluency. An experienced listener—especially one who is familiar with how the speaker is capable of expressing himself in terms of rate, tempo, and syntax—can detect this loss of control in the midst of unstable speech. The clinician may be able to key into the brief pauses or slightly sticky moments present in the unstable speech. Although there are no clear-cut signs of overt stuttering, there will be subtle signs that the individual is not in control. There is a slight hesitation prior to the onset of a word. The clinician notices a momentary prolongation or stickiness during the initial portion of a word. The client selects a word that is close to—but does not quite provide—the meaning the clinician has learned to anticipate. The client's body language (eye contact and movements can be especially helpful) may indicate a brief moment of fear during the production of a word that is not as smoothly articulated as the speaker is capable of producing it. Of course, one of the best ways to identify or confirm these unstable events is to ask the speaker to do so.

One of our adult clients indicated a loss of control in her speech by involuntary rapid eyelid fluttering, both during obvious moments of stuttering as well as during her moments of unstable speech. These eye movements assisted the clinician in identifying each instance when, although the client produced the word fluently in a technical sense, there were obvious surface features that suggested instability. She was slightly constricting her vocal tract, minimally slowing her movements, and using somewhat more effort to produce in sequence the sounds of the word. Furthermore, she consistently agreed with the clinician's assessment that loss of control occurred during each of these events. Other clients have indicated loss of control by such behaviors as loss of eye contact, minimal lip tremor or flaring of the nostrils, and retreating back to an earlier portion of the sentence.

It may be that many of the characteristic differences that have been noted in the acoustics of the "nonstuttered" speech of people who stutter reflect this lack of control. Researchers have observed a number of differences in the fluent speech of stutterers of various ages, including brief pauses (Love & Jefress, 1971), centralized formant frequencies (Klich & May, 1982), fundamental frequency variations (Healey, 1982), vocal shimmer (Bamberg, Hanley, & Hillenbrand, 1990; Hall & Yairi, 1992; Newman, Harris, & Hilton, 1989), voice reaction times (Cross, Shadden, & Luper, 1979; Reich, Till, & Goldsmith, 1981), and voice onset, initiation, and termination times (Adams & Hayden, 1976; Agnello, 1975; Hillman & Gilbert, 1977; Starkweather, Hirschmann, & Tannenbaum, 1976). These acoustic characteristics may reflect brief moments where control was lost and unstable speech occurred. If investigators, rather than considering only stuttered or nonstuttered speech, were to consider as a third category a speaker's unstable speech, these acoustic measures may yield even more distinctive results. It may also be that the perceptual effects of unstable speech also indicate a lack of spontaneity and naturalness (see Chapter 10).

In any case, it is important for the clinician to be able to identify these intrinsic aspects of stuttering. Many features of stuttering do not necessarily coincide with the speaker's overt breaks in fluency. This lack of correspondence is obviously the case when a word is avoided, or during the production of unstable speech. This inconsistency is important for the clinician to appreciate during treatment, for although she may think she is reinforcing fluent speech, she may, in reality, be rewarding something far less desirable. If we base our decisions to reward the client only on the surface behavior, we could easily be reinforcing avoidance behavior, word substitutions, and most of all, a profound feeling of helplessness.

Testing the Link Between Control and Fluency

There is another important aspect of the relationship between fluency and control. Just as a stuttering speaker may be wildly out of control as he circumvents possible stuttering moments and manages to sound fluent, it is also possible for him to speak in an overtly stuttered manner and be in complete control. In other words, the clinician can show him that it is possible to stutter on purpose in an open, easy fashion and be totally in charge of his speech mechanism. Being able to voluntarily stutter with complete control serves to break the remarkably strong link between the experience of stuttering and that of helplessness. The speaker begins to consider, usually for the first time, that it is possible to stutter and not feel helpless. It is possible to stutter and not to be afraid. As we will describe in more detail in subsequent chapters, it may even be possible to stutter in a different, easier, more fluent manner.

By attempting a bit of such voluntary stuttering during the assessment process, the clinician may begin to determine the degree of fear associated with the moment of stuttering for this speaker. If the client can follow the clinician into some experimental forms of easy, open stuttering, it suggests the possibility that the client is somewhat desensitized about stuttering and may be reasonably assertive once intervention begins. During the assessment, we can begin to identify the occurrence of these moments of control loss—even the tiny ones—during nonstuttered speech. We need to identify the way that this speaker indicates a loss of control because we want to determine if these moments decrease as a result of treatment. We can consider how the frequency of these subtle moments of stuttering during "fluent" speech correspond to the frequency of the more overt aspects of stuttering. Moreover, we need to factor in the presence of these subtle moments of stuttering in the form of unstable speech as we consider decisions to terminate formal treatment. The client should be able to identify the presence of these events after formal treatment is completed, since they may well be the first sign of an eventual relapse.

Related to the loss of control is the suspicion that people who stutter are more anxious that those who do not. Most adults who stutter do not show levels of anxiety that are clinically different from speakers who do not stutter. Molt and Guilford (1979) and Miller and Watson (1992) found no differences between adults who stutter and a group of controls on either state or trait anxiety. However, Craig and Hancock (1995) found that adults who experienced (self-defined) relapse were three times more likely to indicate higher levels of trait anxiety levels.

Assessing the Speaker's Decision-Making

Perhaps the most important of the intrinsic features of stuttering is the nature of the decision-making by the person who stutters. As we discussed in Chapter 1, these are the choices a person makes based not on the reality, but on the *possibility* of stuttering. Most especially, we want to examine the narrowing of the speaker's options that can take place in the attempt to avoid stuttering. Herein lies the basis of the handicap for many individuals who stutter: the life choices they make, or fail to make, based on the fact that they are people who stutter.

As with the issue of control, it will take several treatment sessions to become calibrated to the client's lifestyle and manner of expressing himself before the clinician can begin to appreciate the client's decision-making paradigm (Hayhow & Levy, 1989). The person who stutters, even after becoming aware of these choices, is not likely to associate some of them with the syndrome of stuttering. It may be that these choices have become a way of thinking about himself. The client may feel that "it's just the way I am." He may explain that he is shy and does not like to talk to strangers: "I don't want to take part in class. I don't like to speak in front of groups. I don't like to use the phone. I'd rather mind my own business and would prefer not to introduce myself to strangers." Indeed, to some degree, all these things may be true, for that may be the case; not everyone who is free from stuttering is a highly verbal or interactive person.

It takes time in treatment and a clinician who appreciates the possible extent of these choices before the client will begin to identify the subtle decisions that are a function of his stuttering. It takes a clinician who will provide security and insight about the problem before the client will feel free to explore this aspect of his stuttering syndrome. Of course, it does little good to ask the client to stop making these choices at this point. The goal during the early stages of assessment and treatment is simply to help the client in identifying and acknowledging that specific choices to hide or avoid the stuttering are being made. As the person comes to understand this aspect of the problem, one reasonable response is to begin gradually making *different* choices in selected speaking situations.

Once the speaker sees the impact of choices he is making in order to avoid the possibility of stuttering, he may begin to make different decisions. It is important to note, however, that as this form of avoidance behavior decreases during treatment, there is also the possibility that the frequency of stuttering will increase. Even though the person is making progress as a result of treatment, the problem (especially as observed by those who do not understand what is occurring) may appear to be increasing in severity. Because the client is now taking part in speaking situations that he previously avoided (asking a question in class or a store, or taking an opposing view in a discussion), there are more opportunities for stuttering to reach the surface. The person is making better choices but, for the moment at least, he may be (overtly) stuttering more. In this instance at least an increase in the frequency of stuttering can be appropriately interpreted as a sign of progress in treatment (see Chapter 10).

MAPPING THE SURFACE FEATURES OF STUTTERING

The surface features of adults who stutter are relatively easy to evaluate. At the most basic level, there are three categories of behavior that may be used to determine the severity of overt stuttering—frequency, duration, and tension.

Frequency

The frequency of fluency breaks is often one of the most obvious aspects of the problem. Sometimes, a greater frequency of stuttering indicates a greater severity of the problem, but sometimes it does not. Although the frequency of the fluency breaks is an aspect of the problem that is relatively easy to tabulate, it is also the feature that can be the most deceiving. For some speakers, the frequency of fluency breaks provides a sound way to evaluate the problem. For other speakers, however, tabulating the frequency of stuttering events may be the least valid way of considering the problem.

One of the most accurate and efficient ways to tabulate the frequency of stuttering is to determine the percentage of stuttered syllables (%SS) or stuttered words (%SW). It is efficient because with relatively little practice it is possible to reliably count the frequency of breaks during both reading and conversational speech. Counts can be obtained by shadowing the syllable production of the speaker and indicating those syllables on which stuttering occurs. Stuttered syllables can be indicated with a keyboard or by hand by marking dots and dashes for fluent and stuttered syllables, respectively. It is a reasonably accurate procedure for indicating fluency because it is generally agreed that the timing of speech movements is closely related to syllable-sized (as opposed to word-based) units (Allen, 1975; Starkweather, 1987; Stetson, 1951).

Although it is advisable to tabulate %SS or %SW during both conversational speech and reading activities, it is good to remember that these values tend to be highly variable for a speaker, depending on the speaking situation and the reading material. For example, speakers who are adept at avoiding or substituting words may have a greater frequency of stuttering when reading because they are less able to avoid or substitute sounds and words. For these speakers, on the other hand, conversational speech provides the opportunity to alter or substitute words, sometimes possibly yielding a smaller %SS value than would otherwise be the case.

Although the frequency of fluency breaks is usually positively correlated with other estimates of stuttering severity, it is important to appreciate that the frequency of these breaks also may be negatively related to the actual severity of the problem. That is, speakers who substitute words, circumlocute portions of sentences, or avoid words and speaking situations may be stuttering severely but simply do not demonstrate their problem in an overt manner. Thus, although the overt frequency of stuttering may be low, the actual handicap may be quite severe. In fact, a speaker may not be producing any obvious fluency breaks. However, he may be continually making choices to alter the words and the manner by

---

 CLINICAL DECISION-MAKING

There are occasions during the assessment of adolescents and adults when little, if any, overt stuttering will occur. This may be the result of the speaker being able to temporarily will himself to override (or possibly avoid) moments of stuttering. This atypical level of fluency may simply be the result of the speaker's having a particularly fluent day. The experience is similar to taking your car into the repair shop and then finding that you are unable to get it to make that "funny sound." Some clients, in frustration, will plead for the clinician to understand that despite the fact that they are speaking fluently, they really do stutter. An appreciation by the clinician for this situation can show the client that you understand the nature of stuttering. The clinician can acknowledge the variability of stuttering and that often, especially in a situation where it is perfectly alright to stutter, stuttering is less likely to occur. Furthermore, a thorough diagnostic interview will confirm patterns of behavior and decision-making that are consistent with what is known about people who stutter. If the clinician is interested in obtaining examples of overt stuttering, all that is usually necessary is to have the client make telephone calls or speak to strangers in or outside of the building.

which he is communicating. Those choices, although they may not indicate that the person is stuttering, many times communicate (or miscommunicate) other aspects about the person. As one adult client who was extremely good at hiding his stuttering by substituting words said: "They never knew that I was stuttering. They just thought that I was weird."

Cooper (1985) has referred to the hazards of viewing stuttering primarily in terms of the number of fluency breaks as the "frequency fallacy." Persons who stutter and who choose not to raise their hand in the classroom in spite of knowing the answer, not to ask for directions or assistance, not to order a particular item in a restaurant, not to use their spouse's name during introductions, not to place or answer a telephone call (especially in a crowded room), or not to use a paging or intercom system at the office, are still stuttering. Unlike the tree falling in the forest, there is no sound. Nevertheless, such choices are examples of real moments of stuttering. These stuttering moments are insidious because they nearly always have a subtle—but powerful—influence on the person's quality of life.

Duration and Tension

The duration and tension of observable stuttering contribute much to the perception of severity. The speaker may exhibit relatively few moments of stuttering. However, if these moments last for several seconds or are associated with considerable muscular tension as well as other nonverbal behavior (Conture, 1990), the ability of the person to communicate can be severely compromised. Often the tension and duration associated with a fluency break are closely related in the sense that greater tension results in longer moments of stuttering. As tension increases, and particularly if it is focused at a particular point in the vocal tract (lips, tongue, or velum), a tremor is likely to occur. Tremors can be profound and unnatural-looking occurrences involving the rapid oscillatory movement of an articulator. The rate of oscillation is generally faster than that of a voluntarily movement. The effect of these tremors is often dramatic and contributes to the cosmetic abnormality of the problem.

With extreme tension there is the possibility of a stuttering "block." If the tension is great enough and the moment of stuttering lasts sufficiently long, the vocal tract may become occluded, and airflow will cease. Closure often takes place at the level of the vocal folds (the source of the periodic modulation of air in the vocal tract) and a natural point of stricture. However, obstruction at any supraglottal point in the tract will result in partial or complete cessation of airflow and, thus, voicing. A good way for the clinician to interpret what is taking place during a moment of stuttering is to consider what is physically occurring in the vocal tract in terms of the source-filter approach to speech production (Fant, 1960; Kent, 1997; Kent & Read, 1992; Pickett, 1980). That is, the clinician asks herself: "What is the speaker doing to disrupt the source of energy, the air supply from the lungs? How is the speaker preventing the modulation of this source of energy at the level of the vocal folds? How is he constricting or occluding his vocal tract so as to adversely affect the resonant characteristics of this system?" An understanding of the anatomy and physiology, as well as the acoustics, of the speech production system enables the clinician to better apply her knowledge in the assessment of what the speaker is doing to make the process of moving from one speech segment to another so difficult.

As treatment progresses, it will become important for the client as well to begin learning about his speech production system. Most likely the structure and function of the speech production system are not even vaguely understood by the client. Thus it will be useful for him to acquire some *basic* anatomical and physiological understanding. By doing so, speech production becomes less of a mystery, and the client begins to understand his system and that he can choose how the system works. He will gradually come to realize that he is not as helpless as he may feel in the midst of a moment of stuttering. In addition, by understanding the nature of this system, he is able to develop a heightened sense of proprioceptive feedback concerning the respiratory, phonatory, and articulatory integration necessary for fluent speech production. As he begins to develop this understanding and, quite literally, a feel for what he is doing (or not doing) with his system, he can begin making decisions that will make the process of speaking (or stuttering) both easier and smoother.

Measurement of tension has been accomplished using a variety of techniques, including galvanic skin response (GSR), electroencephalography (EEG), and—most often—electromyography (EMG) (Van Riper, 1982). Most clinicians are not likely to have access to such equipment. Fortunately, however, it is not usually necessary to have a high level of precision when measuring tension in the clinical setting. The experienced clinician is able to identify the sites and judge rate the degree of tension with reasonably good consistency. Because tension and duration are often closely related, easily made measures of duration can yield an indication of the tension that is occurring. As with tension, measures of duration, such as spectrographic or waveform analysis—while helpful—are not usually necessary for clinical evaluation. The degree of tension and the duration of the fluency breaks also may be reflected in the rate of speech in words or syllables per minute, with lower rates indicating greater severity.

When determining the severity of stuttering, it is important to understand that no single measure will provide the broad-based assessment necessary to capture the nature of this complex syndrome. The tabulation of the most prominent behaviors, as well as frequency, tension, and duration, is a good start but only a beginning. The degree of abnormality shown by the person as he struggles is indicated by both verbal and physical movements prior to—and during—a fluency break. As we discussed in Chapter 2, the multifactorial-dynamic model proposed by Smith (1990, 1999) and Smith and Kelly (1997) indicate that the stuttering event far exceeds the instance of obvious disfluency. Furthermore, the behaviors associated with stuttering, and especially those at the extreme of the person's inventory of overt behaviors, may only be apparent during the most difficult speaking situations. The clinician may rarely see these behaviors in the clinical setting. However, any behavior that at one time or another helped the person to escape from a stuttering moment—including extreme or even bizarre movements of arms, hands, legs, or torso—may be incorporated into the response to a stuttering moment. Virtually nothing should be a surprise to the experienced clinician. Certainly for those speakers whose speech is characterized by such behaviors, the presence of these behaviors must be included in the overall determination of severity.

Fragmentation

One other way to think of the prominent features of stuttering behavior is the degree to which a *word* is fragmented. Fragmentation of the word—a within-word fluency break—is a fundamental feature of nonfluent speech. On occasion, fluent speakers fragment words, especially when they are under communicative or emotional stress. People who stutter tend to do it more often and sooner in response to stress.

Bloodstein describes stuttering in its most basic form as "speech transformed by tension and fragmentation." He even goes so far as to suggest that "without tension there can be no stuttering" (1993, p. 137). Certainly, tension is an obvious feature of stuttering and contributes much to the perception of severity. As Bloodstein points out, the fragmentation of movement tends to occur prior to—or early in the performance of—a difficult motor task. It is a natural aspect of what takes place when speakers who stutter attempt the difficult task of saying a word. Nearly all fragmentation during stuttering occurs during the initiation of a word or a syntactic unit of a sentence or phrase. Speakers who stutter appear to be doing, to a more extreme degree, what nonstuttering speakers do. Why people who stutter respond to the formidable task of language production by fluency failure characterized by tension and fragmentation remains one of the most intriguing questions of the discipline.

Subtle Surface Features

We have discussed the intrinsic features of stuttering in Chapter 2 and in the earlier sections of this chapter. What we will discuss now are those features of stuttering that, although they are mostly on the surface of the disorder, can be extremely subtle. They are subtle enough that it takes an experienced clinician some time to detect them. We may think of these as surface features that are closely associated with the intrinsic decision-making process.

Avoidance

To the degree that a person who stutters successfully uses avoidance behaviors, he can give the appearance of a person with a mild—even nonexistent—fluency disorder. If the speaker is unable to use avoidance behaviors successfully, he will provide a portrait of greater severity.

It takes time and energy for the client to successfully change his response to the feared stimuli associated with past fluency failure. There are people, words, sounds, and environments that create the anticipation of stuttering. It takes effort to scan ahead for these stimuli, and it takes even more effort to elude them as they come along. Some clients come to us feeling tired of the ordeal. These people often show obvious relief when we suggest to them that they "give themselves permission to stutter."

Speakers who are especially adept at avoidance behavior have been referred to as *covert* (Starkweather, 1987) or *internalized stutterers* (Douglass & Quarrington, 1952). It has been suggested that these clients are relatively rare. However, we have seen many clients who are so adept at avoidance techniques that few people with whom they come into con-

---

 CLINICAL DECISION-MAKING

Avoidance behavior can be difficult to identify and especially resistant to change during treatment. Speakers who show a high degree of avoidance behavior are often some of the most difficult clients. They will strongly resist any suggestion to stutter voluntarily. They tend to recoil against treatment procedures that result in more fluency disruptions, such as cancellation or pull-out techniques. They are likely to resist revealing that they are attending treatment or telling anyone about their therapy activities or goals. Because the behavior of avoiding words, sounds, situations, and people can be so subtle, and because is it is such an effective way of covering up the stuttering behavior, clients will want to hold on to these highly self-reinforcing techniques. Once identified, avoidance behavior in all of its forms is a worthy target for treatment activities. Unless clients understand the hazards associated with avoidance, this response to the anticipation of stuttering is likely to persist. As clients achieve the ability to shape the features of their stuttering and achieve fluency-enhancing targets as described in later chapters, avoidance tends to lose some usefulness and appeal. Avoidance may also be decreased by the clinician's reinforcement of voluntary stuttering, wherein increased (rather than decreased) stuttering becomes a treatment goal.

tact suspect they are a person who stutters. They are able to hide the overt nature of their problem, and they do so. It can hardly be stated too strongly that avoidance is a poor strategy for stutterers who have a high frequency of motoric fluency breaks. Because changing to another word often results in stuttering on the new word, there is no advantage to this strategy. In some instances, clients will even find themselves stuttering on extra sounds used as postponements, such as "ah" or "um."

Substitution

Substitutions are a most obvious form of avoidance. In this case, another word is substituted for the feared sound or word, often with a slight change in the meaning of the sentence. Sometimes the meaning changes only a little (dog/poodle, X-ray/radiology, or white/vanilla). Sometimes it changes a lot (tea/coffee, X-ray/radiology, or no/yes). At the very least, substitution results in the utterance of a less precise or appropriate word for the context of the sentence or the situation. To the unsophisticated listener, nothing abnormal has occurred when the speaker adeptly substitutes one word or idea for another—but of course, the stuttering experience has taken place. It appears to be a good prognostic sign when the substitution of words is frustrating to the speaker. If he recognizes the lack of choice, the lack of precision, and the helplessness that are associated with these choices, he may be willing to make different decisions.

The following example illustrates the impact of this form of decision-making can have for a young man who stutters.

🔍 CLINICAL INSIGHT

Several years ago I worked with a college student who described a pattern of avoidance and word substitution. He was the starting running back for a nationally ranked football team. He had always been a good student, and he attended the university on an academic scholarship. During a group treatment meeting, he described a speaking event that took place when he was in junior high school. Rob had taken a quiz in class, which was then graded by a student in the adjoining aisle. His paper was returned, and he saw that he had received a score of 95. The teacher went up and down the rows of desks, asking each student in turn to report his or her grade. When it was his turn, Rob stood and tried to say "ninety-five." After enduring a speech block for several moments, he decided he would be less likely to stutter if he said "eighty-five." He then became stuck on eighty-five. Quickly, he decided to say "seventy-five"! The teacher recorded the grade, and Rob sat down. No one in the room suspected he had stuttered, but of course, a profound moment of stuttering had indeed occurred under the surface.

Postponement

As the person who stutters approaches a feared word or sound, there is often a moment of hesitation. It is a moment much like hesitating prior to making a difficult leap over an obstacle. Sometimes the hesitation is subtle, taking the form of a slight pause. The speaker may be considering alternative words or thinking of different ways to structure the sentence in order to avoid using the feared word. Other times, particularly before uttering words that have resulted in severe stuttering in previous speaking situations, the speaker will use a series of sounds or words to postpone the attempts to initiate the word. Postponements are most likely to occur with words that cannot be easily avoided, such as names, addresses, schools, or places of employment. These events may take the form of formulative fluency breaks—for example, whole word or phrase repetitions or insertions of such words and phrases as "ah" and "you know"—into the flow of speech. While these sounds and words are generally thought of as formulative breaks, in this instance their presence is a result of an upcoming or anticipated motoric break. Many times these sounds or words are produced rapidly, providing an added indication that they are being employed as a postponement rather than as a formulative fluency break. In anticipation of possible stuttering, the speaker is pushing back and postponing the initiation of the feared word.

If the speaker makes frequent use of these postponements and if they include obvious tension, listening to the speaker is made extremely difficult, even unpleasant. These extra sounds and words, while maintaining a continuous flow of sound, severely disrupt the flow of information. They are justifiably called *junk words*, for they can litter the speech of people who are using them to the point that listeners, if given the option, will flee. Often, as a result of treatment, clients are able to decrease the use of such postponements and starters. Even if the speaker shows no change at all in the frequency of stuttering, the perceptual effect of decreasing the use of these junk words is one of enormous improvement. There are fewer postponements, information flow is improved, and the speech is much easier to listen to.

THE CLIENT'S SELF-ASSESSMENT

The perceptions of the speaker who stutters are likely to be one of the most important aspects of any assessment of severity or handicap, particularly for the adolescent or adult. One of the simplest—yet most helpful—techniques for obtaining an initial perspective of the client is to have him respond to a series of questions designed to survey the range of the stuttering behaviors. These questions provide an opportunity to sample behavior and the client's understanding of stuttering. They easily lead to a brief period of trial therapy, also an important aspect of the assessment process.

🔎 CLINICAL INSIGHT

As a young adult, the often subtle aspects of avoidance, substitution, and postponement were some of the most frustrating aspects of stuttering. I would say things less precisely than I was capable of, and sometimes my meaning was distorted. Sometimes my listener could sense that the words did not exactly match the situation or my affect. In addition, I eventually realized how my thought process was inhibited when speaking. When writing, I enjoyed the challenge of finding and using just the right word to convey my meaning. However, when I spoke, I was often limiting my choices. For many years I had things to say, yet I refused to try. On a more basic level, I had things to say and I didn't even know it. I later realized that it was much like typing on a computer screen and not knowing what you think until you type it. The new sentences result in ideas that, in turn, lead to new thoughts that you wouldn't have had otherwise. The same thing was happening when I spoke. Not only was I screening out certain feared words, I was also discarding current thoughts and future ideas.

In preparation for asking these questions, we can draw a simple scale with equal-appearing intervals (Figure 4-1), with 0 off the scale to the left representing "no stuttering," 1 representing "mild" and so on to 8 at the right representing "severe stuttering." We place the scale in front of the person and ask him to indicate the point on the scale that best represents his overall, or average, stuttering (indicated by AVERAGE and its arrow, as an example of a label a speaker or the clinician might place on the such a scale). The act of giving the client the pen and placing the scale in front of him is a first step toward assigning him responsibility for his speech. It may well be the first time he has directly addressed his stuttering in a concrete and objective manner.

Once the client marks the point on the scale associated with what he perceives as his average level of severity, we next ask him to indicate the point on the scale that best represents the sample of speech that we are

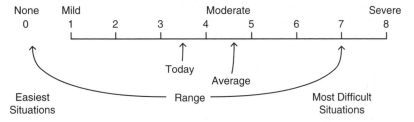

Figure 4-1. Equal-interval scale for determining the current, average, and range of stuttering behavior during the assessment of adolescents and adults.

hearing at the moment. Although these points may, of course, be identical, often they are not. For example, Silverman, (1975) found that older children and adults judged their stuttering severity in a clinical environment to differ from their typical fluency level in extra-treatment situations. By asking these two questions, the clinician is able to demonstrate to the client that she understands the highly variable nature of stuttering and that the behavior observed during the evaluation does not always represent the nature or scope of the problem.

We then ask the client to indicate the extent of his stuttering behavior. How far up and down the scale does his stuttering range? What point on the scale indicates the quality of his speech in the best of speaking situations? For some speakers, this point represents no stuttering at all, a zero (0) on the scale. We then ask him to indicate the point on the other end of the scale that represents his speech in his most difficult or feared speaking situations.

Once he has identified a range of behavior, we can make some observations about his speech and begin a short period of trial therapy. We can determine, for example, whether our view of the surface features of his stuttering coincides with his perception of severity. If it does not, and if the client perceives his stuttering to be very different than does the clinician, it may indicate that some time should be spent during treatment explaining the nature of stuttering and putting the client's stuttering into a broader perspective. Most people who stutter, unless they have attended group therapy or are a member of a self-help group, have not had the opportunity to observe a wide range of severe stuttering behavior. Therefore, it is not surprising when a client has a view of the problem that is more restricted than that of the clinician.

Assuming that the client has indicated a range of severity on the scale, we are able to inform him that, in many ways at least, his stuttering is typical and reasonably normal behavior for someone who stutters. That is, because of the variability and the nature of his stuttering, he is not likely to be stuttering because of some deep-seated psychological problem. Of course, before issuing such a statement, the person's case history should be reviewed and his overall response to the examiner's evaluations should be considered. However, by explaining this to the client, we provide an important service to someone who, for many years, may have regarded himself as being far from normal emotionally. Depending on what he may have read or been told about stuttering as a psychological problem (see Chapter 2), he may have had some doubts about his psychological well-being.

Next, using this information, we conduct some brief trial therapy. We ask the person to follow our lead and stutter along with us. This is very likely to be the first time he has been asked to do this fearful behavior on purpose. The very act of asking the client to willingly stutter demonstrates an unafraid, assertive, and investigative attitude on the part of the clinician. It also shows a willingness to lead the way that can be highly motivating to many clients. In any case, it provides the first opportunity to explore and vary, a behavior that for too long has seemed fearful and uncontrollable.

If the client has been stuttering during the evaluation, we already have an example of his stuttering at the moment. However, we would also like to know what is his speech is like during a less stressful period. Is he able to demonstrate several examples of mild stuttering? Many clients will initially respond to the request "Show me what your mild stuttering looks and sounds like" by describing what they do when they stutter. Instead, we want an *example* of the behavior stuttering. Can he willingly produce this behavior? Finally, can the person demonstrate, perhaps on his own or following our lead, examples of more moderate or possibly severe examples of his stuttering? Is he able to replicate his stuttering to the point that voluntary stuttering changes to real, "out-of-control" stuttering?

The degree to which the person can follow the clinician into stuttering speech tells us much about the client's levels of anxiety and motivation. These activities provide a preliminary indication of how much effort and time will be required for him to accept, become desensitized to, approach, experiment with, and eventually manipulate his stuttering behavior. How difficult is it for the speaker to step away from the moment of stuttering and describe some of his behaviors. The accuracy with which he is able to describe, or better yet, pantomime, moments of stuttering indicates his levels of anxiety and inhibition. Can he correctly identify occurrences and types of stuttering? Can he discriminate between the physical and emotional characteristics of real versus voluntary stuttering? Is he willing to venture with us across the threshold of control to see that that he is able to survive a *deliberate* moment of real stuttering? If the person is unable to follow us in our attempts to experiment and vary his stuttering in this fashion, the process of treatment is likely to be more arduous. Alternately, it may suggest that a different treatment strategy will be necessary. These relatively simple activities provide valuable information about the nature of stuttering as well as the person who stutters.

DETERMINING THE CLIENT'S DESIRE FOR CHANGE

Virtually all clinical authorities agree that the motivation of the person who stutters is a key feature of a successful treatment outcome (Van Riper, 1973). Motivation can also be regarded as a covert aspect of stuttering, for—as with the loss of control—motivation can be difficult to identify and quantify. The person's commitment to change and growth should be assessed prior to—as well as throughout—the process of treatment. Depending on past successes and the client's response to new and difficult challenges, motivation will vary greatly between and within clients.

One thing that does not accurately—or at least completely—reflect a person's level of motivation is the statements made during assessment or treatment sessions. Many clients make sincere and honest statements of commitment. They say things that lead us to believe they are highly motivated. These are similar to the announcements we make when deciding to do things like diet or train for an event such as a marathon or triathlon. While it may be pleasant to hear these declarations of commitment during the assessment interview, if we place too much importance on such statements, we are likely to be deceived. In fact, our advice is to be cautions of statements that indicate that the person is overly committed. It is one thing to talk about making an arduous journey and quite another to take each difficult step along the way.

It is both natural and necessary to be motivated at the outset of treatment. As the process gets underway, there are many interesting things for the client to learn about the nature of stuttering and about his history of attempting to deal with the problem. The fact that the person has come to a treatment center for evaluation is an important step in acknowledging the problem. Moreover, there is some indication that even taking that first step results in desirable changes in both the surface and deep structure of the problem. In determining a person's level of motivation, we first need to appreciate that entering into treatment can be a frightening experience. It is similar to the reaction of anyone who is challenging themselves to take a new class, start a new job, or push the envelope of their lives in any sense. There is an element of risk as well as the possibility of partial or complete failure. In order to consider such challenges, we must reach some level of self-esteem and security. One thing we may do well to consider when evaluating a potential new client is a quality of "mental toughness" and a degree of "psychic energy" (Cooper, 1977) that is present. Often, of course, this is not the case. It is typical for someone to have doubts and anxiety when initiating treatment for stuttering. As clinicians, we need to acknowledge this possibility to the client. This is not to suggest that we only enroll highly motivated people in treatment, but the client's true level of motivation— whatever that may be—does provide an indication of the progress we can expect once treatment is initiated.

It is easy to be motivated before the trek begins, but it often becomes more difficult once you begin climbing. As clinicians, we should take some time during the initial meeting with the client to provide a clear picture of the journey. The assessment process is an ideal time for the clinician to explain an overall picture of the treatment process, both to the client and interested others. The client may be overly enthusiastic, in part because he does not understand the nature of treatment. He may not yet understand that you are unable to cure him of his problem and that, indeed, he is the one who must run the laps and do most of the sweating. Once he begins to appreciate the effort it will take to change his behavior and the way he views the problem, the initial high level of motivation may fade somewhat. Of course, we do not want to deplete the level of motivation, for the client will need to draw upon this reserve. We do, however, want to provide the potential client with a realistic view of the journey.

One practical suggestion for determining a person's level of motivation is to describe examples of the more difficult tasks he will be asked to complete during treatment. These can be explained in some detail or demonstrated during a short period of trial therapy. In addition, there are questions that the clinician can ask to tap into a potential client's level of motivation: questions which will force a realistic consideration of his current priorities. For example, we can ask the person how much treatment is worth to him. Aside from the fees associated with the treatment center, how valuable—in real money—is this service for him at this time? Would he be willing to pay $5, $25, $50, or $80 per hour? How far would he be willing to drive to receive treatment: 5, 50, 100 miles each way? Such questions at first appear to be contrived, possibly even unethical. However, we have found that these thresholds of money or distance often provide an indication of the eventual level of motivation that clients demonstrate once in treatment.

One reason why persons who stutter often experience rapid change during an intensive, residential treatment program is the motivation necessary in order to attend. Not only may the cost of these programs represent a reasonably large financial commitment, but the person also must often make significant social, educational, or vocational adjustments in order to attend. If someone is serious enough to take his vacation time, spend a portion of his savings, and move some or all of his family to the location of an intensive treatment for several weeks, it is probably a good indication that he is highly motivated.

Another important consideration when assessing motivation is where the client may be in the stages of development and change in his life. As with many aspects of life, the timing is crucial. As anyone knows who has attempted to convince a junior high school student who stutters to enroll in treatment, some people just do not want help—or at least they do not necessarily want it when we want to give it to them. The timing of when the path of a life crosses ours can be decisive. Successful treatment is not simply a result of doing more or different things, but of doing the right things at the right time. The moments when people come to us for

---

✓ CLINICAL DECISION-MAKING

The cost of treatment is a major consideration for nearly every client. The usual charge for individual treatment sessions varies widely according to many factors, and the cost for one hour of individual treatment is likely to range from $40 to more than $100 depending on the location. University-related clinic services are going to be less expensive, and private therapy with professional clinicians more expensive. If the client is attending more than one session per week, the cost can quickly increase. Some individuals simply cannot afford professional help unless the services are covered by insurance (which is not typically the case for fluency disorders) or are available at a reduced rate. Many people who stutter would like to be able to speak more fluently but are not willing or able to spend the money it will take to make this change. In order to help clients to realistically consider the cost of treatment, it may be necessary to explain that treatment, especially for adolescents and adults who stutter, is not typically of short duration. Stuttering is a reasonably complex human problem that takes time to change. Whether clients are seen intensively on a daily basis for several weeks or once or twice a week over a period of several months or years, the process will likely involve at least 90 to 100 hours. For example, whether the treatment program is an intensive program lasting approximately three weeks or a nonintensive program of individual treatment sessions once or twice a week for one or two years, total cost can easily approach or go beyond $5000. While this is a significant amount of money by any standard, the impact on the lives of the client can be momentous, even life-altering. Furthermore, many people routinely are willing to spend similar amounts of money for computers and vacations, or considerably more money for a new car every three to five years.

---

help can provide insight into their motivation and readiness for change. Where they are in the process of changing is critical for successful intervention. Recent research regarding the process of self- and assisted change suggests that a person's location on a continuum from self-reevaluation/contemplation of change to action/maintenance of change is a powerful factor in predicting a successful treatment outcome (DiClemente, 1993; Prochaska, DiClemente, & Norcross, 1992). (See Chapter 6 for more detail concerning the change process.) It is often a good idea to ask the client questions such as: "Why are you here today and not six months ago? Or why not a year from today? What is it that prompted you to ask for help at this time?"

The answers to such questions are important in the overall determination of motivation and especially the client's readiness for change. Sometimes people refer themselves for treatment when they finally realize that their speech is preventing them from career advancement. Frequently they come for help when they are facing a major speaking event such as a presentation or a ceremony in which they must take part. In some instances adults come to us at times when they experience landmarks events during their life cycle. That is, as a person comes to the conclusion of a period of his or her life, such as high school or college, schooling, a job, a career, or a marriage, the person tends to stand back and consider the current options that are now available (Sheehy, 1974). They now may have an opportunity to do something about a problem that they have put into the background for much of their lives. Even without the occurrence of a landmark event, such reassessments are likely to occur in middle age. As Newgarten indicates, middle age is characterized by "self-awareness," "heightened introspection," and "restructuring of experience" (cited in Kimmel, 1974, p. 58). Moreover, as Sheehy (1974) suggests, mid-life is often characterized by a reexamination, whereby a person questions many views of the self and others. At this time, he or she is more likely to readjust old responses to lifelong problems (Sheehy, 1974; Vailant, 1977). Adopting new approaches to old problems is possible at any time during the life cycle, of course, but it seems to be most frequent during the decades of the forties and fifties. It could be that if individuals in that age range are interested in treatment, significant progress can result. It would seem that, even if there were no significant change in the vocational or social aspects of their lives, there is the potential for a significant improvement in the quality of life.

On the other hand, there is little information available about older individuals who stutter (Manning & Shirkey, 1981). Manning and Monte (1981) suggest that few people who stutter beyond the age of 50 desire treatment. Manning, Dailey, and Wallace (1984) found preliminary evidence indicating that, in most instances, these people who stutter have learned to adjust to their problem and, although the problem does not appear to diminish in terms of traditional measures of severity, it represents less of a handicap for older speakers. The authors obtained the attitude and personality characteristics of 29 adults who stuttered, ranging in age from 52 to 82. Although these speakers scored approximately the same as young adults who stutter on scales assessing approach and performance speaking behaviors, the large majority of the older individuals who stuttered perceived their stuttering as less handicapping now than when they were young adults. While a few subjects indicated the desire for treatment, most responded by indicating that stuttering had become less of a problem with increased age. In view of the volumes written on the topic of stuttering, the lack of knowledge concerning the nature of stuttering in older speakers is unfortunate. It would seem that in order to completely understand the nature of this communication problem, it is necessary to appreciate the development of the disorder throughout the life cycle. A qualitative study such as that conducted by Corcoran and Stewart (1998) described earlier in this chapter could provide worthwhile information about stuttering in the later years of life.

FORMAL MEASURES OF SEVERITY

When evaluating young children, many of the initial questions focus on whether the observed fluency breaks are unusual or stuttering-like, because of the natural variability of stuttering and because—as we have described—people who stutter sometimes attempt to disguise their stuttering as other communication problems, as this can sometimes be the case with adults. In most cases, however, the diagnosis of stuttering is not terribly difficult to determine. The more basic question is the severity of the problem in terms of affective, behavioral, and cognitive characteristics. Depending on how the person has dealt with stuttering at each of these levels, the handicapping effects of stuttering will vary greatly across individuals. There are a number of assessment devices that the clinician may use to obtain a formal measure of the nature and severity of stuttering (see alphabetical listing in Appendix A). In the following section we will describe some of the assessment instruments that seem to be particularly useful.

Stuttering Severity Instrument (SSI-3)

Perhaps the most used of all scales for determining stuttering severity, this scale was originally developed in 1972 by Glyndon Riley. The newest (third) edition (SSI-3) provides scale values for stuttering severity for both children and adults (Figure 4-2). Speakers who can read are asked to (1) describe their job or school and (2) read a short passage. Nonreaders are given a picture task to which they respond. Scoring is accomplished across three areas. The frequency of the fluency breaks tabulated and the percentage of stuttering are converted to a task score (range, 4–18). The duration of the three longest stuttering moments (fleeting to more than 60 seconds) is tabulated and converted to a scale score (range, 2–18). Last, physical concomitant across four categories is scaled on a 0-to-5 scale (0 = none, 5 = severe and painful looking) and totaled (range, 0–20). The total overall score is computed by adding the scores for three sections. Percentile and severity equivalents are provided for preschool children, school-age children, and adults. The scale is attractive because it can be used with virtually all age ranges and is easy to administer and score (Item 35, Appendix A).

SSI-3

Stuttering Severity Instrument–3

TEST RECORD AND FREQUENCY COMPUTATION FORM

Identifying Information

Name _____

Sex M F   Grade _____ Age _____

Date _____ Date of Birth _____

School _____

Examiner _____

Preschool ___ School Age ___ Adult ___ Reader ___ Nonreader ___

FREQUENCY Use Readers Table or Nonreaders Table. not both.

READERS TABLE				NONREADERS TABLE	
1. Speaking Task		2. Reading Task		3. Speaking Task	
Percentage	Task Score	Percentage	Task Score	Percentage	Task Score
1	2	1	2	1	4
2	3			2	6
3	4	2	4	3	8
4–5	5	3–4	5	4–5	10
6–7	6	5–7	6	6–7	12
8–11	7	8–12	7	8–11	14
12–21	8	13–20	8	12–21	16
22 & up	9	21 & up	9	22 & up	18

Frequency Score (use 1 + 2 or 3) ☐

DURATION

Average length of three longest stuttering events timed to the nearest 1/10th second		Scale Score
Fleeting	(.5 sec or less)	2
Half-second	(.5– .9 sec)	4
1 full second	(1.0– 1.9 secs)	6
2 seconds	(2.0– 2.9 secs)	8
3 seconds	(3.0– 4.9 secs)	10
5 seconds	(5.0– 9.9 secs)	12
10 seconds	(10.0–29.9 secs)	14
30 seconds	(30.0–59.9 secs)	16
1 minute	(60 secs or more)	18

Duration Score (2 – 18) ☐

PHYSICAL CONCOMITANTS

Evaluating Scale

0 = none
1 = not noticeable unless looking for it
2 = barely noticeable to casual observer
3 = distracting
4 = very distracting
5 = severe and painful-looking

DISTRACTING SOUNDS	Noisy breathing, whistling, sniffing, blowing, clicking sounds	0 1 2 3 4 5
FACIAL GRIMACES	Jaw jerking, tongue protruding, lip pressing, jaw muscles tense	0 1 2 3 4 5
HEAD MOVEMENTS	Back, forward, turning away, poor eye contact, constant looking around	0 1 2 3 4 5
MOVEMENTS OF THE EXTREMITIES	Arm and hand movement, hands about face, torso movement, leg movements, foot-tapping or swinging	0 1 2 3 4 5

Physical Concomitants Score ☐

TOTAL OVERALL SCORE

Frequency _____ + Duration _____ + Physical Concomitants _____ = ☐

Percentile _____

Severity _____

Figure 4-2. The Stuttering Severity Instrument-3 (SSI-3). From Stuttering Severity Instrument for Children and Adults—Third Edition (Test Record and Frequency Computation Form, pp. 1–2 by G. D. Riley, 1994, Austin, TX: PRO-ED. Copyright 1994 by PRO-ED. Reprinted with permission.

Modified Erickson Scale of Communication Attitudes (S-24)

This popular and easy-to-administer scale has been used in many clinical studies (Figure 4-3). Clients respond to a series of 24 true/false statements

TABLE 2
Percentile and Severity Equivalents of
SSI-3 Total Overall Scores for Preschool Children (*N* = 72)

Total Overall Score	Percentile	Severity
0– 8	1– 4	Very Mild
9–10	5–11	
11–12	12–23	Mild
13–16	24–40	
17–23	41–60	Moderate
24–26	61–77	
27–28	78–88	Severe
29–31	89–95	
32 and up	96–99	Very Severe

TABLE 3
Percentile and Severity Equivalents of SSI-3
Total Overall Scores for School-Age Children (*N* = 139)

Total Overall Score	Percentile	Severity
6– 8	1– 4	Very Mild
9–10	5–11	
11–15	12–23	Mild
16–20	24–40	
21–23	41–60	Moderate
24–27	61–77	
28–31	78–88	Severe
32–35	89–95	
36 and up	96–99	Very Severe

TABLE 4
Percentile and Severity Equivalents of
SSI-3 Total Overall Scores for Adults (*N* = 60)

Total Overall Score	Percentile	Severity
10–12	1– 4	Very Mild
13–17	5–11	
18–20	12–23	Mild
21-24	24–40	
25–27	41–60	Moderate
28–31	61–77	
32–34	78–88	Severe
35–36	89–95	
37–46	96–99	Very Severe

Figure 4-2. continued

according to whether the statements are characteristics of themselves. The S-24 was modified by Andrews and Cutler (1974) from the original 39-item Erickson S-Scale (1969). Designed for use with older adolescents and adults, the total score is obtained by tabulating one point for each item that is answered as a person who stutters would respond. Individuals who stutter average a total of 19.22 items scored in this manner, while nonstuttering individuals average a total score of 9.14 (Item 4, Appendix A).

Perceptions of Stuttering Inventory (PSI)

This inventory, developed by Woolf (1967), is designed to determine the client's self-rating of his degree of avoidance, struggle, and expectancy for older adolescents and adults who stutter. The subject responds to each of 60 statements according to whether or not he feels they are "characteristic of me." Statements that the person feels are not characteristic are left unmarked (Item 51, Appendix A).

Locus of Control of Behavior (LCB)

This 17-item Likert-type scale (Figure 4-4) was developed by Craig, Franklin, and Andrews to "measure the extent to which adults perceive responsibility for their personal problem behavior" (1984, p. 174). This scaling procedure is designed to indicate the ability of a person for taking responsibility for maintaining new or desired behaviors. Subjects are asked to indicate their agreement or disagreement to each of the 17 statements about personal beliefs using a six-point scale. The scale has good internal reliability and scores are not influenced by age, gender, or social desirability of responses. The scores of the 17 statements are summed to yield a total LCB score (items 1, 5, 7, 8, 13, and 16 are scored in reverse order). Higher scores on this scale indicate a perception of external control (externality), while lower scores indicate the perception of greater internal control (internality). Since all forms of intervention for stuttering in one way or another ask the client to gradually assume responsibility for changing his speech, the locus of control concept is intuitively appealing. As Boberg, Howie, and Woods (1979) have suggested, individuals who continue to rely on the clinician and the clinical environment for reinforcement and who fail to take the necessary responsibility for their fluency are more likely to relapse once formal treatment is completed. Craig, Franklin, and Andrews (1984) found LCB scale scores averaged 32.0 for adults who stuttered and 27.0 for nonstuttering adults. This difference was found to be statistically significant. We have found that scores for adults who would be regarded as severely stuttering often have LCB scores as high as 44 to 55. Nonstuttering speakers generally score in the high teens to low 20s. An example of decreases (improvement) in LCB scores for an adult client with severe stuttering can be found in Chapter 10 (Item 15, Appendix A).

Modified Erickson Scale of Communication Attitudes (S-24)

Name: _____ Date: _____ Score: _____

Directions: Mark the "true" column with a check (√) for each statement that is true or mostly true for you and mark the "false" column with a check (√) for each statement which is false or not usually true for you.

	TRUE	FALSE
1. I usually feel that I am making a favorable impression when I talk.	___	___
2. I find it easy to talk with almost anyone.	___	___
3. I find it very easy to look at my audience while speaking to a group.	___	___
4. A person who is my teacher or my boss is hard to talk to.	___	___
5. Even the idea of giving a talk in public makes me afraid.	___	___
6. Some words are harder than others for me to say.	___	___
7. I forget all about myself shortly after I begin a speech.	___	___
8. I am a good mixer.	___	___
9. People sometimes seem uncomfortable when I am talking to them.	___	___
10. I dislike introducing one person to another.	___	___
11. I often ask questions in group discussions.	___	___
12. I find it easy to keep control of my voice when speaking.	___	___
13. I do not mind speaking before a group.	___	___
14. I no not talk well enough to do the kind of work I'd really like to do.	___	___
15. My speaking voice is rather pleasant and easy to listen to.	___	___
16. I am sometimes embarrassed by the way I talk.	___	___
17. I face most speaking situations with complete confidence.	___	___
18. There are few people I can talk with easily.	___	___
19. I talk better than I write.	___	___
20. I often feel nervous while talking.	___	___
21. I find it hard to make talk when I meet new people.	___	___
22. I feel pretty confident about my speaking ability.	___	___
23. I wish that I could say things as clearly as others do.	___	___
24. Even though I knew the right answer, I have often failed to give it because I was afraid to speak out.	___	___

I. Answers

Score 1 point fore each answer that matches this:

1. False	7. False	13. False	19. False
2. False	8. False	14. True	20. True
3. False	9. True	15. False	21. True
4. True	10. True	16. True	22. False
5. True	11. False	17. False	23. True
6. True	12. False	18. True	24. True

II.   Adult Norms

	Mean	Range
Stutterers	19.22	9-24
Nonstutterers	9.14	1-21

Figure 4-3. Erickson S-24 Scale of Communication Attitudes. Andrews, G., and Cutler, J. (1974). Stuttering therapy: The relation between changes in symptom level and attitudes. *Journal of Speech and Hearing Disorders, 39,* pp. 312–319. Copyright 1974, American Speech-Language-Hearing Association.

LCB SCALE

Name: Age: Date:

Directions: Below are a number of statements about how various topics affect your personal beliefs. There are no right or wrong answers. For every item there are a large number of people who agree and disagree. Could you please put in the appropriate bracket the choice you believe to be true. Answer all of the questions.

0	1	2	3	4	5
Strongly disagree	Generally disagree	Somewhat disagree	Somewhat agree	Generally agree	Strongly agree

1. I can anticipate difficulties and take action to avoid them. ( )

2. A great deal of what happens to me is probably just a matter or chance. ( )

3. Everyone knows that luck or chance determines one's future. ( )

4. I can control my problem(s) only if I have outside support. ( )

5. When I make plans, I am almost certain that I can make them work. ( )

6. My problem(s) will dominate me all my life. ( )

7. My mistakes and problems are my responsibility to deal with. ( )

8. Becoming a success is a matter of hard work; luck has little or nothing to do with it. ( )

9. My life is controlled by outside actions and events. ( )

10. People are victims of circumstances beyond their control. ( )

11. To continually manage my problems I need professional help. ( )

12. When I am under stress, the tightness in my muscles is due to things outside my control. ( )

13. I believe a person can really be the master of his fate. ( )

14. It is impossible to control my irregular and fast breathing when I am having difficulties. ( )

15. I understand why my problem(s) varies so much from one occasion to the next ( )

16. I am confident of being able to deal successfully with future problems. ( )

17. In my case, maintaining control over my problem(s) is mostly due to luck. ( )

Figure 4-4. Locus of Control of Behavior Scale.

Self-Efficacy Scaling for Adult Stutterers

Based on the work of Bandura (1977) with perceptual self-efficacy scaling, the Self-Efficacy Scale for Adult Stutterers (SESAS) (Ornstein & Manning, 1985) is designed to measure the confidence that an adult who stutters can both approach and maintain a level of fluency in 50 specific, extra-treatment speaking situations (Figure 4-5). During the first section of the scale (SESAS approach), clients respond by indicating the likelihood that they could enter into each of the speaking situations by using a decile scale from 10 to 100. The 50 speaking situations are ordered in a hierarchy, from easy to more difficult. Subject responses are averaged over the 50 situations to obtain the SESAS approach score.

The same 50 speaking situations are presented again for the second section of the scale (SESAS performance). For this section, clients are asked to indicate confidence that they could maintain a client-selected "level of fluency" based on their treatment program and current progress. (See Chapter 10 for the most recent modification to this section of the scale.) Again, subject responses are averaged over the 50 speaking situations to obtain the SESAS performance score.

Ornstein and Manning (1985) administered the SESAS to 20 adults who stuttered and a matched group of control subjects. The authors found the SESAS total score to correlate with the Erickson Scale of Communication Attitudes (Erickson, 1969) at −0.71 (sign in the expected direction) and with the Perceptions of Stuttering Inventory (Woolf, 1967) at −0.52 (sign in the expected direction). In addition, test-retest reliability for the SESAS for 10 of the experimental subjects averaged +0.95 and +0.84 for the SESAS approach and performance scales, respectively.

Ornstein and Manning found that the stuttering subjects scored significantly lower on both approach (66.2) and performance (55.8) portions of the SESAS than nonstuttering subjects. Interestingly, the fluent speakers had scores of 94.2 and 98.0 for the approach and performance scales, respectively, indicating that they were less confident about approaching situations than about speaking fluently once they were in a situation. The stuttering subjects, on the other hand, were more confident about approaching speaking situations than about maintaining fluency once they entered the situation. Subsequent investigation (Manning, Perkins, Winn, & Coles, 1984) indicated that with treatment, adults who stutter demonstrate increasingly higher scores. In addition, stuttering subjects began to normalize their approach and performance scores, in the sense that performance scores were slightly greater than approach scores.

A validation study by Saltuklaroglu and Kully (1998) provided both criterion and construct validity for the approach portion of the SESAS. Moderate but significant correlations between SESAS Approach scores and %SS (−0.305) and global severity ratings (−0.279) were obtained for 160 adolescent and adult subjects (age range 14–74 years) prior to formal

A SELF-EFFICACY SCALE FOR ADULT STUTTERERS
(SESAS)

Name _____ Date _____

Date of Birth _____ Gender _____ Race _____

Occupation _____

Years in School _____ Months in Therapy _____

You will be presented with two lists of 50 speaking situations which commonly occur. While you may not typically find yourself in each of these speaking situations, indicate how you believe you would perform in each situation. Please answer all questions. For the first set of 50 questions ask yourself whether or not you would enter each situation. Under the column CAN DO, check the situations you expect you would enter if you were asked to do them now. Then, for the situations you check under the column CAN DO, mark in the column CONFIDENCE how confident you are that you would enter each particular situation. Rate your degree of confidence by recording one of the following numbers from 10 to 100 using the scale below.

10	20	30	40	50	60	70	80	90	100
QUITE UNCERTAIN				MODERATELY CERTAIN					VERY CERTAIN

To familiarize you with the rating form note the following example:

Situation	CAN DO	CONFIDENCE
1. Lift a 25 pound box above your head	__X__	100
2. Lift a 35 pound box above your head	__X__	90
3. Lift a 50 pound box above your head	__X__	80
4. Lift a 65 pound box above your head	__X__	70
5. Lift a 80 pound box above your head	__X__	50
6. Lift a 100 pound box above your head	__X__	30
7. Lift a 200 pound box above your head	_____	___

Now complete the following example to practice using the rating scale.

Situation	CAN DO	CONFIDENCE
1. High jump 1 foot	_____	_____
2. High jump 2 feet	_____	_____
3. High jump 3 feet	_____	_____
4. High jump 4 feet	_____	_____
5. High jump 5 feet	_____	_____
6. High jump 6 feet	_____	_____

Figure 4-5a. The Self-Efficacy Scale for Adults who Stutter. (Ornstein, A., & Manning, W. (1985). Self-efficacy scaling by adult stutterers. *Journal of Communication Disorders, 18,* 313–320.) *Reprinted with permission.*

APPROACH ATTITUDE:

If you are sure that you understand the task, please complete the following list of 50 situations by (1) checking whether you feel you would enter each situation and (2) your confidence in that belief. Please make these judgements honestly with respect to your present ability, not according to what you want to do or think you should do. Rate your degree of confidence by recording one of the following numbers from 10 to 100 using the scale below. If you do not feel that you would enter a situation, do not mark that item.

10	20	30	40	50	60	70	80	90	100
QUITE UNCERTAIN				MODERATELY CERTAIN					VERY CERTAIN

WOULD YOU. . .:   <u>CAN DO</u>   <u>CONFIDENCE</u>

1. Talk with a family member during a meal.
2. Request help in an uncrowded department store.
3. Talk to a close friend while walking down the street.
4. Talk to a family member on the phone.
5. Talk with your clinician while standing in line for a movie.
6. Talk to a fellow worker that you meet in a store.
7. Call up a friend on the phone.
8. Order food at McDonald's when there are no other customers.
9. Talk with your physician in a store.
10. Answer the phone at home.
11. Talk with a fellow worker at work.
12. Ask a friend to drive you to the airport.
13. Talk to a telephone operator on the phone.
14. Introduce two friends at a shopping mall.
15. Talk with your boss at a social gathering.
16. Ask a policeman for directions.
17. Call a member of the opposite sex on the phone.
18. Talk to a group of friends in a noisy bar or restaurant.
19. Talk with your instructor after class.
20. Make a long distance phone call.
21. Tell a joke in front of five people.
22. Answer questions during a group discussion.
23. Call the information operator on the phone.
24. Approach your boss and initiate a conversation at work.
25. Initiate a conversation with a stranger of the
    opposite sex at a party.

Figure 4-5b.

WOULD YOU . . .: (continued)   CAN DO   CONFIDENCE

26. Answer a phone in a crowded room.   _____   _____

27. Ask questions during a group discussion.   _____   _____

28. Order food from your car through a speaker at McDonald's   _____   _____

29. Make a phone call to say that you will be late.   _____   _____

30. Introduce yourself to a stranger.   _____   _____

31. Order a drink from a bartender at a noisy, crowded bar.   _____   _____

32. Talk to your boss on the phone.   _____   _____

33. Get in a long line at McDonald's to order food.   _____   _____

34. Request help in a crowded department store when all the
    salespeople seem busy.   _____   _____

35. Telephone your clinician to cancel a therapy session.   _____   _____

36. Introduce yourself to a group of strangers.   _____   _____

37. Volunteer to present a talk on your work or hobby to
    a group of 20 school-age children.   _____   _____

38. Talk to your boss at work about a work-related error that
    you have made.   _____   _____

39. Ask for directions over the phone.   _____   _____

40. Order food in a restaurant when the waitress is obviously
    in a hurry.   _____   _____

41. Initiate a conversation with the person sitting next to you
    on an airplane.   _____   _____

42. Give an important 30-minute presentation at work or school.   _____   _____

43. Volunteer to present a talk on your work or hobby to a group
    of 25 adults.   _____   _____

44. Order a pizza over the phone.   _____   _____

45. Ask for a raise at work.   _____   _____

46. Complain about the lack of service to your waiter/waitress.   _____   _____

47. Call a stranger on the phone to tell him or her about a meeting. _____   _____

48. Volunteer to go on a T.V. or radio talk show.   _____   _____

49. Order exactly what you want in a restaurant even though
    you might stutter on the words.   _____   _____

50. Call up the telephone company to question a bill.   _____   _____

Figure 4-5c.

FLUENCY PERFORMANCE:

For the second set of 50 questions ask yourself whether or not you could achieve fluent speech in each situation. Please define fluency as speech that would be so fluent in a given situation that, in your opinion, a listener would not recognize that you had a history of stuttering. Again, under the column marked CAN DO, place a check if you believe you could achieve fluency in that situation. Then mark in the column CONFIDENCE, how confident you are that you could achieve fluency. Please make these judgements honestly with respect to your present ability and not according to how you would like to perform or think that you should perform. Rate your degree of confidence by recording one of the following numbers from 10 to 100 using the scale below. If you do not believe that you can achieve fluent speech in a given situation, do not mark that item.

10	20	30	40	50	60	70	80	90	100
QUITE UNCERTAIN				MODERATELY CERTAIN					VERY CERTAIN

If you are sure that you understand the task, please complete the following list of 50 situations by (1) indicating whether you feel you could achieve your fluency level in each situation and (2) your confidence in that belief.
COULD YOU ACHIEVE YOUR FLUENCY LEVEL WHILE. . .:

COULD YOU. . .:   CAN DO   CONFIDENCE

1. Talk with a family member during a meal.
2. Request help in an uncrowded department store.
3. Talk to a close friend while walking down the street.
4. Talk to a family member on the phone.
5. Talk with your clinician while standing in line for a movie.
6. Talk to a fellow worker that you meet in a store.
7. Call up a friend on the phone.
8. Order food at McDonald's when there are no other customers.
9. Talk with your physician in a store.
10. Answer the phone at home.
11. Talk with a fellow worker at work.
12. Ask a friend to drive you to the airport.
13. Talk to a telephone operator on the phone.
14. Introduce two friends at a shopping mall.
15. Talk with your boss at a social gathering.
16. Ask a policeman for directions.
17. Call a member of the opposite sex on the phone.
18. Talk to a group of friends in a noisy bar or restaurant.
19. Talk with your instructor after class.
20. Make a long distance phone call.
21. Tell a joke in front of five people.

Figure 4-5d.

WOULD YOU . . .: (continued)   CAN DO   CONFIDENCE

22. Answer questions during a group discussion.   _____   _____

23. Call the information operator on the phone.   _____   _____

24. Approach your boss and initiate a conversation at work.   _____   _____

25. Initiate a conversation with a stranger of the opposite
    sex at a party.   _____   _____

26. Answer a phone in a crowded room.   _____   _____

27. Ask questions during a group discussion.   _____   _____

28. Order food from your car through a speaker at McDonald's.   _____   _____

29. Make a phone call to say that you will be late.   _____   _____

30. Introduce yourself to a stranger.   _____   _____

31. Order a drink from a bartender at a noisy, crowded bar.   _____   _____

32. Talk to your boss on the phone.   _____   _____

33. Get in a long line at McDonald's to order food.   _____   _____

34. Request help in a crowded department store when all the
    salespeople seem busy.   _____   _____

35. Telephone your clinician to cancel a therapy session.   _____   _____

36. Introduce yourself to a group of strangers.   _____   _____

37. Volunteer to present a talk on your work or hobby to
    a group of 20 school-age children.   _____   _____

38. Talk to your boss at work about a work-related error that
    you have made.   _____   _____

39. Ask for directions over the phone.   _____   _____

40. Order food in a restaurant when the waitress is obviously
    in a hurry.   _____   _____

41. Initiate a conversation with the person sitting next to you
    on an airplane.   _____   _____

42. Give an important 30-minute presentation at work or school.)l. _____   _____

43. Volunteer to present a talk on your work or hobby to a group
    of 25 adults.   _____   _____

44. Order a pizza over the phone.   _____   _____

45. Ask for a raise at work.   _____   _____

46. Complain about the lack of service to your waiter/waitress.   _____   _____

47. Call a stranger on the phone to tell him or her about a meeting. _____   _____

48. Volunteer to go on a T.V. or radio talk show.   _____   _____

49. Order exactly what you want in a restaurant even though
    you might stutter on the words.   _____   _____

50. Call up the telephone company to question a bill.   _____   _____

Figure 4-5e.

treatment. The somewhat modified scale (42 versus 50 speaking situations) resulted in a mean approach score of 53.8. The 20 subjects in the Ornstein and Manning (1985) study had received an average of 9.4 months of treatment and averaged 66.2. Pearson correlations of SESAS approach items showed significant relationships for all items and the total SESAS score, indicating that all items were a representative measure of speaking situations, a finding that strengthened the construct validity of the measure. Finally, factor analysis indicated identified five underlying constructs contained in the scale: 1. speaking to multiple listeners, 2. speaking to one familiar listener, 3. speaking to one unfamiliar listener, 4. speaking to an important listener, and 5. speaking situations in social settings. Manning and Hillis (1998) are currently developing a multidimensional assessment procedure for self-efficacy scaling that includes the effects of both speaking task and the communication situation (Item 33, Appendix A).

The SEA-Scale: Self-Efficacy Scaling for Adolescents Who Stutter

Developed by Manning (1994), this scale is also based on the word of Bandura and his colleagues and—like the SESAS for adults—is intended to indicate their confidence for entering into and speaking in a large variety of extra-treatment speaking situations (Figure 4-6). Clients are asked to assign a whole number value (1 to 10) to each of 100 communication situations. Speaking situations are divided into 13 subscales (based on the work of Watson, 1988). The overall alpha level for the entire scale was 0.98, with subscale alphas ranging from 0.74 to 0.94. Forty adolescents who stuttered scored significantly (p < .001) lower (mean = 7.21; SD = 1.8) than a matched group of nonstuttering control subjects (mean = 8.65; SD = 1.2). Scores are averaged across all 100 situations with individual averages possible for the 13 subcategories of speaking situations (Item 30, Appendix A).

Crowe's Protocols: A Comprehensive Guide to Stuttering Assessment

This new protocol provides a combination of extremely comprehensive assessment options for children, adolescents, and adults who stutter. Using three- and seven-point scaling procedures, sections of the protocol provide forms for obtaining case history and cultural information as well as client self-assessment. Other components include assessment of affective, behavioral, and cognitive features; speech status, stimulability and measures of severity. Several sections and forms are designed to provide

SELF-EFFICACY FOR ADOLESCENTS SCALE
(SEA- Scale)

Name _____   Date _____

Date of Birth _____   Gender _____

Grade _____   Months in Treatment _____

Clinician _____   School _____

Instructions

You are asked to consider a list of 100 speaking situations. Even though you may not typically find yourself in some of these situations, indicate how confident you are about entering into and speaking in each situation by placing one of the following numbers after each situation.

1	2	3	4	5	6	7	8	9	10

No Way, I would be too uptight to speak	I would be very uncomfortable speaking	Unsure	I would be somewhat comfortable speaking	No Problem, I would be confident speaking

EXAMPLE:

SITUATION	CONFIDENCE
1. Lift a 5 pound box above your head.	10
2. Lift a 15 pound box above your head.	9
3. Lift a 25 pound box above your head.	7
4. Lift a 40 pound box above your head.	6
5. Lift a 50 pound box above your head.	1
6. Lift a 80 pound box above your head.	

Please complete the following practice items:

PRACTICE:

SITUATION	CONFIDENCE
1. Jump over a fence 1 foot high.	____
2. Jump over a fence 2 feet high.	____
3. Jump over a fence 3 feet high.	____
4. Jump over a fence 4 feet high.	____
5. Jump over a fence 5 feet high.	____
5. Jump over a fence 6 feet high.	____

Figure 4-6a. Self-Efficacy Scaling for Adolescents (SEA-Scale).

If you are sure that you understand what you are to do, please respond to the following 100 speaking situations by indicating your degree of confidence in your ability to enter into and speak in that situation. When ranking your confidence use a number from 1 to 10. If you do not feel that you can do a particular speaking task, do not enter a number.

SITUATION	CONFIDENCE
1. Talking with a parent about a movie you recently saw together.	____
2. Talking to a brother or sister at the dinner table.	____
3. Talking with a brother or sister about what TV program you would like to watch.	____
4. Talking with three friends your own age during lunch at school about a movie	____
5. Asking a friend to come to your house after school.	____
6. Asking a parent if a friend can spend the night at your house.	____
7. Arguing with a brother or sister.	____
8. Asking a parent if you can spend the night at a friend's house.	____
9. Asking a friend to help you with your homework after school.	____
10. Talking with a group of friends as you have lunch at school.	____
11. Talking about your homework to the people who go with you to school.	____
12. Asking a parent for permission to study with a friend.	____
13. Asking a parent for permission to go to see a movie with friends.	____
14. Asking a friend to come to your birthday party.	____
15. Talking with three friends at school about a new student in your class.	____
16. Talking with a group of classmates during a meeting at school.	____
17. Telling a new friend the names and ages of your brothers or sisters.	____
18. Giving your locker number to a teacher.	____
19. Telling a parent that you do not deserve to be grounded.	____
20. Giving your place and date of birth to an official of your school.	____
21. Calling your best friend on the telephone just to talk.	____
22. Asking a parent for permission to stay out one hour later than usual.	____
23. Telling your teacher at school your name and address.	____
24. Talking with a grandparent on the telephone.	____
25. Explaining how to play a new game to a group of friends.	____
26. Talking with two new people in your class who just began attending your school.	____
27. Talking on the telephone with a classmate about your homework assignment.	____
28. Telling your parent the allowance you are given is not enough.	____
29. Asking a librarian for help in finding a book.	____

Figure 4-6b.

SITUATION   CONFIDENCE

30. Asking a sales clerk about the cost of an item in a store. ____

31. Telling a police officer your home address. ____

32. Telling one of your classmates that he or she picked up your pencil by mistake. ____

33. Asking a sales clerk if a particular item is in stock. ____

34. Calling a store clerk to see what time the store opens. ____

35. Arguing with a friend about who gets to go first in a game. ____

36. Calling a theater to see when a movie starts. ____

37. Talking to other students at a new school. ____

38. Talking on the telephone with relatives who live in another city. ____

39. Arguing with a friend about who gets the last piece of candy. ____

40. Arguing with two friends about which movie you should see. ____

41. Taking a telephone message for a brother or sister. ____

42. Talking with a group of four new students in your class the first week of school. ____

43. Arguing with another student because you let a friend cut in line in front of you. ____

44. Telling a parent that you have to stay after school because you were disruptive
    in class. ____

45. Asking a stranger where the nearest telephone is located. ____

46. Confronting someone who cuts in front of you in line. ____

47. Raising your hand and asking your teacher for permission to leave the room. ____

48. Arguing with an older, larger, friend about who gets the last coke. ____

49. Arguing with a friend about a boy/girl that you both like. ____

50. Answering a question in class. ____

51. Asking a question in class. ____

52. Raising your hand in order to give an answer before the teacher calls on
    someone else. ____

53. Telling the teacher you were not the one who was talking in class ____

54. Introducing yourself to a group of new students at your school. ____

55. Asking someone in a group of five people the correct time. ____

56. Asking a coach of a sports team at school how to join the team. ____

57. Beginning a conversation with a group of three strangers at a party. ____

58. Going to a fast food restaurant with your family and ordering a sandwich. ____

59. Introducing yourself to a group of five students at a new school. ____

60. Telling a parent that you just broke your neighbor's window with a ball. ____

61. Accusing a friend because you believe he or she copied your homework. ____

Figure 4-6c.

SITUATION   CONFIDENCE

62. Asking a stranger for directions to get to a restaurant.   ____

63. Taking your turn ordering when you are having dinner in a restaurant with your family.   ____

64. Telling a group of friends that you will not smoke with them.   ____

65. Telling your teacher you do not understand an assignment.   ____

66. Talking on the phone with a teacher about attending a class party.   ____

67. Answering the telephone at a friend's house.   ____

68. Telling a friend that he or she tore a pair of jeans they borrowed from you.   ____

69. Asking for directions from someone who is in a hurry.   ____

70. Telling an usher at a movie theater that you are old enough to see a particular movie. ____

71. Asking your classroom teacher to move your desk to the front of the classroom.   ____

72. Talking on the telephone with a classmate of the opposite sex.   ____

73. Questioning a teacher about letting the same student always be first in line.   ____

74. Telling a parent about a bad report card.   ____

75. Introducing yourself to a new teacher.   ____

76. Talking to a teacher about something that is bothering you.   ____

77. Going to a party when the only person you know is the one giving the party.   ____

78. Explaining to a teacher why you are late to class.   ____

79. Giving directions to a group of adults who are driving by your home in a car.   ____

80. Explaining to a teacher why you were absent from school.   ____

81. Asking an adult if this is the house where your friend lives.   ____

82. Ordering something at a fast food restaurant when they are very busy.   ____

83. Telling a joke to group of friends at a party.   ____

84. Leaving a message on someone's telephone answering machine.   ____

85. Walking door to door and asking unfamiliar neighbors to buy items you are selling.   ____

86. Reading aloud to a group of seven classmates.   ____

87. Explaining to the school principal why you are in the hall during a class.   ____

88. Asking a girl/boy to dance at a school party.   ____

89. Taking part in a spelling contest.   ____

90. Explaining to your school principal why you were sent to the school office.   ____

91. Reading a paragraph from a book to the people in your class at school.   ____

92. Introducing a speaker to a club or religious group.   ____

93. Asking a person in your school to go with you to a school dance.   ____

94. Giving a book report in front of the class.   ____

Figure 4-6d.

SITUATION   CONFIDENCE

95. Reading aloud to a group of seven adults.   _____

96. Reciting a poem in your English class.   _____

97. Being videotaped when giving a report to your history class.   _____

98. Taking a speaking part in a school play.   _____

99. Making a five-minute speech in a school assembly.   _____

100. Reading an announcement to everyone in your school over the intercom. _____

OVERALL AVERAGE: _____

Note: The overall SEA-Scale score is obtained by averaging the scores for all 100 items.
         Items not checked are scored as a zero.

Clinical Notes:

Figure 4-6e.

Sub-scale items and Alpha scores

Overall Alpha = 0.98

SUBSCALE 1   Telephone Conversations
10 Items: 21 24 27 34 36 38 41 67 72 84   Alpha = 0.88

SUBSCALE 2   Argument or Conflict with a Friend or Family Member
13 Items: 7 19 35 39 40 44 48 49 60 61 64 68 74   Alpha = 0.85

SUBSCALE 3   Argument or Conflict with a Stranger
4 Items: 32 43 46 90   Alpha = 0.73

SUBSCALE 4   One-to-One Conversation with a Family Member
3 Items: 1 2 3   Alpha = 0.88

SUBSCALE 5   One-to-One Conversation with an Authority Figure
7 Items: 31 66 75 76 80 81 87   Alpha = 0.86

SUBSCALE 6   Group Conversation with a Known Group (Informal)
7 Items: 4 10 11 15 16 25 83   Alpha = 0.85

SUBSCALE 7   Group Conversation with an Unknown Group (Formal)
8 Items: 26 37 42 54 57 59 77 79   Alpha = 0.91

SUBSCALE 8   Formal Presentation
11 Items: 86 89 91 92 94 95 96 97 98 99 100   Alpha = 0.94

SUBSCALE 9   Questioning a Friend/Family Member for Information/Action
9 Items: 5 6 8 9 12 13 14 22 28   Alpha = 0.83

SUBSCALE 10   Questioning a Stranger for Information or Action
8 Items: 29 30 33 45 55 62 88 93   Alpha = 0.82

SUBSCALE 11   Questioning an Authority Figure for Information or Action
10 Items: 47 51 53 56 65 70 71 73 78 85   Alpha = 0.89

SUBSCALE 12   Situations Involving Time Constraints
4 Items: 52 63 69 82   Alpha = 0.84

SUBSCALE 13   Situations Involving Memorized or Unchangeable Content
6 Items: 17 18 20 23 50 58   Alpha = 0.80

Figure 4-6f.

information for counseling during treatment. Forms are designed to be completed by the client or by the clinician through respondent interview. An abbreviated protocol is also provided (Item 16, Appendix A).

ASSESSING ATYPICAL FLUENCY PROBLEMS

The large majority of adolescents and adults who are evaluated for fluency problems are people who have a history of developmental stuttering. They have been described by Van Riper (1971, 1982) as following Track I of stuttering development. They have essentially normal histories of speech, language, neurological, and psychological development. Van Riper and others have described another related category of people with fluency problems, defined as Track II. These individuals not only have something less than normal fluency, they also have difficulty in one or more areas of speech and language ability. Thus they display a variety of other concomitant problems. Blood and Seider (1981) noted that 68% of 1,060 children being treated for stuttering in elementary schools had other speech, language, hearing, or learning problems. Articulation

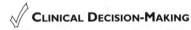 **CLINICAL DECISION-MAKING**

With so many assessment measures available (see also Appendix A) for adolescent and adult speakers, the clinician may wonder which one(s) would be the best to use. The most basic part of any assessment is the clinician's understanding of the client's behavioral and cognitive features of the person's problem, an understanding that can occur as we come to appreciate the client's story. That being said, the scores from formal measures do provide quantitative information that assist the clinician in supporting clinical decisions and verifying progress. Despite inconsistencies of scoring, these measures enable clinicians in different locations to be on "the same page" regarding the general severity and overall characteristics of clients. Of course, there is one measure that will do the job in every case. The utility of any measurement device will be influenced by such client characteristics as motivation, honesty, intellectual ability, and educational background. The choice of a scale will also be determined by the treatment strategy being used. For example, clinicians using a counseling-based therapy program are more likely to seek information about the speaker's locus of control or self-efficacy. On the other hand, clinicians using a behavioral program, emphasizing expansion of fluent intervals of speech, are likely to spend little or no time obtaining such information. Undoubtedly, many clinicians have their favorite scales and adopt measures that are not excessively time-consuming and relatively easy to administer.

disorders were the most frequently reported concomitant problem. Just how these other communication problems relate to the onset or maintenance of fluency disorders is unclear.

Although the large majority of people who stutter show one of the two major developmental patterns, there are other speakers with somewhat less common characteristics. The title of this text includes the words "fluency disorders" rather than the more typical "stuttering" because of the variety of speech and language disorders (other than stuttering) where disordered fluency is a characteristic. Although far less common than developmental stuttering, it is not unusual for clinicians to encounter clients with these atypical fluency problems. Of course, distinguishing these less common disorders of fluency from the more common developmental stuttering is a first step in the helping process.

Acquired Stuttering

The next two forms of fluency problems have often been referred to as "acquired stuttering" because they tend to appear for the first time long after the usual period of childhood developmental stuttering. Although far less common than developmental stuttering, more recent reports suggest that acquired neurogenic and psychogenic stuttering are probably more common than the earlier literature suggests. The speech-language pathologist plays a central role in the diagnostic process because of how speech and language problems reflect the overall health of the speaker. As Braumgartner (1999) and others suggest, the SLP is often able to detect the presence of neuropathology (including possible sites of lesion) as well as provide critical diagnostic evidence based on trial therapy.

As we will see, differential diagnosis of these forms of acquired stuttering can be difficult, not only because they are unusual in most clinical locations (with the exception of medical settings), but because they may occur together—particularly with neuropathologies related to closed head injuries and medications. In the following paragraphs we will discuss the characteristics of these forms of acquired stuttering, as well as speaker characteristics that assist the clinician in differentiating between the two.

Neurogenic Stuttering

The fluency problems of this group of people have been referred to as *organic stuttering* (Van Riper, 1982), *cortical stuttering* (Rosenbek, Messers, Collins, & Wertz, 1978), and *neurogenic stuttering* (Helm, Butler, & Canter, 1980; Silverman, 1992). Other terms such as *neurogenic acquired stuttering, acquired stuttering, neurological stuttering,* and *stuttering of sudden onset* have also appeared in the literature. Recently, Helm-Estabrooks suggested a definition that includes a new term:

Stuttering associated with acquired neurological disorders (SAAND) is an acquired or reacquired disorder of fluency characterized by notable, involuntary repetitions or prolongations of speech that are not the result of language formulation or psychiatric problems. (1999, p. 257)

In speakers with SAAND, stuttering is a result of injury to the central nervous system but is not associated with it. The onset may be sudden—following head trauma, strokes, cryosurgery, drug usage, or anoxia—or the symptoms may develop slowly—as in degenerative disorders, vascular disease, dementia, viral meningitis, or dialysis dementia (Helm, Butler, & Canter, 1980; Helm-Estabrooks, 1986). Neurogenic stuttering does not appear to be associated with a particular site of lesion. One or both hemispheres may be involved, although the left hemisphere appears to be the more likely to be implicated (Rosenbek, Messert, Collins, & Wertz, 1978). Findings by Van Borsel et al. (1998) and Fox et al. (1996) suggest the possible involvement of the supplementary motor area. Although there may be a variety of other language and speech disorders associated with these speakers (e.g., dysarthria, apraxia, and aphasia), Rosenbek et al. suggest that this form of stuttering need not accompany other speech or language problems.

The fluency breaks of these speakers are different in both number and type. Although these speakers stutter on an unusually high percentage (sometimes nearly all) of their syllables, they demonstrate relatively few secondary escape behaviors. The occurrence of stuttering tends to be consistent regardless of such factors as the speaking situation, time pressure, and grammatical complexity (Rao, 1991). Unlike developmental stuttering, fluency breaks occur not only on initial sounds and syllables, but also in medial and final positions of words: for example, "gre-e-en" and "sto-o-ore," although exceptions to this pattern have been reported (Van Borsel et al., 1998). Compared to developmental stutterers, who are more likely to have fluency breaks on content words, neurogenic stutterers are equally likely to stutter on function and content words. They do not show improved fluency with successive readings of a passage (referred to as the *adaptation effect*). While these speakers may be annoyed about their lack of speech fluency, they are not as likely to show the levels of anxiety or fear as the developmental stutterer. That is, compared to more typical persons who stutter, they share some of the same surface features but fewer of the intrinsic features. Another unique characteristic of these speakers is the lack of fluency that is likely to result from fluency-enhancing conditions that tend to immediately eliminate stuttering, such as choral speaking, rhythmic speech, singing, prolonged speech, whispering, and silent speech (Andrews et al., 1983). For example, Perkins (1973) noted that of over 100 people who stuttered, the only person who did not show a reduction in stuttering under such conditions was a woman who was later diagnosed as suffering from a neurological disorder.

Certainly this subcategory of individuals with fluency problems does not represent a homogeneous group, for there are wide varieties of speech characteristics, etiologies, and psychological and physiological influences—as well as speech-language disorders—associated with the stuttering. Partly because these patients are likely to have so many problems and partly because they are not typically referred to the speech-language pathologist, it appears that these speakers may be more common than is suggested by most of the literature (Helm, Butler, & Canter, 1980; Rosenbek, Messert, Collins, & Wertz, 1978).

Psychogenic Stuttering

There is convincing evidence indicating the clinical value of attending to self-concept and self-esteem, interpersonal interaction, and role changes if we are to assist people in becoming less handicapped by stuttering, especially if long-term success is our goal. Nevertheless, the large majority of people we assess for stuttering are fairly normal and do not differ psychologically from a matched group of nonstuttering speakers (Goodstein, 1958; Sheehan, 1958). However, there is a relatively uncommon subcategory of stuttering called *acquired psychogenic stuttering*.

As Van Riper (1979) suggested, only a handful of emotionally ill people come to us with the complaint of stuttering. To be sure, many of the people we will see are deeply troubled by what they correctly perceive as an extremely frustrating problem. The responses that provide avoidance and escape from the experience of stuttering moment are far from normal and can be neurotic and compulsive. However, as Van Riper (1982) suggests, these behaviors are most appropriately interpreted as a result of the fact that the person happens to be, for whatever reasons, someone who stutters. That is, these behaviors are not likely to be the symptoms of some deep-seated conflict. They are learned, often maladaptive responses to the fear of stuttering.

There are, however, some people with more pronounced emotional problems in any randomly selected group of people. Acquired psychogenic stuttering occurs with roughly equal frequency in men and women (Braumgartner & Duffy, 1997). In some instances, the client will have a history of emotional problems and may be currently receiving professional help for this condition. It is also important to note that, even in the absence of a serious and long-standing emotional problem, it is possible for people to experience a temporary reaction to the normal stresses of life and that—on occasion—disrupted fluency is a symptom. As Aronson (1992) suggests, speech and voice disorders may be caused by distress or "psychologic disequilibrium."

As one with considerable experience with acquired psychogenic stuttering, Baumgartner (1999) disagrees with the ASHA Special Interest Division technical paper (1999) which suggests that the term "psychogenic stuttering" should apply only to people who have been diagnosed with a psychopathology. He provides a convincing argument that, at least in many cases, such a diagnosis is not necessary for the speech-language pathologist to determine that a speech disorder is psychogenic. Furthermore, waiting to begin therapeutic intervention until a formal psychiatric diagnosis is forthcoming negates the valuable information that may be gained through trial therapy. Furthermore, as Baumgartner indicates, psychopathology is not always present in psychogenic stuttering: the symptoms may be a natural response to either the anticipation or the experience of life events.

As with organic stuttering, the onset of stuttering behavior is likely to be relatively sudden, and the person comes to us without any previous history of fluency problems. There may be, however, a history of psychological problems, neurological problems, or both (Baumgartner, 1999). Baumgartner and Duffy (1997) found that when a diagnosis of psychopathology does take place, the most common classifications are conversion reaction, anxiety, and depression. Other diagnostic categories were reactive depression, personality disorder, drug dependence, and posttraumatic neurosis, and some patients were placed into more than one category.

When acquired stuttering behaviors are first noticed, they tend to be well developed rather than showing the gradual increase in complexity and severity typically seen in children who stutter into adulthood. One of the more striking aspects of this form of fluency disorder is the stereotypical nature of the fluency breaks. Some people with psychogenic stuttering tend to "hold onto" their stuttering, in the sense that both the frequency and the form show little change, regardless of the speaking situation or speaking task. It is almost as though they have chosen a particular "brand" of stuttering and for a time, at least, that is the way they are going to speak. However, Baumgartner (1999) indicates that disfluencies may vary across speaking situations, certainly more than would be expected with neurogenic stuttering.

Another characteristic of both neurogenic and psychogenic stuttering is the lack of an adaptation effect. However, if stuttering becomes more severe with successive readings of a passage, it is a strong indicator of psychogenic stuttering (Braumgartner & Duffy, 1997). Typically, persons with acquired psychogenic stuttering are unable to achieve fluency even during such fluency-enhancing activities as unison speech, singing, speaking alone, or speaking with a unique rhythm, intensity, or dialect. In contrast—fluency—or at least nonstuttered speech—is relatively easy to elicit from even the most severe speakers with developmental stuttering.

Several years ago we had the opportunity to interview a woman in her early 30s who complained of a sudden onset of severe stuttering. Approximately three weeks prior to our assessment, she had been raped. One week following the attack, she lost her ability to speak, and when she began speaking again approximately three days later, she demonstrated well-developed stuttering. She reported no personal or family history of stuttering. At the time of the assessment interview, she was stuttering on nearly every word and showed a high level of anxiety. The frequency of her fluency breaks was uniform throughout the interview and consisted almost entirely of tense prolongations of whole words. We were unable to elicit any periods of fluent speech through using a variety of fluency-enhancing activities.

We also had the opportunity to interview a 41-one-year-old man who complained of a sudden onset of stuttering. As was the case with the woman described earlier, this man also had no previous history of fluency disorders. In this instance, however, there appeared to be no single traumatic event preceding the onset of his disrupted fluency. He had been receiving ongoing inpatient treatment at a local Veterans Administration hospital for a variety of emotional disorders for several years. We were also unable to get this man to produce fluent speech using a variety of fluency-enhancing activities. The frequency of his stuttering was consistent throughout the entire two-hour assessment interview. His fluency breaks consisted of relatively easy, one- and two-unit repetitions produced at the same rate as the rest of his speech, rather than at a relatively more rapid pace more characteristic of stuttering. Although he explained that he was very concerned about his fluency problem, he showed no struggle or tension during his fluency breaks, nor did he report any avoidances or fear associated with this problem. Perhaps the most interesting aspect of his stuttering was the way he watched listeners as he stuttered. He constantly maintained eye contact, and while we cannot say for sure that he "enjoyed" watching his listeners for their reactions, he clearly did not appear embarrassed or upset by his disfluency. He appeared to remain detached from his stuttering, sometimes smiling as he both stuttered and closely watched the interviewer. As with the woman, it was apparent to us that stuttering was not his most important problem—a characteristic response that the clinician is likely to have when interviewing such clients. However, while the woman's speech seemed to indicate a somewhat temporary emotional reaction to a specific trauma, this man's speech appeared to be one of many symptoms related to a more general and longer-term emotional problem.

Distinguishing Between Neurogenic and Psychogenic Stuttering

Determining whether a client who experiences the sudden onset of stuttering is an example of neurogenic or psychogenic stuttering is one of the more difficult diagnostic decisions a clinician can face. There is considerable overlap between the symptoms for both etiologies, as noted by Baumgartner and Duffy (1997), and the two groups of patients cannot be distinguished based only on the nature of the fluency breaks (Helm-Estabrooks, 1999; Brumgartner, 1999). In a retrospective study of 69 patients diagnosed at the Mayo Clinic for *psychogenic* stuttering, 20 patients were found to have confirmed neurologic disease. One potentially helpful fact is that many more cases of neurogenic stuttering have been reported in the literature than psychogenic stuttering (Helm-Estabrooks & Hotz, 1998). These authors report that since 1978, over 50 cases of neurogenic stuttering have been described. To complicate this clinical decision, however, is the fact that neurological trauma—a known cause of neurogenic stuttering—is often accompanied by psychological trauma, a proposed cause of psychogenic stuttering.

While obtaining case history is always an important first step for the assessment of any communication problem, it is particularly important in the assessment of these forms of acquired stuttering. Helm-Estabrooks (1999) indicates that the first step in diagnosing SAAND is ruling out aphasia using a standardized exam. Depending on the etiology of SAAND, there may also be other memory, attention, or cognitive problems that will impact diagnostic and treatment decisions. Following assessments of these abilities, the clinician may then consider whether the client has any of the following characteristics commonly associated with neurogenic stuttering described by Helm-Estabrooks, (1993, 1999). Finally, there are additional diagnostic decisions that will influence the efficacy of treatment, such as whether or not the person's stuttering presents a significant communication handicap, is the person motivated to take part in a speech rehabilitation program, and whether the patient has a rapidly progressing neurological disorder (Helm-Estabrooks, 1999).

 CLINICAL DECISION-MAKING

Six Features of Patients with Neurogenic Stuttering

1. Fluency breaks are produced on grammatical as well as substantive words.

2. The speaker may appear annoyed but does not appear anxious about the stuttering.

3. Repetitions, prolongations, and blocks are not restricted to initial syllables.

4. Secondary symptoms such as facial grimacing, eye blinking, and fist clenching are rarely associated with the fluency breaks.

5. Fluency does not improve with repeated readings of a passage (adaptation effect).

6. The patient stutters regardless of the nature of the speech task.

Baumgartner (1999) recommends a very careful and systematic "psychologic interview" process in order to determine events that may indicate a temporal relationship between the patient's speech problems, evidence of CNS impairment, and sources of emotional stress in the person's life. Baumgartner suggests that the clinician look for possible patterns of unexplained problems and communication difficulties in the near or distant past. In order to achieve this goal, it is critical that the clinician approach this interview by creating a setting that allows the client to describe these events as well as their reaction to them. As Baumgartner describes:

> The skilled interviewer creates an atmosphere that encourages and supports discussions of feelings, fears, and information not previously disclosed (very possibly to anyone). It is not enough to find out what has happened in an individual's life. The truly successful interview explores how people feel about these things, how they have dealt with them, and whether they would "really like" to do something else about them. (p. 272)

If the clinician is able to create such an exchange of information and the speaker is experiencing acquired psychogenic stuttering, speech fluency is likely to show an immediate change, either by becoming more or less severe. In some cases, stuttering may disappear (Baumgartner, 1999). This is usually taken as a clear diagnostic sign: "Symptom resolution, or a marked disclosure of emotionally sensitive information, is powerful evidence in support of psychogenicity and argues strongly against organicity" (Baumgartner, 1999, p. 272). Clearly such an approach lays the groundwork for subsequent treatment and counseling activities.

Baumgartner (1999) also suggests a series of tasks to further define the nature of the problem with these speakers. Ruling out the possibility of apraxia of speech, nonverbal apraxia as well as dysphagia should occur early in assessment. In addition, the possibility of coexisting neurogenic communication disorders should be considered. The quantity and form of fluency breaks has little etiological value, since these closely parallel those in speakers with developmental stuttering. Although disfluencies are more variable than those of neurogenic speakers, a pattern of worsening of symptoms during the performance of *less difficult speaking tasks* are a clear sign of psychogenicity. In addition, bizarre (non-compensatory) movements that are *unrelated to speech production* are a sign of psychogenicity.

Baumgartner and Duffy (1997) provide several additional features that usually distinguish these patients (see following page).

Cluttering

A final form of fluency disorder that we will discuss is *cluttering*. The term itself distinguishes such speakers from the groups of people who stutter that we have discussed previously. The term also provides a

---

✓ **CLINICAL DECISION-MAKING**

Four Features of Patients with Psychogenic Stuttering

1. The patient often shows rapid and favorable response to just one or two sessions of behavioral treatment.

2. The patient shows (sometimes bizarre) struggle behaviors and other signs of anxiety.

3. There may be intermittent or situation-specific episodes of stuttering.

4. The speaker produces unusual grammatical constructions, e.g. "Me get sick." And bizarre speech, such as multiple repetitions of nearly all phonemes with simultaneous head bobbing, facial grimaces, and tremor-like movements.

---

functional description of the speech and language abilities of these individuals: their language and speech are cluttered and chaotic. Their speech is difficult to understand—sometimes unintelligible—not so much because of the fluency breaks but because the speech is so unorganized, mispronounced, and often produced at an extremely rapid rate (a condition known as *tachylalia*). In addition, these speakers tend to include words that are out of place, superfluous or meaningless—termed *maze behaviors* by Loban (1976). An underlying but key feature that seems to pervade all aspects of expressive language, including both speech and writing, is a nearly complete unawareness of the problem. It is not unusual for clients to deny the presence of this problem that is so apparent to listeners and fail to understand why someone would request that they seek help.

For years, cluttering has been discussed in the European literature (Weiss, 1964). Following a 30-year lapse of interest in this complex communication disorder throughout the world, there was a renewal of interest in the 1990s (Daly, 1992, 1993; Daly & Burnett, 1999; Myers & St. Louis, 1992; Silverman, 1992; St. Louis, 1986; St. Louis & Myers, 1995). Because we tend to find what we are looking for, and because few clinicians have been looking for people with symptoms of cluttering, few clients have been identified by speech-language pathologists. However, as awareness is increasing, more people with this syndrome are being discovered. As Daly suggested in 1986, clinicians in this country are beginning to consider cluttering as a clinical entity, and the problem is beginning to receive more attention. In 1992 Daly reported that approximately 5% of the clients he had seen for treatment for over 20 years demonstrated a pure form of cluttering—without features characteristic of stuttering. When he tabulated those clients who showed a combination of both cluttering and stuttering features, the occurrence increased to 35 to 40%.

Several definitions of this disorder have been offered that emphasize slightly different views of the etiological and behavioral aspects of the problem. All authors agree that the problem is complex and involves many aspects of perception, learning, and expression (both verbal and written). Weiss (1964, 1967) considered cluttering to be the consequence of a central language imbalance that affected all language modalities. Luchsinger and Arnold (1965) described cluttering as an inability to formulate language, with associated organic, familial, and aphasic-like symptoms. St. Louis and Rustin (1992) describe the problem as a speech-language disorder, characterized by abnormal fluency that is *not* stuttering and a speech rate that is rapid, irregular, or both. The definition found in the American Psychiatric Association's *Diagnostic and Statistical Manual of Mental Disorders, Third Edition-Revised* (DSM-III-R) (1987) states:

> The essential feature of Cluttering is a disturbance of fluency involving an abnormally rapid rate and erratic rhythm of speech that impedes intelligibility. Faulty phrasing patterns are usually present so that there are bursts of speech consisting of groups of words that are not related to the grammatical structure of the sentence. The affected person is usually unaware of any communication impairment. (pp. 85–86)

Finally, Daly (1992) provides a behavioral description that includes the most basic features of the problem:

> Cluttering is a disorder of speech and language processing resulting in rapid, dysrhythmic, sporadic, unorganized, and frequently unintelligible speech. Accelerated speech is not always present, but an impairment in formulating language almost always is. (Daly, 1992, p. 107)

Of the groups of people who stutter that we have discussed, clutterers appear to be most like the neurogenic stutterers, in that a pattern of "organicity" runs through the constellation of behavioral symptoms. Weiss (1964) and Arnold (1960) suggest a genetic basis for the disorder. In addition, several authors have pointed out that the symptoms have much in common with learning disabilities (Daly, 1986; St. Louis & Hinzman, 1986; Tiger, Irvine, & Reiss, 1980).

Extensive lists of cluttering features have been provided by Weiss (1964) and St. Louis and Hinzman (1986). A review of the literature by St. Louis and Hinzman (1986) resulted in a list of 65 different characteristics. Many of these listed features overlap with one another and tend to provide a confusing picture of the receptive and expressive problems that characterize these clients. In addition, although there are many key differences, there also are many similarities between the behavior of people who clutter and those who stutter.

However, there are certain distinguishing characteristics that tend to be unique to people who clutter. Daly (1992) suggests five basic features that describe the essence of the disorder:

➤ excessive rate of speaking
➤ inattention to grammatical details
➤ delayed speech and language development
➤ poor reading comprehension
➤ unorganized writing

Daly and Burnett (1999) stated that they have yet to evaluate a person who clutters who did not exhibit at least one disturbance in each of the following five dimensions:

1. Cognitive—People who clutter demonstrate a near-total lack of awareness of their inability to communicate. They characteristically have poor self-monitoring abilities, inadequate thought organization, poor attention span, verbal and nonverbal impulsivity, and show signs of perceptual deficits (auditory or visual processing or poor auditory memory).
2. Language—These individuals show some form of language difficulties that are expessive, receptive, or both. This may be related to their poor auditory memory, attention deficits, and inability to concentrate. They are often poor readers and show little interest in music and literature.
3. Pragmatics—Clutterers are notoriously poor at turn-taking as well as the introduction, maintenance, and termination of topics. In addition, they fail to recognize subtle nonverbal signs indicating turn-taking, and lack of interest or attention.
4. Speech—The fluency breaks of people who clutter are characterized by irregular rate, accelerations, sporadic bursts of speech, variable intensity, and overall poor rhythm. Some fluency breaks are typical of stuttering. Daly and Burnett (1999) also report the occurrence of transpositions such as "The Lord is a shoving leopard."
5. Motor—People who clutter tend to be clumsy and uncoordinated and demonstrate impulsive motor movements. The client may appear to be physically immature. Lack of coordination also may be reflected in the poor legibility of handwriting, which tends to disintegrate during the writing of a paragraph. There is often a lack of ability to imitate a simple rhythm or to sing.

These characteristics are presented as major components of a "linguistic disfluency model" provided in Figure 4-7. Linguistic disfluency is characterized by Daly and Burnett (1999) as "frequent verbal revisions

Cluttering

Cognition	Language	Pragmatics	Speech	Motor
Awareness - listener perspective - self-monitoring Attention span Thought organization - sequencing - categorization Memory Impulsivity	Receptive - listening/directions - reading disorder Expressive—Verbal - thought organization - poor sequence of ideas - poor story telling - language formulation - revisions and repetitions - improper linguistic structure - syllabic or verbal transpositions - improper pronoun use - dysnomia/word finding - filler words, empty words Expressive—Written - run-on sentences - omissions and transpositions of letters, syllables, and words - sentence fragments	Inappropriate topic introduction, maintenance, termination Inappropriate turn-taking Poor listening skills; impulsive responses Lack of consideration of listener perspective Inadequate processing of non-verbal signals Verbose or tangential Poor eye contact	Speech disfluency - excessive repetition of words/phrases Syllabic or verbal transpositions Prosody of speech - rate (rapid or irregular) - poor rhythm - loud, trail off - lacks pauses between words - vocal monotony Slurred articulation - omit sound(s) - omit syllable(s) - /r/ and /l/ Dysrhythmic breathing Silent gaps/hesitations	Poor motor control Slurred articulation Dysrhythmic breathing Speech disfluencies, - excessive repetitions of sounds or words Silent gaps, hesitations Prosody problems - rate (rapid or irregular) - poor rhythm Clumsy, uncoordinated Poor penmanship Impulsivity

Figure 4-7. The Linguistic disfluency model for individuals who clutter, indicating possible impairments across five broad communicative dimensions. [From Daly, D. A. & Burnett, M. L. (1997). Cluttering: Traditional views and new perspectives. In R. Curlee (Ed.), *Stuttering and Related Disorders of Fluency* (2nd Edition, pp. 222–254). New York: Thieme Medical Publishers, Inc.] Reprinted with permission.

and interjections, excessive repetitions of words or phrases, poorly organized thoughts, lack of cohesion in discourse, and prosodic irregularities" (p. 226).

Given that the problem involves the inability to process language, it is not surprising that the writing of people who clutter tends to be disorganized and illegible. Daly (1986) recommends procedures for obtaining written writing samples during the diagnostic interview and suggests (1992) that seeing cluttering in written form exemplifies the problem. Williams and Wener (1996) describe the handwriting of a young man in his 20s who was diagnosed with both stuttering and cluttering behaviors. His writing was composed of simple declarative sentences with short, simple words. Of 148 words, 54 were stricken due to grammatical errors or misspellings. Legibility was poor and there were many punctuation errors, particularly misused commas.

Both during writing and in speaking, these clients seem to lack the ability to attend to the details of a task; indeed, this is reflected in all aspects of their expressive communication. It appears that they are taking a gestalt view of communication; they have difficulty, for example, describing individual aspects of an activity or event. Only with concentrated effort are they able to attend to the individual words or punctuation on a page of text. Their oral reading sounds as though they were demonstrating speed-reading aloud: it is as if they were attempting to produce the entire page of text in a single utterance. Their speech tends to be explosive. The speaker may begin with rapid bursts and louder than normal intensity at the outset of an utterance and conclude with a murmur. In addition, the already rapid rate of speaking often accelerates as they produce longer sentences (Daly, 1986).

To the listener, the initial and most prominent feature of cluttering is often a rapid rate of speech. The speaker seems to be in a hurry—even driven—often displaying a compulsive and tense behavior. There are few if any pauses between words or sentences: the punctuation is disregarded. The speaker pauses only long enough to take a breath—and then only because he must breathe—and then moves swiftly onward. Sounds and syllables are omitted, seemingly as a function of the urgency to produce the utterance. Sounds are sometimes added and misarticulated, particularly /r/ and /l/ (Daly, 1993). Although the fluency breaks are a prominent feature, they appear to be the result of the speaker's rapid rate of speaking rather than an attempt to avoid moments of stuttering. Finally, the tense and compulsive demeanor may also be the case even when the person is not speaking.

The intrinsic features of the person who stutters—which include loss of control, helplessness, and fear—do not appear to be operating here. In fact, as previous mentioned, a primary characteristic of the disorder is the speaker's unawareness that there is any problem at all (Bloodstein, 1987; Daly, 1992; Weiss, 1964). Unawareness does tend to be a characteristic of pure cluttering. It is important to point out, however, that for those clients who appear to present a combination of both cluttering and stuttering symptoms, fear of specific sounds and words as well as avoidance behavior may be present, making it more difficult to distinguish between stuttering and cluttering.

As we have indicated, individuals diagnosed as clutterers and those diagnosed as stutterers have several features in common. In fact, as we have indicated, there are a number of speakers who display both stuttering and cluttering characteristics (Daly, 1986; St. Louis and Hinzman, 1986). This combination of speech behaviors occurs most often in children (Bloodstein, 1987). Indeed, Weiss (1964) suggested that stuttering often is the result of the child's attempts to stop cluttering. However, while whole-word and phrase repetitions are present in the speech of people who clutter, the majority of the breaks take the form of rapid repetitions of one-syllable words and the first sound or syllable of polysyllabic words. Moreover, in contrast to the fluency breaks of people who stutter, for those who clutter, there does not seem to be greater tension associated with the repetitions than is already occurring during their nonrepeated speech.

When the overall patterns of speech, affective behavior, and cognitive nature of the client are considered, the differences between these two groups of speakers become even more obvious. The clutterer's tendency to be unaware of his problem is perhaps most unique. In fact, to the degree that a person who clutters becomes aware of his problem, he is likely to deny any abnormalities in his speech. This response, along with other personality characteristics, makes these clients difficult to work with. They tend to be intolerant of interruptions (Van Riper, 1992b), particularly suggestions to monitor their production, an essential ingredient of treatment strategies. In addition, they may have immature responses, a short temper, and a history of emotional problems. As Daly (1992, 1993) points out, they provide a challenge to our ability and especially our patience.

Another difference between these fluency problems will become apparent during a short period of trial therapy. People who stutter, especially early in treatment, typically have more fluency breaks when asked to monitor their speech. The more attention that people who stutter pay to how they are speaking, the more difficulty they are likely to have. On the other hand, if people who clutter are able to monitor how they are speaking, there is often an immediate improvement. In most cases, as long as they monitor their output, they are able to speak slowly, clearly, and without fluency breaks, even when under communicative pressure. The problem is that their ability to closely monitor their production is short-lived and usually can be maintained for only a few minutes. Much of the treatment for cluttering centers on getting the speaker to monitor his speech production. The person who stutters, on the other hand, must learn to not only monitor but also to modify his behavior.

A final difference between people who clutter and whose who stutter concerns the disrupted flow of information in the speech of clutterers. For people who clutter, sound may be flowing, albeit at an excessive rate. However, information flow is absent, or nearly so. The information is disorganized, and speech is characterized by hesitations, repetitions, use of poor grammar, and a profound lack of smooth and flowing muscular coordination. They demonstrate word-finding difficulties consistent with problems in formulating language. Daly and Burnett (1999) provide examples of transpositions such as "at this plant in time/at this point in time" and "taking/talking." Although it is certainly the case that people who stutter sometimes demonstrate what appear to be word-finding difficulties, this behavior is often a form of word avoidance, substitution, circumlocution, or recoil behavior, as they back away from feared words or pause as they pretend to think of the word.

It is likely that a greater awareness of all the various forms of fluency disorders would result in a greater proportion of people who stutter falling into these categories of "atypical stuttering." While such speakers compose a relatively small percentage of the total population of people with fluency problems, it is important to identify them in order that the most appropriate intervention strategy be initiated.

Daly and Burnett (1999) provide a revised 36-item checklist for the Identification Cluttering (Figure 4-8). Based on their earlier 33-item list (Daly & Burnett, 1996), they suggest that a score of 35–55 indicates cluttering-stuttering, and a score of 55 or higher indicates a diagnosis of cluttering. Each of the 36 items is rated on a four-point scale by ranking to what degree each feature is characteristic of a speaker (0 = not at all; 1 = just a little; 2 = pretty much; 3 = very much).

Because of the large number of language problems these speakers present with, it will be necessary to obtain a wide range of information from individuals suspected of cluttering. Evaluations commonly include assessment of attention, auditory processing, and motor and educational characteristics.

Spasmodic Dysphonia as a Fluency Disorder?

Finally, although not typically classified as a disorder of fluency, there have been a few authors who have suggested that spasmodic or "spastic" dysphonia (SD) and stuttering share some of the same characteristics. Because of these similarities, Silverman (1996), in his text *Stuttering and Other Fluency Disorders,* includes comments concerning the etiology, diagnosis, and treatment for this unique and complex disorder. In an earlier publication, Silverman and Hummer (1989) proposed that SD should be classified as a disorder of fluency rather than voice.

Spasmodic dysphonia is a disorder of laryngeal motor control and has received increased interest by researchers in recent years. SD is a poorly understood disorder of laryngeal motor control affecting speech production. (Comprehensive descriptions of this problem are found in Aronson, 1992; Brodnitz, 1976; and Cannito, 1991). Because of the uncertainty about the etiology as well as the unique characteristics of this disorder, there is debate over whether it should be classified as a fluency disorder.

The most obvious aspect of the disorder is reflected in the spasmodic functioning of the vocal folds. The speaker's speech is characterized by abductor or adductor spasms that result in a breathy, effortful, and

Client's Name _____ Date _____

Instructions: Please respond to each descriptive statement below. Your answer should reflect how accurately you believe the statement is true for the client.

Statement True for Client	Not at all	Just a little	Pretty much	Very much
1. Repeats words or phrases	0	1	2	3
2. Started talking late; onset of words and sentences delayed	0	1	2	3
3. Never very fluent; fluency disruptions started early	0	1	2	3
4. Language is disorganized; confused wording	0	1	2	3
5. Silent gaps or hesitations common	0	1	2	3
6. Interjections; many filler words	0	1	2	3
7. Little or no tension observed during disfluencies	0	1	2	3
8. Rapid rate (tachylalia) or irregular rate; speaks in spurts	0	1	2	3
9. Compulsive talker; verbose or tangential	0	1	2	3
10. Respiratory dysrhythmia; jerky breathing pattern	0	1	2	3
11. Slurred articulation (deletes, adds, or distorts speech sounds)	0	1	2	3
12. Speech better under pressure (during periods of heightened attention)	0	1	2	3
13. Difficulty following directions; impatient/disinterested listener	0	1	2	3
14. Distractible, attention span problems, poor concentration	0	1	2	3
15. Poor language formulation; storytelling difficulty; trouble sequencing ideas	0	1	2	3
16. Demonstrates word-finding difficulties resembling anomia	0	1	2	3
17. Inappropriate pronoun referents; overuse of pronouns	0	1	2	3
18. Improper linguistic structure; poor grammar and syntax	0	1	2	3
19. Clumsy and uncoordinated, motor activities accelerated or hasty, impulsive	0	1	2	3
20. Reading disorder or difficulty reported or noted	0	1	2	3
21. Disintegrated and fractionated writing; poor motor control	0	1	2	3
22. Writing shows omission or transposition of letters, syllables, or words	0	1	2	3

Figure 4-8. Checklist for Identification of Cluttering-Revised [Daly, D. A. & Burnett, M. L. (1997). Cluttering: Traditional views and new perspectives. In R. Curlee (Ed.), *Stuttering and Related Disorders of Fluency* (2nd Edition, pp. 222–254). New York: Thieme Medical Publishers, Inc.] Reprinted with permission.

Statement True for Client

	Not at all	Just a little	Pretty much	Very much
23. Initial loud voice, trails off to a murmur; mumbles	0	1	2	3
24. Seems to verbalize prior to adequate thought formulation	0	1	2	3
25. Above average in mathematical and abstract reasoning abilities	0	1	2	3
26. Poor rhythm, timing, or musical ability (may dislike singing)	0	1	2	3
27. Variable prosody; improper/irregular melody or stress patterns in speaking	0	1	2	3
28. Appears, acts or sounds younger than age; immature	0	1	2	3
29. Other family member(s) with similar speech problem(s)	0	1	2	3
30. Untidy, careless, or forgetful; impatient, superficial, short-tempered	0	1	2	3
31. Lack of awareness of self and/or communication disorder(s)	0	1	2	3
32. Inappropriate turn-taking	0	1	2	3
33. Inappropriate topic introduction/maintenance/termination	0	1	2	3
34. Poor recognition or acknowledgement of non-verbal signals	0	1	2	3
35. Telescopes or condenses words (omits or transposes syllables)	0	1	2	3
36. Lack of effective/sufficient self-monitoring	0	1	2	3

DIAGNOSIS _____   TOTAL SCORE _____

Clinician _____

Figure 4-8. Continued

strained vocal quality (sometimes associated with vocal tremor). The laryngospasms correspond perceptually to severe abnormalities of voice quality, prosody, and fluency (Aronson, Brown, Litin, & Pearson, 1968; Wolfe, Ratusnik, & Feldman, 1979). Because of vocal stoppages and the tremor activity, spasmodic dysphonia has been likened to "laryngeal stuttering" or "stammering of the vocal cords" (Aronson, 1973; Luchsinger & Arnold, 1965; McCall, 1974; Salamy & Sessions, 1980). For example, Aronson (1978) described the speech of people with SD as "staccato or stuttering-like, intermittent, jerky, grunting, squeezed, groaning, and effortful" (p. 533). On the other hand, Ludlow, Naunton, and Basich (1984) suggested that the disfluency characteristics of SD speakers represent a disorder separate from spastic dysphonia.

Based on perceptual judgments of naïve listeners, Silverman and Hummer (1989) proposed that spasmodic dysphonia be reclassified as a fluency disorder rather than a voice disorder. On the other hand, Cannito and Sherrard (1995) used traditional clinical measures to determine rate and fluency characteristics of 20 adult females diagnosed with spasmodic dysphonia. Although these subjects, on average, spoke significantly more slowly and produced more fluency breaks than a matched group of normal speakers, they exhibited a wide range of fluency phenomena. Cannito and Sherrard concluded on the basis of their data that the observed differences in fluency were but one associated feature among of a group of heterogeneous symptoms. In addition, the distribution of fluency breaks exhibited by their subjects was uncharacteristic of stuttering, in that part-word repetitions were often in syllable-final position, and prolongations occurred not only within syllables but also between syllables and words. These authors indicated that spasmodic dysphonia is easily differentiated from traditional stuttering. Their findings coincide with those of Salamy and Sessions (1990), who also concluded that spasmodic dysphonia and stuttering are distinctively different disorders.

More recently, Cannito, Burch, Watts, Rappold, Hood and Sherrard (1997) used a visual analog scaling method for judging speech characteristics of 20 adult female speakers with SD and a matched group of controls. These authors concluded that disfluency is a common characteristic of many speakers with SD and that it was a significant determinant of clinician's ratings of severity. Disfluency was not, however, a defining feature of the disorder for all speakers with SD.

One final similarity between stuttering and spasmodic dysphonia is the use of botulinum toxin injections to relax the vocal folds. Used with some success for patients with spasmodic dysphonia, such injections have also been suggested for enhancing the fluency of individuals who stutter (Brin, Stewart, Blitzer, & Diamond, 1994; Ludlow, 1990; Stager & Ludlow, 1994). The effect of these "biotox" injections is to paralyze the muscle and thereby reduce laryngeal tension, a condition that has often been associated with airflow and fluency. Although short-term fluency enhancement has been demonstrated (Ludlow, 1990; Brin et al., 1994), Stager and Ludlow (1994) found that 19 adult participants with chronic stuttering did not benefit from the injections. Furthermore, as described in Chapter 2, while there are instances where increased laryngeal tension is associated with stuttering events, there is little support for the assumption that excess laryngeal tension plays a primary role in causing stuttering.

CONCLUSION

Because of the developmental nature of stuttering, its occurrence in adolescents and adults is typically much more obvious than it is in younger children. Generally—but not always—the problem becomes more severe with age, as the speaker enters into more competitive speaking situations in educational, social, and work-related settings. Nevertheless, the variability of fluency and associated responses across speaking situations remain a hallmark of developmental stuttering. For most speakers, assessment is an ongoing procedure that is likely to continue well into the initial stages of the treatment process.

The severity of stuttering, as indicated by such surface features as frequency, duration, tension, and avoidance, usually fails to indicate the full extent of the problem as experienced by the speaker. Thus, the clinician's sensitivity for determining and appreciating the features of the problem that are under the surface—such as the client's helplessness and loss of control associated with the stuttering experience—is crucial. Much of the disability and handicap of the disorder is manifested by these features of the problem. Most assessment devices tend to focus on the surface features of stuttering, although some assessment tools are available for determining the speaker's response to his situation. Analyzing the quality of the client's nonstuttered speech is also important, for it may be smooth and easy or characterized by many elements of instability. Finally, an assessment of the speaker's motivation and readiness for change is crucial for the success of what is likely to be, at the very least, an arduous adventure.

Atypical fluency disorders present a somewhat rare and unique challenge to the clinician. Neurogenic and psychogenic stuttering are primarily characterized by sudden onset later in life and stereotypical patterns of fluency breaks. However, the differentiation of these two forms of fluency disorders can be difficult. In addition, although pure stuttering and cluttering are different in many respects, a significant number of speakers appear to demonstrate the characteristics of both disorders. The majority of the differences between stuttering and spasmodic dysphonia suggests that these two problems are distinctly different problems.

STUDY QUESTIONS

➤ How does the variability of stuttering make it difficult to obtain a valid assessment of stuttering?

➤ How does the variability of stuttering affect both the listener and the speaker?

➤ What are examples of the intrinsic features of the stuttering experience?

➤ Prepare several sentences that you can ask as you telephone at least 15 commercial establishments. Conduct all the telephone calls in one session. Perform realistic stuttering with moderate repetitions and prolongations in selected words as you have rehearsed. Make notes of listener responses as well as your cognitive and emotional reactions to the experience.

➤ Prepare a list of questions you will ask at local establishments. With a colleague, take turns stuttering with moderate repetitions and prolongations and mild-to-moderate physical struggle behavior with at least 20 people. Make notes of listener responses—see if you are able to elicit "The Look." Note also your cognitive and emotional reactions (including avoidance behavior).

➤ What are examples of things that people who stutter often avoid? Make a list of activities, people, and situations you avoid.

➤ What are the steps for taking a client through the process of self-assessment and trial therapy as described in Figure 4-1?

➤ What can you do to determine a client's level of motivation?

➤ What are at least three basic characteristics of acquired neurogenic and acquired psychogenic stuttering?

➤ How can you distinguish between acquired neurogenic and psychogenic stuttering? What activities would you ask a client to do in order to distinguish between these two forms of acquired stuttering?

➤ Why is cluttering viewed as a broad-based linguistic disfluency (see Figure 4-8)?

➤ What are at least five basic characteristics of someone who displays the classic signs of cluttering?

➤ Explain why you think that spasmodic dysphonia should (or should not be) classified as a fluency disorder.

RECOMMENDED READINGS

Baumgartner, J. M. (1999). Acquired Psychogenic Stuttering. In R. Curlee (Ed.), *Stuttering and Related Disorders of Fluency* (2nd Edition, pp. 269–288). New York: Thieme Medical Publishers, Inc.

Corcoran, J. A., & Stewart, M. (1998). Stories of stuttering: A qualitative analysis of interview narratives. *Journal of Fluency Disorders, 23,* 247-264.

Daly, D. A., & Burnett, M. L. (1999). Cluttering: Traditional views and new perspectives. In R. Curlee (Ed.), *Stuttering and Related Disorders of Fluency* (2nd Edition, pp. 222–254). New York: Thieme Medical Publishers, Inc.

Helm-Estabrooks, N. (1999). Stuttering associated with acquired neurological disorders. In R. Curlee (Ed.), *Stuttering and Related Disorders of Fluency* (2nd Edition, pp. 255–268). New York: Thieme Medical Publishers, Inc.

St. Louis, K. O. (Ed.). (1996a). Research and opinion on cluttering: State of the art and science. *Journal of Fluency Disorders, 3-4.*

CHAPTER

5

ASSESSING FLUENCY DISORDERS IN CHILDREN

> *I think that inside my mouth there is something wrong with me. And that is why I'm going to speech therapy to help my speaking. I have to take my time and be brave. I think my body is ready to talk but my mouth isn't. If I take my time I think I will be all right. But it is very hard because I want to be like everybody else. It's hard being different from everyone else. I'm lucky that I have such supportive parents and friends to help me get through my problem. I've learned that real friends do listen and I love them for it.*
>
> Lester L., 10 (nearly 11), Philadelphia, PA

PRELIMINARIES TO ASSESSMENT WITH CHILDREN

The majority of people who stutter begin to do so during the early childhood years, at any time from the preschool period—when children begin to produce combinations of words—to the point where they are about to enter formal schooling. Until recently, the onset and development of stuttering was thought to be gradual, and for most children this is the case. That is, when first noticed—usually by the parents—the breaks in the child's fluency are characterized by brief and relatively easy repetitions and slight prolongations. Then over the next several months or years these fluency disruptions gradually become longer and are associated with greater awareness and struggle behavior. However, as discussed in

Chapter 3 and in this chapter, there are also a significant number of children who, at the outset of their stuttering, present with markedly overt fluency disruptions and high levels of struggle.

Making use of the suggested criteria for distinguishing usual from unusual fluency breaks described in the previous chapters, the clinician must first make a judgment about the nature of the child's fluency and whether or not it is within reasonably normal limits. As a result of clinical research and subsequent refinements in clinical practice, clinicians have be able to increase their ability to distinguish children who are stuttering from those who are not (Conture, 1997). However, because there is no absolute standard for differentiating normal from pathological levels or types of fluency breaks, this judgment can be somewhat tenuous. Further complicating this question is the natural variability of fluency in a young child as well as indications that fluency and acceptance of disfluencies vary considerably across cultures (Cooper & Cooper, 1993; Culatta & Goldberg, 1995; Van Riper, 1971).

Because children are in the process of maturing neurologically, physiologically, emotionally, and linguistically, they tend to have greater variability of performance for all behaviors, including speech and language. This is unquestionably the case for speech fluency. A few authors have found that nonstuttering children do not tend to show much variability in fluency across speaking situations (Martin, Haroldson, & Kuhl, 1972a,b; Wexler, 1982). On the other hand, the variable nature of fluency in young speakers who do stutter has been frequently demonstrated and discussed (Bloodstein, 1995; Conture, 1990; Starkweather, 1987; Van Riper, 1982; Yaruss, 1997a). Such variability suggests some good news and some bad news. The good news is that because it is generally easier to change behavior that is variable and relatively new, treatment is likely to be successful (Starkweather, 1992, 1999; Starkweather, Gottwald, & Halfond, 1990). The bad news is that this same variability can make obtaining a valid sample of fluency more complicated than it is with older speakers.

If the clinician concludes that the child's fluency breaks are unusual or abnormal, she will then need to make a second, even more difficult decision: Will these abnormal fluency breaks be a temporary or a permanent characteristic of the child's speech? Conture (1997) concludes that while clinicians may be reasonably good at identifying abnormal or stutter-like fluency breaks, they are not particularly good at predicting whether or not a child will continue to stutter or the possible benefit of intervention. Given this uncertainty about the chronicity of stuttering, the clinician will need to devise a response that—depending on such factors as the child's age, length of time since onset, family history of stuttering, cognitive development, and language and speech performance—will range from informal monitoring of the child's speech to formal and direct therapeutic intervention.

Before discussing the details of the diagnostic process with young children, it is important to appreciate that this initial meeting with the child and the parents is the first opportunity for the clinician to show her understanding about both the general nature of stuttering and the impact it can have on the child and his family. This is the first chance for her to begin making the problem less mysterious, to respond to some of the myths or misinformation that the family may associate with the problem, to alleviate the feelings of guilt that usually accompany stuttering, and to begin to provide an overview about the direction of treatment. As Conture (1997) suggests, the clinician's ability to orientate the family to the true nature of the problem may be the main benefit that the child and the family receive from the diagnostic meeting(s).

DECISION 1: DETERMINING WHETHER OR NOT THE CHILD IS STUTTERING

Eliciting Fluency Breaks

During the assessment of children, there will be occasions when the very behaviors the clinician wants to observe and evaluate are not present. Although this also may occur during the assessment of adults who stutter, it is more often the case with children. On the day and time of the evaluation, the child may fail to exhibit the behaviors that concern the parents or the teacher.

On such occasions the clinician may choose to elicit these behaviors. That is, the clinician assessing the young child must be prepared to introduce various forms of communicative stress during the assessment. She must be uninhibited enough and unafraid of stuttering in order to elicit these fluency breaks. Moreover, she must understand that by eliciting such breaks, she is not going to hurt the child. Furthermore, minimal examples are all that are usually required. Of course, as it becomes necessary to elicit fluency breaks from children in this fashion, parents or others who may be observing the evaluation should be informed of the purpose and intention of these activities so they will have an understanding of what is taking place.

There are many benign techniques the clinician may use to elicit fluency breaks in children. Essentially, what we are doing is creating a speaking situation where, temporarily at least, the demands we are placing on the child exceed his ability to use his speech production system. The clinician may, for example, turn away as the child is describing an event or activity. Loss of the listener's attention has long been known as a powerful technique for eliciting fluency breaks in children (Johnson, 1962; Van Riper, 1982). The clinician may ask the child to respond quickly to a series of questions or ask him to answer somewhat abstract or difficult-to-answer queries (Guitar & Peters, 1980), such as, "How far is it from here to your home and how do you get there?" "What does your mother (or father) do when they go to work?" Depending on the age of the child, he or she could be asked to read from books that are somewhat above his grade level (Blood & Hood, 1978) or asked to describe a series of pictures which are presented at a rapid rate so that he is unable to formulate a complete response. The clinician can also, of course, interrupt the child's response prior to completion, although this is not often necessary. Other listeners may be brought into the room or additional listeners can take the role of distracting or interrupting the child. Typically, only one of these activities is necessary to elicit examples of fluency breaks.

Obviously, these techniques must be performed with appropriate understanding and sensitivity by the clinician as well as others who are involved. On occasion, the clinician may need to use several forms of communicative stress in order to elicit fluency breaks. It is not necessary to elicit many of these breaks. Once a few examples have been obtained, the clinician can consult with the parents to determine if these behaviors are indeed the behavior they have observed and are concerned about. The clinician cannot assume that the fluency breaks that occur are of the same form and degree that the parents have seen before.

Support for the importance of observing children in a variety of speaking situations was noted by Yaruss (1997a) in a study of 45 preschool children undergoing diagnostic evaluations for stuttering. Frequency counts were obtained for both more and less usual disfluency types for each of the children as they took part in three to five of the following situations during the evaluation session. Reliability measures using video recordings for 15% of the speech samples indicated no significant differences and high positive correlations between the original and recalculated observations.

1. Parent-Child Interaction—The child interacts with the parents (usually the mother) while playing with figures or games.
2. Play—The child and the clinician play with objects in a natural, free-play situation.
3. Play with Pressures Imposed—The clinician gradually increases conversational pressure by asking questions, breaking eye contact, interrupting, or increasing time pressure (e.g., speaking faster).
4. Story Retell—The child retells a familiar story while using a picture book.
5. Picture Description—The child describes pictures with minimal input from the clinician.

Yaruss found that these children who stuttered showed significantly more variability across the speaking situations than within any single situation. He also found that children who produced a higher overall frequency of less typical disfluencies also exhibited greater variability

(r = 0.88; p < .001). No significant correlation was found for the more typical fluency breaks. Finally, the "Play with Pressure" situation resulted in the greatest number of disfluencies, although this was not the case for all the participants, as many children exhibited highly individualized patterns.

Based on these results, Yaruss (1997a) suggested that sampling of a child's fluency in a single speaking situation is unlikely to result in a representative sample of behavior, particularly for children who exhibit a greater number of stuttering-like disfluencies. He also noted that approximately 19 of the children evaluated had fewer than 3% stuttering-like fluency breaks in at least one situation and that 18 of these children produced more than 10% stuttering in another situation. In other words, if the common guideline of 3% disfluencies has been used as a threshold, approximately 40% of the children would not have been correctly identified as stuttering. Of course, as Yaruss points out, a single metric of stuttering frequency would not be used alone to indicate the presence of stuttering. However, the results do point out the potential problem of placing too much importance on the frequency of stuttering, especially during a single speaking situation.

In some instances, despite our best attempts within several speaking situations and environments, we are unable to obtain samples of the fluency breaks that the child is apparently producing at home. It is usually possible to reschedule another assessment during a time when the child is experiencing more difficulty, or we may observe the child in a more natural setting at home or in school. An alternative is to ask the parents to make an audio- or videotape of the child at home as he is experiencing the fluency breaks they are concerned about. This step may be recommended even before the formal assessment, so that some preliminary analysis of the child's speech can be started prior to the initial meeting.

In any case, consultation with the parents, grandparents, teachers, or other concerned persons who were involved in making the referral is a fundamental part of the assessment procedure. In addition to the activities discussed earlier in this section, we can explain the process of speech and language acquisition to begin to help the parents to differentiate between normal and abnormal fluency breaks. Several booklets and video tapes that may be helpful in this regard are listed in Appendix C.

The Nature of the Fluency Breaks

When we discussed the nature of the onset and development in Chapter 3, we presented the characteristic surface behaviors that tend to differentiate between normal and less normal fluency breaks. We will now present some additional criteria that have been proposed for distinguishing the speech-related behavior for preschool children who stutter.

Yairi (1997) recommends a speech sample of at least 500 syllables. The child is both audio- and video-recorded over two separate days to account, at least to some degree, for the variability of stuttering. The following guidelines are based on a per-100-syllable disfluency metric. *Stuttering-like disfluencies* are indicated as SLD and *short element repetitions* (syllable and word repetitions) are indicated as SER.

Behavior	Preschool Children Who Stutter
1. Total number of disfluencies per 100 syllables	Average of 16
2. Number of SLD per 100 syllables	Minimum of 3; mean of 11
3. Percent SLD to total disfluencies	Range of 60% to 75%
4. Number or SER per 100 syllables	Mean of 6 to 8
5. Number of units per instance of SER	Mean of 1.5
6. Percent of SER containing two or more extra units	Mean of 33%
7. Number of SER containing two or more extra units per 100 syllables	Mean of 3
8. Percent of disfluencies occurring in clusters	Mean of 50%
9. Number of disfluencies per cluster	Mean of 3
10. Number of face and head movements per disfluency	Mean of 1.5 to 3
11. Duration of disfluencies in msec	Mean of 750
12. Duration of interval between repetition units	Mean of 200 msec
13. Proportion of silent interval to total duration of SER containing one extra unit	Mean of 1/4 to 1/3

Conture (1997) also suggests that clinicians consider a number of subtle signs (which tend to be additive) that may help to distinguish the possibility of stuttering:

➤ Within-word disfluencies that average 3 or more per 100 words (minimum of 300 word sample)
➤ Sound prolongations in 25% or more of the children's number of fluency breaks
➤ An average difference of two or more syllables per second in the speaking rates of the mother and children during conversational speech, increases in the occurrence of simultaneous-talk by the child and parent, and greater amounts of parent-child interrupting behaviors
➤ The presence of stuttering-stuttering clusters in the child's two-element speech disfluency clusters

➤ Eyeball movements to the side, eyelid blinking during stuttering, or both
➤ Clusters of two or more within-word breaks on adjacent sounds, syllables, or words within an utterance.

Indicators of Awareness

An important difference between the assessment of fluency in younger children and adults is the child's lack of ability to describe the frustration and anxiety related to his fluency failure. Some children seem to be completely unaware of their fluency breaks. Others are keenly aware of their speech difficulty, but may not know how to verbalize their helplessness, frustration, and anxiety. We cannot assume a lack of these intrinsic features simply because a child is unable to express them. Using a unique videotape of puppets—one of whom stuttered—Grinager, Ambrose and Yairi (1994) found that 20 children who stuttered (aged two to five years) identified more with the disfluent puppet, while control children identified with the fluent puppet. Their findings indicated that a child's lack of overt reactions to stuttering indicate a lack of awareness of speech difficulty. They also noted that awareness of stuttering was not related to stuttering severity (as indicated by an 8-point stuttering severity scale).

Based on their experience with many young children, Rustin and Cook (1995) point out that some preschool children are able to be very clear about the difficulties they experience. There are ample research findings indicating that young children who stutter develop a negative attitude toward communicating (DeNil & Brutten, 1991; Riley & Riley, 1979), as well as fears and avoidance behaviors (Conture, 1990; Peters & Guitar, 1991; Williams, 1985). Bloodstein (1960) observed that parents reported consistent difficulty on specific sounds or words as early as 2.5 years.

For many years clinicians chose not to intervene directly with a child if he or she did not express a complaint (Cooper, 1979). However, although young children may not verbalize their speech difficulties, their feelings will be reflected in such behaviors as pitch rise, tension, prolongations, schwa substitutions, a high rate of part-word repetitions, and cessation of airflow and voicing (Adams, 1977a; Throneburg & Yairi, 1994; Van Riper, 1982; Walle, 1975). When a child demonstrates such behaviors, it can be assumed—to some degree at least—that he is aware of his problem, and is searching for ways of coping. The child is attempting to overcome the helplessness and loss of control inherent in the experience of stuttering. He may be ready to try nearly anything to avoid that experience. In such a case, regardless of the child's age or ability to verbalize his feelings, the decision to intervene is clearly appropriate.

Another possible indicator of awareness on the part of the child may be in the form of associated physical movement. Johnson and his colleagues (1959) noted long ago that young children who stutter tend to display tense body movements. These movements have often been referred to as "secondary behaviors" or "secondary characteristics" and sometimes provide the clinician with a indication of awareness. A number of studies by Conture and his associates (Schwartz & Conture, 1988; Schwartz, Zebrowski, & Conture, 1990; Conture & Kelly, 1991), as well as Yairi, Ambrose and Niermann (1993), indicated that young children who stuttered exhibited more non-speech behaviors—including head, eye, torso, and limb movements—during stuttering. Children who stuttered averaged 1.48 movements during stuttered words and 0.63 movements during nonstuttered words (Conture & Kelly, 1991). Yairi et al. (1993) found that 16 young children who were within three months of stuttering onset demonstrated averaged 3.18 (range of 0.8 to 5.9) head and neck movements per moment of stuttering. During follow-up testing, the authors found that the movements were found to decrease as the occurrences of stuttering decreased.

Determining a Child's Level of Anxiety About Speaking

Interest in investigating levels of anxiety in children began to occur in the 1990s. Although research to date does not suggest that stuttering is caused by anxiety, it is more reasonable to assume that anxiety is a consequence of stuttering. Two types of anxiety have been identified and have been the focus of this research. Trait anxiety (indicated as *A-Trait*) has to do with the person's *general level of anxiety* and is obtained by having the client respond to self-report scales containing questions about how he or she generally feel (I feel happy "hardly ever, sometimes, or often"). Measures of state anxiety (indicated as *A-State*) are intended to indicate a measure of a person's *anxiety response at a specific moment* as he or she react to specific situational stimuli. A frequently used measure of anxiety is the State-Trait Anxiety Inventory for Children (STAIC) developed by Spielberger, Edwards, Luschene, Montuori, and Platzek (1972). Scores on both State and Trait sub scales range from 20 to 60, with higher scores representing greater anxiety. Using the STAIC, Craig and Hancock (1996) found no significant differences between 96 (untreated) children who stuttered and 104 children who did not stutter (age range of 9–14 years). This was the case for both State and Trait sub-scales. In addition, the authors found no significant association between stuttering frequency and state anxiety.

Parent Participation in Assessment

In the sections of this book where we discuss the treatment of young children (Chapter 5) and suggestions for counseling (Chapter 7), much will be said about the importance of parent participation in the treatment of young children. Assessment procedures should include some measure of parent interest in actively participating in the treatment of their child. Unfortunately, there will be occasions when parent involvement during assessment or treatment will be nonexistent. The motivation for initiating treatment may be minimal if the family physician or friends and family members suggest that the problem will likely go away by itself (Ramig, 1993c). In contrast to Rustin, who is reluctant to recommend treatment without parent involvement (1987; Rustin & Cook, 1995), Ramig contends that even in cases where parents cannot or will not become involved in treatment, the clinician should enroll the child. In our experience, while some children may benefit from increased understanding about the nature of their problem and some practice with basic therapeutic techniques, real long-term changes are unlikely to occur without the involvement of at least one dedicated parent.

Rustin and Cook (1995) provide several questions the clinician can use to discover the nature of the family and of parent-child interaction. Though the questions themselves are important, the most important aspect of the interview process is the clinician's style and ability to be flexible and creative as she interacts with the parents. As Caruso (1988) describes, the intent is to follow the parent's lead, all the while probing for areas of interest and concern. As Rustin and Cook indicate:

> In the interview, we learn about the rules and regulations in the child's life, the parents' attitudes toward child rearing, pertinent issues within the parental relationship, the problem-solving strategies employed, and the place the disfluency problem holds within the family. The interview is structured in such a way that the basic and noncontentious case details are gathered in the early stages of the process, with a gradual move toward more sensitive and emotional material as it progresses. (1995, p. 129)

Many inventories, scales, and procedures have been developed for evaluating the quality of both the surface as well as the deep structure of the syndrome (see Appendix A). Many of these measures are helpful for obtaining both data-based and criterion-referenced information for assessing fluency disorders. However, the variety of surface behaviors and intrinsic features that come together in stuttering do not always lend themselves to a realistic or valid analysis. Individual speakers rarely fit the descriptions, situations, and categories associated with any single measure. Many of these scales do provide helpful information that will prove useful as we make decisions concerning the initiation of treatment, the selection of a treatment strategy, and the phasing out or termination of formal treatment. However, assessment must go beyond all these procedures. No matter how many formal measures we administer or what we are able to discover during the initial meeting, we must recognize that we are viewing the speaker and his problem through a small window. As much as with any other human communication disorder, the assessment of fluency disorders is an ongoing process.

The process of assessment—while most intense during the initial stages of treatment—continues through treatment and into the posttreatment period, when the speaker may experience relapse (Silverman,

1981). In order to continue making good clinical decisions, the clinician must continue to obtain data concerning all aspects of the syndrome. The data obtained by using any number of assessment protocols are no substitute for the clinician's ongoing observation of the child's daily behavior in naturalistic settings.

Examples of Assessment Measures

There are several measures for assessing children. The SSI-4 (Figure 4-1) is one popular instrument. Another is the Communication Attitude Test-Revised (CAT-R) (Figure 5-1). The CAT-R was developed by Brutten and his colleagues (Brutten & Dunham, 1989; DeNil & Brutten, 1991) and most recently revised in 1997. This self-administered measure asks the child to respond to 35 true-false statements (e.g., "I like the way I talk" and "My words come out easily"). One point is scored for each response that corresponds to the way a child who stutters is likely to respond. De Nil and Brutten (1990) found that the average score for 70 children who stuttered was 16.7, while the scores for 271 children who did not stutter averaged 8.71.

Another scale designed for use with young children is the A-19 Scale for Children Who Stutter (Guitar & Grims, 1977) (Figure 5-2). Guitar and his colleagues have found that once a secure and trusting relationship is established, this 19-item scale helps to distinguish between children who stutter and those who do not. Once the clinician is assured that the child understands the task, the scale is administered by the clinician, who asks the child a series of questions concerning speech and related general attitude. One point is assigned for each question that is answered as a child who stutters might respond. In an unpublished study of 28 children who stutter and a group of matched control children, Andre and Guitar found that the average scores of K through 4th grade children who stutter was 9.07 (SD = 2.44), while the nonstuttering children averaged 8.17 (SD = 1.80).

The Component Model:
One Comprehensive Diagnostic Approach

For more than 20 years, Glyndon and Jeanna Riley have been developing and successfully applying a model for helping young children who stutter. The most recent description of this model is found in a recent publication (Riley & Riley, 2000). Because this model provides a comprehensive approach to both diagnosis and the assessment of young children, we will present portions of this approach in this chapter (the diagnostic implications) as well as in Chapter 9 (treatment recommendations).

Name _____ Age: _____
                                        Sex: _____
                                        Grade: ____

Read each sentence carefully so you can say if it is true or false <u>for you</u>. The sentences are about talking. If <u>you</u> feel that the sentence is right, circle true. If you think the sentence about your talking is not right, circle false. Remember, circle false if <u>you</u> think the sentence is wrong and true if <u>you</u> think it is right.

1.	I don't talk right.	True	False
2.	I don't mind asking the teacher a question in class.	True	False
3.	Sometimes words stick in my mouth when I talk.	True	False
4.	People worry about the way I talk.	True	False
5.	It is harder for me to give a report in class than it is For most of the other kids.	True	False
6.	My classmates don't think I talk funny.	True	False
7.	I like the way I talk.	True	False
8.	People sometimes finish words for me.	True	False
9.	My parents like the way I talk.	True	False
10.	I find it easy to talk to most everyone.	True	False
11.	I talk well most of the time.	True	False
12.	It is hard for me to talk to people.	True	False
13.	I don't talk like other children.	True	False
14.	I don't worry about the way I talk.	True	False
15.	I don't find it easy to talk.	True	False
16.	My words come out easily.	True	False
17.	It is hard for me to talk to strangers.	True	False
18.	The other kids wish they could talk like me.	True	False
19.	Some kids make fun of the way I talk.	True	False
20.	Talking is easy for me.	True	False
21.	Telling someone my name is hard for me.	True	False
22.	Words are hard for me to say.	True	False
23.	I talk well with most everyone.	True	False
24.	Sometimes I have trouble talking.	True	False
25.	I would rather talk than write.	True	False
26.	I like to talk.	True	False
27.	I am not a good talker.	True	False
28.	I wish I could talk like other children.	True	False
29.	My words do not come out easily.	True	False
30.	My friends don't talk as well as I do.	True	False
31.	I don't worry about talking on the phone.	True	False
32.	I talk better with a friend.	True	False
33.	People don't seem to like the way I talk.	True	False
34.	I let others talk for me.	True	False
35.	Reading aloud in class is easy for me.	True	False

Score 1 point for each answer that matches these:

1. True	9. False	17. True	25. False	33. True
2. False	10. False	18. False	26. False	34. True
3. True	11. False	19. True	27. True	35. False
4. True	12. True	20. False	28. True	
5. True	13. True	21. True	29. True	
6. False	14. False	22. True	30. False	
7. False	15. True	23. False	31. False	
8. True	16. False	24. True	32. True	

Figure 5-1. Communication Attitudes Test-Revised (CAT-R). Copyright by G. Brutten, 1985. Reprinted with permission.

A-19 Scale for Children Who Stutter

Susan Andre and Barry Guitar
University of Vermont

Establish rapport with the child, and make sure that he or she is physically comfortable before beginning administration. Explain the task to the child and make sure he or she understands what is required. Some simple directions might be used:

"I am going to ask you some questions. Listen carefully and then tell me what you think: Yes or No. There is no right or wrong answer. I just want to know what you think.

To begin the scale, ask the questions in a natural manner. Do not urge the child to respond before he or she is ready, and repeat the question if the child did not hear it or you feel that he or she did not understand it. Do not re-word the question unless you feel it is absolutely necessary, and then write the question you asked under that item.

Circle the answer that corresponds to the child's response. Be accepting of the child's response because there is no right or wrong answer. If all the child will say is "I don't know" even after prompting, record that response next to the question.

For the younger children (kindergarten and first grade), it might be necessary to give a few simple examples to ensure comprehension of the requited task:

a.	Are you a boy?	Yes	No
b.	Do you have black hair?	Yes	No

Similar, obvious questions may be inserted, if necessary, to reassure the examiner that the child is actively cooperating at all times. Adequately praise the child for listening and assure him or her that a good job is being done.

It is important to be familiar with the questions so that they can be read in a natural manner.

The child is given 1 point for each answer that matches those given below. The higher a child's score, the more probable it is that he or she has developed negative attitudes toward communication. In our study, the mean score of the K through 4th grade stutterers (N = 28) was 9.07 (S.D. = 2.44), and for the 28 matched controls, it was 8.17 (S.D. = 1.80).

Score 1 point for each answer that matches these:

1. Yes	11. No
2. Yes	12. No
3. No	13. Yes
4. No	14. Yes
5. No	15. Yes
6. Yes	16. No
7. No	17. No
8. Yes	18. Yes
9. Yes	19. Yes
10. No	

Figure 5-2. A-19 Scale, Directions, and Responses

A-19 SCALE

Name _____   Date _____

1. Is it best to keep your mouth shut when you are in trouble?		Yes	No
2. When the teacher calls on you, do you get nervous?		Yes	No
3. Do you ask a lot of questions in class?		Yes	No
4. Do you like to talk on the phone?		Yes	No
5. If you did not know a person, would you tell your name?		Yes	No
6. Is it hard to talk to your teacher?		Yes	No
7. Would you go up to a new boy or girl in your class?		Yes	No
8. Is it hard to keep control of your voice when talking?		Yes	No
9. Even when you know the right answer, are you afraid to say it?		Yes	No
10. Do you like to tell other children what to do?		Yes	No
11. Is it fun to talk to your dad?		Yes	No
12. Do you like to tell stories to your classmates?		Yes	No
13. Do you wish you could say things as clearly as the other kids do?		Yes	No
14. Would you rather look at a comic book than talk to a friend?		Yes	No
15. Are you upset when someone interrupts you?		Yes	No
16. When you want to say something, do you just say it?		Yes	No
17. Is talking to your friends more fun than playing by yourself?		Yes	No
18. Are you sometimes unhappy?		Yes	No
19. Are you a little afraid to talk on the phone?		Yes	No

Figure 5-2. Continued. A-19 Scale Items.

The approach for assessing children who may be in the early stages of stuttering evolved from the Rileys' clinical observations of subgroupings of children based on risk factors for stuttering onset and development. Using a correlation approach that included many components and the results of diagnostic information from 54 children, they developed an assessment model that included what they felt to be the most important components. Of the nine components included in their original model, five were found to be most common among children who stuttered: Attending Disorders, Auditory Processing Disorders, Sentence Formulation Disorders, Oral Motor Discoordination, and High Self Expectations. Children were defined as being disordered if they scored in excess of the normal expectations for performance on a standardized measure of each component.

The basic premise of this model is that the onset of stuttering is related to a "vulnerable system" in a young child. The purpose of the model is to identify those components that contributed to the vulnerability of their speech production system and resulted in stuttering. In many ways, of course, this model is comparable to the demands and capacities model. Those components or capacities of the child's system that were low were identified for treatment. Components or demands that may be taxing the child's vulnerable system were also identified. Treatment, as we will describe in more detail in Chapter 9, emphasizes improving the child's areas of vulnerability and reducing those components that are stressing the system. These procedures are accomplished prior to focusing on the enhancement of the child's fluency.

As the Rileys developed instruments designed to assess the various components and tested the model on additional children, they also revised their model. Currently the Revised Component Model (RCM) includes three generic factors with associated subcategories:

I. Physical Attributes
   A. Attending Disorders
   B. Speech Motor Coordination
II. Temperamental Factors
   A. High Self-Expectations
   B. Overly Sensitive
III. Listener Reactions
   A. Disruptive Communication Environment
   B. Secondary Gains
   C. Teasing/Bullying

Although readers are directed to the recent article by the Rileys (2000) for greater detail, a summary of the diagnostic procedures is provided in the following paragraphs. The factor of *Physical Attributes* is subdivided into components of Attending Disorders and Speech Motor Coordination. Attending Disorders were identified by using the Poor Impulse Control Scale (e.g., can't control self, is implusive) and Poor Attention Scale (e.g., easily distracted, cannot finish things) of the Burks' Behavior Rating Scales (BBRS; Burks, 1976), the Hyperactivity Index from the Conner's Parent Rating Scale (Conners, 1998) and the clinician's judgment that the child has a reduced attention span and was distractible. The Rileys found that 36% of the children in the original study (1979) presented with either severe (20%) or moderate (16%) attending disorders. In the more recent study, 26% of the 50 CWS were found to have severe (18%) or moderate (8%) attending disorders. Speech motor control problems were identified using the Oral Motor Assessment Scale (OMAS, Riley & Riley, 1985). This measure determines—among other areas—the child's accuracy of voicing, coarticulatory movements between syllables, and rate—including diadochokinetic rate for syllable production. In the original study, 69% of the CWS indicated oral motor disorders (36% severe and 33% moderate), and 33% had moderate or severe articulation disorders. The more recent sample of 50 children yielded 68% of the CWS with speech motor difficulties (50% severe and 18% moderate), compared to levels in the non-CWS population of 2% severe and 8% moderate. Moderate or severe articulation or phonological disorders occurred in 50% of the more recent sample.

The next generic category of *Temperamental Factors* includes the components of High Self-Expectations and Overly Sensitive. Overly high self-expectations were determined by parent report (e.g., the child appears perfectionistic, is cautious, and has low threshold for frustration), clinician observation, and the child's performance on three subtests of the BBRS: Excessive Anxiety Scale (e.g., appears tense, worries too much) and Excessive Self-Blame (e.g., blames self if things go wrong, upset if makes a mistake). The Overly Sensitive components are determined by scores on the Excessive Suffering subtest of the BBRS. In 1979 the authors found that 89% of the children assessed had abnormally high self-expectations; the more recent study indicated that 70% of the CWS had either severe (13%) or moderate (57%) levels of unusually high expectations.

The *Overly Sensitive* component is reflective of children who appear to overly react to their environment. The Excessive Suffering Scale of the BBRS (e.g., feelings easily hurt, appears unhappy) is used along with parent reports and clinician judgment of the child's tendency to be easily upset, shy, or withdrawn to determine whether children are unusually sensitive. This component was not measured in the earlier model (1979), but this component occurred in 73% of the 50 children most recently studied (30% severe, 43% moderate).

The final factor is termed *Listener Reactions* and is described by three components: Disruptive Communication Environment, Secondary Gains, and Teasing/Bullying. Disruptive Communication Environment is determined by parent reports that the child has a difficult time obtaining the parent's attention, family members tend to rush the child's speech, interruption by the family members, teasing about the child's speech, and observations of critical or negative comments about the child's speech. This component occurred in 53% of the children in the 1979 sample and 61% of the families in the more recent sample (32% severe, 29% moderate).

Secondary Gains indicate that the child is able to manipulate family members as a result of his stuttered speech (e.g., obtaining special privileges, not being told "no" due to fear of placing stress on the child, ability to dominate family conversations). This form of manipulative behavior was found in 25% of the 1979 sample and 35% in the more recent sample (9% severe, 26% moderate).

The final component of this factor is Teasing and Bullying and is iden-tified by both parent and child report concerning the amount and type of these negative reactions that the child has experienced. Children in the most recent sample were found to have experienced these listener responses in 31% of the cases (9% severe, 22% moderate).

This comprehensive diagnostic approach for children as described by the Rileys is similar to other multi-factor assessment approaches that the clinician may decide to use (e.g., Starkweather & Givens-Ackerman, 1997; Stocker, 1980; Wall & Myers, 1995).

DECISION 2: DETERMINING THE LIKELIHOOD OF CHRONICITY

Assuming that the young child's fluency breaks are considered to be unusual or abnormal, the next clinical decision is whether this pattern is likely to continue developing: Will this manner of speaking and respond-ing become chronic? Given all this information, the clinician will make a decision about whether or not to initiate treatment. Finally, the clinician will make a choice about the degree of intervention. As we will discuss in subsequent chapters, intervention can be implemented at many levels. Intervention can take the form of prevention that seeks to keep the early stages of the syndrome from developing into more complex and habitual stuttering. The goal, of course, is to keep stuttering from reaching its fully developed state, and—as much as possible—to avoid the impact of the associated handicapping effects. Because treatment has been shown to be quite successful with young children who are still in the early stages of stuttering, a wise decision at this point is critical. Everything else being equal, the longer one waits (considering, of course, the results of studies concerning spontaneous recovery in young children), the longer it will take to treat the child, and the possibility of a successful long-term treatment outcome swiftly decreases.

If a preschool child presents with part-word repetitions (especially if they are rapid), prolongations with tension, obvious restriction, or even complete blockage of airflow or voicing, the diagnosis and the decision to intervene would seem to be obvious. However, the severity of the overt stuttering does not always predict whether or not the child will recover. Nonverbal signs of struggle in the form of eye, head, or general body movement may also indicate the need for intervention. However, if these signs are less evident, the best clinical choice is questionable. A family history of stuttering and the parents' concerned response to the child's disrupted fluency may suggest intervention as the clear choice. Parental judgment of a child's speech difficulty should be considered a fundamental part of a diagnosis of stuttering (Conture & Caruso, 1987; Onslow, 1992; Riley & Riley, 1983). On the other hand, if there is no family history of stuttering (or recovery from stuttering) and the parents and other caregivers are unconcerned about the child's speech, it *may* be advisable to monitor the child for approximately three months, as investigations by Yairi, Ambrose, and Niermann (1993) suggest that there is a tendency for children to recover within three months following onset. Still, the ideal window for intervention will contract, and it may be that intervention—even in the absence of great parental concern—is the best choice.

Conture (1990) proposes that intervention is called for if there is a pattern of within-word fluency breaks on predictable parts of speech. The pattern of disfluency, even though cyclical, should persist over a period of several months and be associated with certain sounds, syllables, words, or speaking situations. The clinician also will want to assess and consider the possible effect of other aspects of the child's speech, language, and oral-motor proficiency (Riley & Riley, 1986).

Information is obtained from many sources during the evaluation of young children. Case history information about the child's general development, family history, speech and language history, academic performance (if the child is of school age), and social and emotional status are all important for assessing the trade-off between the child's capacities and demands for fluent speech. Speech samples will hopefully be obtained during the formal evaluation, assuming the child will cooperate. Additional speech samples from representative situations outside the clinic setting can also be obtained either prior to or following the evaluation in the form of audio- or videotapes. A reasonable goal is to obtain a 300- to 500-word sample produced in a natural setting. Frequency counts of fluency breaks can be obtained in either percent syllables stuttered (%SS) or percent words stuttered (%WS) and the type of fluency breaks analyzed. Andrews and Ingham (1971) suggest that %WS can be converted to %SS by multiplying %WS by 1.5.

Fluency Breaks That Signal Chronicity

Without treatment, an adult who stutters is not likely to significantly change his level of fluency. For the young person who stutters, however, there is a real possibility that the stuttering behaviors will decrease and even cease. This decrease has been termed spontaneous recovery, unassisted recovery, and natural remission. Although the estimated number of these young speakers who obtain fluency without intervention varies widely from approximately 32% to more than 80% (Andrews & Harris, 1964; Bryngelson, 1938; Cooper, 1972; Curlee & Yairi, 1997; Kloth, Kraaimaat, Janssen, & Brutten, 1999; Panelli, McFarlane, & Shipley, 1978; Starkweather, 1987; Van Riper, 1982; Yairi & Ambrose, 1992a; Young, 1975), it is certain that a significant number of children do "recover." Some authors have suggested that these relatively high rates of spontaneous recovery have come under question (Martin & Lindamood, 1986; Ramig, 1993a).

Determining which young children who are stuttering will someday spontaneously recover is even more difficult than determining whether a young speaker is, in fact, stuttering. In attempting to determine whether a young child's stuttering will become chronic, we are attempting to predict the future. In making the decision about chronicity, we have somewhat fewer data on which to draw than we have to distinguish between normal and abnormal fluency breaks.

One important consideration is the gender of the child. Andrews et al. (1983) report that from 5 to 10 times more males than females stutter. Certainly this would seem to be the case based on the ratio of males to females who come to treatment centers. Recent data suggests, however, that gender may be more of an indicator of recovery from—rather than occurrence of—stuttering. That is, recent studies of young male and female children (ages 2 to 2 1/2 years old) indicate that the gender ratio is 50-50: Young boys and girls are equally as likely to demonstrate abnormal fluency breaks. However, as Starkweather (1987) points out, by the ages of 7 or 8 a clear difference begins to emerge: More boys than girls continue to manifest difficulties with fluency. Recovery, even without formal intervention, appears to be likely during the preschool years.

Some early information about the timing of spontaneous recovery from stuttering is suggested by the classic longitudinal study of English children living at Newcastle-on-Tyne reported by Andrews and Harris (1964). One-thousand children were followed for 15 years and examined for a variety of health problems, including stuttering. Most of the children studied began to stutter by the age of 5. No child began stuttering after the age of 11. Approximately one third of the children demonstrated nonfluency from ages 2 to 4. Another third began to stutter at an average age of 7.5 years but continued to do so for only two years. The final third of the children began stuttering during the age range of 3 to 6, and children continued to stutter. Following a review of these data, Starkweather (1987) observes that:

> The children who became chronic stutterers, however, were all stuttering between the ages of five and one-half and six and one-half. In other words, a child who begins stuttering during the preschool period has a reasonable chance, about 50 percent, of recovering soon. The same is true of a child who begins stuttering later, after age seven. But if a child begins stuttering at a young age, and the problem persists into the five and one-half to six and one-half year range, there is a good chance that it will become a chronic disorder. It looks as though there is a critical period, somewhere between age five and age seven, during which the patterns of speech become automated or habituated so firmly that it is difficult later to change. And if stuttering is present during this period of time, it too will be difficult to change later on.

In order to assist clinicians in determining the likelihood that a child would continue to stutter, Cooper (1973) developed a chronicity prediction checklist (Figure 5-3). This checklist is scored on the basis of the number of "yes" responses to questions concerning the historical, attitudinal, and behavioral aspects of stuttering in children. Based on the findings of McLelland and Cooper (1978), two to six "yes" responses are indicative of possible recovery, 7 to 15 "yes" responses indicate the need for continued monitoring of the child, and 16 to 27 "yes" responses are predictive of chronicity. Essentially, it appears that the more abnormal the speech in terms of tension and fragmentation (Bloodstein, 1960, 1987; Schwartz, Zebrowski, & Conture, 1990), the less likely the chance that the child will recover from stuttering. In addition, the Stuttering Prediction Inventory (SPI) (Riley, 1981) was developed in order to determine the likelihood of chronicity (Figure 5-4). These may be valuable adjuncts to the diagnostic procedure with young children, but to date there have been no longitudinal investigations that allow for the accurate prediction of future fluency.

Making the Decision to Intervene

Evidence of whether or not verified stuttering is likely to persist in young children has been obtained in a series of longitudinal investigations by Yairi and his colleagues (1996). After following more than 100 preschool children who stuttered from the outset of their stuttering, Yairi et al. (1996) compared children who stopped stuttering within 36 months following onset with those who continued to stutter during this period. The authors found that the children who recovered were younger when they began stuttering (prior to the age of three), were female, and had fewer relatives with chronic stuttering. Interestingly, they also had more relatives who had stuttered and recovered. Furthermore, the frequency of part-word and monosyllabic word repetitions and dysrhythmic phonations (stuttering-like disfluencies or SLDs) decreased by 12 months post-onset for all of the children who stopped stuttering. Recall that Yairi et al. (1993) found that children who recovered from stuttering continued to produce (or even increased their production of) other types of fluency breaks (revisions, interjections, phrase repetitions, and other between-word or formulative fluency breaks).

In contrast to traditional views of the relationship between stuttering severity and chronicity, the severity of stuttering near onset *failed to* differentiate the children who recovered from those who did not. In fact, as Yairi et al. point out, the initial level of SLDs in the children who recovered was higher than that of the children who continued to stutter. In addition, the presence of accessory or secondary physical behaviors at outset also failed to differentiate the two groups of children. That is, the presence of head and facial movements did not predict chronicity with this sample of

Instructions: To be completed for children ages three to eight. Answers to questions require the assistance of the child's parents. Each item should be explained and discussed with the parents. Place a check (√) on the appropriate blank.

		Yes	No	Unknown
I.	Historical Indicators of Chronicity			
	1. Is there a history of chronic stuttering in the family?	____	____	____
	2. Is the severity (frequency, duration, consistency) of the disfluencies increasing?	____	____	____
	3. Did the disfluencies begin with blockings rather than with easy repetitions?	____	____	____
	4. Have the child's disfluencies persisted since being observed (as opposed to being episodic with long periods of normal fluency)?			
	5. Has the child been disfluent for two or more years?	____	____	____
II.	Attitudinal Indicators of Chronicity			
	1. Does the child perceive himself or herself to be disfluent?	____	____	____
	2. Does the child experience communicative fear because of the disfluencies?	____	____	____
	3. Does the child believe the disfluency problem to be getting worse?	____	____	____
	4. Does the child avoid speaking situations?	____	____	____
	5. Does the child express anger or frustration because of the disfluencies?	____	____	____
III.	Behavioral Indicators of Chronicity			
	1. Do sound prolongations or hesitations occur among the disfluencies?	____	____	____
	2. Are the repetitions more frequently whole word or phrase repetitions rather than part-word repetitions?	____	____	____
	3. Are part-word repetitions accompanied by visible tension or stress?	____	____	____
	4. Do part-word repetitions occur more than three times on the same word?	____	____	____
	5. Is the rapidity of the syllable repetitions faster than normal?	____	____	____
	6. Is the schwa vowel inappropriately inserted in the syllable repetition?	____	____	____
	7. Is the air flow during repetitions often interrupted?	____	____	____
	8. Do prolongations last longer than one second?	____	____	____
	9. Do prolongations occur on more than one word in a hundred during periods of disfluency?	____	____	____
	10. Are prolongations uneven or interrupted as opposed to being smooth?	____	____	____
	11. Is there observable tension during prolongation?	____	____	____
	12. Are the terminations of the prolongations sudden as opposed to being gradual?	____	____	____
	13. During prolongations of voiced sounds is the airflow interrupted?	____	____	____
	14. Are the silent pauses prior to the speech attempt unusually long?	____	____	____
	15. Are the inflection patterns restricted and monotone?	____	____	____
	16. Is there loss of eye contact during the moment of disfluency?	____	____	____
	17. Are there observable and/or distracting extraneous facial or body movements during the moment of disfluency?	____	____	____

Total "Yes" Responses ____

Instructions: Place a check on the appropriate blank.

Predictive of Recovery: 0 – 6   ____
Requiring Vigilance: 7 – 15   ____
Predictive of Recovery: 16 – 27   ____

Caution: The categorization of scores used on this checklist is based on an interpretation of data reported by McClelland and Cooper (Journal of Fluency Disorders, 1978) and on clinical observation. It is not based on longitudinal studies. Judgments as to probably stuttering chronicity should not be based solely on the scoring of this checklist.

Figure 5-3. The Cooper Chronicity Prediction Checklist (Eugene B. Cooper. *Personalized fluency control therapy.* Austin, TX: Pro-Ed. Reprinted with Permission.)

Stuttering Prediction Instrument
For Young Children
by Glyndon D. Riley, Ph. D.

TEST FORM

NAME _____   SEX   M F GRADE _____

SCHOOL _____   DATE OF BIRTH _____

EXAMINER _____   DATE _____   AGE _____

SECTION I: HISTORY

BACKGROUND

1. When did your child first exhibit disfluencies? _____

   What were the related circumstances? _____

   _____

2. Is the severity of the stuttering increasing? _____

   Is the severity of the stuttering decreasing? _____

3. Does the stuttering come and go? _____

   Is today's speech more or less disfluent than usual or is it about average? _____

FAMILY HISTORY OF STUTTERING

4. Have any family members ever stuttered?

   a. The biological father?   Yes _____   No _____
      From age ____ to age ____

   b. The biological mother?   Yes _____   No _____
      From age ____ to age ____

   c. Any biological siblings?   Yes _____   No _____
      From age ____ to age ____

   d. Any other relatives?
      Grandfather   Yes _____   No _____
      Grandmother   Yes _____   No _____
      Aunt   Yes _____   No _____
      Uncle   Yes _____   No _____
      Cousin   Yes _____   No _____
      Other _____

Figure 5-4. *The Stuttering Prediction Instrument for Young Children,* Glyndon D. Riley. Austin, TX: Pro-Ed. Reprinted with Permission.

SECTION II: REACTIONS

5. Does the child's disfluency make you feel:

   a. unconcerned (Score 0)
   b. concerned (Score 1)
   c. very concerned (Score 2)   Score

6. Has your child been teased about his stuttering?

   a. never observed (Score 0)
   b. observed to a mild degree (Score 1)
   c. observed to a moderate or severe degree (Score 2)   Score

7. Does your child get frustrated when he cannot get the word out? (e.g., cries, stamps foot, hits himself, or asks, "Why can't I talk right?")

   a. never observed (Score 0)
   b. observed to a mild degree (Score 1)
   c. observed to a moderate or severe degree (Score 2)   Score

8. Does your child sometimes change a word because of a fear of stuttering?

   a. never observed (Score 0)
   b. observed to a mild degree (Score 1)
   c. observed to a moderate or severe degree (Score 2)   Score

9. Does your child avoid some situations because of a fear of stuttering?

   a. never observed (Score 0)
   b. observed to a mild degree (Score 1)
   c. observed to a moderate or severe degree (Score 2)   Score

10. Are there any observable and/or distracting extraneous facial or bodily movements during stuttering?

   a. never observed (Score 0)
   b. observed to a mild degree (Score 1)
   c. observed to a moderate or severe degree (Score 2)   Score

                                        Subtotal Score

Figure 5-4. Continued.

SECTION III: PART-WORD REPETITIONS

number:	none	1-3	4 or more	
score:	0	1	3	Score

Transcribe the most severe abnormalities   ____   ____   ____   ____

Abnormality of repeated syllables	normal	mild	mod.	sev.	
(e.g., schwa, tension, abruptness)	0	1	2	4	Score

Subtotal Score

SECTION IV: PROLONGATIONS

Record only the highest score obtained, i.e., A or B or C but *not* the total.

A. Vowel Prolongations

duration:	less than 1.5 secs.	1.5-2 secs.	2-4 secs.	4 secs. +
score:	0	2	4	6

B. Phonatory Arrest

duration:	none	.5-1 secs.	1-3 secs.	3 secs. +
score:	0	4	8	12

C. Articulatory Posturing

duration:	none	.5-1 secs.	1-3 secs.	3 secs. +
score:	0	4	8	12

Subtotal score

SECTION V: FREQUENCY

percentage:	0	1	2-3	4	5-6	7-9	10-14	15-28	29 +
score:	0	2	3	4	5	6	7	8	9

Subtotal Score

Add subtotal scores for Sections II-V to arrive at the total score.   **Total Score**

Figure 5-4. Continued.

SECTION VI
TABLE IV

Distribution of *SPI* scores for 85 children ages 3-8 who stutter.

Stanine	Total Score	Percentile	Severity
1	10-11	0-4	Very mild
2	12-13	5-11	Mild
3	14-17	12-23	
4	18-19	24-40	
5	20-24	41-60	Moderate
6	25-28	61-77	
7	29-30	78-89	
			Severe
8	31-35	90-96	
9	36-37	97-100	Very Severe

Median = 21
Mean = 22.2
Sd   = 7.01

SECTION VII
TABLE V

Distribution of *SPI* scores for 17 children whose disfluencies had not become chronic.

Stanine	Total Score	Percentile	Severity
1	0-1	0-4	
2	2	5-11	
3	3-4	12-23	
4	5	24-40	Sub-clinical
5	6	41-60	
6	7-8	61-77	
7	9	78-89	
8	10	90-96	Very Mild
9	11-13	97-100	Mild

Median = 6
Mean = 6.17
Sd   = 3.13

Figure 5-4. Continued.

children. Another important finding was that the children who continued to stutter for 12 months following onset had an increased risk of stuttering for another two years or more. Finally, although the scores of both chronic and recovered children were within normal limits on measures on phonological, language, and nonverbal intelligence measures, the children who continued to stutter performed more poorly overall, especially in phono-logical skills, than did those who stopped stuttering.

A recent series of longitudinal studies sheds additional light on the nature of unassisted recovery in early childhood stuttering. Yairi and Ambrose (1999) obtained extensive and multiple speech samples from 84 preschool children who were followed closely for a period of at least four years after onset of stuttering. None of these children received treatment for stuttering. Recovery was indicated by a series of clinician and parent ratings (e.g., clinician severity ratings of less than 1 [borderline stutter-ing], no stuttering present for a minimum of 12 months). The authors found what they felt to be conservative estimates of 74% recovery and 26% persistency rates. Recovery occurred gradually over a period of three and sometimes four years following onset. Females were more likely to recover than males with a male-to-female ratio of 4.50:1 for the chil-dren who continued to stutter and a ratio of 1.82:1 for the children who recovered. The authors point out that claims of successful therapeutic intervention with young children must take these high levels of unas-sisted recovery into account.

Determining the probability of chronic stuttering can be particularly difficult in young speakers. Given the high rates of nonassisted recovery by young children who stutter noted by Yairi and his associates, the deci-sion about whether to intervene can be especially troublesome. Yairi and Ambrose (1992a) conducted a two-year follow-up of 27 young children who had spontaneously recovered and found no instances of relapse. Their data, along with their 1999 findings from a different group of chil-dren, make a strong case for continued recovery from stuttering during the early childhood years, a trend that is counter to a good deal of think-ing about the developmental nature of the problem. Not only do such results seriously confound studies of treatment efficacy with this popula-tion of young stuttering children, they suggest caution concerning inter-vention decisions.

For decades, parents of children who stutter have been told to take a wait-and-see approach in the hope that the problem would go away. This advice is a common response of pediatricians (Yairi & Carrico, 1992). Following a review of the literature concerning the high levels of sponta-neous remission in young children, Curlee and Yairi (1997) argued against the necessity of intervention for all children who are stuttering, particularly those who have only been doing so for one of two years fol-lowing onset. Given the large number of young children who stutter who are likely to recover on their own, the authors question the argument that withholding or delaying treatment could be unethical and clearly incon-sistent with current information about unaided remission from stutter-ing. They suggest that close monitoring of preschool children during the first 12–24 months following the onset of stuttering permits the unaided remission of stuttering for most children and does not adversely affect later treatment. They also suspect that much of the treatment success frequently noted with young children is probably influenced by the high levels of spontaneous recovery in this age group. Finally, they argue that there is insufficient evidence to support the efficacy of early intervention in all cases of early childhood stuttering.

In response to these suggestions, Zebrowski (1997) pointed out that although we may find many factors that appear to be related to the chronicity of stuttering, each child who comes to us for an evaluation is completely unique and that—in many cases—knowledge of these factors does not allow us to predict the future. Furthermore, as we shall see in Chapter 8, there is a wide continuum of intervention, ranging from indirect modeling by the parents or the clinician to more direct behavioral treatment. It may be that, following the initial evaluation, parents follow the suggestions and information that is provided and facilitate what is then seen as "unaided" remission. Zebrowski also suggests that, based on the likelihood of children recovering without intervention, the clinician many want to consider one of several "decision streams" according to the characteristics of the child and the family. As shown in Figure 5-5, children are placed in one of four streams based on the time interval since onset. The clinician's response (Plans A–E) are based on factors that have been identified in the literature, most recently by Yairi and his colleagues, as indicating remission or chronicity of stuttering. Points are assigned when children possess the factors listed within each stream. For example, children stuttering for fewer than six months are placed in stream I. Children demonstrating all of the five characteristics associated with this stream are assigned a score of five points, and the clinician would respond with Plan A as described below. Children with a score of 4 or less would undergo Plan B.

Plan A: (Stream I children who have all five recovery factors)

These children have a high probability of recovery. Treatment consists of information-sharing and bibliotherapy. The clinician provides parents with information about (1) normal speech and language development, (2) their child's speech and language relative to a normal child, (3) information about what we do and do not know about causal factors for stuttering in children, and (4) the prognosis for recovery for their child given all the information accumulated at that point. In addition, parents are provided with reading material (Appendix C). Clinicians can make monthly contact with the parents via telephone follow-up or e-mail to further explain the information and answer questions. Parents can monitor changes in frequency or type of fluency breaks. Particular attention is given to whether there is a gradual decrease in the repetitions of sounds, syllables, monosyllabic whole-words, and sound prolongations—fluency breaks that Yairi and colleagues found to lessen during the first 6 to 12 months post-onset. The parents may request a formal re-evaluation if they are unable to monitor their child's fluency breaks or record good examples of their child's

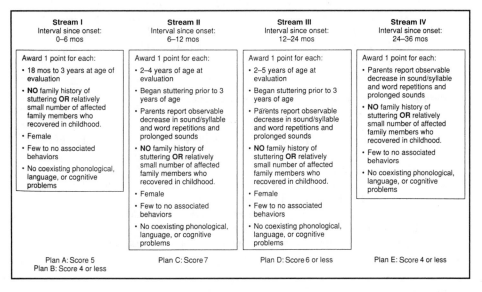

Stream I Interval since onset: 0–6 mos	Stream II Interval since onset: 6–12 mos	Stream III Interval since onset: 12–24 mos	Stream IV Interval since onset: 24–36 mos
Award 1 point for each:	Award 1 point for each:	Award 1 point for each:	Award 1 point for each:
• 18 mos to 3 years at age of evaluation	• 2–4 years of age at evaluation	• 2–5 years of age at evaluation	• Parents report observable decrease in sound/syllable and word repetitions and prolonged sounds
• **NO** family history of stuttering **OR** relatively small number of affected family members who recovered in childhood.	• Began stuttering prior to 3 years of age	• Began stuttering prior to 3 years of age	• **NO** family history of stuttering **OR** relatively small number of affected family members who recovered in childhood.
• Female	• Parents report observable decrease in sound/syllable and word repetitions and prolonged sounds	• Parents report observable decrease in sound/syllable and word repetitions and prolonged sounds	• Few to no associated behaviors
• Few to no associated behaviors	• **NO** family history of stuttering **OR** relatively small number of affected family members who recovered in childhood.	• **NO** family history of stuttering **OR** relatively small number of affected family members who recovered in childhood.	• No coexisting phonological, language, or cognitive problems
• No coexisting phonological, language, or cognitive problems	• Female	• Female	
	• Few to no associated behaviors	• Few to no associated behaviors	
	• No coexisting phonological, language, or cognitive problems	• No coexisting phonological, language, or cognitive problems	
Plan A: Score 5 Plan B: Score 4 or less	Plan C: Score 7	Plan D: Score 6 or less	Plan E: Score 4 or less

Figure 5-5. Decision streams for intervention (Zebrowski, 1997).

speech. If there are many of these and no decrease is noted, a follow-up visit may be indicated.

Plan B: (Stream I children who have four of five recovery factors)

These children also have a high probability of recovery. Treatment consists of all the components of Plan A, with the addition of language intervention, phonological intervention, or both, if appropriate for the child. The degree of intervention would vary depending on the child's age and the severity of the problem. In addition, family members with a positive history of stuttering are provided with counseling, given the likelihood of greater concern about the child. Although Zebrowski does not suggest it, such counseling may be appropriate for family members even if there is no family history of stuttering.

Plan C: (Stream II and III children with a score of seven recovery factors)

Recovery is less likely for the child who has been stuttering longer. These children began stuttering before the age of three and have been doing so for six months to two years. If these children are female, have no family history or a family history of recovery, have few or no associated behaviors or concomitant problems, and demonstrate a decrease in symptomatology, they are more likely to recover. As the child continues to stutter two years post-onset, recovery becomes less likely. Treatment consists of all the components of Plan B with the addition of counseling for parents about how they verbally interact with their child. Parents are counseled about ways to indirectly enhance fluency of their child by practicing such activities as rate reduction, longer turn-switching pause durations, and avoiding interrupting. Children could also enroll the child in a parent-child group designed to facilitate fluency.

Plan D: (Stream II and III children with a score of six or fewer recovery factors)

This plan contains all the components of Plan C that are applicable plus monthly visits to the clinic or the parent's home for monitoring. Taped speech samples are analyzed for the quality of the child's fluency (disfluency form types, speed of repetitions, duration of stuttered moments, and reactions of the child as well as associated behaviors). In addition, during the visits to the clinic or the home, parents can be counseled about the possibility that their child may not recover from stuttering as well as the many emotions that accompany the acceptance that their child has a handicap (see Chapter 6).

Plan E: (Stream IV children with a score of four or fewer recovery factors)

These children have been stuttering from two to three years post-onset and are the least likely to recover. Treatment consists of all the factors included in the above plans plus direct intervention according to treatment protocols described in this and other texts.

Although authors agree that many speakers recover from stuttering, few have questioned whether these same speakers are more likely to begin stuttering again later in their adult years. As we described in the previous chapter, it is relatively rare to find speakers who begin to stutter as adults. Most often, stuttering is a gradually developing phenomenon beginning in the early years of speech and language development. It may be, however, that some people who begin stuttering later in life are those people who also stuttered as children, more or less spontaneously recovered, and later—apparently in response to one or a combination of factors—again began to experience breaks in their fluency. We have seen a few such adults with whom a reoccurrence of stuttering seems to be a central component for what appeared to be a "late onset" of stuttering.

USING AT-RISK REGISTERS

Another possible strategy that has been suggested for improving the clinician's decision-making process concerning intervention is the use of an "at-risk" register (Adams, 1977b; Onslow, 1992). These authors suggest that such a strategy will decrease the occurrence of the false positive and false negative errors in the identification of young stuttering children, who may or may not be showing the early signs of chronic stuttering. A false positive decision occurs when a normally speaking child is incorrectly identified as a child who stutters. A false negative decision occurs when a child who stutters is incorrectly identified as a normally speaking child. The goal of any such process, of course, is to make accurate choices—true positive identifications of the disorder. While decreasing the likelihood of either type of the two possible errors is desirable, a false negative identification is a more serious error. That is, a false positive identification could result in a child receiving some less-than-vital assistance in producing fluent speech, something that should be no great cause for concern—at least according to Onslow, (1992). As we have indicated, other authors (Yairi, 1997; Curlee & Yairi, 1997) suggest that this decision does represent a more serious error. On the other hand, a false negative decision would likely be an error of even greater consequence, given the evidence that treatment for more advanced stuttering is considerably more time-consuming and prone to failure and relapse (Bloodstein, 1987; Conture, 1996; Costello, 1983; Onslow, 1992). Thus as Onslow recommends, the process leading to negative identification should be conservative, while the process resulting in positive identification should be relatively liberal. It has been suggested that the negative identification of communication disorders may result in the inefficient use of health care services (Andrews, 1984). However, Onslow comments that this view is not held for other communication disorders and questions both the logic and the ethics of withholding treatment from young children who stutter. In addition, he suggests that clients who are seen in the clinical setting may be more severely affected than nonclinical cases and less prone to recovery without intervention. Finally, he points out that because of the overall inefficiency in treating cases of advanced stuttering, accurate early identification may actually improve the overall efficiency of service delivery.

The development of an at-risk register is described by both Adams (1977b) and Onslow (1992) and is depicted in Figure 5-6. This strategy involves three basic elements: the at-risk register and both negative and positive identification components. When stuttering is suspected, the parents bring the child to a clinic for a formal evaluation. The parents are requested to bring audio- or videotapes of their child's speech made in a natural environment, indicating the fluency characteristics of concern. The identification of a problem is based on the perception of stuttering by the clinician (or clinicians) and the parents. If a parent considers that a child is stuttering but the clinician fails to perceive stuttered speech in the clinic or in the recording, the child is listed in an at-risk register. In an instance where a clinician perceives stuttered speech but a parent does not, positive identification occurs if a second clinician perceives stuttered

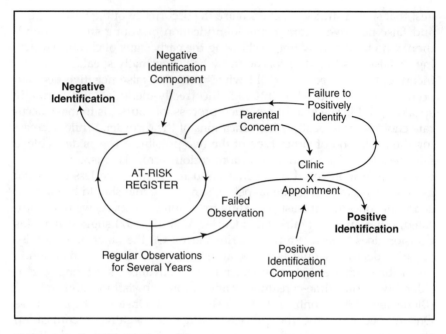

Figure 5-6. Onslow's (1992) At-Risk Register.

speech. If the second clinician does not perceive stuttered speech, then the child is placed in an at-risk register (Onslow, 1992, p. 25).

Those children listed in the at-risk register are observed on a regular basis for a period of months or years. Onslow suggests that ongoing evaluations can take a variety of forms, including telephone conversations, face-to-face interviews with parents, or questionnaires mailed to the home. Another tactic is to have the parents periodically call the clinic and respond to a series of questions that might indicate forms of speech fragmentation, tension, or struggle. Those children who pass the ongoing evaluations will continue being included on the register until a negative identification is made. How long this process should continue is a primary question, but based on Bloodstein's (1987) literature review, Onslow suggests a possible upper limit of 12 years. A child is moved to the positive identification component if at any point a parent becomes concerned, and a formal evaluation is again scheduled. A child who is routed to the positive identification component but fails to be positively identified is moved back to the register.

The use of an at-risk strategy places no pressure on the clinician to make either a positive or a negative identification. If there is uncertainty concerning the diagnosis, the child is listed on the register and, if necessary, will remain there until a decision is made. However, as we suggest on several occasions in this text, if the clinician is in doubt, intervention is likely to be the safest decision in the long run.

CONCLUSION

Fluency is often highly variable, particularly for children and especially for children with fluency disorders. The assessment of stuttering in young children may be more complicated, since these children are maturing neurologically, physiologically, emotionally, and linguistically. Clinicians typically need to obtain examples of speech in a variety of conditions and, on some occasions, elicit the fluency characteristics that the parents or others are concerned about. Parents and significant other caretakers play an important role in the assessment process, providing both historical and developmental information, as well as indicating patterns of interpersonal communication.

Clinicians have two major clinical decisions when assessing young children as they determine (1) whether the fluency breaks of the child are unusual and stutter-like and (2) given the reported levels of spontaneous recovery for young speakers, the possibility that stuttering behaviors will diminish. Although early intervention is reported to be highly successful with young children, part of this success may be attributable to the process of maturity of the speech production system and related components. The clinician's decision about whether or not to initiate treatment involves the determination of factors such as age since onset, frequency and clustering of disfluencies, the quality of the fluency breaks, occurrence of nonverbal behaviors, gender of the speaker, family history of stuttering, and recovery from stuttering. Strategies for tracking children for a period of time following onset, based on factors that seem to predict recovery, allow for monitoring and eventual intervention before stuttering develops to the point where a successful outcome becomes less likely.

Because stuttering is most likely best thought of from a multifactorial perspective, an example of a comprehensive assessment approach is provided in the form of the Rileys' (2000) Revised Component Model. This model assumes that a vulnerable speech production system is influenced by several components that place a young speaker at risk for fluency disruption. Assessment consists of identifying those components that contribute to the vulnerability of a particular child's speech production system as well as the components of the child's system that need to be enhanced in order to facilitate fluent speech. The information identified during one or more assessment interviews will enable the clinician to formulate treatment strategies that are most appropriate for each child.

STUDY QUESTIONS

➤ Describe three activities that would be likely to elicit fluency breaks in the speech of a young child.

➤ What are both verbal and nonverbal behaviors indicating that young children are aware that they are having a difficult time speaking?

➤ Differentiate between trait and state anxiety. How do children who stutter differ from nonstuttering children on these measures?

➤ Which of the assessment measures and procedures described in this chapter do you feel provides the best picture of a child's affective and cognitive response to the stuttering experience?

➤ What factors did Yairi et al. (1996) suggest as distinguishing children who would be likely to recover from stuttering? What factors suggest that children will not recover?

➤ What are your thoughts concerning whether you would intervene with a young child who is showing the initial stages of stuttering development? What strategy would you take for making this decision?

➤ How closely does the Rileys' Revised Component Model compare with the Capacities and Demands model described in Chapter 2? What features are similar and which ones are different?

➤ What are your views concerning the efficacy and the ethics of using "at risk registers"?

RECOMMENDED READINGS

Riley, G., & Riley, J. (in press). A revised component model for diagnosing and treating children who stutter. *Contemporary Issues in Communication Sciences and Disorders.*

Yairi, E., & Ambrose, N. G. (1999). Early childhood stuttering I: Persistency and Recovery Rates. *Journal of Speech, Language, and Hearing Research, 42,* 1097–1112.

Yaruss, J. S. (1977a). Clinical measurement of stuttering behaviors. *Contemporary Issues in Communication Science and Disorders, 24,* 33–44.

Zebrowski, P. M. (1997). Assisting young children who stutter and their families: Defining the role of the speech-language pathologist. *American Journal of Speech-Language Pathology, 6,* 19–28.

CHAPTER

6

FACILITATING THE CHANGE PROCESS

> *Nothing in this world can take the place of persistence.*
>
> *Talent will not; nothing is more common than unsuccessful people with talent.*
>
> *Genius will not; unrewarded genius is almost a proverb.*
>
> *Education will not; the world is full of educated derelicts.*
>
> *Persistence and determination alone are omnipotent.*
>
> *The slogan "press on" has solved and always will solve the problems of the human race.—Calvin Coolidge*

INTRODUCTION

Before beginning our discussions of how to facilitate change for our clients, some comments about the nature of change may be beneficial. On the surface of the change process we are discussing behavioral changes, actions we want our clients to take and things we want them to do differently. We want them to develop new ways of considering themselves and their choices. For younger speakers, particularly preschool and early school-age children, change, pliability and growth are natural. In Chapter 5 we noted some of the important affective and cognitive aspects of the stuttering experience that may impact even these young speakers. As we have seen, even during the early years, the experience of stuttering can be much more than the surface features, and some children recognize and react with frustration and struggle to their inability to speak. For these children, however, modeling of fluency-enhancing techniques by the clinician and both guidance and support by the parents can result in relatively brief and successful intervention. As the child begins formal schooling and reacts to the effects of socialization, there is likely to be an increase in the negative response to his nonfluent speech. For these older children who have begun to define themselves as someone who stutters, and certainly for adolescents and adults, the process of change becomes considerably more elaborate. As we will describe, change for these people is often more strenuous and perhaps best thought of as a process that occurs in stages. It is usually possible to assign a beginning to the process, but—in most cases—there is no end stage, since the person will continue to evolve. If the clinician is particularly good, the process of change can also be creative and exciting.

THE NATURE OF CHANGE

As clinicians we often have a vision of what our client can be and where he may be able to go. We sometimes take a role of pushing and prodding in order to nudge this person in directions we believe that he or she is capable of going. However, using a wonderful phrase, Zinker (1977, p. 23) explains that we cannot "push the river" in the creative process of therapy. As much as we would like to, we cannot *fix* the client and we cannot make the client do what he is not ready to do. This means that for many clients who stutter, we cannot pour fluency into a vessel that is not ready to hold it. Sometimes we can lead our younger clients toward fluency by modeling techniques such as easy and slow speech, and many times they will follow. With these young children, often we can create the fertile soil where fluency may grow. For most adolescents and adults who have been stuttering for many years, we are facing a multi-layered and complex problem whose true solution will defy simplistic solutions. This is why we include both this and the following chapter on counseling as it relates to fluency therapy. We do not make it happen—rather we are preparing the client for change and when he is ready, he will. With another colorful phrase, Zinker (1977) suggests that much of therapy involves "priming the canvas" (p. 24).

Ideally, the clinician reading this chapter will see how information on the change process folds into the description of clinician characteristics found in Chapter 1, the principles of counseling found in Chapter 7, and the many treatment approaches to be discussed in subsequent chapters. As such understanding becomes the case, it becomes clear that comprehensive treatment for adolescents and adults involves so much more than simply "fixing the stuttering" and making people fluent. It is much bigger than that and far more exciting. In many ways we are "people-making" and enabling them to live life in a broader and deeper manner as we help them to become "unstuck," not only from their speech but from a life of restricted decision-making. In that sense doing therapy is, as Zinker suggests, like making art, and the medium is a human life (p. 37). Experienced clinicians do not work on fluency techniques in one session and the next day focus only on a client's negative and positive self-talk. It's all part of the same process.

THE LIKELIHOOD OF SUCCESS

Successful treatment for stuttering and related fluency disorders must take place with an acceptance on the part of the clinician that she is attempting to help people who have a complex problem. As we have discussed, the problem is complex because it involves many layers, including—but not limited to—the quantity and quality of a person's speech. If the person has been stuttering for many years, patterns of behavior and thinking become established. Helping people to move from their current state of speaking, thinking, and functioning with a severe communication problem that impacts virtually all aspects of life is no simple process. It should not be surprising, therefore, that stuttering is a communication problem that takes time—often years—to change. This is especially true for adults who have been stuttering for many decades (Manning, 1991b).

On the other hand, it is also important to appreciate that this syndrome is probably no more enigmatic than many other problems that humans can have. Andrews, Guitar, and Howie (1980) provide one of the few positive comments suggesting that stuttering, although complex, is reasonably well understood and not so terribly difficult to treat. Using meta-analysis, these authors compared the results of 42 treatment investigations and found treatment for stuttering to be effective and the results stable over time. Craig et al.'s. (1995) 12-month post-treatment outcome data on children who were treated for stuttering with a smooth speech procedure indicated that 70% of the children maintained fluency levels of less that 2% SS. In addition, Howie, Tanner, and Andrews (1981) followed 36 adults for up to 18 months post-treatment and found that adult clients have a 70% chance of gaining substantially improved speech as well as increased speaking confidence. Indeed, some adults who have experienced successful treatment for stuttering are able to achieve high levels of spontaneous fluency. On occasion, these speakers score higher than nonstuttering adults on measures of approach behavior in difficult speaking situations (Hillis & Manning, 1996). As a result of treatment, they are likely to have learned much about the speech mechanism and the nature of speech and language and to have gained considerable experience in speaking in a large variety of individual and group situations. If the person continues expanding these experiences following treatment, it is not surprising that some clients are able to become above-average speakers.

Another note of optimism is that working with children and adults who stutter can be enormously enjoyable. As we mentioned in Chapter 1, as the client grows often the clinician grows also, for the most effective clinicians are nearly always learning. They are making real-time decisions about the needs of the client as these needs become apparent. Thus while the treatment process for fluency disorders can be complex and even messy, it can also be dynamic and exciting.

If it is done well, fluency treatment can result in degrees of positive change in the client's perspective of the problem, level of fluency, and—in many cases—improvement in the client's relationships and overall approach to life. It is also important to appreciate that the process of growth goes well beyond specific treatment techniques and behavioral changes. Therapy involves helping to create a better future—as well as much improved communication—for the person we are helping. Important cognitive and affective changes occur. Just as most athletic activities are much more than the sum of many individual skills, the process of treatment is much more than the application of techniques to be mastered. In fact, it may be argued that the consequences of overemphasizing therapeutic microskills leads to ineffective treatment.

MATCHING TREATMENT TO CLIENT STAGES OF CHANGE

Prochaska, DiClemente, and Norcross (1992) propose that individuals usually go through several stages as they change. Although their work generally focused on individuals with addictive behavior, their ideas have many applications to the treatment of other complex behavioral problems, including stuttering. Their stage model of change can be summarized as follows:

1. Change is cyclical through the stages.
2. There is a common set of processes that facilitate change.
3. It is possible to integrate the stages and processes of change.

The success of treatment is closely tied to the ability of an experienced clinician to determine a client's readiness for change and adjust treatment techniques accordingly. Thus the utility of the techniques depends on the clinician's ability to apply the right technique(s) at the right time. The first part of the model suggested by Prohaska et al. is composed of the five stages of change as described by Prochaska and colleagues (1992).

Precontemplation

Individuals are generally unaware of their problem during this initial stage. Even with some awareness and a wish to change, the person has no intention of doing something about their problem in the immediate future (i.e., the next six months). Some people may have enough awareness of their problem to be defensive, but they generally feel that it is under control. Because others often see the problem, when people in this stage come for treatment, they often do so as a result of pressure from others. In such cases, the client may be capable of change as long as the pressure is on but is likely to cease treatment once the threat is past. A hallmark of people in this stage is their *resistance to either recognizing or modifying the problem.*

Contemplation

As they enter this stage, persons have become aware of their problem and are actively beginning to consider the possibility of change (i.e., during the next six months). Although they often begin seeking information about the problem, they have no formal plan to take action. Even with this increased awareness and concern about their problem, some may stay in the contemplation stage for years. After weighing the pros and cons of their behavior and the time, effort, and money it will take to change, they begin *serious consideration of the possible ways to resolve the problem.*

Preparation

People in this stage are ready to change and intend to take action during the next month. However, while they may begin to demonstrate some small behavioral changes, they have not yet taken effective action. The important aspect is that they are *now making decisions in terms of goals and priorities.*

Action

In this stage people are now beginning to modify specific behaviors, their environment, or both. They use newly acquired skills to make overt changes. Because behavioral changes have now become obvious, they are apt to receive recognition by others. A key element of this stage is that the person's *altered behavior is defined by the achievement of specific criteria.*

Maintenance

In this final stage people are beginning to stabilize their behavioral and cognitive changes. Because it takes a long time to reduce the occurrences of old behaviors, attitudes, and cognitions and replace them with new ones, this period lasts from six months to an undetermined period of time. A marker of this stage is *the appearance of new and incompatible behavior in real-life situations.*

All those involved in treatment need to understand that progress throughout the stages is not usually linear. A spiral or cyclical pattern of change is more likely to occur. Individuals may choose to move through these stages with professional assistance, or the changes may be self-initiated. As Prochaska et al. indicate, people often move from the action stage and into maintenance and then back to precontemplation. As clients learn from their mistakes, they again advance to the next stage of change. Furthermore, relapse at any point in the change process is the rule rather than the exception.

It is also important to appreciate that relatively few people who have a chronic or long-standing problem are actually ready to make changes. Summary data obtained on smoking cessation by Prochaska et al. (1992) illustrates this point. They noted that 50–60% of smokers are in the pre-contemplation stage and 30–40% in the contemplation stage. Only 10–14% of this population can be categorized as being in the action stage. A key implication of this stage model is that people in different stages of change need to be matched with different treatment processes, or change will be less likely to take place. This way of considering the process of treatment coincides with the client-centered approach advocated by many clinicians.

Processes of Change

The second part of this trans-theoretical model is how the processes of change are linked to clients' stages of change. DiClemente (1993) described 10 categories of processes that facilitate change. Gathered from various clinical approaches to psychotherapeutic intervention, these processes are grouped together regardless of the theoretical construct in which they typically used.

1. *Consciousness raising:* These processes involve helping clients to increase information about themselves and the problem. This is accomplished using such techniques as observation, confrontation, interpretation, and bibliotherapy (the client obtains educational materials addressing the problem).
2. *Self-reevaluation:* These are processes that help clients to assess how they feel and think about themselves with respect to their problem behaviors. This self-assessment is accomplished by techniques of value clarification, imagery, corrective emotional experience, and challenging beliefs and expectations.
3. *Self-liberation:* Such processes involve helping clients to choose and commit to taking action. Clients also may need help to increase their belief in their ability to change. Action taking can be accomplished by decision-making therapy, developing resolutions, logotherapy and commitment-enhancing techniques.

4. *Counter-conditioning:* These processes enable clients to substitute alternatives for the anxiety related to problem behaviors. Anxiety reduction may be accomplished by techniques of relaxation, desensitization, assertion, and positive self-statements.

5. *Stimulus control:* These processes help persons to avoid or counter stimuli that elicit problem behaviors. Such techniques include restructuring the environment, avoiding high-risk cues, and fading techniques.

6. *Reinforcement management:* These processes involve showing clients how to reward themselves or create rewards from others for the changes they make. Rewards can be created by contingency contracts and overt and covert reinforcement for self-reward.

7. *Helping relationships:* These processes help clients to be open and trusting about problems with people who care. Trust may be enhanced by the development of therapeutic alliances, increased social support, and association with support groups.

8. *Emotional arousal and dramatic relief:* These processes have to do with helping clients to experience and express feelings about their problems and possible solutions. Greater insight can be achieved by techniques such as psychodrama, grieving losses, and role playing.

9. *Environmental reevaluation:* These processes enable clients to evaluate how a problem affects their personal and physical environment. Understanding can be accomplished by using techniques of empathy training and documentaries.

10. *Social liberation:* These are processes that help clients to increase alternatives for non-problem behaviors that are present in society. Such involvement can be accomplished by advocating for rights of the repressed and empowering policy changes and interventions.

Prochaska et al. (1992) suggest that stage/process mismatches by clinicians may prevent or impede successful change by clients. This commonly occurs, for example, when clinicians select processes associated with the contemplation stage (e.g., consciousness-raising, self-evaluation) at a time when a client is moving into the action stage. Becoming more aware and gaining insight, alone, do not bring about behavioral change, so these are not efficient processes at this stage of change. Such mismatches may explain some of the criticisms directed at counseling and non-directive approaches for changing behaviors. Another common mismatch is using action-oriented processes (e.g., reinforcement, stimulus control, and counter-conditioning) with clients in the contemplation or preparation stages of change. Accordingly, modification of behaviors without clients' awareness have been a frequent criticism of radical behaviorism. In addition, behavioral changes achieved in the absence of insight are likely to be temporary, according to Prochaska et al. (1992).

DIFFICULTIES IN INITIATING AND MAINTAINING CHANGE

For all the positive things that treatment can be, both for the client as well as the clinician, the process can also be difficult. It is difficult for many reasons, but often because it usually requires hard work. In most cases the speaker has learned many inefficient and maladaptive behaviors that tend to call attention to the fact that he is stuck. Patterns of denial, fear, shame, and avoidance are powerful and complex. Some ways of thinking and living that have become habitual will have to be altered. At times it can be difficult to separate the individual from the person who stutters. It may be difficult to understand whether or not numerous missed opportunities and unused potential are related to stuttering.

The process of getting people unstuck and moving in a better direction may be complex and messy. Getting people to the point where they no longer need our guidance and support involves time and learning. It is a daunting task to help another person work toward constructive change, and often we are faced with our lack of power to make things happen. Clinicians who are new to the task of helping people who stutter do these things need to appreciate the difficulty of what they are asking our clients to do. As we indicate throughout this book, especially for adolescents and adults, most of the time treatment is far more than showing people how to do techniques that enhance fluency. With timing that is often uncertain, we try to assist them to understand, monitor, and eventually change the many levels of stuttering across gradually more difficult speaking situations.

Successful intervention also requires continued commitment and motivation by the client. Therapy can be frustrating. It may take more than a little time and money. Although Peck (1978) is reflecting on the nature of psychotherapy in his book, *The Road Less Traveled*, his comments easily apply to any treatment that requires behavioral as well as cognitive change. He suggests that of the choices one may have in dealing with a problem, treatment is usually the most difficult path. This is so, he argues, because each of us is always working against entropy: the tendency for things, including programs of change, to fall apart. Peck sees entropy manifested as laziness. Peck indicates that as many as 9 out of 10 patients who begin psychotherapy (or other therapies) stop long before the clinician believes that the process has been completed. Sometimes, after the client experiences success and a corresponding lessening of the problem, the cost-benefit ratio decreases and further change is no longer worth the effort. The price for continuing change is too high. Unfortunately, this can also the case for clients with fluency disorders.

It is also worth noting that there are some influential forces against which the clinician and the client must work during treatment. For example, there are old ways of seeing the problem and oneself. In order to change, there may be a period of holding on to the old perceptions and the old self. This is more likely, of course, with adults. We show them new ways of viewing themselves and the problem which, although often attractive, also suggest that the old view of life may be in error. Many authors (Egan, 1998; Emerick, 1988; Hayhow & Levy, 1989; Peck, 1978) acknowledge that giving up the old way of doing things, particularly the loss of the old belief system, is a blow to the client. For example, Kuhlman (1984) suggests that a "mourning process" may be necessary. New insights about the shortcomings of the old system of beliefs can be a blow to a client's self-esteem. This is not always a major problem during treatment, but it is likely to occur to some degree and thus to provide some resistance to change.

Egan (1998) describes what he terms the "shadow side" of change. He suggests that even as we respond to a client's request to help him change, what is in many cases, a limited lifestyle, we are precipitating a degree of disequilibrium or disorganization. We are asking those we are trying to help to give up a way of functioning (surviving) in a fluent world. For some, the loss of functioning can create a crisis. Such idiopathic responses may be thought of as a natural part of the change process. After years of denial, such a response should not be surprising to the experienced clinician.

Starkweather (1999) also discusses the various forms denial that people who stutter may use as a means of survival. As Starkweather points out, denial is difficult to see, even for adults. Clients will deny that many of their decisions and their behaviors are a function of stuttering. Crowe (1977b) cites Kubler-Ross (1969) in suggesting that an individual's tendency to rely on denial as a defense against life's pressures increases the possibility of this response with an illness or disability. As Crowe points out, although clinicians should understand that denial is a natural reaction to unwanted situations, denial should gradually lessen to the point that the client is able to move forward in the treatment process. If denial does not lessen, it could be a function of the clinician moving too quickly into action-oriented processes when the client is still in the contemplation or preparation stage of change.

Some people will show a reluctance to get started, or once started, they tire of the rigor necessary for completing the tasks they have agreed to do. Egan (1998) also describes several reasons why clients fail to change. He suggests that much of the art in helping people change has to do with overcoming these forms of reluctance without pushing our clients too much and turning reluctance into resistance. Some clients have a *passive lifestyle* and clinicians, beyond listening and understanding, must act as agents of change to help their clients take responsibility for their own change. Sometimes a client's inability to change presents as "learned helplessness," and a clinician may find ways of increasing the person's resourcefulness for changing specific aspects of one's life. These clients may also be minimally depressed. Their self-talk, what they tell themselves about themselves and about their stuttering, often provides a window for understanding their current view of their situation.

Because it often requires a long journey to change behaviors and belief systems developed over many years, some people will choose not to change. They may begin to understand some of the basic characteristics of their speaking problem and may have a good idea of what it will take to change their situation. For some, this understanding and acceptance of their situation may be enough. As Egan (1998) explains, they feel that "The price of more effective living is too high" (p. 333).

Perhaps the most important ingredient for success, as it is with many things, is that of persistence. Many of us have had the experience during our freshman year of college of looking around the room at the faces and being told that many of these people would not be there by the senior year. There is no shortage of these occurrences throughout life. Many factors including innate intelligence, talent, and good fortune play a major role in achieving success. However, as suggested at the opening of this chapter, the most critical factor is usually persistence.

LEADING FROM BEHIND

Conducting treatment with fluency disorders is similar to many other relationships, both therapeutic and otherwise. Certainly, as clinicians we must have a clear direction where treatment is leading. However, it is also true that if we too closely control the relationship, we may narrow the possibilities for change and growth. Unquestionably, the clinician must have an overall plan and a direction for treatment and must be familiar with many associated treatment techniques. However, we cannot control all aspects of the other person and make him into our own image of him. Our goal is to help him to self-manage his situation, and we can help direct that process. However, sometimes it is clear that we have to lead from behind, following the client where he needs to go and helping him to get there. We can assist him in developing new views of himself and new options concerning his fluency. With the right timing in response to changes by the client, we can help him to make better choices and to become less handicapped. We can also acknowledge that while we provide direction, insight, and information, the person who must ultimately take the lead in repairing the problem is the client. The clinician must know the choices that are available in terms of overall treatment strategies and associated applications. However, the mark of an experienced clinician is not knowing what strategies or techniques to use. Every clinician should have that information. The mark of an effective clinician is reflected in her clinical insight about *why* and *when* to employ it.

THE GOALS OF TREATMENT

Of course, it is necessary to have a good idea of where we want to go during treatment. One of the first objectives during the initial treatment sessions is to demonstrate our sense of direction to the client by providing a map of the journey (See Cooper, 1985; Guitar, 1998; and Maxwell, 1982 for excellent examples of pretreatment orientation statements). It is important for the client to have a clear understanding of the treatment process, and success is more likely to occur if both the client and the clinician share a similar view. At the outset of treatment the client's concept of his fluency disorder itself is apt to be ambiguous. The clinician who is able to help the client decrease the mystery and understand the lawfulness of the stuttering syndrome provides a valuable service to the client. Before the client can begin to accurately monitor and self-manage himself and his speech, he must begin to appreciate the nature of the problem in general and the dynamics of his own specific response to his situation.

Levels of Fluency

Speakers who are regarded as normally fluent demonstrate a wide range of fluency across different situations. As discussed in Chapter 3, this range of fluency is greatest in speakers who stutter. When considering the goals of treatment, authors have found it useful to distinguish at least three levels of fluency (Guitar, 1998).

Spontaneous fluency can be thought of as ideally normal speech. The speech is smooth and may contain only sporadic fluency breaks, which are formulative in nature. Speech flows easily with little apparent effort, and virtually no attention is paid to how the speech is produced. The speaker as well as the listener are able to attend to the message, and the speaker's fluency does not detract from the information being delivered. Although relatively rare, it is possible for some clients who stutter, even adult clients, to eventually achieve this level of spontaneous fluency in all speaking situations.

Controlled fluency is nearly normal speech production, but with the price of increased effort on the part of the speaker. Although the speaker must attend to his manner of speaking in order to maintain fluency, the speech moves forward with few obvious fluency breaks. There is a price to be paid in the form of vigilance and self-management of those fluency breaks, which could otherwise go out of control. This effort, to the degree that it is perceived by the listener, may detract somewhat from the message. Thus the method and the message of speaking may carry nearly equal weight. Depending on the ability of the speaker to apply techniques that facilitate the smooth coordination of respiration, phonation, and articulation, this type of fluency may be perceived as *unstable speech*. In many ways, this type of fluency is similar to that of a normal speaker who is placed in a speaking situation that contains a high level of communicative or emotional stress.

Acceptable fluency takes the level of monitoring and self-management of the speaker to another stage. Now the effort to maintain fluency is increased, and the method of producing speech may be slightly more obvious than the content of the message. Even though stuttering events are occurring, the speaker is actively changing the form of these events. This is far less than ideal fluency but much preferred to the client's old automatic, reflexive form of stuttering. Although stuttering is taking place, because these events are undergoing modification or smoothing it is possible for the speaker and the listener to achieve a high degree of satisfaction and contentment. Although more research is needed, there is some suggestion in the literature that people who do something about their problems are regarded more positively than those who do not (Blood & Blood, 1982; Collins & Blood, 1990; Hastorf, Windfogel, & Cassman, 1979; Silverman, 1988a). Most importantly, however, it is possible for the speaker—despite the presence of some stuttering—to make decisions that result in a significant decrease in the handicap of the fluency disorder.

Achieving Spontaneous Fluency

Even for the most severe clients, the quickest way to reduce the frequency of stuttering is to have the speaker use a number of techniques or devices that result in nearly instantaneous fluency. It is well known that immediate, if temporary, fluency can be achieved by having most clients sing, read, or speak in unison with another person; speak in a loud or whispered voice; use a dialect or bouncy intonation; or speak while rhythmically moving a finger, arm, or leg. In addition, devices that provide for auditory masking of the speaker's voice production, a pacing tone (e.g., a metronome), or an audio delay in the speaker's speech also tend to result in less frequent—or at least less severe—stuttering events. The fluency-enhancing effects of these activities have been attributed to both the rhythmic effects (Van Riper, 1973) and the modification of phonation (Wingate, 1969).

These fluency-enhancing activities can provide highly dramatic results, and such instantaneous improvements tend to have the effect of making anyone who uses them an "expert" on how to help people who stutter. Although many early stuttering and stammering schools were built around some of these efforts, the effects on the speaker's fluency are generally short-lived (Silverman, 1976). In instances where the speaker has been unable to achieve lasting benefit from other treatment methods, such devices have been advocated. For chronic stutterers (Cooper, 1986a) such devices may provide the only way to effectively communicate. Although these devices are helpful, it is usually best if the speaker can systematically wean himself from their use.

The achievement of *spontaneous* fluency is often the primary outcome many of our clients ask of us. However, should the achievement of spontaneous fluency be held as the only criterion for successful treatment? Spontaneous fluency is more likely to be a reasonable goal for young children. Something approaching complete fluency is also attainable for the infrequent adult who, as a result of emotional trauma, has experienced a sudden onset of stuttering in adulthood. As the underlying or associated problems become resolved, these speakers may be able to achieve their previous levels of fluency.

High levels of posttreatment fluency may also occur for adults after taking part in an intensive residential program. However, because of logistic or financial reasons, that is not where many clients are able to find help. In addition, the difficult transition from the focused and supportive clinical environment of an intensive program back to the client's home and work environments usually has an adverse effect on the gains made during formal treatment. It has been suggested that rapid and dramatic improvements that can occur in an intensive program may result in a fluent speaker who is unsure what he did to accomplish change (Boberg, 1986; see p. 491). Prins (1970) indicated that intensive residential programs may produce *disfluency overkill* and provide the client with the notion that stuttering will not occur as long as he follows the techniques he has mastered. Kamhi (1982) cautions clinicians who suggest to clients that the use of fluency-shaping techniques will result in error-free speech on all occasions. Perhaps the best statement in this regard was Sheehan's (1980) comment that producing stutter-free speech is no more realistic than playing error-free baseball. He reasoned that because the person possesses the capacity to function in an error-free manner it does not follow that this will always be the case.

Thus for most adults who have stuttered since childhood, some fluency breaks are the rule. The question is not so much whether the client will stutter, especially in more difficult speaking situations. In many instances he will. The more basic question is *how* he is going to stutter and what he is going to do about each stuttering event. As Van Riper often stated, the speaker may not always have much of a choice about when he is going to stutter, but he certainly can have a choice about how he is going to stutter (Van Riper, 1990).

Certainly it is possible for a client to achieve fluency levels approaching 100% both within and outside the treatment setting. However, it is not necessarily realistic to expect such levels of fluency before dismissing the client from treatment. Using a stringent criterion of 100% fluency is problematic for other reasons. First of all, this measure of success places far too much emphasis on a single surface feature of the syndrome, the frequency of stuttering. Decreasing the occurrence of overt stuttering events is clearly one of the things clinicians can target during treatment. For many speakers, however, it provides a compressed view of progress and success.

It is not surprising that the surface features of the stuttering syndrome will be the first to change. A client will often demonstrate rapid improvement in his level of fluency prior to or during the initial days or weeks of treatment. Much of this change is a result of the client's acknowledging his problem and adapting to the clinician, the treatment setting, and the client's understanding of his role during treatment. The client's fluency improves as he understands what is expected of him and what challenges he is asked to meet. Certainly, an increase in fluency is reflective of change. However, it may not necessarily indicate progress. That is, the increased fluency in the treatment setting may have little relationship to the client's level of fluency in his daily environment. Even complete fluency in a clinical environment can provide an unrealistic indication about the probability of such success in extra-treatment speaking situations. It is one thing to hit 10 out of 10 shots when playing basketball alone, but the real question is how many shots will be successful during competitive game conditions, when the pressure is great and performance counts. It is not unusual for a clinician to unexpectedly meet a client outside the therapy situation and find examples of severe stuttering that have never been observed in the clinic.

As obvious as overt fluency breaks may be and as much as they get in the way, there is much more to the syndrome of stuttering than these surface events. It is tempting to focus the majority of the diagnostic and treatment efforts on the surface features while failing to consider changes in the intrinsic features of the syndrome, which are nonetheless important, both for a comprehensive diagnosis and for lasting therapeutic change. Most authors suggest that, at least with adolescents and adults, a truly comprehensive treatment strategy should be multidimensional (Hillis, 1993; Prins, 1970; Van Riper, 1973). With a multidimensional approach the criterion of success in treatment is considerably broader than a relatively simplistic measure of the number of fluency breaks in the form of percent syllables or words stuttered. Assuming that the syndrome of stuttering involves not only surface behaviors but also attitudinal and cognitive features, it will be necessary to promote changes across these features as well.

Although spontaneous fluency is both a reasonable and an attainable goal for some clients, many people tire of treatment before such levels of fluency are reached. They reach the point where they are less handicapped and the fluency breaks, although still present, no longer present a large threat to the quality of life. In addition, there are some clients, especially those with chronic stuttering, who are unable to make lasting progress toward high levels of fluency. Even speakers with frequent fluency breaks can learn to revise features of their stuttering and adjust to listener reactions in order to become less handicapped.

The Importance of Modeling

Modeling by the clinician and others is discussed throughout this text. Because modeling is such an important aspect of the change process, we will take a moment to discuss this aspect of treatment. Modeling of different attitudes and behaviors can have a profound impact on some clients. Examples of alternative and possibly better ways of doing and thinking about things can be modeled by the clinician as well as other people in the client's environment. If we want our clients to give themselves permission to take risks and experiment with new ways of doing things, we should probably model such behavior. Observing people as they successfully perform athletic, singing, writing, or speaking activities can be a critical and motivating influence for those who desire to perform these activities. The experience often helps to increase the observer's self-expectations and willingness to invest the effort to undertake difficult tasks. Our expectation of our client's ability to change is confirmed by our willingness to lead the way by challenging ourselves and changing aspects of our own lives. Our modeling of attitudes and behaviors can provide a way to challenge, disrupt, and eventually alter the client's current belief system and behaviors.

VARIABLES IN CHOOSING A TREATMENT

There are several basic treatment characteristics that are influenced by such things as the clinical setting and the client's needs and capabilities. These characteristics often require the clinician to make decisions about the form that treatment will take. In some instances, the choices are already made for the clinician according to the nature of the treatment setting or the options that are available because of such issues as time and expense (Starkweather, St. Louis, Blood, Peters, & Westbrook, 1994).

The Timing and Duration of Treatment

There is considerable variation here, ranging from intensive, residential programs lasting six or more hours each day for one or more weeks to treatment in public schools, which may take place as little as one hour or less each week. Generally, adolescents and adults who stutter require a longer time in treatment. Preschool clients require a shorter time and often make faster progress. Treatment that is less intensive disrupts the client's everyday life less, but the change involved can be slow and the client may become discouraged. On the other hand, intensive treatment often results in more rapid change (Prins, 1970), with the likelihood of greater problems when it comes time to transfer the gains made in the clinical setting to the speaker's everyday life. The duration of treatment also can be influenced by such factors as the complexity of the fluency disorder, other coexisting communication problems, and especially the client's motivation. For adult speakers, formal treatment lasting one year with at least one individual and one group meeting each week seems to be regarded as a minimum (Maxwell, 1982; Van Riper, 1973).

The Complexity of Treatment

A client's degree of handicap across the social, educational, and vocational aspects of his life will be a major factor in determining the course and length of intervention. Furthermore, the client's personality and emotional characteristics such as defensive behaviors, coping strategies, resistance to change, anxiety, inhibited behavior, or even—on occasion—depression or sociopathic behavior can also increase the length and complexity of treatment. In such instances, treatment may require the use of many strategies and techniques as well as other professional clinicians in areas such as counseling, psychology, or psychiatry.

The Cost of Treatment

This important aspect of treatment also varies widely. Because of the typical length of treatment and the usual lack of reimbursement by insurance companies, the cost of successful treatment can quickly become prohibitive for many clients. Fees for diagnosis and treatment are generally lower when there are restrictions on the intensity of service, as in some training programs. Service in these settings can be secondary to the academic and clinical training requirements of the program. The level of service can also be compromised somewhat in public or private school settings, where caseload requirements may vary widely.

The Treatment Setting

The treatment that is provided is often determined in large measure by the setting. In this regard, St. Louis and Westbrook (1987) provide an insightful comment explaining that the choice of treatment may not be made with the client as the primary consideration.

> It seems plausible that typical delivery models for stuttering therapy evolved as much to suit clinicians' tastes; administrators' desires; school, university, or hospital schedules; or physicians' prescriptions as they did to provide the maximum benefit to stutterers. (p. 250)

The treatment strategies and techniques the clinician selects may or may not coincide with the available environment. That is, the clinician may want to schedule the client for several sessions each week, but multiple sessions may not be possible due to the logistics of the client's work schedule and distance from the treatment center. The clinician may consider parent participation to be critical for success, but the parents may be employed in one or more jobs and unable or unwilling to attend sessions. Individual treatment may be necessary, yet the caseload in the clinical facility (particularly in the public schools) will only allow for group treatment, sometimes including clients who possess a variety of other communication problems.

In addition, the opportunity for monitored practice outside the clinic or school setting is essential. Often, however, because of logistic, legal, insurance, or time constraints, the clinician may be unable to go with the child or adult to more realistic speaking situations in offices, restaurants, or shopping malls. This is an important feature, for as the Guidelines for Treatment by ASHA's Division 4 (Appendix D) suggest, treatment settings that fail to create such experiences also may fail to provide realistic indications of change or progress. At the very least, the clinician should create opportunities to monitor the client's performance in the form of direct observation, interviews with the client following practice sessions, or monitoring with audio or video recordings of extra-treatment practice. The logistics of distance, cost, and location of the treatment setting may prevent many desired features of treatment from occurring. At the very least, however, the client should be made aware of any important limitations of treatment.

CONCLUSION

Getting humans to change behavior, particularly something as complex as stuttering, requires more than a quick fix of the surface features of the disorder. It is also important to realize that, as clinicians, we cannot *make* it happen. Sometimes, we can facilitate the often long process of change for a client who is ready to take the journey. Great success is possible for many people who stutter, even if they have done so for many years. The timing of the clinical relationship is probably critical in terms of that person's readiness to change and his or her position within the stages of change (Precontemplation, Contemplation, Preparation, Action, Maintenance).

Facilitating change requires that we recognize where the client is across stages of change and employ clinical processes that are most appropriate for assisting our clients at that stage. It is not unusual for clinicians to run up against a variety of obstacles as we attempt to facilitate change in our clients. Often we are asking them to think about things and do things they have denied or avoided for years. The process is not linear, and sometimes it is far from tidy. We can help the client to identify realistic goals, we can model different ways of thinking and speaking, and we can help our client to assess the variables that may facilitate successful intervention.

STUDY QUESTIONS

➤ What are the three basic assumptions of Prochaska et al.'s change model?

➤ Briefly explain the five stages of change as described in this chapter.

➤ Write (for yourself) a short description of how you interpreted events or responded with behaviors that may be examples of denial on your part.

➤ Provide three examples of how it would be possible for a clinician to create a mismatch between the five stages of change and one of the 10 therapeutic processes.

➤ Explain some of the factors that make it difficult for people to initiate and maintain change. Write a brief story about how one or more of these factors explain why it was hard for you to change some aspect of your behavior or thinking.

➤ What does Egan mean by the "shadow side" of change?

RECOMMENDED READINGS

Prochaska, J. O., & DiClemente, C.C. (1992). Stages of change in the modification of problem behaviors. In Herson, M, Eisler, R, & Miller, P. (Eds.), *Progress in behavior modification* (pp. 184–218). Sycamore, IL: Sycamore Publishing Company.

Prochaska, J. O., DiClemente, C. C., & Norcross, J. C. (1992). In search of how people change: Applications to addictive behaviors. *American Psychologist*, 47(9), 1102–1114.

Zinker, J. (1977). *Creative process in Gestalt therapy*. New York: Random House.

CHAPTER

7

COUNSELING STRATEGIES AND TECHNIQUES

All clinicians should also train themselves in the subtle skills than enable them to sense the hidden feelings of their clients. These are not to be found in textbooks or classrooms. They must be mastered in the situations of intimate human encounter. Some of my students and clients have felt that I had an uncanny ability to read their thoughts—and at times I have indeed experienced something akin to clairvoyance—but only after I had observed and identified closely with the person long enough. . . . It is the result of very careful observation, uninhibited inference making, and the calculation of probabilities. It comes through empathy. (pp. 107-108)
    Charles Van Riper (1979). A career in speech pathology.
                    Englewood Cliffs, NJ: Prentice-Hall.

At a certain point in this self-generated event, the client experiences an Aha! He says, "Now I understand how I am," or "Yes, that's how I feel," or "Now I know what I need to do, how I need to act to get what I want in this situation." He is his own teacher. (p. 125)
        Joseph Zinker (1977). The Creative Process in Gestalt Therapy. New York: Random House.

235

INTRODUCTION

In this chapter we contend that counseling skills are a basic characteristic of an effective clinician and that counseling techniques are a basic part of the therapeutic change process. As we will see, there is a notable history of counseling in our field in general and in the area of fluency disorders in particular. If the recent increase of texts and chapters devoted to counseling is an indication (e.g, Bloom & Cooperman, 1999; Crowe, 1997; Shapiro, 1999), the appreciation of this aspect of the change process is increasing.

We will also suggest that because the relationship of the client and the clinician are at the center of the change process, counseling activities are taking place (either directly or indirectly) regardless of the approach that is chosen for the treatment of stuttering. Crowe (1997a) provides a helpful definition of counseling. He cites Hinsie and Campbell (1970) who differentiate counseling and psychotherapy. Counseling is seen as a type of psychotherapy for the purpose of support or (re)education for behavioral problems *not* associated with mental illness. As Crowe explains, counseling is intended for assisting those people with less severe interpersonal (v. intrapersonal) problems. Psychotherapy, on the other hand, is intended for persons with mental illness related to basic problems in personality development and personal adjustment. Although communication disorders often result in serious problems on many levels, in most cases we are not working with people who have chronic life-adjustment problems.

EGAN'S THREE-STAGE SKILLED-HELPER MODEL

In the first edition of this text, this chapter on counseling contained several references to the fourth (1990) edition of Gerard Egan's book *The Skilled Helper: A Systematic Approach to Effective Helping*. The current chapter, along with other references from the literature on counseling, contains additional information from Egan's sixth edition of *The Skilled Helper: A Problem-Manage Approach to Helping* (1998), a text that is reported to be the most widely used counseling text in the world. In this most recent edition, Egan provides a model for helping people who have a wide variety of problems. In the following chapter, and to some degree throughout this book, Egan's model is interpreted and adapted for helping individuals who have the specific problem of stuttering. Because only the most basic features of Egan's model are included in this chapter and because it offers guidance that is helpful for all clinicians, readers are urged to obtain the most recent edition of this text.

Egan's three-stage model presents an interactive approach for helping people to clarify their problem(s) and to systematically select a plan of action for changing their situation. As we will describe, this model is not designed to fix or solve problems but rather to help people cope with and manage their situation. Egan proposes that the two primary goals of counseling are to (a) help the person live more effectively and develop unused opportunities more fully and (b) help clients become better at helping themselves in their everyday lives. An overview of the model is summarized in Figure 7-1.

Stage I is designed to help both the clinician and client begin to understand the current state of affairs. This is accomplished by enabling the client to tell his story with enough detail in order for the clinician (as well as the client) to fully understand the current scenario. Once the current problem situation is understood, the client is helped to identify "blind spots" that prevent the client from more clearly and objectively seeing the problem as well as unused opportunities. Finally, given a possible range of behavioral and cognitive features associated with the problem, the client is helped to select the features that have a major impact on his current situation.

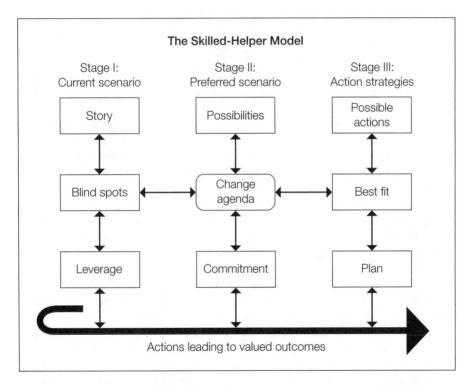

Figure 7-1. Egan's (1998) three-stage Skilled-Helper Model (Egan, G. (1998). *The skilled helper: A problem-management approach to helping* (6th edition), Pacific Grove, CA: Brooks/Cole Publishing Co.) Reprinted with permission.

Stage II is intended to identify the preferred scenario: the things that the client wants and needs in order to live a better life. This stage is about the preferred *outcomes* of therapy. The client's preferences are identified by helping the person imagine the possibilities for a better future. What would a different life look like? The clinician then assists the client in developing a "change agenda" for determining realistic and challenging goals necessary for achieving the new scenario. Finally, in this stage, the clinician helps the client in developing the courage and persistence for accomplishing the work necessary for achieving the desired goals. The client considers whether or not the selected outcomes are worth the effort it will take to achieve them.

Stage III is focused on developing strategies for taking action and the *activities* the client will need to do to get what he wants. The clinician and the client brainstorm possible actions for achieving what they want. Egan points out that one reason "clients are clients is that they are not very creative in looking for ways of getting what they want" (p. 275). Next, the clinician helps the client to choose the best plan given the talents, resources (e.g., support groups and family members), and style of the client. It is important to remember that, in general, simpler plans are usually better. Finally, the clinician assists the client in creating a specific plan for accomplishing the goals. This final stage can be long and arduous. Clients will need guidance in formulating small steps, help in developing discipline, support when they are feeling overwhelmed, assistance in developing procedures for realistically evaluating success, insight in being flexible, and help in dealing with unanticipated problems.

The bi-directional arrows shown in Figure 7-1 indicate that although the overall direction of change generally proceeds from Stage I through Stage III, there is the likelihood of returning to a previous stage. That is, sometimes action will precede understanding, and strategies may be refined as the result of attempts to implement change. This, of course, is similar to the interpretation of the change process described for the transtheoretical model in the previous chapter. Contemplating the possibility of what things could be like (Stage II) may highlight aspects of the client's current situation (Stage I) and help to identify blind spots not yet considered.

In the final analysis clients must act in their own behalf and choose to take action to change their situation. Thus, the "Action Arrow" begins at the outset of therapy and underlies all stages of the model. Egan stresses throughout his text that change does not occur unless action is taken. The Action Arrow also represents transition as clients move from their current state to their preferred scenario. This transition can bring with it a degree of disruption and anxiety, as clients begin to give up familiar but often dysfunctional behavior and ways of viewing themselves and their world.

Lastly, the activities of the model are delivered and filtered through the developing relationship between the clinician and the client. The central nature of this relationship and factors that may influence it will be discussed later in this chapter.

The primary features of Egan's model have much in common with the specifics of treatment for stuttering. Regardless of the treatment approach the clinician selects for a child, adolescent, or adult who stutters, the clinician must understand the client and his story. Unlike the situation in the field of counseling, we generally (but not always) know that the problem is stuttering. Nevertheless, as in Egan's Stage I, we want to begin treatment by understanding the client's history of stuttering, his awareness of his behavior and his success or failure in negotiating within the world of fluency. It is essential to find out why is the client coming to us for help at this time. We will want to discover possible blind spots the client has about his situation. We want to know of his motivation and determine a good starting point in therapy.

Clinicians working with people who stutter typically may not consider Stage II issues. That is, we might assume that our clients know what the preferred scenario would be—we want our clients to stop stuttering and live the life of a fluent speaker. However, as we've said, a multidimensional problem such as stuttering requires multidimensional outcomes. Some clients have only a single focus—they want to be fluent. They don't recognize the larger view of the stuttering phenomenon and certainly don't want to spend time with activities that don't result in the rapid cessation of stuttering. On the other hand, there are many people who do not necessarily want or expect perfect fluency. Many adults are not able to achieve spontaneous levels of fluency in order to be successful or happy. Many adults who stutter do not need to achieve such fluency in order to become good communicators. As we shall see in later chapters, fluency brings with it many adjustments of the speaker and many people with whom the person interacts. Different clients may select different agendas for change, and not everyone will be able to define both realistic and challenging goals. Finally, we need to determine the client's ability to implement the activities of Stage III and be sure that they appreciate the energy and time they will need to invest in order to achieve realistic outcomes.

The activities of Stage III can be based on the talents and resources of the client rather than the dogma of a particular stuttering treatment package. Although there are many treatment programs that provide activities that clients will find helpful, the treatment team of the client and clinician may benefit from brainstorming from among many programs and associated techniques. Ideally, rather than the clinician telling the client what to do, the client can play a significant role in formulating a plan for implementing one or a combination of stuttering treatment activities. This would, of course, require many decisions by the client as well as the clinician. Many clients simply want the clinician to tell them what to do rather than having to choose from among several options. Whatever the plan, the clinician will necessarily play a major role in supporting and guiding the client during the long process of change both within and outside of the treatment setting.

HOW TO "DO COUNSELING"

Telling someone how to conduct counseling is like telling someone how to have a relationship. How you do it "depends." It depends on the people who are involved and on the issue that brought the person to counseling to begin with. How to counsel also "depends" because counseling is client-centered, and each client is unique. Of course, it is also hard to tell someone how to counsel because counseling is a hands-on, dynamic experience rather than an academic exercise.

A few years ago I had the opportunity to read through a manual that was on display at a national professional meeting of speech-language pathologists. Because the focus of the manual was on counseling people who stutter and their families, it caught my eye. On the first few pages of the manual the authors promised that upon reading this manual, the reader would know *exactly* what to say to parents who are concerned about their young stuttering child, *exactly* how to respond to the spouse and family of an adult who stutters, and *exactly* how to counsel an adolescent or adult who stutters. No doubt the manual gave some common responses to the questions that parents and clients typically ask and provided the clinician a measure of help. However, as we mentioned in Chapter 1, following a preprogrammed approach does not permit a dynamic, client-based approach for dealing with the many layers of stuttering. Although such a manual may provide a measure of comfort to a beginning clinician, it represents a technical approach to counseling and is far from the interactive and dynamic nature of a professional, therapeutic relationship.

Responding to a question such as "How do you do counseling?" reminds me of questions I am sometimes asked when giving workshops on fluency disorders. Often someone in the audience will ask me how I would respond to one of their clients during a particular treatment situation. When that happened early in my career, I immediately became role-bound. I felt that I had to assume the role of the expert clinician who had come from some far-away city to enlighten all those in attendance. For years I tirelessly tried to provide a worthy list of suggestions. I no longer do that. Now when someone asks such a question I am more likely to elicit a puzzled look from the audience by saying, "You know, I have absolutely no idea!" Of course, for the moment at least, I don't come across as much of an expert.

It is difficult for the clinician to *know* what to do at a given moment during treatment until a relationship is established. Establishing that relationship normally takes at least three or four sessions. Before I can make accurate and reasonable clinical decisions, I need to know how motivated the client is. I must know his story and begin to understand his situation in order to develop empathy for this person. I need to have a sense about his personality before I can probe and challenge him. Moreover, I need to get a feeling about how tough he will be when asked to apply his treatment techniques in the real world.

THE NECESSITY OF COUNSELING

Ackoff (1974) calls human problem solving "mess management." Clients as well as clinicians tend to be unsystematic and irrational in their decision making (Egan, 1990). The information on which we act is often incomplete, incorrect, or colored with emotion. The information we use to make our decisions tends to be distorted and far from objective. We must accept uncertainty and inconsistency. Clearly, this is also the case with our clinical decisions, based as they are on a combination of facts (or what seem, at least, to be facts) and the intuitive feelings achieved from the clinician's experience and insight. Although this collection of less-than-accurate information may be complex and even confusing at times, as Egan (1990) points out, it also reflects the richness of the human condition.

Should speech-language pathologists even be dealing with counseling issues? Should issues such as affect, emotions, and cognitive change be left to the professions of psychology, psychiatry, or counseling? If we find ourselves working with clients who have chronic life-adjustment problems, the answer is most likely yes. However, the vast majority of our clients are ordinary people experiencing a normal reaction to a communication disorder (Luterman, 1991). Serious communication disorders create genuine stress and anxiety. As Luterman indicates, such people are generally experiencing normal emotions in the face of an important problem. Clearly then, speech-language pathologists should be doing counseling with their clients. Actually, we have no choice but to counsel them if our goal is to provide truly comprehensive treatment.

Many things are good for people. Exercise is one of them; having a network of good friends is another. There is no question that counseling is also beneficial for humans, especially those of us who have specific problems. Counseling is valuable for communication disorders in general and fluency disorders in particular.

In the field of counseling, research has shown (Egan, 1990, 1998) that success rates typically have more to do with the therapist than the type of treatment. When reading through the current literature in counseling, the word that comes up more than any other is *relationship*. As Backus proposed in 1957, the learning and the substance of what goes on in the therapeutic relationship between the client and clinician are more essential than the materials. That relationship is also likely to be more crucial than the treatment strategies or techniques that are employed. In a review of research findings, Goleman (1985) discovered that the best predictor of success in the helping process—a better predictor than the therapy used, the attributes of the clinician, or the problems of the client—is the quality of the relationship between the client and the clinician. Patterson (1985) stated that counseling not only *involves* the relationship; it *is* the relationship.

As a participant in the counseling relationship, the clinician plays a pivotal role. In order to be an effective counselor, the clinician must be well trained and clever. However, the clinician must also be wise. As Egan (1990) states, we clinicians must understand the limitations of our profession, the shortcomings of the treatment strategies and techniques, and the strengths and weaknesses of both the clients and ourselves. We must recognize that the dogma of treatment approaches and book learning can filter and, on occasion, bias what we would otherwise understand about the person we are trying to help. Egan (1990) cautions that learning must be sifted through experience in order for the person to be wise.

Although as clinicians we learn about counseling strategies and techniques primarily in order to help our clients, it does not take long to realize that we can apply these same techniques to ourselves and the relationships in our own lives. For example, as a part of his rational emotive behavioral therapy (REBT), Ellis (1977) provides a list of irrational ideas to which most of us adhere. Obviously, we would be healthier and happier if we could change our attitude about the following issues:

➤ It is a dire necessity for an adult human to be loved or approved of by virtually every "significant other" in his community.
➤ A person should be thoroughly competent, adequate, and successful in all possible respects if he is to consider himself worthwhile, and he is utterly worthless if he is incompetent in any way.
➤ Certain people can be labeled bad, wicked, or villainous, and they deserve severe blame or punishment for their sins.
➤ It is awful or catastrophic when things are not the way an individual would very much like them to be.
➤ Human unhappiness is externally caused, and individuals have little or no ability to control their sorrows and disturbances.

➤ If something is or may be dangerous or fearsome, one should be terribly concerned about it and should keep dwelling on the possibility of its occurrence.

➤ It is easier to avoid certain life difficulties and self-responsibilities than to face them.

➤ An individual should be dependent on others and needs someone stronger than himself on whom to rely.

➤ A person's past history is an all-important determinant of his present behavior, and because something once strongly affected his life, it should continue to do so.

➤ An individual should become quite upset over other people's problems and disturbances.

➤ There is invariably a correct, precise, and perfect solution to human problems, and it is catastrophic if this perfect solution is not found.

In order for us to become the best possible clinicians it will be necessary that we not only continue to grow professionally but that we approach such was of thinking in ourselves. As Egan argues, in order to move from "smart to wise" we must recognize the shadow side of ourselves (e.g., tendencies to be selfish, lazy, or even predatory) as well as the messiness of the helping process (e.g., misuse of models and techniques, receiving payment for treatment although it is ineffective, not giving your best effort during treatment). These issues are rarely discussed but as Egan suggests, "If helpers don't know what's in the shadows, they are naïve" (1998, p. 19).

COUNSELING IN PSYCHOLOGY

Counseling is an everyday experience. Indeed, we counsel others in an informal manner as we help our friends and colleagues deal with life's problems. Egan provides a particularly useful suggestion when he states that the goal of professional counseling falls somewhere on a continuum between telling the client what to do and leaving him to his own devices. The ideal location on the continuum is a point where we are able to help our clients make their own decisions and act on them (Egan, 1990).

One helpful way to characterize professional counseling is to say that the primary focus is on the person and the secondary focus is on the problems. Along with the problems the individual may be facing are emotions associated with them. Another issue in counseling that especially applies to clients with communication disorders is the concept of missed opportunities. These may not be directly tied to a decreased ability to communicate per se, but have to do with situations of daily living that the client suspects could be handled better. In many instances, counselors are asked to help with both issues: specific problems and missed opportunities.

Another useful way to consider the nature of counseling is to think in terms of "stuckness." People go to counseling because they are stuck (Ivey, 1983; cited in Egan, 1990, p. 270). Often, along with being stuck, clients feel helpless to do anything constructive about their situation. As Ivey (1983) submits, it is the responsibility of the counselor to get them unstuck. Often there is no distinct way to accomplish this. It takes experience and wisdom on the part of the clinician to assist the client to progress from the stuck and helpless feelings to better ways of dealing with the situation. However, as Ivey (1983) indicates, it is not an easy task to describe the "possible self" one can imagine and become.

At its most basic level counseling requires the clinician to respond with nonjudgmental respect for a client's unique differences and a willingness to listen instead of prescribe (Luterman, 1991). Furthermore, to be a counselor one must go beyond being a technician. The effective counselor is one who frequently does much more than the traditional requirements of the job.

One of the most misunderstood—but at the same time, more helpful—insights concerning counseling is that the goal of counseling is not to make people feel better. Rather, the primary purpose is to enable the client to separate his feelings from his nonproductive behavior (Luterman, 1991). Moreover, although the problem or the pain may not go away (as with the loss of a loved one or the realization of a son's or daughter's handicap), with successful counseling the client should be better able to manage the situation (Egan, 1990). As Egan states: "Helpers are effective to the degree that their clients, through client-helper interactions, are in a better position to manage their problem situations and develop the unused resources and opportunities of their lives more effectively" (1990, p. 5). Experiencing emotional pain in the face of great difficulty is normal. As Peck (1978) states in the first sentence of his book, *The Road Less Traveled,* "Life is difficult" (p. 15). It is normal and acceptable for people to feel sad when undesirable or bad things happen to them. The goal of counseling is to help the client disengage the feelings from behavior that is self-defeating.

It is not the task of the clinician to "rescue" clients (Luterman, 1991). In other words, the purpose of counseling is not necessarily to "solve" anything. In the case of fluency disorders, we are not necessarily solving or curing stuttering. Although it is possible, especially with young children, to essentially do away with most or all the behaviors associated with stuttering, it is not possible to "cure" attitudes or ways of thinking about a problem. Accordingly, counseling is not something that clinicians *do* to clients. Rather, it is a collaborative process between the people involved. As Egan (1990) suggests, in many ways counselors stimulate clients to provide services to themselves. We help them to have "more degrees of freedom" for making choices in their lives (Egan, 1990, p. 6).

Of course, it is true that as a result of counseling, clients sometimes feel better. However, it is even better if what the client is feeling good about are his accomplishments outside the counseling setting. Feeling good about a counseling session is of some benefit and such feelings may be thought of as the "perceived" gain (Egan, 1990). It is also possible, of course, that the counseling sessions prove painful. Sessions can be difficult simply because changing and growing are often painful.

However, in order to be effective, the counselor must help the client translate his choices into *action*. Thinking—even clear, creative, healthy thinking—will not change anything. It is the taking of action by the client that will result in more effective living. As Egan consistently indicates, counseling is not about talking—it is about acting. If people want to manage their lives in a better way, they usually have to act differently.

Contemplating the situation is fine, but too much thinking can paralyze a person (too much analysis leads to paralysis!). When counselors fail, Egan suggests, they most often do so by not helping their clients to act, for counseling can too easily become a process of too much talking and too little action. We all know people who frequently talk about losing weight, running a marathon, taking a trip, or writing a grant and yet never get around to actually doing any of those things. Wonderful things often take place during the treatment or counseling session, but this is of little consequence if no action takes place, especially outside of the treatment setting.

The counselor plays a critical role by providing the security and insight necessary for the client to explore new possibilities, go into action, and take risks. Support by the counselor makes it possible for the client to move into a future of his own creation. As Egan eloquently states, at the conclusion of successful counseling the clinician may be able to say about the client:

> Because I trusted him, he trusts himself more; because I cared for him, he is now more capable of caring for himself; because I invited him to challenge himself and because I took the risk of challenging him, he is now better able to challenge himself. Because of the way I related to him, he now relates better both to himself and to others. Because I respected his inner resources, he is now more likely to tap these resources. (Egan, 1990, p. 59)

Trust is understandably an essential part of a successful and therapeutic relationship and may be particularly important when working with adolescents (Daly, Simon, & Burnett-Stolnack, 1995).

COUNSELING IN COMMUNICATION DISORDERS

Many of the counseling principles we have discussed obviously apply to clients with communication disorders. In the case of fluency disorders, the "problem" is usually apparent. What may not be so obvious, however, is the client's response to his situation.

In the field of communication disorders, there is cause for concern that few of our students receive adequate preparation for counseling our clients. McCarthy, Culpepper, and Lucks (1986) found that only one third of the programs in communication disorders require a course in counseling. These authors noted that only 12% of clinicians who responded to their survey felt that they were adequately prepared to counsel their clients. According to Luterman (1991), far too many clinicians, although knowledgeable about the field, are clinically and interpersonally inept.

It is understandable that students are apt to feel uncomfortable taking on the role of a counselor. After all, most students are likely to be in their early twenties and should feel cautious, or at the very least sensitive, about counseling adults and parents who have considerably more life experience than the student has had the opportunity to obtain. Although the new clinician can appreciate that she is not an expert in all areas, she is in the process of becoming an expert in communication disorders. Gregory states it nicely:

> Because we are the specialists in communication disorders, no one else can counsel in this area as well as we. The first requisite of counseling is to understand the nature of the problem, and no other professional group knows as much about stuttering as the speech-language pathologist. (1995, p. 198)

To many clinicians, counseling means giving information and advice. However, as Luterman cautions, counseling by informing or persuading is a seductive model. It presents the view that "I as a professional have all of this information and experience. You as clients are ignorant of so many things that you need to know; therefore, I can make a better decision for you than you can for yourself" (1991, p. 3). Not only is this information-giving approach likely to result in the clinician "playing the role" of a counselor, but over time, it results in the job becoming a bore for the clinician and contributes to burnout.

Luterman (1991) suggests that a better approach is learning how to relate to our clients. By listening and valuing the client's story, we allow more affect to enter into the relationship. If the client is viewed as possessing the inherent wisdom to ultimately make good decisions for himself, we are less likely to take a role of lecturer, providing information that we assume will be helpful to this person. By listening and valuing, however, the counselor is more apt to assign the responsibility for change and action to the client. This strategy also increases the client's control, as well as his options.

EMOTIONS ENCOUNTERED DURING TREATMENT

Emotions are brought to the treatment session not only, of course, by the client, but also by parents, spouses, and friends. Because clinicians working with fluency clients tend to believe their clients are so fragile that any mistake might do damage or at least result in increased stuttering (Cooper and Cooper, 1985b; 1992), clinicians tend to be careful about exposing their own feelings.

According to Luterman (1991), an underlying principle when counseling is that emotions are neither good nor bad; they just are. Emotions (generally of the client but, on occasion, also those of the clinician) need to be acknowledged and accepted rather than judged. This, of course, is not necessarily an easy thing to do. There is often deep pain in those involved in a communication disorder (Luterman, 1991). In many cases, that pain is not going to go away. It is appropriate to acknowledge it for what it is—a normal reaction to an unwanted situation. In any case, as Luterman points out, it is always a mistake in any relationship to tell people that they should not feel a particular way. No matter how you do it, it is likely to make them feel guilty about their feelings.

There are several sources of emotions during treatment. The emotions of everyone who may be involved in the treatment process—including the client, the clinician, parents, spouses, siblings, and friends—all come into play. Luterman (1991) describes several of these emotions.

1. **Grief**: Grief may be more likely to be associated with a communication problem if there is a relatively sudden onset, such as with a stroke or traumatic brain injury. However, grief also exists for other problems, including fluency disorders. Clients and parents may move through the stages of grief: denial, anger, bargaining, depression, and acceptance. However, as Luterman (1991) suggests, the process is likely to be cyclical without set boundaries separating the stages. Participants will find themselves back in stages of grief that they have visited before. Luterman (1991) cites a wonderful story by the parents of a handicapped child who describe how they accepted the realization that they will spend a lifetime dealing with the fact that their child, although lovely and special, is not the child they expected. By recognizing and confronting grief and loss, one is able to slowly appreciate the goodness that is nonetheless available. Similarly, although it can be helpful to accept the grief associated with having a fluency disorder, the client can, nonetheless, continue to strive to self-manage his situation.
2. **Inadequacy:** There is great frustration in being unable to "fix" a problem. Clinicians as well as parents feel a great need to help the person with an obvious problem. However, Luterman (1991) calls

attention to what he terms the Annie Sullivan syndrome (referring to the teacher, counselor, and caretaker of Helen Keller). There is a danger in *rescuing* the client. There is a profound difference in taking charge of the situation (and the client) rather than empowering the client or the parents to manage it themselves. Luterman makes a convincing case for keeping ourselves from rescuing the client and thus making him codependent on a clinician. As in parenting, the ultimate goal in treatment is for the client to become independent. The clinician needs to be aware of her own need to be needed, and the client must be aware that his situation is his responsibility to handle.

3. **Anger:** Anger has many sources, one of which is a violation of expectations. Clients, parents, and spouses have many expectations about themselves and each other. Clinicians and clients also have expectations of each other. When these expectations and hopes are not realized, anger is a common result. Communication problems typically restrict many options for the client and his family, which can be extremely frustrating for all involved. Moreover, as we see every day, when people are frustrated sufficiently often, anger will surface. Another source of anger is loss of control. As Luterman (1991) compassionately illustrates on several occasions throughout his book, having a loved one, especially a child or a spouse, hurting in some way makes one angry. Ask yourself how you feel when your choices or options are taken away. What is your response when you feel that you no longer have complete control over your life? Anger is not the only response, but it is certainly a basic one. The real danger is that such anger eventually can be displaced to others or turned inward to become depression.

   One way not to be angry is not to care, to become numb. This is a well-known response of people who are unable to escape chaotic or threatening situations and is a common topic for support groups such as Al-Anon or Al-Ateen. Of course, however, it is generally better to recognize anger. For example, professionals have the right to be angry at clients. If the client means enough to the clinician, a behavior that provokes frustration and eventually anger—such as not completing a clinical contract—should be acknowledged. In some cases, anger can be healthy, for as Luterman (1991) points out, there is a great deal of caring and energy therein; the energy contained in anger can become the fuel for change.

4. **Guilt:** Along with anger, guilt is another common emotion experienced by families of clients. As parents verbalize their feelings about their child's stuttering, they may also experience a form of secondary guilt as they feel bad about feeling sorry or embarrassed for their child. They may express guilt for having waited so long to seek help. Some of this guilt may abate as parents learn about the nature of stuttering. Acknowledgement and acceptance of these naturally-

occurring feelings during support group meetings of parents can be an important step in lessening guilt.

Luterman (1991) makes the observation that guilt is often a statement concerning power. It says, "I have had some power to influence or cause this bad result." Feeling guilty about something (or worrying) implies that the person can control the situation. It is a little like worrying about the weather or your safety before leaving for a trip. Obviously, it is possible to do appropriate and judicious planning for the weather or a trip, but worrying will not control the situation or save you from harm.

Luterman also points out that guilty parents may overprotect their children. Such people can be the ideal parent for the clinician or teacher to work with. Although they are usually able to work well with younger children, difficulties typically arise when the child is a teenager and the parents face the prospect of letting go. On the other hand, guilt can fuel a commitment to rectify the problem and to undertake creative and demanding solutions.

5. **Vulnerability:** We are all vulnerable. Luterman states, "If we live long enough something bad will happen to us, and if we don't live long enough then something bad has already happened" (1991, p. 62). Speakers who stutter can be especially vulnerable in social settings. The ability to separate the problem (stuttering) from the client's reaction to the problem (feelings of vulnerability) is one measure of progress. Fortunately, vulnerability is usually easier to deal with than guilt and can actually be a positive force. Once our vulnerable and finite nature is acknowledged and even accepted, we are free to take action to do what we can to improve our situation.

6. **Feelings of Confusion:** Communication disorders can be not only anxiety-producing, but confusing, especially for parents. It is difficult to know what to do and whom to turn to for assistance. By giving information-based counseling, the clinician can add to feelings of confusion by providing information before the client is ready to receive it. On the other hand, such information can function to establish the credibility of the clinician at the outset of treatment. In any case, confusion on the part of the client can become a motivating force for learning.

In summary, the clinician's task is not to change, but to acknowledge and accept all these emotions. They are, for better or worse, part of the syndrome and a component of the treatment process. While we will not always be able to make our clients feel better, we can help them by preventing the many emotional components of the problem from developing into inappropriate behaviors and secondary, negative feelings such as feeling guilty about feeling guilty or being depressed as a result of anger.

COUNSELING STRATEGIES

As we mentioned in Chapter 1, the experienced clinician should "beware the person of one book" because such a narrow and dogmatic view tends to close the possibilities of new and unique ideas. The focus of treatment is not a particular strategy, but the client.

Several years ago, I attended a professional meeting of a state association of speech-language pathologists. During the meeting I was a member of a panel that was asked, along with the audience, to view a series of videotapes of children and adults with fluency disorders. The panel's task was to react to these hypothetical clients and discuss the strategies and techniques we speculated might be appropriate to use with them. As we took our turns offering suggestions about each tape segment, it became apparent that one member of the panel was giving the same response each time. Regardless of the client's age, severity, or nature of the fluency breaks, this clinician would take the microphone and say something like: "I believe strongly in the —————— method and have found it to be a wonderful approach. I feel that this approach would be ideal for this client. I have seen this method work for many clients and would use this approach with this person."

Regardless of the possible efficacy of this particular method, we were all witnessing a clear example of a "one book" approach to helping clients. Just as in any treatment, the choice of a counseling strategy *must* be driven by the needs of the client rather than the dogma from a book. As discussed in Chapter 1, if you want to be a technician, you may make your clinical decisions according to the treatment manual. If you want to be a professional, however, you will base your decisions primarily in response to the client.

Just as there is no one ideal treatment strategy for the treatment of stuttering, there is no experimental evidence supporting the superiority of any one counseling strategy (Luterman, 1991). Often, an approach is chosen because it coincides with the personality of the clinician and her view of reality. Webster (1966) suggested that the risk of hurting a client may be heightened by using a prescriptive approach with a non-accepting and non-compassionate clinician. If in doubt about what strategy to employ, she recommended a less direct approach since she believes it is virtually impossible for the clinician to damage a client by listening and trying to understand what his world looks like. On the other hand, Luterman (1991) indicates that the safest approach is not a nondirective approach, because this can generate client anger when it violates expectations of what the clinician should provide. He suggests that the safest choice is a cognitive approach that advises clients to restructure the view of their situation. People can survive bad advice, he suggests, for we have been doing it for most of our lives.

Luterman (1991) describes four general approaches to counseling: behavioral, humanistic, existential, and cognitive.

Behavioral Counseling

Behavioral counseling can be an attractive strategy, especially for new clinicians. It provides a distinctive structure whereby the clinician can break down the behavior to be changed into a series of subtasks, each with successive approximations toward the desired goal. This approach is relatively easy to teach because of the concrete nature of the techniques and the specific, overt criteria for moving on to a new level.

Humanistic Counseling

This approach was developed by Carl Rogers (1951) and Abraham Maslow (1968). The underlying concept of this strategy is that humans have an innate drive toward self-actualization (e.g., the true Buddha is within oneself). The basic elements of this approach include the concepts of congruence (bringing into parallel the parts of the self, particularity the intellectual and emotional components), empathy, self-actualization, and unconditional positive regard for the client. Without labeling him, the clinician attempts to release the client's self-actualizing drive so that he can take appropriate actions to solve his problems. Luterman (1991) points out that, because of the abstract nature of the basic concepts involved, this approach can be difficult both to teach and to learn. Furthermore, the responsibility for change rests almost completely on the client, and—for some clients—it is difficult to accept that the self-actualizing drive will take effect. According to Luterman, this approach does not work well with severely involved adults and children or those with limited abilities.

Existential Counseling

This approach comes from the French intellectual movement of the mid-1800s and the work of the Danish philosopher Søren Kierkegaard. This view holds that many human problems are a result of anxiety due to the facts of our existence. That is, we must die, we have freedom to make choices, we are alone, and life is meaningless. This view is different from traditional psychoanalytic theory, where the source of anxiety results from the conflict between the id (the pleasure drive) and the superego (social restrictions). In existential theory, there is no clinical value in understanding the client's past history or behavior.

For individuals whose response to life is to avoid the basic facts of human existence, there are some interesting results.

> ➤ *Death:* Existentialists hold that anxiety resulting from our eventual death can result in the avoidance or postponement of activities or decisions. Furthermore, it can result in a decreased ability to appreciate our everyday existence. By not recognizing the boundaries of our

existence, we are likely to miss the beauty of the commonplace. The greater this death anxiety, the more one is likely to experience a restricted and unfulfilled life. The recognition that nothing is permanent enables us to value what we have been given while we can.

➤ *Responsibility:* Each of us is responsible for our own actions. Whether we admit it or not, in many respects, at least, we are in charge. Because of this, the clinician should not feel sorry for the client with a problem. The client has a choice about what to do about his situation and about what to tell himself about his circumstances. If he chooses, his problems can be approached as challenges, as opportunities to grow. Virtually every writer in counseling agrees that the starting point of therapeutic change is the *assumption of responsibility* by the client and a decision to change (DiClemente, 1993). However, acknowledging this responsibility frequently results in anxiety. As Luterman (1991) points out, the assumption of responsibility by the client implies that we ought not to play the role of the rescuer. Rather, the clinician ought to empower clients to assume the major responsibility for their situations. To the degree that we rescue clients, they will continue to feel powerless.

➤ *Loneliness:* As Luterman states, "We are alone and that crushing fact is central to existential thought" (1991, p. 19). We are all lonely at times, but clients with communication disorders are apt to be uncommonly so. By confronting our loneliness, we are able to generate an unconditional regard for humanity in general.

➤ *Meaninglessness:* As if loneliness were not difficult enough to face, existentialists propose that there is no extrinsic meaning to the world, which cannot be judged good or bad. The world just is. Nevertheless, as Luterman (1991) points out, it is possible to find meaning in the solution of a problem, a strategy that often results in success for families or individuals.

Existentialist philosophy suggests that it is the counselor's mission to help the client face these facts of existence and find more appropriate and nonpathological ways of managing his life situation.

Cognitive Counseling

This view of counseling holds that many human problems are, in many important ways, a function of how we think about the problem. The clinician helps the client to identify specific misconceptions and unrealistic expectations that underlie his situation and his behavior. In one way or another, the client is challenged to examine the underlying assumptions that are reflected in his language and his actions. Ellis's (1977) list of irrational thought processes presented at the outset of this chapter and his rational emotive behavioral therapy (REBT) compose a good example of inaccurate assumptions. Another example of this approach is Personal

Construct Theory (PCT). Fransella (1972) and others (Botterill & Cook, 1987; Dalton, 1987, 1994; Evesham, 1987; Fransella & Dalton, 1990; Hayhow & Levy, 1989; Williams, 1995) have adapted the work of Kelly (1955a,b) and adapted the therapeutic principles of PCT to individuals who stutter. Basically, PCT holds that as a person experiences life, he develops a system of personal constructs that allow him to anticipate future events. These constructs become the person's reality. Change, particularly as a result of therapy, requires a person to develop alternative constructs (reconstrue), a process that is difficult because it means letting go of accepted and safe views and attempting new ways of thinking and acting. As applied to people who stutter, the clinician helps the client to consider and experiment with alternative views (constructions) of themselves, their stuttering, their responsibility for their situation, and the nature of speech modification techniques. The client is taught to problem-solve as he considers a set of alternatives about interacting and speaking and to experiment with alternative ways of responding, ways that may appear unique or often threatening. In the area of fluency disorders, there are a number of authors who advocate the use of these and related techniques with clients (Bryngelson, Chapman, & Hansen, 1944; Emerick, 1988; Johnson, 1946; Manning, 1991; Maxwell, 1982; Van Riper, 1947, 1982; Williams, 1979).

EXAMPLES OF COUNSELING TECHNIQUES

According to Luterman (1991), good counseling technique flows from personality. He suggests that specific techniques should not be easily apparent to the person being counseled or to an observer. "If clients know they are being counseled, the counselor is probably doing it poorly" (Luterman, 1991, p. 87). Ideally, the techniques become congruent with the personality of the clinician and blend into the treatment process. If the clinician acts mechanically, the technique is likely to fail because it will be discontinuous with the authenticity of the relationship.

Moreover, although specific counseling techniques are helpful in and of themselves, they are not counseling. For example, Rogers (1980) spoke against the appalling consequences of overemphasizing microskills during counseling. Rather, to be effective, the clinician must approach counseling as a *fully human endeavor*. The clinician's counseling skills must become extensions of the helper's humanity, not just bits of technology.

A good example of this idea is the use of silence during treatment. Less-experienced clinicians are often uncomfortable with silence. Silence can be embarrassing for the client as well as the clinician, and its intensity will eventually force the inexperienced clinician to act. Luterman (1991) suggests that silence forces inexperienced clinicians to become role-bound. The clients, meanwhile, sit back and watch. Actually, silence can be a powerful technique to facilitate change, for where there is silence, there is often growth. Indeed, silence can be a powerful motivator for client action.

Silence is not a void, but a part of the process. As in Oriental ink drawings, the open spaces are an intentional and important part of the overall composition. The deepest feelings in a relationship can take place in silence, for there is companionship in thoughtful silence. Observe couples who are congruent. There is much communication during the silence. This is observable also in the process of a dynamic clinical relationship. As a clinician with whom I worked years ago used to say, "I knew we were friends when we could share the silence."

NONVERBAL BEHAVIORS OF THE CLINICIAN AND THE CLIENT

Most clinicians today are aware that the use and appropriateness of many nonverbal behaviors are culture-specific. The array of just what is and is not considered appropriate across the categories of age, gender, race, and nationality makes for fascinating study and interesting accounts (see Leith, 1986). It can also make a clinician inhibited, for even the most cursory study of cultural traditions makes one acutely aware of the sometimes serious consequences of misreading clients from various cultures. While race has to do with the biological and anatomical attributes of a group, culture is about the behavior, beliefs, and values of a group (Battle, 1993). The cultural experience of the client and the family will influence the effectiveness of counseling and treatment activities. For example, the cultures of individuals from some cultures are taught to closely guard family values and practices, to regard eye contact between different ages or genders inappropriate, to feel that speaking in a "loud" voice is unsuitable, or to regard any form of touching (e.g., patting on the head) as inappropriate.

The potential for failed communication is further complicated by the fact that many individuals within a cultural group also vary according to their values and beliefs. That is, it is easy to stereotype all members of a group as responding the same way, when in fact they do not. Cooper and Cooper (1993) cautioned that it is all to easy to create additional stereotypes as we identify cultural influences that may influence diagnostic and treatment decisions. Similarly Cole (1989) stated that "care must be taken to avoid over-generalizing or over-emphasizing such differences to the point that they interfere with effective service delivery" (p. 68). Finally, add into the mix the (typically negative) stereotypes that each culture tends to assign to people who stutter, and the opportunity for ineffective communication is increased.

It is difficult, if not impossible, for the clinician to fully understand all the possible microcultures present in a pluralistic society. We must, of course, continue to learn as much as we can about the populations we are likely to encounter in our clinical practice. As Culatta and Goldberg state:

> Speech-language pathologists cannot be expected to be experts in anthropology. Nor can we be expected to be intimately aware of all the microcultural variables of each cultural subgroup in our country. Sensitivity toward the existence of differences within a pluralistic society, however, is critical. (1995, pp. 116–117)

With all this in mind, we will refer to Egan (1990), who provides the following recommendations for facilitating interpersonal communication. With an awareness of these behaviors, the clinician should be able to monitor her nonverbal reactions to clients' comments in terms of such responses as defensiveness, anger, surprise, and encouragement. Egan uses the following acronym to recall the relevant behaviors: SOLER.

S Face the client *Squarely*, with a straightforward posture.
O Adopt an *Open* posture; do not cross your arms or legs, as the open posture indicates confidence and involvement.
L At times, *Lean* toward the client; leaning forward or backward indicates the degree of involvement and the equilibrium during a discussion.
E Maintain good (appropriate) *Eye* contact.
R Be relatively *Relaxed* or natural.

Another aspect of nonverbal behavior involves calibrating yourself to the client. A good way to think of this process is that the clinician should be doing something well beyond what a tape recorder could do. Rather than merely recording the client's words, you are observing and interpreting cues, such as his posture, facial expressions, movement, tone of voice, and general grooming. As Egan (1990) suggests, a person's nonverbal behavior has a way of *leaking* messages to others. In addition, Egan suggests that nonverbal behaviors can serve to punctuate verbal statements, to confirm or enhance, to reveal inconsistencies, and to send controlling or regulating messages to others.

VERBAL BEHAVIORS

The verbal behaviors of the clinician combine with nonverbal actions of the client and the clinician to indicate the status of the therapeutic relationship. The clinician has several options for verbally responding to the client's questions and circumstances. Luterman (1991) provides some general categories of verbal responses from which the clinician can choose.

The Content Response

The content response is the most commonly used. Such responses tend to keep the relationship at an expected and predictable level. Content responses are most likely used at outset of treatment, especially if the participants anticipate that the treatment will be short-term. The client may ask such questions as "What are the best ways to respond when my child stutters?" or "What is the likelihood of relapse following treatment?," to which the clinician will provide the answers.

The Counterquestion Response

Luterman (1991) points out that most people do not really want advice. What they seek is confirmation for a decision they have already made. Although their statement may take the form of a question, what they are asking for is not an answer, but a confirmation of a decision they have already made. Luterman points out that people do not learn from (or even listen to) advice. If the advice works, the client will come back for more, while if it does not, he may be angry. Luterman suggests that the most productive response one can give to a confirmation question is a counterquestion. The client may ask, "Am I making progress in therapy?" and the clinician may respond, "What behaviors and attitudes have you changed?" or "How are people responding to you at the office?"

Early in the therapeutic relationship, before trust has evolved, there are apt to be many questions (Luterman, 1991). With the development of a secure relationship, there tend to be fewer questions and more observations and statements. Luterman suggests that the counterquestion can be a powerful tool for moving a relationship beyond the initial stages.

The Affect Response

The affect response by the clinician is also helpful for building the counseling relationship. Rogers (1951) called this empathetic listening. Examples of this type of response would be comments by the clinician such as, "I can understand that it must be frightening to speak in front of the class" or "It must make you must feel extremely frustrated when that occurs."

The Reframing Response

This response takes the form of restating the client's question in a different context: "Why should I have a stuttering problem?" to "Why do you believe that you shouldn't have a problem such as stuttering?" This response involves reconstructing the situation (problem) as a chance to learn and grow. Luterman (1991) suggests that this is a powerful tool for anyone in an undesirable situation.

The Sharing-Self Response

The sharing-self response may be more natural for some clinicians. On the other hand, this response is less likely to come from a professional who has a need to be in control at all times. By sharing our own doubts and uncertainties, we become more genuine (see Chapter 1). The clinician is free to honestly answer a question by saying something like, "At the moment I don't have any idea what would be best for you [or your child]." The clinician may acknowledge that the process of treatment is difficult or that she is uncertain about the next therapeutic step. Luterman (1991) indicates that it is permissible to ask the client if he has any ideas about what to do next (a form of assigning responsibility and independence and increasing the internal control of the client). According to Luterman (1991), it is not advisable for the clinician to do this too early in treatment, for she may lose credibility if she has not yet proved herself. Once the client has achieved a higher degree of self-esteem, such sharing responses can emerge, however.

The Affirmation Response

In this response the clinician affirms the client and provides a sounding board for the client to explain and ventilate the emotions associated with his situation. The clinician listens to the speaker and *nonverbally* indicates that the client is free to express himself. In a wonderful comment, Luterman suggests that "It often shows a fine command of language to say nothing" (1991, p. 94). Of course, in order to know which of the possible responses may be best, the clinician must actively monitor both the client's verbal and nonverbal messages.

ACTIVE-LISTENING TECHNIQUES

Active-listening techniques are essential for facilitating the development of any relationship. In a clinical relationship, active listening is vital if the clinician is to effectively probe and challenge the client. It is one of the primary ways that we are able to learn the client's story. Listening actively implies something beyond understanding the client's verbal and nonverbal messages. It involves "being with" the client, both physically and psychologically, in order to communicate empathy (Egan, 1990).

In the active-listening process, the clinician uses both verbal and nonverbal cues to recognize the client's core messages and cognitive patterns.

The clinician continually asks the question, "What is it that the client wants me to understand?" The task takes persistence and concentration. Furthermore, the clinician must be aware of possible cultural biases. As Egan (1990) suggests, if the clinician's cultural filters are strong, there is a greater likelihood of bias and distorted understanding. He also cautions that (as discussed earlier) book learning can distort perception. It is important to keep academic theories in the background and the client in the foreground. In addition, it is helpful for the clinician to keep from rehearsing a possible response to the client before he has completed what he has to say. Rehearsal puts a stop to active listening by the clinician. Finally, interrupting the client can be permissible if it is done appropriately, especially for clarification. However, it must not be done simply because the clinician has something to say.

Expressing Empathy

The clinician who is able to express empathy has a way to get inside another's world. As Egan (1990) explains, "being with" the client is temporarily living another's life as a means to viewing the person without labels, interpretation, or categories. Rogers suggested that empathy is in and of itself a healing agent. "It is one of the most potent aspects of therapy, because it releases, it confirms, it brings even the most frightened client into the human race. If a person is understood, he or she belongs" (1986, p. 129).

Egan (1990) indicates that while listening to the client helps the clinician get in touch with the client's world, empathy helps the clinician to understand that world. He noted that clients rate understanding as the thing they find most helpful during counseling. Unfortunately, the clinician's ability to indicate empathy is not a skill that comes naturally. Of course, the clinician must first *be* empathetic before empathy can be expressed (often without words but rather with a glance or touch). The expression of empathy involves the clinician's shared understanding of the client's experiences, behaviors, and feelings. It is important to distinguish empathy from sympathy. Sympathy denotes agreement, whereas empathy denotes *understanding* and *acceptance* of the person.

Virtually all authorities agree that active listening and expressing empathy are affirming and highly therapeutic for the client. Furthermore, such involved listening with understanding allows the clinician to establish a cognitive map that describes the client's experience of himself (Zinker, 1977). It is from this map—this understanding of the client—that the clinician can begin to formulate the direction(s) of change that will assist the client through the treatment process.

The clinician's perception of the client should be as accurate as possible. Furthermore, in order to be helpful, the clinician's understanding of the client must be presented to the client, and the clinician must be assertive enough to act when the time is right. Egan (1990) suggests that once the clinician has formulated an accurate understanding of the client's situation, the clinician can try the formula, "You feel _____ because _____." Egan indicates that the client will help the clinician stay on track by responding with silence, correcting her, or restating her understanding. If, on the other hand, the clinician is accurate in her perception, the client will often respond by moving on. Other helpful suggestions for responding with empathy include allowing yourself time to reflect on what the client said, using short responses (i.e., do not give speeches), and being yourself in your choice of words and style.

Probing the Client

The purpose of probing is to highlight the client's blind spots about his situation. Egan (1990) describes probes as verbal tactics that help the client talk about himself and define his problem in terms of specific *experiences, behaviors*, and *feelings*. The goal of probing is not to identify a single, momentous piece of information but rather to increase understanding. This is usually accomplished by asking the client to become more specific. With accurate probing there should be an increase in the quality of the information the client can use in making better decisions. The speech-language pathologist working with a client who stutters is not likely to probe as often or as deeply as the psychologist who is working with a client with a personality disorder. Nonetheless, on many occasions

---

🔍 CLINICAL INSIGHT

Several years ago I was working with a colleague who was both insightful and gentle. She rarely said anything negative about anyone. One day, after working with one of our young graduate students and an adult who stuttered severely, she turned to me and said something that surprised me. "You know, I don't think that some of our students have had the opportunity to suffer enough to be able to relate to our clients!" Her comment rang true, for I had experienced the same feelings about some (thankfully few) other clinicians. I have smiled over the years when students would ask questions such as "Is grief going to be on the test?" or "How much do we need to know about suffering for the final?" Of course, there are many possible explanations for why this young person had difficulty relating to the suffering her client had experienced. Whether or not this clinician had not yet suffered enough, they did not appear to have learned from the experience, or at least they were not able to use their experience of suffering in relating to another person.

throughout treatment, clinicians need to obtain more specific information concerning a client's behavior, motivation, and cognitive processes.

Egan (1990) provides some guidelines for probing:

➤ Do not assault your clients with too many questions; don't grill them.
➤ Ask questions that serve a specific purpose. Use questions that challenge the client to think—questions that have teeth but not fangs.
➤ Ask open-ended questions that get clients to discuss specific experiences, behaviors, and feelings.
➤ Keep the focus on the client; keep placing the ball in his court.
➤ Keep in mind the value of using nonverbal communication to prompt the client.
➤ Consider the possibility that if you ask two questions in a row, it may well be that they are poor questions.
➤ Think of verbal probes as the spice of the communication process. They should remain condiments.

Challenging the Client

Closely related to probing techniques is the skill of challenging the client. This is similar to challenging and pushing the client, as described in Chapter 1. As the clinician determines the client's strength and resilience, it is often necessary to push him into attitudes and behaviors that he is likely to resist. It is possible, of course, to challenge someone and still be "for" that person. Challenging another person signifies that you take him seriously enough to respond when his choices are not in his best interest. It also indicates the clinician's belief in the client's potential. As Fisher and Ury (1981) suggested, it is best to be soft on the person and hard on the problem.

Using Humor

As discussed in Chapter 1, humor can play an important part in the clinical relationship. Humor allows the clinician to challenge the client and discuss things that would otherwise be risky. Humor involves aspects of distancing oneself from a problem, conceptually shifting one's view of the situation, and mastering events and situations that were previously avoided or anxiety-producing. As Rusk (1989; cited in Egan, 1990) suggests, deliberate self-change requires a willingness to (a) stand back from yourself far enough to question your familiar beliefs and attitudes about yourself and others, and (b) persist at awkward and risky experiments designed to increase your self-respect and satisfy your needs. Not only can humor facilitate such self-change, but for the clinician, humor provides a window for viewing the cognitive changes associated with a problem.

CLIENT RESPONSIBILITIES

At the core of the helping process is the assumption that, within limits, people are capable of making choices and controlling their destinies. Egan (1990) argues that many people adopt a deterministic view of life without realizing it. Moreover, while it is true that many limits are imposed on us by social, political, economic, and cultural forces, accepting responsibility for one's own life is at the heart of self-respect and happiness. Egan cites Farrelly and Brandsma (1974), who suggest a view of the client that is both encouraging and probably accurate.

➤ Clients can change if they choose to do so.
➤ Clients have more resources for managing problems in living than most clinicians assume.
➤ The psychological fragility of clients is overrated both by themselves and others.
➤ Maladaptive attitudes and behaviors of clients can be significantly altered, no matter how severe or chronic.
➤ Effective challenge can provide in the client a self-annoyance that can lead to a decision to change.

Often we need to hit an emotional bottom in order to move on with the coping process. As a result of growth, we begin to recognize that denial is not the best response to a situation. It really is possible to accept the associated pain and move along with it. The goal of counseling may not be a matter of going exactly where we think we should go or even reaching what we may think of as normalcy. *Rather, the goal is to live life to the fullest in the face of the situations with which we are presented.*

METALINGUISTIC ISSUES: CHANGING HOW THE CLIENT DESCRIBES THE PROBLEM

As we will describe in Chapter 10, how a person describes himself and his situation reflects his condition and whether or not things are changing. Clinicians may find it useful to listen closely to the client's self-talk as an indication of his current condition. However, suggesting changes in the way the client talks about himself need to be made gently. Encouraging such changes is less appropriate early in treatment, for it may be all the client can do to accurately tell his story and describe his situation. Furthermore, as Ellis (1977) indicates, trust in the clinician must be high, or suggestions by the clinician to change this self-talk will be seen as interfering and annoying. Ellis provides some recommendations for changing the way we talk about ourselves and our situations.

As Luterman (1991) suggests, these ideas can be of great help in both professional and personal interactions.

➤ *Should* and *ought* may be changed to *want to* or *not want to*, as in changing "I should use my new fluency modification techniques" to "I want to [or do not want to] use my new fluency modification techniques."

➤ *Have to* can be changed to *want to* or *choose to*, as in changing "I have to stay home and not speak to people" to "I want to stay home" or "I choose to stay home and not risk a stuttering moment."

➤ *We, us, society* may be changed to *I*, as in changing "We are unhappy with this treatment program or technique" to "I am unhappy with this approach [therefore, I can do something about it if I choose to]."

➤ *To be* verbs can be modified from "I am a dumb person" to "Although I did a dumb thing, I am still a smart person."

➤ The word *but* can be changed to *and*, as in changing, "I want to speak in public but I am afraid" to "I want to speak in public and I am afraid."

More accurate and appropriate ways of using language to describe a situation can force the person to take responsibility for his behavior and the associated self-talk concerning it.

CHOOSING A FUTURE

According to Lindaman and Lippitt (1979), in order to shape a future, we need to hold in our minds an image of what it is that we truly want. Imagination is one way for the client to propel himself into the future. Egan (1990, 1998) points out that the use of imagery is slowly moving back into the mainstream of counseling after many decades of disfavor. He suggests that the use of conscious and creative imagery can help to overcome inertia. Egan asserts that inertia tends to permeate life and influence our decisions and is one of the principal mechanisms for keeping individuals, organizations, and institutions mired in the *psychopathology of the average* (Maslow, 1968).

Some procedures for realistically defining the future include having the clients find new models for configuring their own lives. Egan recommends using as a model biographies of current or previous clients, keeping in mind issues of confidentiality. Clients can be asked to write about a desired future or construct their own epitaph. Based on his experience, Egan points out that many clients are much better writers than most people realize and can use this ability to define a new future.

CLINICIAN CHARACTERISTICS

This chapter began with a discussion of the importance of the clinical relationship. The characteristics of the clinician have a primary impact on the nature of that relationship. We discussed many of the characteristics of the clinician in Chapter 1 and will include a few additional qualities here as they relate specifically to the counseling relationship. As Luterman (1991) comments, if the literature on the desirable personality characteristics of the ideal counselor were examined, the only ones who might conceivably have a chance to qualify would be some of the more outstanding saints. However, as Egan (1990) argues, it is not necessary for the effective clinician to be an entirely self-actualized person. It is critical, he states, for the clinician to be a person who has a deep interest in people and a sensitivity to others. The competent counselor needs to be a caring individual who does not impose his or her beliefs on others, who maintains a constant awareness of self, and who does not hide behind the role of professional. Luterman states:

> I think the key to counseling is the congruence of the counselor. As I become more congruent, technique slips away or, more accurately, becomes incorporated into everything I do. I think the most important thing a counselor brings to the helping relationship is self. The importance of the congruent professional far exceeds the value of any diagnostic test or specific techniques in counseling. (1991, p. 180)

In a similar manner, Egan indicates that for a clinician to be an effective counselor, it is essential that she understand herself, including her own assumptions, beliefs, values, standards, skills, strengths, weaknesses, idiosyncrasies, style of doing things, foibles, and temptations. She needs to appreciate how her characteristics will be apt to influence her interactions with her clients. To begin the process of introspection, Egan suggests the following questions (1990, p. 25):

➤ How did you decide to be a helper?
➤ Why do you want to be a helper?
➤ With what emotions are you comfortable?
➤ What emotions—in yourself or others—give you trouble?
➤ What are your expectations of clients?
➤ How will you deal with your clients' feelings toward you?
➤ How will you handle your feelings toward your clients?
➤ To what degree can you be flexible, accepting, and gentle?

One critical characteristic for an effective clinician and counselor is her overall competence. Whatever true competence may be for each professional, it is likely to be a lifelong pursuit. Particularly in the areas of human behavioral science, competence means more than simply understanding models, strategies, and techniques. It means being able to "deliver the goods" to the people you are trying to help. All effective counselors must continue to learn—it is basic for counseling and for life. Beyond learning, the effective counselor must model the things she challenges her clients to do. More than learning and thinking must be modeled: Action must be modeled as well. As Egan (1990) suggests, if the clinician wants her clients to act, she must be active in her own life in regard to her own problems. Berenson and Mitchell (1974) forcefully suggest that only those counselors who are committed to living fully themselves deserve to help others.

Being competent does not mean having solutions to all the problems you will face. Difficult cases will, as Luterman (1991) suggests, cause the icy finger of possible failure to threaten and test our confidence. Nonetheless, if the clinician is learning, if she is a truly responsible professional, she should be operating on the *fringes of incompetence*. Effective counselors, clinicians, and people in general should take risks and occasionally make mistakes, or they will not grow.

At the conclusion of his 1990 edition, Egan has a wonderful paragraph discussing the need for the counselor to go beyond the technology of helping and move toward becoming authentic. He indicates that our clinical and other life experiences can be either a teacher or a tyrant.

> Going through these experiences provides us with the opportunity to recognize and accept the shadow side of ourselves, our clients, and the world. To do so without becoming a victim is crucial but not the reward of the experience. The events of each life need to be wrestled with, reflected on, and learned from. Only then can these events become our teacher and friend. Wrestling with our self, our colleagues, our friends, our demons, and our God will provide us both pain and comfort. It is that struggle that will help the skilled helper become the wise helper. (1990, p. 409).

CONCLUSION

Even though clients with fluency disorders do not tend to have chronic life-adjustment problems, they experience real and normal reactions to a serious and handicapping communication disorder. To influence how clients respond to this fact is the goal of counseling. If clinicians are to provide a comprehensive response to their clients, they have no choice but to provide some form of counseling. Although there are many possible counseling strategies for assisting clients, Egan's three-stage model for the skilled helper provides a set of guidelines for assisting the client to take action and move from the current to the preferred scenario.

As clinicians, we are not able to fix the problem or make unwanted emotions go away. At the center of the counseling process is the relationship of the client and the clinician. The clinician can enhance this relationship, not by playing the role of a counselor, but by providing a nonjudgmental response and actively listening to the client's story. How much of a role we will play in directing change will be determined by the needs of the client, and an ideal response is likely to fall somewhere between telling the client what to do and having him make his own decisions. Although the goal of counseling is not to make clients feel better, people will usually feel better as a result of the *actions* they take as a result of treatment.

The emphasis of Egan's and other counseling models is to help people to take action that will enable them to design a new future for themselves. The goal is to deal more effectively with the situations with which they are presented. To the degree that the clinician can model this response to problems, the client is more likely to modify his own behavior. The client's manner of changing and adjusting to his communication disorder will determine the long-term success of treatment and the possibility of relapse.

STUDY QUESTIONS

➤ Differentiate the three main stages of Egan's skilled-helper model.

➤ How do you explain the counseling role of the speech-language-pathologist?

➤ Why is it important for a clinician to understand counseling strategies and techniques when working with children or adults who stutter?

➤ Briefly describe the emotions that the clinician is likely to encounter from clients and parents of children during the process of assessment and treatment. What is the clinician's role in responding to these emotions?

➤ Which one (or more) of the counseling strategies seems to be most congruent with your personality?

➤ Recount one or more recent discussions with a friend or family member and describe how your nonverbal signals communicated information about you and your feelings.

➤ Explain the difference between sympathy and empathy. Provide a good example of a truly empathetic response you had during a recent discussion with a friend.

➤ Give at least three examples of how you have humorously interpreted a previous event or circumstance.

RECOMMENDED READINGS

Albach, J., & Benson, V. (Eds.). (1994). *To say what is ours. The best of 13 years of letting GO* (3rd ed.). San Francisco, CA: National Stuttering Project.

Crowe, T. A. (1997). Counseling: definition, history, rationale. In T. A. Crowe (Ed.), *Applications of counseling in speech-language pathology and audiology* (pp. 3–29). Baltimore: Williams & Wilkins.

Egan, G. (1998). *The Skilled helper: A problem-management approach to helping* (6th edition). Pacific Grove, CA: Brooks/Cole Publishing Co.

Luterman, D. M. (1991). *Counseling the communicatively disordered and their families* (2nd ed.). Austin, TX: Pro-Ed, chs. 1 ("Counseling by the Speech Pathologist and Audiologist," pp. 1–8), 4 ("The Emotions of Communication Disorders," pp. 49–76), 8 ("Working with Families," pp. 135–166), and 9 ("Counseling and the Field of Communication Disorders," pp. 167–180).

Webster, E. (1966). Parent counseling by speech pathologists and audiologists. *Journal of Speech and Hearing Disorders, 31,* 331–345.

CHAPTER

8

TREATMENT FOR ADOLESCENTS AND ADULTS

> *When I was climbing, my partner and I were giving each other advice about which way to go and which rock might be the best one to go to next. In learning to manage my stuttering, I have found that I need to find the things that work for me. I need to use my own best words to express myself, find my best chances or opportunities to talk, and discover which tools work best for me. Other people can guide me, but I have to find my own "right rocks."*
>
> Brad Sara, age 14 (1999, April), Letting GO, The National Stuttering Association Newsletter.
>
> *"We must do the thing we think we cannot do."*
>
> *Hellen Keller*

INTRODUCTION

Earlier in this text we discussed the nature of stuttering onset and development. Although to this point we have not described the specifics of treatment, it should be apparent that understanding stuttering behavior, and particularly the characteristics of the person who is doing the stuttering, is the essential first step for successful intervention.

Understanding the intrinsic nature of the person who is asking for help is fundamental to making wise clinical decisions. Silverman puts it well when he says, "The better able you are to understand the problems your clients will encounter as they try to change, the better able you will be to help them do so" (1996, p. 170).

It is good to begin with a note of optimism regarding treatment for adolescents and adults who stutter, for there is plenty of literature that is confusing or not so encouraging. Because of the volume of information and the many uncertainties about the important issues of etiology, treatment, and relapse, the literature can be discouraging for clinicians interested in helping speakers with fluency disorders. It is no secret that many clinicians are unsure of general strategies and specific techniques to employ with clients who come to us with fluency disorders. Students graduating with a master's degree are no longer required to receive specific training in fluency disorders. They are required, however, to receive experience with a wide variety of communication disorders (e.g., language and learning disabilities, aphasia, motor-speech problems, dysphagia, neurogenics, augmentative communication, and multicultural aspects of diagnostics and treatment). Fluency disorders, an area that for many years was at the core of the academic and clinical experience of students, is often omitted from the student's program or given far less than adequate emphasis. As a result, many clinicians actively avoid—or at the very least are anxious about—the possibility of working with children and adults with fluency disorders (Conture, 1990; Silverman, 1992). Over the years I have spoken with students who had been told by their instructors that treatment for fluency disorders was rarely successful and that the student would be well advised to concentrate on those clients who were more likely to make progress.

Adults who have stuttered for several decades are likely to have become sophisticated travelers within the culture of stuttering. By the time we are able to see them, they have a lengthy history of thinking about their speech and about themselves as someone who stutters. They have made many life choices and important decisions based on the fact that they are a person who stutters. They have learned much about how to survive, and because of the shame and stigma associated with stuttering, they have learned subtle ways to hide and avoid revealing themselves (Bennett & Chemela, 1998; Murphy, 1999). It is not unusual for the original fluency breaks to be so well-disguised that their stuttering behavior is not apparent even to sophisticated listeners.

THE SPECIAL CASE OF ADOLESCENTS

Although it was probably recognized long before, in 1971 Van Riper commented that adolescents are often the most difficult cases to treat. In

1995 Daly, Simon, and Burnett-Stolnack suggested that this age group is particularly challenging, because adolescent years are typically characterized by emotional conflicts, fears, and frustrations that interact with the anxieties and negative feelings associated with stuttering. Blood (1995) also acknowledged the special nature of this population. He noted that the extensive treatment some adolescents experienced during elementary school tends to reduce their motivation to continue working on the problem. Blood proposed that in many cases an adolescent's many social and school activities leaves little time for treatment. Teasing or peer pressure may be problems, and there may be limited parental or school personnel involvement. The 1997 survey of 287 school-based clinicians by Brisk, Healey, and Hux (see also Chapter 1) found that school-based clinicians felt that they had fewer successes with adolescents who stutter than with any other student age group. Finally, Manning (1991) expressed the view that any clinician who is able to convince a teenage speaker who stutters to enroll in treatment should probably receive a large bonus. The bottom line is that achieving success with this population requires understanding at least as much about adolescence than it does about treating stuttering.

Relatively few adolescents are motivated enough to initiate and continue with treatment. On the other hand, the handicap associated with

---

🔍 CLINICAL INSIGHT

As a young man in college, on those occasions when someone would ask me where my hometown was, I would do nearly anything to avoid saying the name "Williamsport." Instead, I would often say "Well, I'm from a small town in Pennsylvania." If they inquired further, as of course they often did, I would say "Well, it's in central Pennsylvania" or "It's a city about 85 miles north of Harrisburg." "Lock Haven" they would respond. And I would say, "Well, it's a little east of Lock Haven." "Bloomsburg?" they would query. And I would respond, "No, it's actually west of Bloomsburg." Sometimes we would go on for awhile, gradually narrowing down the possibilities, until they were able to correctly guess the name of the city. I would do whatever it took, including acting as though I had no idea where I lived, in order to hide my stuttering. During these exchanges I certainly appeared to be, at the very least, a little strange or, at most, not very bright. I frequently did the same thing when asked about such things as the schools I attended, the names of my teachers or classes, or my street address. The problems presented by stuttering went far beyond my speech. Stuttering was a way of making choices and a way of living.

stuttering sometimes becomes greater in junior high/middle school as a result of academic and social pressures. Avoidance and substitution often become more frequent during the early teenage years. Following several years of adaptation to the handicap, the deep structure of the disorder—the cognitive and affective features—become further refined and sophisticated.

Priorities during teenage years are not likely to be conducive to getting adolescents into treatment. That is, although stuttering may be a major problem, it is not usually seen as the most pressing one. Other issues take higher priority, including sports, social activities, cars, and work. There is often the hope that facing the problem can be postponed or that it will go away with time and maturity. It may be difficult to get teenage clients to commit to the arduous tasks involved in treatment in order to achieve the long-term goals of changing the many levels of their stuttering. In some instances, adolescents begin treatment but soon find it difficult to take responsibility for treatment activities. Completion of assignments outside of treatment becomes inconsistent. If we are unsuccessful in convincing teenage clients to pursue treatment at this stage of their life, we may be able to provide them with two basic messages: (1) There are qualified professionals who enjoy working with people who stutter who will be willing to help them when they are ready. (2) It is possible to have a happy and very productive life even though you stutter.

The activities and techniques that are part of any treatment strategy tend to set the speaker apart from his peers, an important issue with teenagers. Some teenagers are not particularly good at confronting emotions, often assigning responsibility or blame to others, including clinicians, parents, and teachers. Teenagers sometimes want to separate from the family and are less likely to enter into a trusting, intimate clinical relationship with adults. Finally, although parents can play a significant role in the treatment process, the desire by teenagers to be independent may frustrate parents and make it more difficult for them to take part. Conversely, sometimes it becomes necessary to convince parents that there is a problem, for the child may not demonstrate overt stuttering when they are around their parents.

Treatment is more likely to be successful for adolescents if they are able to locate a clinician who specializes in stuttering. The Special Interest Division 4 of the American Speech-Language-Hearing Association and groups such as the National Stuttering Association and the Stuttering Foundation of America have lists of such specialists. It is also important for teenagers who stutter to have the opportunity to share their experience with other teenagers who also stutter. In the security and privacy of his own room, the adolescent can make contact with others around the country and the world via the Internet. The isolation of being a person with a handicap such as stuttering can be lessened by contact with other people and self-help groups that provide important sources of information and support (see Chapter 10). The teenager will be able to see that he is not alone and is, in fact, far from the only person with this problem. The National Stuttering Association (NSA) workshops for teenagers are one example of such an opportunity. Reading materials and videos from NSA and the Stuttering Foundation of America (SFA) are available that may set the stage for future treatment. This information can educate and desensitize the teenager so that he can someday move into formal treatment procedures. In addition, information via the Internet can also facilitate learning, sharing, and educating in a non-threatening way. Several stuttering networks allow like minds to share information and feelings.

There are also some interesting gender issues that may be apparent with adolescent clients. For example, adolescent males who stutter—and of course there are more males who do—may have some hesitancy about being seen by a female clinician. Although this is more likely to be a problem at the outset, as treatment progresses the difference in genders may provide a learning experience for expanding the client's knowledge of male-female relationships and social issues in general.

Many people who stutter find that many things, including fluency, improve considerably as they get older (Manning & Shirkey, 1981). The clinician may also want to communicate this possibility to a teenage speaker who may not be able to envision many social or career options because of his stuttering. You don't have to stutter to realize that many things get better with age, especially if you are able to develop some history of successes in a variety of skills. As teenagers are able to develop a broader understanding of relationships, social skills, and life in general, they are more likely to develop greater confidence in themselves, even if they happen to stutter.

A few years ago a teenager with more insight than most prepared a brief article describing the common themes he noted as he simultaneously learned to rock climb and to work through treatment for his stuttering. His name is Brad Sara, and he was 14 years old when he wrote the following article that appeared in the National Stuttering Association Newsletter *Letting GO* in April, 1999 (see also the NSA web site).

CHOOSING A TREATMENT STRATEGY

When reading through the literature on treatment strategies, it is possible for the clinician to get the feeling that what is being contrasted is the doctrine of political or religious groups. Writers may invite the reader to take a stand concerning the treatment of this problem, offering a sure

LESSONS I LEARNED WHILE ROCK CLIMBING

My name is Brad Sara, and I am a 14-year old eighth grade student who stutters. Last year I attended a monthly "speech group." I have also been learning to rock climb. In indoor rock climbing, there are two people; one who is climbing while the other is holding the rope that is connected to the ceiling. So if you fall, that person will catch you. The lessons I learned about rock climbing were many, but they also taught me about speech. Here's how they are similar.

You have to learn and then practice. In rock climbing, we had to practice over and over before we could even get on the wall. This is just like in speech, where you have to practice speech tools in order to get better at them.

You have to take on more responsibility. As we paired up for climbing, I remember thinking that I had not expected to be in charge of another person's safety. This meant that I had to be really responsible. This reminded me of how I used to feel about working on speech. I have learned that dealing with stuttering is my responsibility, and I have to accept more and more of it as I get older.

You have to trust the other person. While climbing, I needed to trust that my partner would not drop me. With stuttering, you have to trust listeners, teachers, friends, your speech therapist, and your parents that they will listen to you and say positive messages. You also have to trust yourself to follow through on your goals.

Effective communication is essential. When people are rock climbing, they have to talk to each other for safety. In speech, the most important thing is to get your point across, whether you stutter or not. The message is more important than how you say it.

You have to conquer your fear. When we started up the wall I think we were all afraid at first. But we faced it because we trusted the person hanging onto our rope. I also had trust in my training, and got less afraid by watching others being successful. So I went up and climbed, too. When I speak in front of a large group, I get afraid. Fear has a big deal to do with speech. If you don't face it, you will hold yourself back. If you conquer your fear, you will learn to be less afraid each time.

It's OK to make mistakes. One thing is very obvious to me. It's OK to make mistakes. Because if we felt we had to climb perfectly all the time, we were most likely to do worse. If you stutter, it's not the end of the world. If you say it's not OK, you're putting too much pressure on your speech to be perfect, and then if you do make a mistake, you will discourage yourself.

LESSONS I LEARNED WHILE ROCK CLIMBING (*CONTINUED*)

It's OK to get frustrated; eventually you will get it. There were many times while climbing that we got frustrated. Just like in speech, you keep on trying and you are going to "get it" someday. Have faith in yourself.

It's OK if you fall. You catch yourself and start from there. Sometimes on the wall, I would slip and then catch myself. I just started again from where I was. If you stutter, it's OK and you can pick up your message from where you left off.

If you fall all the way down, start over again. When I fell a long way down while climbing, I started from the bottom, but knew I had learned the skills I needed to begin again. We have bad spells in our speech, sometimes. It's OK. We have learned what to do, and can start again.

Remain calm. I thought of this because one of our speech teachers is afraid of heights. When she got to the top, she was very scared to start down again, and we all talked to her to help her remain calm. In dealing with stuttering, I have had to learn how to deal with fear and to calm myself down when I am nervous so that I can manage my speech better.

When you're facing the edge, have faith in your support. When we got to the top of the wall, we had to stand on a ledge and then lean out to start going down again. We had to really have faith in the person who was supporting us. When I am real anxious and nervous about my speech, I have faith in the people who are behind me and who support me in whatever I do or say.

You just have to find the right rocks. When I was climbing, my partner and I were giving each other advice about which way to go and which rock might be the best one to go to next. In learning to manage my stuttering, I have found that I need to find the things that work for me. I need to use my own best words to express myself, find my best chances or opportunities to talk, and discover which tools work best for me. Other people can guide me, but I have to find my own "right rocks."

road to success to the exclusion of other possibilities. There are many therapeutic approaches that have been shown to help people who stutter. To be sure, the logic and techniques associated with most intervention strategies provide the clinician with a framework and a sense of direction about the syndrome and its treatment. Each strategy comes with its own doctrine. Each of these approaches can provide something of value for the clinician and her client, depending on such variables as the needs of the client, the stage of treatment, and the talent and experience of the clinician. As Bloodstein (1999) commented, "Almost any therapy has the power to eliminate stuttering in someone, sometime, someplace." Sometimes simply having the client tell his story and understand the basic dynamics of speaking or stuttering more easily, along with decreasing patterns of avoidance, is enough to bring about progress.

Treatment strategies are reasonably straightforward and relatively easy to understand. Treatment for stuttering is not, after all, rocket science. On the other hand, while the concepts themselves are not difficult to grasp, it is considerably more difficult to put them to use with a specific person. It is one thing to be able to remember textbook information for an examination and quite another to respond to a person with an appropriate and perceptive clinical decision *during* treatment. Despite what may be written in a text or treatment manual, the most appropriate clinical choice is not always obvious, even to the experienced clinician. Whatever the structure of the treatment program, the process of change is far more than the use of the dogma of a treatment method and associated criteria. Real intervention for human communication problems is dynamic. At its finest, treatment is the clinician's astute and precise response to the *person* who has come for help. These responses become more likely as treatment progresses and the clinician becomes calibrated to the client. Depending on the client, the clinician may use a variety of techniques and possibly more than one overall treatment strategy. Even if a single overall strategy is used, the application will never be quite the same with each client, for individuals often respond differently to identical techniques.

Whatever treatment strategy and associated techniques are used, it is undoubtedly a good idea for the clinician and the client to be in agreement. During the past few years there has been increased interest in determining the efficacy of our intervention strategies for fluency disorders (Ingham, 1993; Prins, 1970; Curlee, 1993). However, plugging clients into different forms of treatment and then asking which program might, by some criteria, be the best one is the wrong question. Such a question is analogous to questions about which car, religion, or political party is the best. Prochaska and DiClemente (1992) have referred to research in behavioral therapy that has concentrated on trying to determine which treatment is best for a particular problem as "horse race research." In some cases a particular approach won, and in another investigation another method finished first. Most cases, however, indicated "a disappointing abundance of ties" (p. 204). In addition, they propose that one of the major research issues for the future is how those interested in modifying human behavior can more effectively match treatment strategies and techniques to people. Thus, a better question to ask is, What behavioral processes are best for whom and when? It is the wise clinician who is in a position to make this decision.

The first decision for the clinician when initiating treatment is the choice of a general intervention strategy. There are many paths for the clinician to follow, each with something to offer. We will begin by simplifying the situation and discussing the most fundamental paths currently being taken: *fluency modification* and *stuttering modification*. We will also discuss a third, less frequently used strategy, which may be called *cognitive restructuring*. To take the possibilities a bit further, the *Guidelines for Practice* found in Appendix D describe a total of 10 treatment goals involving a variety of treatment choices.

The essential difference between fluency modification, stuttering modification, and cognitive restructuring is best illustrated by considering the relative emphasis placed on the surface and intrinsic features of the syndrome. Fluency-shaping approaches tend to focus on the surface features of the syndrome. That is, the physical attributes of stuttering in terms of the normal or dysfunctional use of the respiratory, phonatory, and articulatory systems are central to the treatment process. This approach might be thought of as *physical therapy for the speech production system*. The primary goal with this treatment strategy is to modify the surface features of the syndrome and not (as Emerick, 1988, explains) to deal directly with such intrinsic features as the client's cognitions about loss of control or attitudes of fear or anxiety associated with stuttering. A basic assumption of the fluency-modification strategy is that once the

---

 CLINICAL DECISION-MAKING

We have consistently argued for the concept that as clinicians, we should generally be leading from behind and guiding the client in directions that he or she needs or wants to go. At times the goals of the client and clinician coincide, and sometimes they do not. A common example is the client who is in urgent pursuit of a "cure" and is unwilling to take part in tasks that do not immediately yield improved fluency. The client is unwilling to take part in activities that are likely to result in more overt stuttering such as decreasing avoidance and word substitution behaviors or voluntary stuttering. My usual preference is to begin by helping the client in understanding his stuttering behavior and to become desensitized to many aspects of the stuttering experience before asking him to begin specific stuttering or fluency modification techniques. However, for speakers who need some immediate "success," we are more likely to begin with activities that result in some instantaneous fluency. As the client is able to gain confidence in us as well as to alter specifics components of his speaking mechanism and his ability to achieve fluency, we can begin to consider a broader landscape of therapy activities.

client has learned new ways of producing fluent speech, he will eventually show a corresponding change in the cognitive and affective features of his problem. Relatively little counseling in a traditional sense takes place. It is interesting to note, as have others (McFarlane & Goldberg, 1987; Ratner & Healey, 1999) that fluency-shaping approaches tend to be favored by clinicians with no personal history of stuttering. Stuttering-modification approaches, on the other hand, tend to be the treatment of choice by clinicians who themselves have experienced stuttering.

The stuttering-modification strategy is, by nature, more cognitive in nature in that the treatment requires the client not only to evaluate and change behavioral characteristics, but to self-monitor and self-manage cognitive and attitudinal features of the syndrome as well. Informal counseling in some form is typically an integral part of this approach.

With the third generic path, which we have termed cognitive restructuring, the intrinsic features of the syndrome become the major focus of treatment. With this approach, relatively little effort is directed toward the direct modification of surface behaviors and the speaking mechanism. The primary goal is to change the way in which the client considers himself and his stuttering and how he interprets the events of stuttering. By decreasing avoidance behavior and becoming more assertive, the speaker is often able to make significant changes in the handicapping nature of his stuttering. Rather than fighting his speech blocks, he may be asked to stutter more openly. Although the frequency of stuttering moments will stay the same or even increase, the quality of the fluency will improve. In addition, and most important, the quality of the client's communication, as well as his lifestyle, will often change for the better.

Rational emotive behavioral therapy (REBT) (Ellis, 1977) may be the best known of the cognitive psychotherapies (Emerick, 1988). The basic premise of this approach is that a person's belief systems are not always logical, rational, or realistic. Thus a restructuring of a client's internal verbal statements (and, hence, his belief systems) may result in a corresponding reorganization of the individual's problem. Although there are relatively few practicing clinicians who have advocated such a cognitive approach for the treatment of stuttering (Fransella, 1972; Hayhow & Levy, 1989; Johnson, 1946; Shapiro 1999; Williams, 1979), there is much to be gained by incorporating some of the techniques associated with this strategy into the process of treatment, particularly for many adults who stutter.

Although there are obvious differences between these three generic treatment strategies, they are far from mutually exclusive. For example, the consistent contact between the clinician and the client that is required during any treatment approach is, by nature, interpersonal and offers the likelihood of some form of supportive counseling. In addition, during the later stages of stuttering-modification treatment, many of the fluency-initiating techniques used during fluency modification coincide with and complement the stabilization and maintenance activities. Each of these treatment strategies requires the client to monitor and self-manage many aspects of his surface and intrinsic behaviors. Each strategy dictates that the speaker systematically learn and practice techniques, first within the treatment setting and then—gradually—outside the security of the clinic, in real-world speaking situations. Each method places great emphasis on the client taking primary responsibility for his own self-management. By beginning from somewhat different perspectives, each approach can result in increased fluency, as well as increased assertiveness and risk-taking behavior. Finally, each approach can result in a significant reduction of the client's handicap associated with his fluency disorder.

Which of these approaches is preferred by professional clinicians? Although there are no recent data, in 1987 St. Louis and Westbrook reported the results of a survey of 30 treatment intervention studies that were published from 1980 through 1986. These authors found that the reported treatment of choice for the majority of adults who stutter was a form of prolonged speech- or rate-control procedure, both forms of fluency modification. Furthermore, St. Louis and Westbrook pointed out that few of the authors of the studies listed activities such as the modification of stuttering moments, client counseling, or desensitization as a significant part of treatment.

Whether these reports accurately reflect the treatment approaches that were being used in the many clinical centers throughout the country is open to question. Whether or not stuttering modification, counseling, and desensitization techniques are highlighted as the major focus of treatment, there is little question that such aspects of treatment are used in some form. The very nature of a clinician working closely with an individual and guiding him through the many components of treatment provides the client with a degree of support and insight about his problem. Therapy, by definition, is always personal, for treatment involves one person assisting another in order to define and manage the problem (Emerick, 1988). Any systematic analysis and subsequent self-management of attitudes and speech behaviors will provide a degree of desensitization during treatment. Whether or not counseling is identified as a basic or formal goal of treatment, in some form it is taking place if the client is being listened to, encouraged, motivated, and challenged. If, on the other hand, the only changes that are emphasized during treatment have to do with the client's speech rate and the related improvement in fluency, it may explain the reasonably high occurrence of relapse with this treatment strategy (Silverman, 1981). Moreover, if, following treatment, the client's speech sounds and feels unnatural and lacks spontaneity, the long-term effects of these changes are not likely to last (Boberg,1986; Kalinowski, Nobel, Armson, & Stuart, 1994; Schiavetti & Metz, 1997). As the field of fluency disorders continues to mature, there is the possibility that clinicians are more likely to prefer a treatment approach that is eclectic, one that incorporates elements from each of these three generic strategies according to the capacities and needs of the client.

SOME SPECIFICS OF
FLUENCY-MODIFICATION STRATEGIES

It is not usually difficult to invoke fluency in even the most severely stuttering speakers. Bloodstein (1949, 1950) researched a variety of conditions where stuttering was reduced or absent. He found that there were as many as 115 conditions that decreased stuttering markedly. Such circumstances included activities such as speaking alone or during a relaxed state; speaking in unison with others; talking to an animal or an infant or in time to a rhythmic stimulus; singing; using a dialect; talking and simultaneously writing; speaking during auditory masking, in a slow, prolonged manner under delayed auditory feedback; and shadowing another speaker. Many of these fluency-producing activities involve combinations of altered vocalization (Wingate, 1969) or enhancement of the speaking rhythm (Van Riper, 1973).

Originally, fluency-modification approaches, because they were based on behavior modification, placed little or no emphasis on the intrinsic features of the stuttering syndrome. Although this has changed somewhat in recent years, the major focus of these approaches continues to be on managing the surface features and achieving a high level of fluent— as well as natural-sounding—speech.

Fluency-modification approaches are also referred to in the literature as *fluency shaping*. Many of the techniques used with this approach are similar to fluency-enhancing procedures that have been used for many years to elicit fluent speech. With the addition of operant-conditioning and programming principles in the latter part of the 20th century, these techniques were organized into systematic approaches for fluency enhancement.

The essence of fluency modification is the establishment of fluent speech in a controlled clinical setting. Once fluent speech is attained, it is shaped and expanded so that the speaker can gradually maintain fluency in conversational speaking situations both within and outside the clinical setting. Clinicians using the fundamental form of this strategy typically do not deal directly with the speaker's attitude, fear, and avoidance behavior. Nevertheless, this treatment often results in more assertive attitudes and a reduction of avoidance behavior as the speaker's fluency increases. Examples of such fluency-shaping programs are described by Cordes and Ingham (1998), Costello (1983), Ingham (1984), Perkins (1973), Ryan (1980), and Webster (1974).

Because—as mentioned previously—fluency-modification treatments tend to be behavioral and highly structured, they can be easier to teach than stuttering modification or—especially—cognitive restructuring strategies. However, as Conture (1990) points out, being able to modify aspects of fluent or stuttering behavior does not mean that we are necessarily changing all, or even the most, critical aspects of the syndrome. After many years of conducting behavioral studies in fluency disorders, Siegel (1970) provided a perceptive review of the problems and unresolved issues inherent in the behavioral-modification approach. More recently, Prins and Hubbard (1988) pointed out some of the potential problems associated with this strategy. After more than four decades of intense research, behavior-modification strategies have not come any closer than the more traditional stuttering-modification approach to solving the problem of stuttering. There is no question, however, that behavior modification techniques have provided valuable insight about the techniques that clinicians can use to modify many of the surface features of the disorder.

One of the best examples of a fluency-modification program is the Precision Fluency Shaping Program (PFSP) developed by Webster (1975). This program has been used more than any other in a wide variety of settings around the United States and other countries. With this program, stuttering is viewed as a physical phenomenon, and there is usually little or no discussion of emotional or affective features of the syndrome. If the speaker follows the rules of speech mechanics, his speech will be fluent; if he violates these rules, his speech will not be fluent. As incorrect and distorted muscle movements are altered, the speaker is able to achieve fluent speech. The client is carefully taken through five gradations of muscle movements associated with sounds and sound sequences which are less and then gradually more complex. Clients are informed about the basic classes of sounds in English and the associated vocal tract features associated with each sound. Clients are taught new, specific muscle movements associated with each sound and class of sounds. Muscle movement targets related to respiration, phonation, and articulation are provided to the client along with the opportunity to practice the new movement skills. The ability to self-monitor the accuracy of their new skills is emphasized. Clients are provided with systematic opportunities to feel and control their new skills in a wide variety of treatment and extra-treatment settings. Eventually, the client becomes completely responsible for self-managing his speech.

A concise description of a typical fluency-modification approach is provided by deNil and Kroll (1995):

> The basic premise of this approach is that stuttering is a physical behavior that can be modified by systematic exposure to a series of rules for fluent speech. The specific and observable behaviors of speech that are reconstructed include those related to speech rate, respiration, voice onset, and articulation. Clients are provided with specific instructional sets for individual response units initially taught in isolation. These responses are then transferred gradually to more complex sequences and ultimately to conversational speech. During the first sixty hours of the program, clients work at establishing fluent speech skills both during individual and group learning sessions. Target behaviors are established by strict adherence to detailed and sequenced exercises under close clinician supervision. The final third of the treatment procedure involves the transfer of newly acquired fluency skills to everyday settings. Transfer activities are structured such that clients progress gradually from simple, one-message questions to complex conversational dialogues in natural settings. Following the three week intensive program, clients are scheduled for a one-year follow-up program consisting of weekly group sessions for the first month, followed by groups sessions every other week for the next two months, and monthly group sessions for the remainder of the year. Each year, a refresher course, which is open to all former participants in the program, is organized.

SOME SPECIFICS OF STUTTERING-MODIFICATION STRATEGIES

The stuttering-modification strategy is also referred to as the *traditional, Van Riperian,* or *nonavoidance* approach. It is based on the concept that a large part of the problem is the speaker's struggle and avoidance of the core moment of stuttering. Whatever the reason for the motoric break in the first place, there is no question that the problem becomes dramatically expanded when speakers begin avoiding feared sounds, words, and situations and increase their struggle, fear, and tension associated with the stuttering moment.

A primary focus of the stuttering-modification strategy involves the reduction and management of fear and avoidance, typically via desensitization and assertiveness training. In addition, treatment focuses on modifying the surface features of the stuttering into intentional, open, smooth, and relaxed forms, which are intended to replace the old, out-of-control, and reflexive stuttering. The result of this treatment can be a form of easy, less handicapping, even acceptable stuttering. In contrast to a common misconception concerning this treatment strategy, clients are not just trained to be "happy stutterers." In some instances, clients can achieve speech that is completely and spontaneously fluent. If not, at least the speaker learns to exert control over previously uncontrolled stuttering moments and to make decisions that are less influenced by the possibility of stuttering. Examples of this approach can be found in Luper and Mulder (1964), Sheehan (1970), Van Riper (1973), Guitar (1998), and Williams (1971).

Stuttering-modification strategies also have as a goal the achievement of fluency, but with greater emphasis on the client's self-perception of the stuttering experience. That is, while a gradual improvement and the eventual attainment of fluency are obviously one indicator of progress, the nature of the fluency breaks are of primary concern. Progress is noted as the types of stuttering events change from those with higher levels of tension and fragmentation of syllables and words to fluency breaks that are characterized by less effort and increased smoothness. As stuttering events are systematically identified, varied, and modified, the speaker is able to incorporate the various techniques in conversational speech during treatment as well as in extra-treatment speaking situations.

Stuttering-modification approaches tend to be somewhat eclectic and therefore somewhat difficult for the new clinician to conceptualize and learn. While being able to observe a model clinician is always helpful when learning any treatment approach, it is especially important when learning treatments that involve the modification of affective and cognitive features of stuttering. The more eclectic the approach, the less opportunity the clinician has to "go by the book" or treatment manual. Stuttering-modification approaches tend to be somewhat more counseling-based and require greater adjustment of the treatment to the individual client. Again, while not usually directly addressed, cognitive and affective changes may also occur during fluency-modification programs, as clients begin to consider new ways of thinking about themselves.

Change often occurs rapidly during the first few treatment sessions. At the outset the client is inclined to be highly motivated, and there are many interesting—even exciting—things to learn about this fluency disorder. The clinician has the opportunity to introduce the lawful aspects of the problem in general and for this client in particular. She can demonstrate that she is unafraid, interested, and excited about exploring how this person manifests the problem in his unique way. The clinician cannot fake an open and interested approach: it must be genuine (see Chapters 1 and 7 concerning clinician characteristics).

The stuttering-modification strategy, as described by Van Riper (1982), takes the client through the stages of Identification, Desensitization, Variation, Modification, and Stabilization.

Identification

Clients are first asked to identify both the surface and intrinsic features of their stuttering. They are asked to identify, analyze, and confront the specifics of their individual patterns of stuttering. With the assistance of the clinician, clients can make a list of "things I do *when* I stutter" to identify the surface features of their stuttering. These are behaviors that can be observed in a mirror, recorded, and identified on video- and audiotapes. Another list, termed "things I do *because* I stutter," can include the less obvious, intrinsic features of the syndrome such as avoidances, anxieties, feelings of fear and helplessness, and the decisions and choices the speaker makes because of the *possibility* of stuttering. The identification of features that occur frequently during treatment is often a good place to begin simply because there are multiple occurrences. Features that are particularly abnormal or distracting may result in increased motivation on the part of the client.

Although the clinician will obviously lead the way during the initial stages of identifying the client's stuttering characteristics, it is important for the client to make this list and write down these features of his stuttering. It is very likely the first time he has been asked to assume the responsibility for this behavior and these feelings. By writing down and analyzing these surface and intrinsic features, he is taking the first step toward self-management of the many aspects of his fluency disorder. Another assignment at the outset of treatment could be to ask the client to prepare an autobiography. The goal is to find out the client's story and, of course, the influence that stuttering has played in the many facets of the life to this point. The assignment may also reveal something about how motivated he is, his general intellectual and linguistic abilities, and his understanding about the nature of stuttering. After some training by the clinician, the client could also analyze tapes of himself or other people who stutter in order to begin categorizing and understanding different surface features of stuttering. Examples of open and easy stuttering moments are especially good behaviors to identify.

Desensitization

The process of identification naturally leads the client toward becoming desensitized to both the overt (surface) and covert (intrinsic) features of his stuttering. It is difficult to critically identify and analyze one's behavior and attitudes without achieving at least some distance and objectivity. Some clients continue to be overwhelmed by the stuttering experience and take considerably longer to reduce their anxiety as they are in the midst of their own stuttering. If the clinician can model a reasonable level of calm during stuttering, the client will be more likely to adopt the same attitude. As the client learns that it is indeed possible to stutter without losing complete control, he will begin to realize that he has some choices that were not apparent before. For example, he has the ability to alter selected features of his stuttering syndrome. He will come to appreciate that he is able to reduce his anxiety during the stuttering event and to realize that some variation of this event is possible. His anxiety does not have to be absent during stuttering, but as he is able to reduce his fear to a manageable level, he will have the chance to accurately identify and analyze his behavior. He will also set the stage for making some variations to his surface behaviors as well as beginning to alter some of the cognitive aspects of his disorder. He may even begin making choices to decrease his avoidance of situations, sounds, and words.

We briefly discussed the idea of stuttering on purpose when describing procedures for self-evaluation in Chapter 4. This technique is often termed voluntary, intentional, or pseudostuttering. As we indicated, the speaker's level of fear associated with this activity provides the clinician with a good indication of the trauma and lack of control associated with the stuttering experience. High levels of fear and avoidance for voluntary stuttering suggests the necessity of focusing on desensitization activities. Until the speaker is able to decrease such fear to manageable levels, he will have little success in the succeeding steps of treatment, which require self-monitoring and variation of specific behaviors. The clinician often begins by asking the client to follow her in producing easy one- or two-unit repetitions and brief (1–2s) prolongations. Later, more elaborate stuttering can be attempted, gradually incorporating the characteristics that are typical of the client during his more severe stuttering moments, including struggle behaviors and blocking of airflow and voicing. This can be done in a variety of treatment (including telephone calls) and extra-treatment settings.

Most—but certainly not all—clients will resist the idea of stuttering on purpose. Because they come to us for help in stopping stuttering, it seems counterintuitive to perform the behavior on purpose. However, with the clinician leading the way, voluntary stuttering opens the door for the speaker to experiment with other ways of stuttering and to become desensitized to the stuttering moment. Perhaps most importantly, it provides a way to break the link between the experience of stuttering and being out of control. As the speaker learns to stay in the moment of stuttering, he will gradually see that instead of being helpless, he has some choices and that there are some good options available.

Variation

As the client becomes able to identify specific behaviors and attitudes and to decrease his automatic reaction of fear and anxiety associated with the moment of stuttering, he will slowly achieve the ability to make some changes in the features of his stuttering, which are no longer things that happen to him but rather aspects of his speech that he is producing: things that he can identify and change. Of course, going from his old, reflexive, and automatic response of stuttering to perfectly fluent speech is an enormous leap and not one that he should be expected to accomplish early in treatment. He has a much greater chance of success if he is asked to simply alter or vary some feature of his stuttering. A small step forward is all that is necessary—or expected—at the outset. Moreover, success is apt to be intermittent. As with identification, secondary or surface behaviors (eye blinks, junk words, postponement devices) that occur frequently and are especially distracting or unappealing are ideal features on which to concentrate. The client is *not* asked to stop performing these features, but rather to vary them in some preplanned manner. That is, the client may select the feature of producing a series of "ahs" prior to a feared word. Rather than attempting to cease production of the "ah" as a postponement or timing device as he anticipates a feared word, he could choose to systematically vary the rate, intensity, number, or vowel segment (e.g., "eh," "oh," or "uh," instead of "ah"). As long as he achieves some measure of control as evidenced by his ability to vary his old automatic utterance of "ah," he is successful.

Another example might involve the slight variation of the especially difficult and scary blocks where airflow and voicing have stopped. At the initial stages of variation, a victory for the adult (or child) is not to move from being stuck to saying the word fluently. A more reachable goal is for the speaker to let some air leak out and achieve primary levels of airflow, and possibly even voicing. Voluntary stuttering is yet another example where the goal is to let some of the stuttering out so that we can help him change it. Of course, some of these activities may result in a decrease in his overall fluency, but the critical issue here is that he has achieved a level of control over his speech that he had not experienced before. The variation of his previously uncontrolled behavior will set the stage for the client to further modify his stuttering moments in even more specific and better ways.

Modification

During this stage the surface features of the client's stuttering that have been identified are further altered. The client is now asked to begin varying some of his behaviors in even more specific and appropriate ways. These changes are, in a sense, closer to the core of the stuttering moment. The goal is to replace the old, out-of-control fluency breaks with a new, smoother utterance which he can completely control.

Changing the well-practiced and stable patterns of these surface features of stuttering is no easy process. The old patterns are not only well-learned, they are comfortable. The new, better ways of speaking will feel awkward and strange, at least until they are practiced enough to become habituated. Smith (1997) proposes a helpful theoretical explanation of what occurs as clinicians assist a person who has stuttered for many years. She suggests that stuttering behaviors may be best considered as hypercoordinated rather than discoordinated behaviors. That is, complex systems have a tendency to self-organize and settle into a mode of behavior that is preferred over other possible modes (attractor states). This also may be the case with a pathology or disease such as stuttering. The more stable the attractor state, the more effort or energy is required to move the system out of that condition. The relative stability-instability of these behaviors should not necessarily be viewed on a continuum of good or bad. However, the process of change may involve helping the system (or person) to re-organize in order to move from a stable mode of functioning to a different mode. Furthermore, because many systems are likely to function in a nonlinear and dynamic manner, it is unlikely that there is one particular approach for facilitating change from one mode to another. Creating or assisting change goes beyond simple cause-and-effect relationships, since there are many levels of functioning and many interactions occurring in such complex and dynamic systems. Finally, there are no particular end-states to be defined for such systems. Rather, the properties of a complex and dynamic system interact and combine to produce new *emergent properties* that are likely to be unique to each system.

What this model means for the process of treatment is that established ways of thinking and behaving are usually stable. Changing from this mode will usually require a great deal of energy and practice in order to reorganize the system. Because people are complex and dynamic, there is no single best strategy for assisting the person in this reorganization. Finally, the end result of successful intervention and reorganization is not necessarily predictable.

The first step in the modification techniques is often termed *cancellation* and has the client approach the moment of stuttering after the event. That is, the client is shown how to perform a post-event modification of his stuttering. Immediately following a stuttered word, the speaker is asked to stop and pause for approximately three seconds. Undoubtedly, this pause can serve as a mild form of punishment for the speaker, since he can no longer continue communicating with the listener. The pause also allows the speaker to highlight the behavior that he just produced. While all clients tend to have some difficulty with this task during reading and especially conversational speech, those speakers who have not achieved a reasonable degree of desensitization often find this task especially difficult. As with many people who stutter, they are somewhat driven to complete the message, and any stoppage both increases the time pressure to communicate and creates the hurdle of having to reinitiate speech.

As the client is able to recognize the stuttering moment and consistently pause following the event, he can now perform an analysis of his stuttered behavior. Following the clinician's lead, he can do this by slowly pantomiming the way he just stuttered the word and examining the physical features of his behavior. He can ask himself how and where he may be cutting off his airflow or voicing. As he rehearses his just-stuttered speech, he can identify points of constriction in the vocal tract, postural fixations he may be using, and inappropriate use of his respiratory or phonatory systems. Once this is accomplished, he is rewarded by being allowed to continue with his message.

Once the client becomes consistently able to stop and accurately analyze his stuttered speech, he will progress to the point where, following a real stuttering moment, he will routinely stop and silently practice a new, smoother, and more open way of stuttering on the word. Although he could easily pantomime a completely fluent version of the word, the task here is to produce a smooth form of "fluent stuttering." Cancellation is usually done during reading, monologue, and conversation, both inside and outside the treatment setting. Following his pantomiming of the new fluent form of stuttering, the client is requested to stop after each stuttered word for a moment and this time produce the new form of fluent stuttering out loud. Again, it is important to note that although the client could likely say the word again completely fluently, the purpose here is not to be fluent, but to replace the old, automatic stuttering with a new form of fluent stuttering.

It is important to point out that the client is not canceling the stuttering event in order to achieve fluency. After all, the addition of yet another moment of (fluent) stuttering following a real stuttering event will result in speech that is even less fluent. However, what is occurring is that the client is not canceling the stuttering so much as eliminating the loss of

---

✓ CLINICAL DECISION-MAKING

The fluency that results from this repair technique is earned fluency to be sure, but it is extremely tenuous. On occasion, especially if additional desensitization to stuttering needs to be done, a speaker will be unable to successfully cancel the stuttered word. That is, as he begins to replace the old stuttering with a smoother, controlled version of stuttering, he will lose control and revert back to his old, automatic, and helpless stuttering. If this happens, the client should attempt the cancellation of the stuttered word again until he regains control of the fluent stuttering. Success is defined by the client indicating that he is in charge of the word. The client can signal to the clinician with his finger whether he is in control of his stuttering. On occasion, it may take several cycles of regaining and losing control before he is able to be completely in charge of the stuttered word. In any case, he should not leave that word and go on to the next one until he has taken charge of that word by successfully canceling it.

control associated with that stuttering event. The sense of power and control that the client is able to achieve with this technique is important for the client to appreciate. Each moment of stuttering, while it may be undesirable, is an opportunity to take charge of the stuttering—a chance at bat. At the outset of treatment, stuttering is scoring run after run while the speaker has not rounded the bases once. Once the speaker begins to achieve control of a large majority of his stuttering moments (something approaching 80%), there is often a flow of fluency and, more importantly, a dramatic increase in the speaker's confidence about repairing the situation. The analogy of rolling back to the surface after an error in paddling a kayak, as detailed in Chapter 9, is an especially good way to describe this experience.

It may be obvious from the previous descriptions that cancellations are usually difficult to perform, particularly during the expectations and time pressure of real-life speaking situations. Listeners tend to interrupt without waiting for the client to go back and work through the stuttered word. Speakers, because they are concentrating so closely on how they are speaking, tend to lose track of their train of thought. Most people who have undergone treatment will indicate that while they often become efficient in using cancellations in the treatment setting and outside of treatment while in the company of the clinician, they choose not to use this technique in most daily speaking situations.

The next step in the modification of the stuttered event is the para-event modification, often called the *pullout*. Now, rather than waiting until he makes it all the way through a stuttered word, the speaker will grab the word and begin to "slide out of it" by enhancing his airflow, altering his vocal tract with articulatory postures, and generally stuttering smoothly through the word. Clients often find that this technique of pulling out of a stuttered moment is a natural progression from the cancellation technique and may begin doing this spontaneously. The pullout is less obvious than the cancellation, and listener reactions tend to be more favorable. Thus clients will want to stop using the cancellation technique. Nevertheless, even though the speaker may gradually improve in accuracy using the para-event modification, it is important to continue practicing the post-event or cancellation technique as well, as there will undoubtedly be many stressful occasions when the speaker will not be able to catch and modify his speech using a pullout. The last line of defense, the final opportunity to catch and take charge of a moment of stuttering, will be the cancellation technique.

The final step in the modification sequence is the pre-event modification or *preparatory set*. As the speaker anticipates an upcoming moment of stuttering and, of course, chooses not to avoid the word, he is able to approach it with a smooth form of stuttering. It is important to understand that just as with the previously mentioned techniques of stuttering modification, the "prep set" is intended to produce a smooth form of easy stuttering. The speaker is preplanning, rather than reacting to, his stuttering. The purpose is not to avoid stuttering and produce completely fluent speech. Many of the fluency-initiating gestures incorporated in the fluency-shaping techniques (full breath, air flow, gradual onset of constant phonation, and light articulatory contacts) are helpful in achieving a smooth preparatory set. Furthermore, if a client's speech contains many very brief fluency breaks that he has difficulty identifying, the preparatory set is one way to eliminate them.

The most difficult thing for both the clinician and especially the person who stutters to understand about these techniques is that the initial goal is *not* to have the client produce fluent speech. That is the long-term purpose. As the speaker begins to gradually modify the form of his stuttering and slowly achieves a measure of command over his speech production system, fluency will follow. The nature of the fluency may be unstable, and it will take additional practice to achieve a natural and spontaneous flow to the movements.

These techniques are often difficult to master, particularly in speaking situations outside of the clinical setting. The vigilance required for closely monitoring one's own speech and producing specific modifications in the way one is speaking require that the speaker is desensitized to the stuttering experience and able to make significant variations to his speech in spite of time pressure to communicate. The cancellation technique in particular, because it asks the speaker to revisit the stuttering and produce another (voluntary) form of smooth and obvious stuttering, is difficult for clients to perform in real world settings. Even when using fluency shaping techniques, listeners are not likely to understand this somewhat unnatural behavior and react negatively to this altered and somewhat unique version of stuttering. Manning, Burlison, and Thaxton (1999) found that nonprofessional listeners reacted less favorably to a speaker who stuttered mildly (SSI = 17) and used the stuttering-modification techniques of cancellation and pull-outs than when the same speaker simply stuttered (see Chapter 11 for additional detail).

As the client is learning each of these techniques, it is often effective for the clinician to coach the speaker through stuttering moments by explaining and demonstrating how stuttering behavior can be altered. The goal at this point is not fluent speech, but rather to help the client to experiment and to "play" with the possibilities for stuttering in a different, usually easier, manner. This form of coaching is vividly demonstrated on videotapes available through the Stuttering Foundation of America (see especially Tapes 76, Do you Stutter: Straight Talk for Teens; 79, Therapy in Action: The School-Age Child Who Stutters; and 83, If you Stutter: Advice for Adults). Such coaching might sound something like the following, as a client is describing a conversation with his supervisor:

Client: "I was trying to tell my su, su, su . . ."
Clinician: (reaching quickly to touch the arm of the client) "Good, ok get

that one. Stay with it. Keep stuttering as you are. Now see if you can gradually begin to slow the rate of your repetitions slightly." The client continues to repeat the syllable "su" but finds that he is able to stay in the stuttering and eventually slow his rate of repetitions.

Clinician: "Now, produce the repetitions more rapidly. Now slowly again." (Client does so.) "Good, now slow down again and slowly move through the word by stretching out the sounds and continue."

In order to be sure that the client understands a technique, the clinician may ask the client to explain the steps of the technique as well as demonstrate it for the clinician and others present in the treatment setting (or at home with a spouse or parents). It may also be instructive to switch roles so that the client guides the clinician through the use of the technique as the clinician makes intentional errors. Of course, it is also important for the client and others to understand the rationale for the technique.

Stabilization

During this stage, the newly learned modification skills are practiced under more stressful conditions both within and outside of the treatment setting, with the goal of having the speaker become more resilient in response to stress and communicative pressure. It is important for the client to understand that in order to withstand the pressures of the real world, techniques must be overlearned, or the speaker will be unable to count on them when communicative demands are swift or serious. As we suggest many times throughout this text, speakers will have to (correctly) practice a technique many *thousands* of times in order to refine this new approach to the stuttering moment and to develop confidence in the technique. Performing a technique in the safety of the clinic, regardless of how many times it is done, provides little indication about how the client will perform in the stressful speaking situations found in everyday life.

This is also a good time to heighten the ability of the speaker to monitor speech production via proprioception, by using devices that create auditory masking or produce delayed auditory feedback (DAF) or frequency altered feedback (FAF). In addition, with the aid of the clinician, the client can bring forth, revisit, and resist old fears and anxieties associated with speaking situations. With practice, he can learn to withstand the old, negative self-talk that he has played in his head many times in the past. The new patterns of speaking and thinking need to be tested in the difficult waters of the real world in some systematic way, gradually working through hierarchies of increasing difficulty. Telephone calls, public speaking, and social introductions are examples of particularly difficult speaking situations, which often need to be systematically confronted.

Most stabilization activities take place away from the clinician and the treatment facility and will continue long after formal treatment is concluded. For continued success, the speaker must continue to push the envelope and challenge himself with new speaking adventures. This is also likely to be an ideal time to expand the practice of voluntary stuttering in some speaking situations, particularly when others put pressure on him for unrealistic or perfect fluency.

COGNITIVE RESTRUCTURING

Regardless of the overall treatment strategy, for the speaker to have long-term success, he must eventually develop fresh ways of thinking about himself and his problem. Over the years many authors have emphasized the merit of speakers experimenting with the role they play as someone who stutters, or alternately, as someone who is able to achieve fluency. This aspect of therapeutic change is most often suggested within the context of Rational Emotive Behavioral Therapy (REBT), Personal Construct Therapy (PCT), or Gestalt Therapy. Each of these therapeutic approaches attempts to assist the client in experimenting with new ways of thinking about himself and developing his own problem-solving responses to speaking and interacting with others—often critical changes that are necessary for long-term success. This aspect of treatment does not always need to be dealt with directly with all clients in order for change to occur. For example, if the clinician is using a classic behavioral modification/fluency shaping approach, which does not typically involve changing the intrinsic features of the syndrome, cognitive changes may spontaneously follow successful changes in the speaker's fluency. Regardless of the approach, the client will sense that new ways of speaking and thinking will sound and feel strange, possibly making him feel that he is standing out even more than he has in the past. The person had spent years adjusting to his speech and the way he interprets himself. Changes in these features of the problem require ongoing adjustment. These cognitive adjustments often become particularly important as the treatment reaches the transfer and maintenance phases. The client who retains self-defeating mental images and negative thoughts and beliefs about speech and his ability to manage it is much less apt to succeed once he is on his own.

Emerick (1988) concludes that clients who have an analytical and introspective orientation at the outset of treatment respond the most favorably to cognitive-restructuring approaches. According to Emerick, the cognitive aspects of treatment involve at least four main phases. *Phase 1* focuses on educating the client about the overall approach of the treatment. Suggesting to the client that he change his orientation to both himself and his problem can pose a threat to his self-integrity and equilibrium. This is not surprising, and Emerick suggests that these changes should be viewed as a challenge for client and clinician alike. Threat or not, the clinician must frequently challenge the client if change is going to occur.

Phase 2 involves having the client identify his self-defeating patterns of thinking analyzing his thoughts before, during, and after speaking situations in general and stuttering events in particular. He is asked to identify his mental constructs about the event, keep a log of his emotions and thoughts, and indicate the outcome of situations. He then categorizes his responses in terms of dependency/helplessness ("I know I will relapse when therapy is over"), irresponsibility ("I just cannot control my feelings"), dichotomizing ("There are good listeners and bad listeners"), catastrophizing ("I know I will fall apart if I am asked to introduce myself") and fantasy ("Most of my problems would be solved if I didn't stutter").

Phase 3 is one of reality testing. The client's task is now to evaluate his mental constructs by asking (a) Does the construct deal with the reality of the situation? (b) Does this construct make unreasonable demands on me? and (c) Does the construct help me accomplish the treatment goals? In addition, the client also contrasts possible negative imagery with positive, self-enhancing imagery. As Emerick says, "It is difficult to think of failing in a speaking situation while at the same time concentrating on positive thoughts" (1988, p. 262). The old, negative cognitions must become cues for the client to tell himself, "Stop." At this point, the clinician can role-play for the client, alternating between the negative and positive self-statements. As these concepts are introduced and practiced with several clients, this form of reality testing can be an ideal activity during group treatment sessions.

The final and *fourth phase* involves having the client substitute self-enhancing language for the traditional negative thoughts. The new, positive affirmations may not always be completely true (e.g., "This may be a difficult situation, but I can deal with it"). Nonetheless, imaging success brings the possibility of success that much closer (Daly, 1994).

Clients can, of course, have problems with cognitive restructuring activities, especially when they continue to view stuttering as something that happens to them rather than something they do (a fairly common perception). According to Emerick (1988), such clients have great difficulty stopping and changing the old negative cognitions. An even greater problem is posed by those clients who are unable to recognize the inaccuracy of their cognitions. Some clients believe that the way they are processing reality is the normal, correct, and most acceptable way. The client may agree intellectually that there are several ways to view something, but still privately believe that his view is the most accurate.

A good example of a program that emphasizes cognitive restructuring along with a stuttering-modification approach is described by Maxwell (1982). The approach is educational rather than curative, with a primary goal of teaching the client better ways of managing his speech. Clients typically attend the treatment program for one individual and one group session each week for approximately one and a half years. Maxwell (1982) summarizes the program in the following steps:

1. *Information giving:* In this initial stage, the client receives verbal preparation and instructions. The purpose of this stage is to provide the client with a map of the treatment process. The client also receives a verbal or written summary of the treatment plan.

2. *Cognitive appraisal:* The client summarizes, in his own words, the objectives and methods of the treatment plan and how the plan will meet his needs. This process establishes a common perception of the treatment process for the client and clinician.

3. *Thought reversal:* The client begins to reduce and eliminate negative cognitions. Essential to this process is the technique of "thought stopping" when negative self-talk occurs. This requires the client to tell himself (initially out loud) to "stop" using the negative ways of thinking about himself and his speech. Later, this stopping process is done silently. The primary goal is for the client to begin disengaging from undesired thoughts and images. Near the end of this stage, the client begins taking steps to utilize positive and productive cognitions. These activities take place within the treatment setting.

4. *Vicarious observation:* Once the client is able to experience some success at disengaging negative (and often self-fulfilling) cognitions, the clinician begins to model positive cognitions. As the client observes the clinician succeed and cope with challenges in her own life, the client's self-efficacy will be enhanced. Such modeling increases the client's hope that he, too, can perform as he desires, despite any setbacks.

5. *Speech modification*: In this initial stage of behavioral change, the client begins to improve his information-processing, decision-making, and problem-solving abilities. Maxwell points out that clients typically are not accurate self-observers. However, even before the client is able to successfully modify specific stuttering events, the fact that he is able to accurately self-monitor his behavior tends to have a positive treatment effect in terms of reduced avoidance and possibly even increased fluency (Cooper, Cady, & Robbins, 1970; Daly & Kimbarow, 1978; Wingate, 1959). Many aspects of the Identification and Termination steps as described by Maxwell are similar to the variation and modification stages of treatment as described by Van Riper (1973). Rather than thinking about his speech as something that happens to him, the client eventually begins to understand the lawfulness of his syndrome. An essential aspect of this modification stage of treatment involves the client describing what he does with his speech production mechanism. With more accurate monitoring of his behavior, the speaker begins to see the lawfulness of his behavior and will be more likely to understand and predict his behavior.

6. *Identification:* The client becomes proficient at identifying specific moments of stuttering, beginning with ten-minute segments using short words and progressing to reading and conversation.

7. *Termination:* The client terminates the old form of stuttering by following a moment of stuttering with a silent pause. The client then gradually replaces the fluency break with cognitive and behavioral skills that are more appropriate. Termination is accomplished first following (as in a cancellation), then during (as in a pullout), and finally before (as in a preparatory set) the stuttering moment. The client uses imagery to see, hear, and feel a new motor plan consisting of fluency-enhancing targets. The client is also asked to identify and modify avoidance or substitution behaviors.

8. *Cognitive restructuring:* As during the third stage of this treatment, the client is asked to "identify maladaptive speech-related emotions, and self-defeating cognitions on which these are based" (Maxwell, 1982, p. 415). This time, however, the client is asked to restructure his thought in more stressful extra-treatment speaking situations.

9. *Coping skills:* The client begins to use positive self-statements and to model imagery techniques to revise negative aspects of his covert verbal behavior. The client's ability to restructure his thinking about himself and his problem is often reflected in self-talk. As Egan (1998) suggests, clients often talk themselves out of things by verbalizing feelings such as "I can't do this. This technique won't work. I'm not good enough to do this yet." This self-talk is often disabling and tends to get the person into difficulty before he has given himself a chance to succeed. Egan indicates that clinicians can add value to the treatment experience by helping clients challenge negative self-talk that prevents them from taking action. With the clinician's modeling, the client reorganizes monologues in preparation for actual speaking tasks. Group sessions using role-playing activities are recommended here.

Maxwell provides a clear example of how a client can alter his thought process about giving an oral report to an art history class. The first paragraph indicates the client's initial thoughts about this task.

> Oh, Lord, here I am in class with all of these people and soon I'm going to have to talk. What if my controls don't work? What if I fall on my face—make a fool of myself? Then, they'll think I'm stupid. Maybe I ought to quietly get up and walk out of here. Maybe there won't be time to get to my report. If I stutter, will they laugh or feel pity? (1982, p. 417)

Following analysis of the nonproductive content of that self-message, the clinician then models a revision of more positive internal monologue, as in this example.

> I am now in class with other students like me discussing the subject of art history. Soon I will be asked to speak on a topic that I know well. I have interesting information to share. When I speak, I plan to use to the best of my ability the controls that I've learned to use well in therapy. What I want to convey is the strong interest I have in my topic. I'll remember to smile, maintain eye contact with my listeners, and try to be open and friendly. (Maxwell, 1982, p. 417)

10. *Self-management:* During this final stage of treatment, the client takes ever greater responsibility for setting his own goals and self-management of the cognitive and behavioral features of his speech. From the outset there must be the recognition that the "majority of therapeutic work takes place between, rather than during, therapy sessions" (Maxwell, 1982, p. 418; see also Kanfer, 1975). The time for dismissal from formal treatment approaches as the client becomes able to self-manage without the assistance of the clinician. Related to the above-mentioned activities are the recommendations of Daly (1992, pp. 135–136) for using positive affirmations for reinforcing and enhancing cognitive changes.

EXPERIMENTAL TREATMENT

A new example of a cognitive treatment for stuttering is currently being developed by Starkweather and Givens-Ackerman (2000). In this client-centered approach, the authors adapt the principles of Gestalt therapy to the treatment of stuttering. Treatment activities are based on four premises. First, "experience is as important as performance." That is, the experience of being someone who stutters is more central to understanding and change than the surface behavior called stuttering. The reader will recall a similar description provided by Smith and her associates in Chapter 2 and her explanation of a the multifactorial-dynamic model. Because the clinician and the client may well have different interpretations of the stuttering experience, some time is spent at the outset of treatment communicating about the nature of the experience and ways to address therapeutic change.

The second premise is that understanding the development of the problem is more important than explaining the possible etiology. That is, from a therapeutic standpoint, it is more beneficial to understand the developing nature of stuttering for a particular client than to focus on the possibilities of the original cause(s). The third assumption is that the client and the clinician need to understand what can be changed and what cannot be changed. That is, the speaker must become aware of his stuttering behaviors as well as ways of thinking about himself. He must become aware of the scope of his stuttering including the difficult-to-change patterns of avoidance behavior.

The final premise is that adults really change from within. Because people resist being manipulated, successful change is much more likely to take place if the client leads the way. It is also important for the client to discover desirable ways to change while still being true to who he is or who he can become.

Another unique aspect of this therapeutic approach is that the clinician, rather than spending the bulk of the treatment session showing the client how to "control" his stuttering, helps the client in creating experiments that will allow the client to explore alternative ways of behaving and thinking. Experimentation is accomplished by following the client's lead and adopting a variety of roles throughout treatment. For example, the clinician *facilitates change*, drawing from her experience and advising the client to choose therapeutic experiments that may be useful and advises against experimenting with techniques that are not likely to be useful. The clinician also becomes an astute *listener*. Starkweather and Givens-Ackerman point out that few people who stutter have had this experience, because listeners tend to respond to the speaker's lack of fluency rather than the content. Listening by the clinician assists in modeling self-listening by the client. The client begins to recognize what he is communicating in terms of emotions and cognitive interpretations of himself and his situation. The client also begins to appreciate the quality of his fluent utterances, how he is capable of producing easy fluency breaks, and how he responds to different ways of speaking. The clinician also takes the role of a *witness*. In this case, the clinician shares in the process of recovery and verifies change by keeping a record of progress and helpful therapeutic experiences. The clinician also witnesses the client's growth and the development of independence from the clinician. Finally, the clinician plays the role of the *experimenter*. At the outset of treatment the clinician takes the lead in designing and selecting experiments that may facilitate change and growth, a role gradually assumed by the client. Experiments are intended to assist the client in increasing his awareness of his stuttering across levels of behavioral, emotional, cognitive, and linguistic functioning. Other experiments are designed to help the person become more accepting of his current situation with an emphasis placed on approaching, rather than avoiding, himself and his stuttering behavior. In addition, experiments are planned that will help the client to accept the changes that take place as a result of his increased awareness and acceptance.

Finally, the basic responsibility for planning and implementing the treatment activities is with the client. That is, the client raises the topics for discussion, suggests directions of treatment, and identifies issues to focus on. Because the process is one of experimentation and exploration, "failures" are no one's fault. Rather, unsuccessful experiments are seen as opportunities that lead to new directions to be explored. This approach to treatment will be described in greater detail by Starkweather and Givens-Ackerman in the next few years.

GROUP TREATMENT

One of the earliest uses of group treatment in the field of communication disorders was the work of Backus (1947), who advocated the use of speech in social situations beyond the usual speech production drills popular at the time (Backus, 1957). The popularity of group treatment for adults increased as a result of World War II. The many men in need of treatment for various psychological and medical problems, in combination with the relative shortage of clinicians, resulted in group meetings taking the place of individual treatment. The decades of the 1970s and 1980s saw some decline in group treatment due to the popularity of behavioral-modification approaches that emphasized individual treatment (Conture, 1990).

The experiences provided by group interaction are a valuable part of a comprehensive treatment program. The group provides an ideal setting for "divergent thinking," as the client observes how others have dealt with similar problems. Divergent thinking (e.g. "lateral thinking," "thinking outside the box") is uncomfortable for individuals who are bound to the idea that there is a single "correct way to approach issues or

---

 CLINICAL DECISION-MAKING

Regardless of the methods of treatment, some clients will make more rapid and more obvious progress than others. It is not always clear how long we should continue to move in a therapeutic direction with particular techniques if relatively little progress seems to be taking place. Formal assessment devices available to the clinician usually provide useful information concerning whether or not the desired changes are taking place. These measures assist us in demonstrating our accountability. Still, the clinician's best source of information about change is the astute observation of the client's behavior in a variety of settings and the client's forthright views of the many changes they desire and are able to bring about. Experienced clinicians are able to rely on their accumulated clinical intuition for many of their decisions and are able to change the game plan as necessary. In the final two chapters of this text, we describe indicators of progress during and following treatment.

problems" (see Egan, 1998, p. 228–231). The many opportunities for activities such as brainstorming, role-playing, and problem-solving make group meetings especially attractive and potentially enlightening for clients.

Luterman (1991) suggests that there are two basic types of groups: therapy groups and counseling groups. Group meetings for clients with fluency disorders typically serve both functions. The group setting provides opportunities for enhancing as well as maintaining change in both the surface and intrinsic aspects of the syndrome. Unless there happens to be a local support group chapter, the group treatment meeting will be the only way for the client to understand that he is not alone. The group provides a social setting where the client can discuss his problem openly. As the client adjusts to the roles and expectations of the group setting, he is more likely to become desensitized to stuttering in general as well as his own stuttering in particular.

Conture (1990) points out that group meetings can also provide social and speaking opportunities for some people who might otherwise go for days or weeks without communicating with others. This group setting is also likely to be the only place where the speaker is permitted to stutter without being penalized. The members of the group can provide an important source of motivation and courage to keep members connected to the overall treatment process.

There are other advantages. The structure provided by a group setting provides the client with the opportunity to practice the techniques learned during individual treatment sessions. Group interaction provides the clinician with an opportunity to monitor the client's progress in a social context (Conture, 1990). When the treatment is taking place in an academic program, the group setting provides an opportunity for student clinicians to observe a broad range of behavior and to note the dynamics of progress in other clients. If the goal of treatment is to help the speaker to change both the fluency of his speech as well as his understanding of himself and his interaction with others, group treatment is essential. Furthermore, group activities are a natural extension of individual treatment (Levy, 1983). It is clear that group treatment permits a greater variety of treatment choices and a more comprehensive treatment approach than would be possible with individual treatment alone.

Determining Group Membership

The selection of those who will take part in the group is a first step in assuring the success of the group. Each individual participant must be committed, motivated, and willing to contribute to the group process. Group treatment is not appealing to all clients, and it can be difficult to get adults who stutter to commit to a group setting. Silverman and

Zimmer (1982) found, for example, that women who seek treatment tend to prefer individual rather than group settings. On occasion, some individuals will express the fear that their problem will become more severe by being exposed to others who stutter. For anyone with a long history of stuttering, even an informal group can be particularly aversive and carry with it the threat of severe social penalty. Thus simply getting a client to attend his first group meeting can be a major success. However, almost without exception, once a reluctant client takes part or observes his first meeting, he will begin to change his mind. Most people are attracted by the interest, support, and energy provided by the other participants.

The initial decision about whom to include in a treatment group is critical. Once an individual is included, it will be difficult to remove him. As Luterman suggests, individuals must have "a willingness to examine their lives and to share their insights with the group" (1979, p. 199). Furthermore, the group will be more likely to be dynamic and self-directed if the members are motivated and share a common interest for introspection and contributing to the success of others in attendance (Luterman, 1979). It makes little sense to attempt to include a client who strongly resists group contact. It may be possible to change his view of the experience through observation via a one-way mirror or by viewing videotapes of group meetings. However, individuals who tend to be argumentative, who consistently attempt to dominate group discussions, or who consistently withdraw from participation are generally not good candidates for group sessions.

Advantages of Group Treatment

The group meeting is likely to be the only place in town where people who stutter can come and feel safe. It is the only place they can come and not be penalized for stuttering. If they are able to stutter openly and easily, they can even be rewarded for stuttering well. Based on my experience both as a client and as a clinician, I think the group treatment experience plays a major role in facilitating change. There can be great support among a group of people striving for similar goals. There is the freedom to practice skills and risk-taking in a supportive environment. The group provides a captive audience for gaining confidence during many activities such a public speaking, making introductions, role-playing, discussion, and even debate. The group setting also allows clinicians to observe additional clients other than the one they are seeing during individual treatment sessions.

Luterman (1991) indicated several characteristics of group treatment that are beneficial.

> *The instillation of hope:* As other members of the group are able to make positive changes in their speech and ways of viewing their situation, the

client can increase his belief that he is also capable of such success. The client can often gain momentum from others in the group who are becoming more assertive and taking risks. Much like being a member of an athletic team, group participation often motivates a client to extend himself beyond his original notions of what is possible.

The promotion of universality: By being a member of a group of individuals who share a common problem, the client comes to recognize that he is not alone. The group provides a means for coping with feelings of isolation and loneliness. The group setting also provides the client with the opportunity to practice recently learned modification techniques in a more realistic setting than alone with the clinician. Speaking in a group situation is a good initial step in generalizing the newly acquired and tenuous techniques to a social, albeit clinical, situation. Using the fluency- or stuttering-modification techniques in a group setting can also provide one means of reducing the client's dependence on his clinician.

The imparting of information: Information is provided not only by the group leader as in individual treatment, but also by the other group members and, in some cases, other clinicians. All members of the group are able to provide examples and advice based on their own, unique experiences, whether or not they stutter. The inclusion of other clinicians, spouses, or friends provides the opportunity for individuals who stutter to understand, many for the first time, that nonstuttering speakers share many of the same fears about speaking in public or formal situations and about risk taking in general.

The provision of altruism: Each group member provides not only information to other members, but also support, reassurance, and insight. Furthermore, as the group members are helping others, they also tend to experience an increase in their own self-esteem.

The enhancement of group cohesiveness: As with most small groups, the treatment group develops its own history and evolves through the stages of "forming," "storming," "norming," and "performing" (Tuckman, 1965). That is, group members discover and adjust to the group protocol, find out how to identify roles and resolve conflicts, become committed to working with each other, and eventually focus on group objectives and goals. As this process occurs, the group as a whole gradually becomes more self-directed, and individual members experience an increased desire to maintain their role in the group and look forward to group meetings. As group unity increases, group activities will be more likely to facilitate growth and change of individual members.

The possibility of catharsis: The group provides a safe place for individual members to release and share feelings and attitudes concerning their own problems. As opinions and views are expressed, there is often a release from the control these feelings have had over the individual. This can be especially obvious during certain aspects of treatment for fluency disorders, as members become desensitized to their long history of fear associated with fluency failure. The group provides a safe place to ventilate feelings of embarrassment, shame, and social failure associated with stuttering. Participants are able to let go of these past experiences by achieving distance and greater objectivity, and perhaps even allowing humor to be associated with past events.

The development of existential issues: The group can provide the opportunity for individual clients and clinicians to deal with questions concerning anxiety associated with daily living, such as feelings of loneliness, dependency, and meaninglessness. The discussions can help reduce anxiety and allow the members to improve the quality of their decision making, including the many interpersonal aspects of their lives.

Of course, group treatment sessions also provide an ideal way to gradually phase individuals out of the more intensive individual treatment schedules. Following the conclusion of formal treatment, clients can return again to the group meetings as they experience signs of relapse (Levy, 1983) or simply feel the need for a booster session.

Potential Problems With Group Activities

As might be expected, there are apt to be a variety of problems with attendance and schedules. Group meetings are not always possible to schedule, particularly for clinicians working in a public school environment. Even when scheduling is possible, it is often difficult to maintain consistent participation by all members. In some settings it can be a major hurdle simply to find a time and a place to meet. Often it is difficult to gather together enough clients to form a group of a critical and consistent mass. Conture (1990) recommends a group size of approximately seven members, while Luterman (1991) suggests an upper limit of 8 to 15 members. A general rule might be that the group should be large enough for a variety of interactions but small enough that members have opportunity to know and trust one another. If clinicians are included (something that is highly recommended for student clinicians), the group can easily become too large. One solution is to break up the larger group into smaller subsets so that all members have the opportunity to participate. At the conclusion of the session, all members can gather together for summary comments.

Achieving diversity among the members is not usually a problem. In most instances clients will be at different stages of change or will have been in treatment for varying lengths of time. Just as social, cultural, and educational diversity provides for learning for clients and clinicians alike, variety in client responses to treatment is usually informative.

Obviously, group members will bring a variety of personalities and experiences to the meetings. As Sheehan (1970b) suggested, a group is only as good as its membership. The group will be less effective if one or more members tend to try and dominate or if members are reluctant to contribute to the group activities or discussions. Some participants may give feedback that is less than constructive, and—in some cases—

members can become dependent on the group as their basic means of socializing (Levy, 1983).

Group leaders can also be a source of problems. The leader serves a critical role, for she provides direction and consistency for the group. However, she must be flexible and facilitate the growth of each participant. If the leader promotes a highly structured group in which she directs all activities, the result may be passive participation by the members. Clients will be less likely to initiate interaction and assume responsibility (Luterman, 1991). On the other hand, groups that lack the necessary leadership tend not to be task-oriented and often lack a direction and purpose for the group meetings. As indicated by Levy (1983), this is especially apt to occur if the leader is unable to convey her understanding of the stuttering experience and therefore lacks credibility. Groups that meet several times a week are more likely to develop their own direction, and the professional clinician may be able to gradually assume the role of consultant rather than that of a group leader. The nature of the group may then begin to evolve from a teacher-student relationship to a integrated group with its own identity and sense of direction.

The Effective Group Leader

The effective group leader is able to establish credibility during the initial group meetings. Credibility can be accomplished by demonstrating both a knowledge of stuttering and people who stutter as well as a genuine interest in the members of the group. Just as the characteristics discussed in Chapter 1 describe the actions of an ideal clinician during the individual treatment, these same features indicate that empathy, warmth, and genuineness are necessary requirements of an effective group leader. Furthermore, the leader should be flexible: She should be able to sufficiently structure the group so that members have a sense of direction but also be prepared to discard prearranged plans when necessary. That is, the leader must provide a sense of mission to the group but at the same time be able to respond to the needs of individual group participants. As in individual treatment, the clinician is likely to be somewhat more directive during the early group meetings. Once the norms of the group become established and the purpose and direction of the group have been defined, the group leader will be less instructive so that there will be more opportunity for the members to be self-directive and interact with one another (Luterman, 1991). Of course, the group is more likely to become self-directed if group attendance remains consistent over several weeks. If the membership of the group is constantly changing, it is more difficult for the group members to assume their own direction.

Establishing Group Norms

Since the goal of the group is to have the individual members interact with one another, it is usually not helpful for the group leader to simply ask or answer questions. In order for the group to become self-directive, the leader must promote the concept that the members should take responsibility for the activities and topics. Another norm or characteristic of the group is one of self-disclosure. The leader and other clinicians can model such disclosure so that the clients gradually become more comfortable about revealing feelings, beliefs, and attitudes. The trick is to do so without eliciting judgmental statements by other members. On occasion, there is likely to be confrontation among members of the group. This is normal and to be expected. Group members should not feel pressure to self-disclose before they are ready. A good guideline is that no one has to talk unless one wants to, and no question *must* be answered. Still, members must feel that their individual needs are being considered. Finally, members must be reassured of the confidentiality of the group's discussions (Luterman, 1991).

Structuring Group Activities

Ideally, group meetings should be held in a large room with comfortable seating. A degree of privacy is preferred (Levy, 1983), and if relaxation and imagery activities are to be conducted, the area must be quiet. It is also useful if the room is large enough for public speaking and can be divided into areas for small-group discussion or role-playing. Some nearby access to outside speaking situations is helpful so that group members can leave the building, conduct brief speaking assignments, and return to evaluate the experience. Of course, arranging the participants in a circle is useful in enhancing conversation as well as promoting eye contact and allowing the clinicians and clients to read each other's body language (Luterman, 1991). Once the group's structural and procedural norms have been established, the group can conduct specific activities.

Relaxation-Imagery Exercises

Many of the activities that are done in group meetings for fluency disorders are useful for all members, regardless of the quality of their speech. This is clearly the case with this category of techniques (Kirby, Delgadillo, Hillard & Manning, 1992). It is not necessary or even desirable to be extremely relaxed in order to produce fluent speech. However, being able to relax in the midst of life's many anxiety-producing stimuli is a valuable skill for anyone. The process can be done anytime during the meeting, but often it works well to begin the meeting with these activities. Assuming the meeting is taking place in a reasonably quiet room with comfortable seating, the lights are dimmed. Playing quiet, relaxing music can be helpful. Each group member closes his eyes and gradually focuses his thoughts on the instructions being delivered by a member of the group. The instructions direct each participant to sequentially relax groups of his skeletal muscles, eventually focusing on the muscles of respiration, phonation, and articulation. The emphasis is on slowing and smoothing breathing, as well as visualizing an open vocal tract with cool air smoothly flowing through and out of the oral cavity. Participants are asked to imagine themselves in a serene and natural setting. Once relaxed, they are led through images of success, which include speaking activities. They are asked to remember the positive feelings associated with each success.

The process usually lasts approximately 10 minutes. Often, a relaxed state is created that carries over into the remainder of the group session. Initially, the responsibility of leading this portion of the session can be directed by a clinician. However, the instructions, which should be delivered slowly and smoothly, provide an ideal speaking situation for clients who have limited experience speaking in front of a group.

Relaxation has been advocated as a way of promoting fluency for many years. In and of itself, relaxation is far from a solution to the problem of fluency disorders. Such techniques can, however, contribute to the learning that takes place during a comprehensive treatment program. The goal is not to promote fluency per se but to teach the client better ways of responding to stress-producing situations, whether giving a presentation to a large audience or having dental surgery. Some members of the group will respond more readily to this experience than others, and some will be better able than others to make use of the relaxation and imagery skills in everyday situations. It takes consistent practice for these skills to be available when needed.

Role-Playing

The acting out of real-life situations is facilitated by group treatment sessions. This exercise is useful in helping the stutterer work through feared moments he has previously encountered. Such situations may include ordering food at a restaurant or drive-through window, taking an oral exam for certification, giving a formal oral presentation, exchanging marriage vows, or dealing with threatening or confrontational situations at home, work, or school. Role-playing activities by the group lend themselves to creativity and role-reversal. It provides an opportunity to become desensitized to past fluency failures and future anxiety-provoking situations. Observers can analyze the interpersonal aspects of the situation and offer constructive feedback and alternative ways of responding to the situation.

Public Speaking

Public speaking is a highly feared situation for nearly anyone, and the group session provides a forum for speaking before a group. Depending on the level of each member's experience and upcoming demands at work or school, public-speaking situations can be created during the session. Clients have the opportunity to experience the preparation of different types of presentations (informative, demonstration, storytelling, extemporaneous) and to practice responding to questions from the audience. Participants also have the opportunity to improve important speaking and organizational skills and to learn to sequence and present their ideas in front of a group. Public speaking can be done in the same room where the group session normally takes place or in a more formal setting such as a classroom or auditorium, sometimes making use of a microphone and amplification system. During the final stages of preparing for a presentation at work or school, the individual or the entire group can meet at the site. Of course, when it comes time for the actual presentation, the group members can share in the success of the event by actually being there or by viewing the presentation on videotape.

Demonstration of Client Skills and Progress

During the group meeting, each client has the opportunity to demonstrate techniques being worked on during the individual treatment sessions. For example, each group member can explain, demonstrate, and respond to questions about the use of specific techniques. Voluntary stuttering is a good example of such an activity. Other activities involve demonstrating examples of decreased avoidance behavior, providing examples of risk-taking activities, and describing humorous situations that occurred as a result of potential or real stuttering.

TREATMENT OF ATYPICAL FLUENCY CASES

As discussed in Chapter 4, the large majority of the people who seek assistance for fluency disorders have a history of developmental stuttering with etiology of unknown origin. While each client has his own story and his own intrinsic and surface features, his physical and psychological characteristics are typically well within normal limits. Although these more typical clients are otherwise normal, healthy people—as we have described in Chapter 4—some clients present with symptoms and etiologies that are considerably less common, and modifications to the typical treatment procedures and additional clinical decisions are required.

Acquired Neurogenic Stuttering

Helm-Estabrooks (1999) provides a comprehensive approach for intervention for patients with acquired neurogenic stuttering. Once the clinician determines that the nonfluent behavior represents a real communication handicap and that the speaker is motivated and able to work on changing the problem, intervention is possible. A wide variety of treatment approaches have been used with these speakers including pharmacological agents, thalamic stimulation, delayed auditory feedback and auditory masking, biofeedback and relaxation, and speech-rate techniques. Helm-Estabrooks reported that each of these approaches has resulted in improvements to the patient's fluency, although some (particularly some pharmacological agents) have resulted in undesirable side effects. Fluency-enhancing techniques such as the initiation of airflow, gradual onset of phonation, easy articulatory contacts, and desensitization are commonly used by clinicians (Market, Montague, Buffalo, & Drummond, 1990; Meyers, Hall, & Aram, 1990; Rousey, Arjunan, & Rousey, 1986). In addition, since word finding has been mentioned as a common problem in neurogenic fluency disorders and may contribute to fluency breaks (Brown & Cullinan, 1981; Meyers, Hall, & Aram, 1990), a slow rate of speech production may also assist the speaker by providing more time for retrieval.

Several authors have reported an improvement of fluency in clients with neurogenic stuttering who have suffered further damage to their central nervous system (Helm, Yeo, Geschwind, Froedman, & Wenstein, 1986; Jones, 1966; Manders & Bastijns, 1988; Van Riper, 1982). The additional trauma apparently resulted in an improvement of function for fluency. These observations suggest that of all the forms of fluency disorders encountered, pharmacological treatment may be most beneficial for this group of clients (Helm-Estabrooks, 1986). Because, as pointed out by Helm-Estabrooks (1999), acquired neurological stuttering is far from a unitary disorder, it is not possible to predict a particular speaker's response to intervention. She has found that Parkinson's patients tend to respond well to several techniques, while stroke patients are more difficult to treat. However, she also points out that acquired stuttering is more likely to be a temporary symptom for stroke patients. Finally, although acquired stuttering is not uncommon for patients with closed head injuries and is sometimes associated with seizure activity, resolution of the seizures may result in improved fluency.

Acquired Psychogenic Stuttering

Because there is a relatively small number of speakers with acquired psychogenic stuttering, there are few empirical studies documenting treatment strategies and the nature of recovery for this population, especially over the long-term. Roth, Aronson, and Davis (1989) recommend "traditional fluency treatment" in combination with counseling from a psychologist or psychiatrist. According to Roth et al., these patients are receptive to both stuttering- and fluency-modification procedures. Reflecting a common theme with such patients, these authors stress the importance of encouragement and optimism concerning a successful outcome on the part of the clinician.

Baumgartner (1999) indicates that because behaviors vary so much across patients and because even the initial assessment procedures may be highly therapeutic, treatment goals should be open-ended. The initial goals of treatment, which can occur during the first (diagnostic) session, are to provide the client with an explanation of the evaluation and the development of an atmosphere whereby "the patient becomes receptive to the idea that these findings are good news and indicate that a total resolution of symptoms is possible" (p. 279). Because many patients with acquired psychogenic stuttering believe that the problem is organic in nature, it is important for the patient to have a positive reaction to the news that no organicity is present and that this an unsurprising result of the evaluation. As Baumgartner explains:

> A "cognitive set" must be achieved so that the lack of organicity is perceived in a positive light by the patient, as is the clinician's belief that this is a reasonable, not unexpected findings. If this is not achieved, a patient may have received indirectly the message that the clinician is surprised or that the findings are somehow mysterious. Worse yet would be the message that a lack of organicity indicates that there is not a real problem. In my opinion, a prerequisite for patients achieving such a cognitive set is the clinician's belief that psychogenicity is a valid concept and that findings pointing to such a diagnosis are reasonable and not uncommon. (1999, p. 279)

Treatment should proceed with the same confidence on the part of the clinician about the possibility of achieving normally fluent speech. According to Baumgartner (1999), it is not uncommon to achieve much improved speech during the first treatment session. If improvement occurs, the patient should be informed that this is a positive sign. On those occasions when this is not the case, the clinician can focus on reducing struggle behavior associated with abnormal movements that are not involved in speech production (e.g., movements of the limbs or torso or bizarre movements of the eyes) and altering aberrant behaviors such as speaking only when lying down or when grasping an object. Baumgartner (1999) recommends that it is often helpful to focus treatment activities on the area of the body that is associated with excessive effort or tension. He has found that touching or manipulating of these areas by the clinician is particularly effective in reducing musculoskele-tal tension (see Baumgartner [1999, 284-285] for a description of this technique).

As pointed in Chapter 4, psychiatric referral is not typically the treat-ment of choice. However, in cases where the patient continues to be affected by environmental stress or if there is little change in the patient's fluency following several sessions, such referrals are in order.

Baumgartner stresses that it is important not to "rush" the patient in these activities, but rather emphasize the fact that he is producing improved speech and that this represents a good prognosis. In other words, changing the patient's "belief system" is more essential than elic-iting fluent speech or practicing speech-related movements. The princi-pal goal of treatment is not so much to achieve fluency as it is to assist the speaker in reducing the effort that is being used to produce speech and to alter the client's belief that certain circumstances must be met in order to speak. As these measures are successful, the clinician can then show the patient how to expand his fluency.

In contrast to the usual prognosis for persons with acquired neuro-genic stuttering, patients with acquired psychogenic stuttering are more likely to demonstrate rapid change in the direction of speech fluency. For example, Baumgartner and Duffy (1997) reported that more than 50% of their patients improved to normal or near normal following one or two sessions of symptomatic treatment. Importantly, many who respond well to treatment show no need for a psychiatric referral (Braumgartner, 1999).

Cluttering

As with the diagnosis of cluttering, treatment for this disorder—especial-ly when it presents in combination with stuttering—can be perplexing. Because the problem is broad-based, involving many linguistic, motoric, emotional, and pragmatic features, treatment can also be complex. St. Louis and Myers (1995) suggest the three principles of (1) slowing rate, (2) heightening self-monitoring, and (3) developing the ability to encode language, including the pragmatics and turn-taking aspects of communi-cation. These authors suggest that a focus on these principles often results in improvement in articulation and intelligibility as well as fluen-cy. St. Louis and Myers (1995) provide a detailed list of treatment activi-ties, particularly for children and adolescents.

Daly and Burnett (1999) advocate a comprehensive and inclu-sive approach to treatment for these individuals where all the problem areas are addressed. In addition, they suggest three basic principles of intervention.

1. Because these clients are unaware of their communication behavior as well as listener reactions, *frequent repetition of therapy goals and rationale* will be necessary.
2. Also because of the speaker's lack of awareness of his communication problems, the clinician should *provide immediate and direct feedback.*
3. Parents and significant others should play a major part in providing feedback, correction, and reinforcement.

One of the most difficult aspects of treatment is the aversive attitude frequently taken by these clients. As Daly (1986) points out, clients can be aggressive and extremely defensive, characteristics that make it difficult to develop a workable clinical relationship. On the other hand, because these speakers are usually oblivious about their communication problem, intelligibility and fluency can often be dramatically improved as these speakers develop the ability to monitor their speech. These speakers need to concentrate almost totally on *how* they are speaking rather than on what they are saying. As the speaker is made aware of his irregular and rapid speech, he will typically be able, at least for brief periods, to make appropriate alterations in his production, often even without specific instruction. As the client is shown techniques for self-managing his speech and the effects on others, his fluency will improve, as will his expressive language and articulation. Unfortunately, without the development of self-cueing strategies, the improvement is often short-lived. Temporary success often occurs rapidly, but many clients quickly lose their motivation for self-monitoring activities. In addition, the person often finds it difficult to tolerate speaking at what seems to him an exceedingly slow rate. The "driven" quality of these clients described in Chapter 4 becomes obvious after even a brief period of speaking at a slower rate.

The essence of treatment with these clients involves varying the rate of speech production and increasing their ability to monitor output. A variety of stuttering-modification and fluency-modification techniques have been found to have a positive effect. Van Riper (1992b) provided a summary of techniques that he found assisted individuals who clutter in modifying their speech.

➤ Read in unison with the client, beginning with a fast rate and systematically changing speed while the client shadows the clinician's rate changes.
➤ Have the client write down the words he wants to say before he utters them.
➤ Have the client repeat phrases using different tempos, altering the stress placed on different words or syllables.

➤ Using recorded samples, have the client analyze the audio- or video-tape and instruct you about his speech, explaining the repetitions, misarticulations, revisions, interjections, and so forth.

➤ Using modeling and signals, have the speaker increase his ability to pause for gradually increasing lengths of time. Use the natural pauses afforded by punctuation and clause boundaries. Practice pausing in reading as well as paraphrasing of pictures of events. Role-playing of extratreatment events can also be useful here.

Other authors (Daly, 1986, 1988; Trotter & Silverman, 1973; Weiss, 1964) have suggested the use of masking devices (Dewar, Dewar, & Anthony, 1976) or delayed auditory feedback (Daly, 1992) in order to heighten the speaker's ability to monitor his speech proprioceptively. The slowed speech rate resulting from these devices also improves intelligibility and fluency. The use of a metronome (or tapping with a finger, pencil, etc.) may also facilitate concentration on how the client is speaking. Using a window-card so that one or a few words are visible to the client or reading backwards one word at a time may help to increase the speaker's ability to tolerate something other than his typical excessive rate. Fluency-modification programs, because of their tendency to incorporate rate variation and control as well as specific alterations of the vocal tract and articulators, are often especially useful with individuals who clutter.

As with the other "atypical" fluency disorders, treatment for cluttering is more appropriately done with a team approach, for these speakers are likely to have other educational, emotional, and learning difficulties. The prognosis for success is not particularly good, but, as always, it is better for children than adults (Daly, 1986, 1993; Luchsinger & Arnold, 1965; Myers & St. Louis, 1992; Silverman, 1995; Weiss, 1964).

A comprehensive treatment approach is provided by Daly and Burnett (1999), who describe a strategy for treatment that they call a profile analysis (Figure 8-1)). Information obtained on the checklist for identification of stuttering (See Figure 4-9, Chapter 4) is converted to the profile. For example, a score of three (3) on the checklist corresponds to a negative three (−3) on the profile analysis, indicating that this characteristic is "undesirably different from normal" (p. 239). A score of two (2) on the checklist is recorded as a negative two (−2), and a score of zero (0) indicates that the speaker's performance on that item is within (or above) normal limits. The profile analysis is intended to facilitate individualized treatment according to the areas where the speaker is in particular need of assistance.

Daly and Burnett (1999) also provide an extensive list of suggestions for helping a client across each of nine common deficit areas. These are found in Table 8-1.

Client's Name _____   Date _____

	Undesirably different from normal		Normal or above
	-3	-2	-1	0

A. COGNITION and LANGUAGE

(12) Speech better under pressure (during periods of heightened attention)

(14) Distractible, attention span problems, poor concentration

(24) Seems to verbalize prior to adequate thought formulation

(25) Above average in mathematical and abstract reasoning abilities

(31) Lack of awareness of self and/or communication disorder(s)

(36) Lack of effective/sufficient self monitoring

(4) Language is disorganized; confused wording

(6) Interjections; many filler words

(13) Difficulty following directions; impatient/disinterested listener

(15) Poor language formulation; storytelling difficulty; trouble sequencing ideas

(16) Demonstrates word-finding difficulties resembling anomia

(17) Inappropriate pronoun referents; overuse of pronouns

(18) Improper linguistic structure; poor grammar and syntax

(20) Reading disorder or difficulty reported or noted

(22) Writing shows omission or transposition of letters, syllables, or words

B. PRAGMATICS

(9) Compulsive talker; verbose or tangential

(32) Inappropriate turn-taking

(33) Inappropriate topic introduction/maintenance/termination

(34) Poor recognition or acknowledgement of non-verbal signals

C. SPEECH and MOTOR

(1) Repeats words or phrases

(8) Rapid rate (tachylalia) or irregular rate; speaks in spurts

(11) Slurred articulation (deletes, adds or distorts speech sounds)

(23) Initial loud voice, trails off to a murmur; mumbles

(27) Variable prosody; improper/irregular melody or stress patterns in speaking

Figure 8-1. Profile analysis for planning treatment with cluttering clients. [Daly, D. A., & Bennett, M. L. (1997). Cluttering: Traditional views and new perspectives. In R. Curlee (Ed.), *Stuttering and related disorders of fluency* (2nd Edition, pp. 222–254). New York: Thieme Medical Publishers, Inc. Reprinted with permission.]

	Undesirably different from normal		Normal or above
	-3	-2	-1	0
(35) Telescopes or condenses words (omits or transposes syllables)				
(5) Silent gaps or hesitations common				
(7) Little or no tension observed during disfluencies				
(10) Respiratory dysrhythmia; jerky breathing pattern				
(19) Clumsy and uncoordinated, motor activities accelerated or hasty, impulsive				
(21) Disintegrated and fractionated writing; poor motor control				
(26) Poor rhythm, timing, or musical ability (may dislike singing)				
D. DEVELOPMENT				
(2) Started talking late; onset of words and sentences delayed				
(3) Never very fluent; fluency disruptions started early				
(28) Appears, acts or sounds younger than age; immature				
(29) Other family member(s) with similar speech problem(s)				
(30) Untidy, careless, or forgetful; impatient, superficial, short-tempered				

Figure 8-1. continued

CONCLUSION

For the clinician who understands the surface behaviors as well as the underlying cognitive and affective components of stuttering, fundamental treatment decisions can become reasonably obvious. In contrast to the young person who stutters, the adolescent or adult client comes to treatment with a well-developed syndrome. Because the older speaker has learned to survive with the problem of stuttering and because his patterns of behavior and his thinking about the problem are often tightly bound together with anxiety and fear, treatment is typically more complex and takes more effort and time. The speaker has made many subtle adjustments to his communication problem that will take even the experienced clinician some time to detect. Furthermore, in addition to acquiring new ways of speaking and thinking, he may have to discard his old patterns and beliefs about himself and his speech.

The experienced clinician recognizes that in many ways, it is the client who will lead the treatment process. What is possible during treatment is often determined by treatment variables such as the availability, setting, and cost of services. Ideally, treatment will result in spontaneous fluency.

Table 8-1. Suggestions for treatment of cluttering (Daly & Burnett, 1999).

Targeted Deficit Areas	Treatment Principles and Activities
Awareness It is important to address awareness as a whole and as it pertains to each deficit area.	-Provide rationale for each task and goal in each session -Utilize video and audio recordings -Provide immediate, direct feedback with positive reinforcement for appropriate performance/behavior -Multisensory feedback; e.g., vibro-tactile feedback, pacing board -Negative practice
Self-Monitoring Tasks for awareness also assist in improving self-monitoring and vice versa. Impulsivity also improves.	-Monitor number of times the client self-corrects (e.g., an articulation error, self-cues to reduce rate, etc.) -Use of Delayed Auditory Feedback -Self-rating for specific task performance (i.e., demonstrating ability to accurately judge correct performance) -Train awareness and accurate response to listener feedback
Attention Span	-Measure time on task (sustained attention) -Tally number of times redirection to task is required -Use time or alarm to indicate task beginnings, endings. -Listening for comprehension and details, following directions; selections of increasing duration -Auditory memory for increasingly longer series of numbers (forward or backward), words (related or unrelated)
Thought Organization/ Formulation Note that each activity may actually address multiple target areas simultaneously.	-Naming attributes within given categories for specific objects -Categorization of items or objects -Detailed description of objects, increase use of descriptors/ adjectives -Describe similarities and difference of two objects -Sequencing activities, such as naming steps to complete a task or giving directions -Story telling; structured with use of picture sequencing cards or unstructured narrative -Writing; same tasks as above with written responses
Semantics, Syntax, and Lexical Selection The activities in the sections above as well as these can be targeted in verbal or written exercises.	-Unscramble words, sentences, paragraphs -Vocabulary building exercises -Naming activities, including confrontation naming and naming to description or category -Cloze activities at sentence or paragraph level -Sentence framing -Combining simple sentences into one complex sentence

Pragmatics/Social Skills

- Listening activities requiring careful follow-through; blind board activities
- Training appropriate means of requesting clarification, questioning
- Building awareness of specific behaviors through direct feedback (verbal, audio or video replay, role-playing)
- Overt practice of social skills (greetings, introductions, salutations)
- Topic-specific discussion; attempt to make all remarks pertain to one topic
- Overt or exaggerated practice of acknowledging nonverbals (reading expressions, body language)
- Practice of turn-taking in activities and conversation; move from highly structured to less structured tasks)
- Appropriately tell jokes (proper sequencing, timing)

Speech Production and Prosody

Many suggestions in this section address speech & motor abilities.

- Rate reduction programs; DAF; deliberate, exaggerated practice decreasing rate and increasing linguistic skills
- Reduce repetitions via use of DAF, deliberate phonation, decreasing rate and increasing linguistic skills
- Emphasize appropriate changes in inflection/intonation; stressing different words to change meaning, statements versus questions
- Breathing modifications for better coordination, with speaking and increased use of pauses; appropriate use of "verbal punctuation"
- Overarticulation and exaggeration of mouth movements; articulation drills if necessary
- Imitation or oral reading of nursery rhymes, poetry

Motor Skills

- Oral-motor skills training (e.g., Riley and Riley)
- Recite tongue twisters
- Address penmanship in written assignments
- Practice various rhythmic patterns (tapped or verbalized)

At the outset of treatment, the clinician, although being realistic about the level of fluency that may eventually be achieved, should include spontaneous and natural fluency as a possibility. For most adult speakers, however, controlled or acceptable fluency is the outcome. More importantly, however, it is possible to reduce the severity of the disability and the handicapping effects of the problem. The person is able to expand the scope of his lifestyle and to gradually make choices that are minimally or not at all influenced by even the possibility of stuttering.

Treatment for adults often includes, of necessity, many features of both stuttering- and fluency-modification strategies. Fluency-modification techniques can help adult clients learn how to use their speech production mechanism more effectively and produce stable fluency in progressively more difficult speaking situations. However, most adult speakers who are able to achieve controlled or acceptable fluency also need to have confidence in using techniques that will enable them to repair their fluency breaks in an efficient and effortless manner. Following the client's lead, the clinician must decide how to sequence and blend the variety of strategies and techniques for each speaker.

Fluency treatment for adults often requires arduous work over many months and often years. The cognitive changes that occur can take some time to catch up to the behavioral changes taking place on the surface. Group meetings can serve as an essential part of treatment, providing information, support, and insight that are otherwise unavailable. The group activities provide the client with an opportunity to practice skills learned during individual meetings, try out new speaking roles, and test new perceptions with others who share the same problem. As a group leader, the clinician must develop the skill to carefully walk the line between giving the group direction and promoting flexibility of discussion.

The less typical forms of fluency disorders represent unique and exciting opportunities for clinicians to help individuals who acquire disordered fluency some time after the usual onset for those with developmental stuttering. It can be difficult to distinguish these adult speakers who have acquired disordered fluency as a result of neurogenic or psychogenic origin from speakers with developmental stuttering. Clients who experience acquired psychogenic stuttering are more likely to have a successful treatment outcome. The unique combination of broad-based problems experienced by those who clutter (or have a combination of cluttering-stuttering features) also present the clinician with unique diagnostic and treatment decisions. These atypical fluency problems have received more clinical and research attention in recent years, and diagnostic and treatment protocols have expanded considerably.

STUDY QUESTIONS

➤ Make a list of three "risk-taking" activities you will perform in the next week. Ideally, they can be related to speaking activities. These will be things that you would typically like to avoid or have avoided for some time. Make brief notes about your reaction to the challenge of taking each risk.

➤ What will you tell your older clients about the possibility of success as a result of treatment?

➤ How will you respond to an adult client who has been stuttering for about 30 years when he asked you, "What are my chances of success?"

➤ What are some basic characteristics of the adolescent years that sometimes make it difficult for teenagers to have a successful therapy experience?

➤ Using Brad Sara's description of rock climbing, prepare a similar set of guidelines for working through success for a challenging activity that you have done or would like to do.

➤ Describe the three to four most basic characteristics of the four main treatment strategies described in this chapter (fluency-modification, stuttering-modification, cognitive restructuring, and experiential treatment).

➤ What are the most common misconceptions that clinicians typically have about the stuttering modification techniques of cancellation, pullout, and preparatory set?

➤ Write for yourself or describe to a friend how you recently used negative self-talk about your anticipated performance in an upcoming event. Indicate whether or not you were able to change your negative self-talk to positive self-talk.

➤ How would you explain the advantages of attending a group treatment meeting to an adolescent or adult client?

➤ Describe the most important characteristics of an effective leader of a group treatment meeting.

➤ What are the one or two primary goals when helping people with acquired psychogenic stuttering?

➤ What are Daly and Burnett's three basic principles of intervention with people who clutter?

RECOMMENDED READINGS

Culatta, R., & Goldberg, S. A. (1995). *Stuttering therapy: An integrated approach to theory and practice.* Boston: Allyn & Bacon. (See especially the chapter "A Synopsis of Approaches to the Treatment of Stuttering.")

Guitar, B. (1998). Advanced stutterer: Stuttering modification and fluency shaping therapies (Ch. 8, pp. 213–234). Advanced stutterer: Integration of approaches (Ch. 9). *Stuttering: An integrated approach to its nature and treatment.* Baltimore, MD: Williams & Wilkins.

Manning, W. H. (1999). Progress under the surface and over time. Chapter 10 (pp. 123–129) in N. B. Ratner and E. C. Healey (Eds.), *Stuttering research and practice: Bridging the gap.* Mahwah, NJ: Lawrence Erlbaum.

Van Riper, C. (1973). *The treatment of stuttering* (2nd ed.). Englewood Cliffs, NJ: Prentice-Hall. See Part 2, "Our Therapeutic Approach."

Williams, R. (1995). Personal construct theory in use with people who stutter. In M. Fawcus (Ed.), *Stuttering: From theory to practice.* London: Whurr Publishers.

CHAPTER

9

TREATMENT FOR PRESCHOOL AND SCHOOL-AGE CHILDREN

> *A lot of times, after I'd been outside playing and had gotten real thirsty, I'd run into the kitchen and ask her to give me a glass of water. I was still stuttering badly, of course, so it took some time. And early on, she would stop washing dishes or whatever she was doing and just reach down, pat me on the back, and encourage me: "C'mon Robert Earl, spit it out now, son." After a while though, whenever I ran in there and started tripping over my words, she'd say the same thing, but instead of patting me on the back she'd take the dishrag and pop me upside my head with it. It didn't' help me "spit it out" any quicker, but I learned to stop asking and get that water for myself, real quick.*
>
> Bob Love (2000). The Bob Love Story.
> *Chicago, IL: Contemporary Books.*

INTRODUCTION

As one spends any time at all reading the literature about preschool and early school age children who stutter, several important findings become obvious. Perhaps most apparent are the results of a number of studies and reviews indicating that younger children can benefit from a variety of forms of indirect and direct intervention (e.g., Bloodstein, 1995; Conture, 1996; Conture & Guitar, 1993; Conture & Wolk, 1990; Fosnot.,1993; Gottwald & Starkweather, 1995; Lincoln, Onslow, & Reed, 1997). The reports of successful treatment are undoubtedly aided (or confounded) by the fact that many children would have recovered on their own during the first two years following onset. The literature indicates that a number of different approaches appear to help the younger child become more fluent. These approaches typically make use of combinations of techniques that help the child to make slower and easier movements for voicing and articulation, decrease sensitivity to the stuttering event, increase self-confidence and problem solving as it relates to speech and communication, and promote an enjoyment of speaking. Depending on the child and the degree of struggle behavior that is present, clinicians also use stuttering-modification procedures such as voluntary stuttering, cancellations, and pull-out techniques. In other words, clinicians tend to employ a multifactorial approach whereby the clinician, often with the assistance of one or more parents, helps the child to improve skills or capacities in a number of areas that facilitate a smooth flow of language and speech. The literature on treatment of young children also indicates that treatment for somewhat older school age children is effective (Conture, 1997; Runyan and Runyan, 1993). However, as children experience the penalty of less than acceptable fluency during the early years of school, treatment tends to become more complex.

This chapter discusses strategies and techniques for helping the younger child who is beginning to stutter. The major focus is the child from approximately age 2 through age 12. There are far more children who stutter than adolescents or adults. As described in Chapter 3, the literature strongly suggests that by the early teenage years, there is a notable decrease in the number of individuals who stutter. As Bloodstein's 1995 review of prevalence studies indicates, stuttering remains consistent through grade 9 and begins to decline during grades 10 through 12. Thus, by far the largest number of potential clients with fluency disorders are to be found among children in their preschool and early school years (Conture, 1990). For years, writers in the field of fluency disorders have suggested that clinicians will have the greatest impact by providing service to this group of clients (Van Riper, 1982).

Although a child's chronological age is a factor influencing the behavioral features and severity of the stuttering syndrome, age is not as meaningful as the length of time stuttering has been taking place. As Conture (1982) puts it, the age of the stuttering is usually more meaningful than the age of the child. Children as young as two or three years old can present with strikingly complex stuttering behaviors and exhibit high levels of tension, struggle, and fear. Furthermore, the longer children have been stuttering, the more likely it is that the problem will become chronic. Chronicity may be especially likely if the child continues to stutter throughout ages of five to seven, which constitute the *critical period* (see Chapter 5) during which stuttering may become habituated.

Both the amount as well as the directness of clinical intervention with preschool children who stutter has clearly increased during the last decades of this century. According to Gottwald and Starkweather (1995), this increase is partially a result of the implementation of federal legislation in 1975 of Public Law 94–142, calling for the education of all handicapped children, and in 1986 of Public Law 99–457, requiring early intervention for children three to five years old. There may be at least one other factor contributing to increased interest in early intervention. The results of research findings with young children by Yairi and his associates have documented many of the characteristics of very early childhood stuttering. Furthermore, Yairi and Ambrose (1992a, 1992b) have noted that 75% of the risk for stuttering onset occurs before the age of three years, five months. The increased understanding of early childhood stuttering, in combination with successful intervention for children who are seen as soon as possible after stuttering onset, has made it clear that such treatment offers the best chance for altering the development of the problem. As we shall see in the following pages, early intervention has been found to be both effective and long-lasting.

BASIC CONSIDERATIONS WHEN TREATING YOUNG CHILDREN

There are, of course, many salient distinctions between intervention with children and with older clients. In earlier chapters it was shown that fluency is often variable with young children, a fact that makes both assessment and therapeutic progress somewhat more difficult to track for this age group. There is always the question of how much behavioral change is due to treatment and how much is due to the natural variability of the behavior. Other important differences when working with younger clients are the following:

1. Children are functioning with neurophysiological systems that are far from adult-like and are still in the process of maturation.
2. Depending on the child's level of awareness and reaction to the stuttering experience, the clinician may select treatment techniques that are less direct than those used with adults.
3. Parents and a variety of other professionals, and particularly the child's classroom teacher, play essential roles in the treatment process.
4. The clinician will more likely place greater emphasis on the evaluation and possible treatment of the child's other communication abilities, including language, phonological, and voice. On occasion, some children will also present with a variety of other learning or

behavioral problems (e.g., Obsessive Compulsive Disorder [OCD] or Tourette's syndrome).

5. The likelihood of achieving spontaneous or automatic fluency is much greater for young children than for adults.
6. There tends to be somewhat less effort needed for helping the child to transfer and maintain treatment gains into extra-treatment environments.
7. Relapse following formal treatment is not usually a serious problem, as it is with adult clients.

Another thing that is unique about children who stutter is the setting where they are likely to be receiving therapy. By far, the largest number of children are seen in a public school setting under conditions that sometimes limit the effectiveness of therapy. It is not unusual for clinicians to be responsible for double or triple the maximum caseload of 25 to 40 children recommended by ASHA direct service itinerant model (ASHA, 1984; Kelly, et al., 1997; Mallard & Westbrook, 1988). The lack of time available for individual treatment often results in children who stutter being seen along with children with other communication problems. In most cases, children are only able to be seen, at the most, twice a week for 20 to 30 minutes each (Kelly, et al, 1997; Healey, 1995). Finally, because children who stutter typically make up only 3%–4% of a clinician's caseload (Blood & Seider, 1981; Kelly, et al., 1997; Slater, 1992), it is usually difficult to organize group therapy for these children with unique problems and treatment goals. All these issues combine to create what are often clearly inadequate services for children who stutter. As I have listened to public school clinicians describe their frustrations concerning these and other conditions that hamper the delivery of quality services for children who stutter, I have been tempted to suggest that the parents of children who stutter should seek services elsewhere. Clearly this is not always the case and there are examples of clinicians and school systems that provide outstanding service to these children and their families, sometimes during after-school or summer programs. However, it is also clear that because of lack of support, ineffectual service in many other settings results in little help for these children and leads to some of the frustration and anger concerning service delivery that one can hear expressed by people at self-help meetings.

One final issue that may not be completely unique to children has to do with how we as clinicians assign value to fluent and nonfluent speech. That is, when we are speaking to younger as well as older individuals who stutter, how do we express ourselves about stuttering and the importance of fluency? If, by our verbal and nonverbal behavior, we consistently indicate that fluency is "good" and stuttering is "bad" (or at least not as good as fluency) we may be compounding the problem and possibly impeding long-term success. As we will describe later in this chapter, we could easily be engendering feelings of shame in the person who already feels as though stuttering is his fault. Regardless of the overall treatment strategy, the effectiveness of many treatment techniques requires that the child be free to experiment with a variety of fluent and nonfluent speech behaviors. An overemphasis on fluent speech as the only goal of treatment can easily lead to the child trying hard not to stutter, something he is already doing. Although it is true that listeners will react negatively to most forms of stuttered speech, one of the clinician's first goals to break up the conceptual dichotomy that all fluent speech is good and that stuttered speech must always mean that the speaker is out of control and helpless.

All these aspects of stuttering in younger speakers combine to produce a number of clinical choices that the clinician must consider with children. One of these is the directness of the intervention process.

Indirect and Direct Strategies

During the first seven or eight decades of this century in the United States, the treatment used with young children who stuttered was indirect. That is, the children themselves were not the recipients of the intervention activities, and no specific instructions were given to the child. Rather, the significant adults in the child's environment—the parents, family members, grandparents, and teachers—were advised concerning procedures for altering the child's environment. The choice of this general approach was due to the many cautions from authorities who strongly recommended that the clinician not do anything to make the child aware of the problems he seemed to be having with his speech. Clinicians were extorted not to bring the child's attention to his disrupted speech or to respond in any way that might associate speech with negative emotion. This view was especially popular during the decades of the 1940s through the 1960s and coincided with the prominence of the diagnosogenic theory of stuttering onset and development (see Chapter 2). A series of quotes from a popular textbook of the time by Eisenson and Ogilvie (1963) reflect the then-current thinking about intervention for the early or primary stages of stuttering. Described by Bluemel in 1932, primary stuttering is seen as a transient phenomenon during which the child does not yet show awareness of his problem or demonstrate special effort during speaking.

> Emphasis in the treatment of the primary stutterer is to prevent him from becoming aware that his speech is in any way different from that of others around him and a cause for concern. (p. 318)

Essentially, therefore, the primary stutterer is to be treated through his parents if he is not of school age. If he is of school age, teachers as well as parents become the recipients of direct treatment. (p. 318)

Parents were instructed to respond in the following ways:

If the child is a primary stutterer or is showing any of the speech characteristics associated with stuttering, it is essential that signs of parental anxiety be kept from him. Do not permit the child to hear the word stuttering used about his speech. Do not . . . do anything that makes it necessary for him to think about speaking or to conclude that he is not speaking well. (p. 323)

Johnson's 1962 "Open Letter" contained this statement:

"Do nothing at any time, by word or deed or posture or facial expression, that would serve to call Fred's attention to the interruptions in his speech. Above all, do nothing that would make him regard them as abnormal or unacceptable" (p. 3).

Finally, Van Riper, in the first edition (1939) of his popular text, *Speech Correction: Principles and Methods,* wrote, "The way to treat a young stutterer in the primary stage is to let him alone and treat his parents and teachers." With such cautions, few clinicians and parents were likely to intervene directly and assist a young child with his communication problems. The fear was that direct intervention could make the stuttering more severe, a fear that permeated the decision-making process for clinicians. Doubtless there continue to be many clinicians who continue to hold such views and are overly cautious when deciding whether treatment is appropriate for young children.

Even if a young child is producing frequent fluency breaks, a less direct strategy is often used during the initial period of treatment. An indirect approach is often the case for the child whose fluency is characterized by relatively easy breaks with low levels of tension or struggle and who is generally unaware of any speaking difficulty. With indirect intervention the clinician takes no direct action to modify specific features of the child's speech. Parents and significant others are counseled and provided with information concerning the developmental nature of language and fluency. The clinician will likely spend as much or more time working with the parents as with the child. The major focus of an indirect strategy is to make speech enjoyable for the child and to adjust those environmental factors that tend to disrupt his fluency. By decreasing demands, desensitizing the child to fluency-disrupting stimuli, and giving rewards for open, easy, and forward-moving speech, the child is guided step-by-step toward increased fluency.

Treatment is likely to be more direct if the child is experiencing tension and struggle behavior or fragmenting multisyllabic or, especially, monosyllabic words. In addition, the child may be exhibiting the nonverbal characteristics of more developed stuttering such as breaking eye contact with the listener (Conture, 1990). For these children, the clinician will be more straightforward in demonstrating specific activities for enhancing fluency and modifying moments of stuttering. A number of authors (Gregory, 1995; Healey & Scott, 1995; Peters & Guitar, 1991) have indicated that fluency modification techniques are more likely to be used at the outset of treatment. Depending on the success of these techniques, stuttering modification techniques may also be employed. A more direct approach to modifying stuttering consists of identifying stuttering events, contrasting both fluent and stuttered speech, and having the child intentionally produce both forms. The clinician will select the most appropriate activities along a continuum of directness according to the needs of the child and his response to treatment.

Regardless of how directly the clinician works to alter the child's speech, treatment for young children who stutter should be characterized by a high degree of reassurance and encouragement by the clinician. Conture (1990) holds that these clinician characteristics cannot be overemphasized. The treatment environment must be highly supportive as the child is guided into the exploration of his speech and himself. The primary targets of communication by the clinician and the parents can be such concepts as (1) stuttering is not the child's fault, (2) stuttering is not the parent's fault, (3) speaking can be easy and fun, and (4) the child is able to be in charge of his speech production system.

The clinician's choice about the directness of treatment depends more on the characteristics of the child's problem than on his age. Although clinicians or parents need not be alarmed or seek immediate help, it is generally agreed that early intervention is an influential factor in the success of treatment (Adams, 1984; Gottwald & Starkweather, 1995; Peters & Guitar, 1991; Starkweather, 1987; Starkweather, Gottwald & Halfond, 1990). Nonetheless, as Conture (1990) points out:

> Unfortunately, some professionals, who do not have enough experience or interest in stuttering, will use up precious time in the early stages of the development of the child's stuttering problem and only refer to a more qualified professional when the child is showing signs of a worsening and, generally, more habituated speaking problem. (p. 126)

The Role of the Parents

Clinicians have known for many years that parents play a central role in the successful management of stuttering with young children (Bluemel, 1957; Wyatt, 1969). Since stuttering is most often a developmental disorder beginning during childhood (Bloodstein, 1987; Conture, 1990; Van Riper, 1982), the problem unquestionably involves the parents. Parents are the most important models for children. Conture (1990) wisely points out that parents need to be rewarded for their insight and courage when they ask for help. The last thing they need is for the clinician to lecture or reprimand them for their previous patterns of parent-child interactions. Parents should be informed at the outset that they have not caused this problem to occur and are not totally responsible for eliminating it. However, as a good deal of research has demonstrated, parents can be shown how to assist in altering the child's environment so that stuttering behavior is not maintained. Parents are significant listeners in the child's environment and have a powerful influence on the child's attitudes and speech behaviors.

Ratner (1993) provides a helpful metaphor that may be used to explain the nature of stuttering to parents. She points out the similarities of stuttering to allergies or juvenile diabetes. "Parental behaviors are not presumed to play a role in the onset of either allergies or juvenile diabetes. However, it is clear that the response of parents to these disorders can either mitigate or aggravate their consequences" (p. 238). To the degree that parents are able to adjust the child's environment in regard to such problems (e.g., exposure to allergens or adjustments in diet), the symptoms will become less severe. As with stuttering, the maintenance of the symptoms, if not the etiology, can be significantly affected by actions taken by the child's parents.

It is the consensus of many clinicians who have achieved success with young children who stutter that parental involvement in treatment is crucial (Conture, 1990; Conture & Schwartz, 1984; Ham, 1986; Peters & Guitar, 1991; Riley & Riley, 1983; Rustin, 1987; Starkweather, Gottwald, & Halfond, 1990). Rustin indicates that, if there is going to be any realistic chance for therapeutic success, the parents must play a major role. She states that "without the involvement of parents, clinicians become powerless to help the child beyond the confines of the clinic room" (Rustin, 1995, p. 125). Likewise, Ramig (1993c) and Bronfenbrenner (1976) state that without the parents' ability to eventually develop the capability to help their child, the effects of treatment will likely deteriorate. Our experiences in running summer programs with children who stutter plainly show that those children whose parents also attend sessions designed to show them how to assist their child make considerably more progress than children whose parents, for one reason or another, do not attend.

Parental involvement not only assists the child in making behavioral and cognitive changes but also permits a form of mental hygiene to occur for the parents. Through counseling and parent group contact, the parents can accumulate the necessary information to become stronger and more confident about helping their child (Rustin & Cook, 1995). Although it may not be necessary for the clinician to spend a great amount of time desensitizing the young child to his fluency breaks, other people in the child's environment—including grandparents and teachers—often receive great benefit from these activities (Silverman, 1992). It is also worth considering that increasing numbers of children from non-traditional families are being seen in clinical facilities. In such cases, the major caregiver may not be the child's parent. Whoever takes on this role, however, will play a central role during the stages of assessment, change, and maintenance.

Lest it sound as thought the author is sitting in an ivory tower rather than a functioning speech and hearing center as this is being written, it should be pointed out that although having active parental involvement is an exemplary goal, it is not always possible. Ramig (1993c) points out that parents have many priorities, including work schedules and financial survival, which may well be regarded as more important than the status of their child's fluency. Particularly in rural or poor urban areas, there may be no way to contact the parents by telephone, the parents may not be able to read or write, or English may be a second language. If there is only one parent in the home, transporting the child to treatment may be difficult, or the single parent may not be able to afford services.

In order to assist the parents in understanding the problem and making good decisions on their own, the clinician can provide behavioral models as well as information. The clinician needs to be cautioned to provide information slowly. As discussed in Chapter 7, when counseling parents it is easy to provide too many recommendations too quickly (Conture, 1990; Luterman, 1991). As a result, parents can become overwhelmed and discouraged. Rather than lecturing the parents, it is more effective to follow their lead by listening to their questions and responding to—and expanding on—the issues they want to know about. Once they have an opportunity to read informative pamphlets, see instructional videotapes, and observe treatment being conducted with their child, they will be much more likely to provide many insightful ideas and suggestions. As we will discuss in more detail later in this chapter, Logan and Yaruss (1999) provide a variety of helpful suggestions that the clinician can use for helping parents respond to the attitudinal and emotional features of stuttering in their young child.

Stages of Parent Involvement

Ramig (1993c) suggests three possible stages of parent involvement during fluency treatment for young children: facilitating communicative interaction, educational counseling, and involving parents as observers and participants.

Educational Counseling

During this stage the clinician explains the difference between normal disfluencies and not-so-normal fluency breaks by discussing the surface characteristics of the child's behavior (see Table 2–1). Parents can be informed that although the etiology of stuttering is not completely understood, a great deal is known about the dynamics of the problem and much can be done to influence the increase or decrease of associated features. As parents begin to understand the problem, they will become less anxious. The clinician's early role during treatment is to demystify an undesirable situation and give the parents something concrete to do beyond simply feeling helpless. The booklets listed in Appendix C will provide answers to many of their questions. For some parents, the increasing access to information about fluency disorders on computer Internet systems is likely to be appealing (see Appendix C).

Through informed and reasonable counseling, parents will come to understand that, with a minimum of care, they are not likely to "do any damage" to their child. The child's parents will eventually become less inhibited and more likely to do reasonable and helpful things. Moreover, they will learn it is generally much better to acknowledge the obvious rather than behave as though the child's stuttering were something too awful to discuss openly and frankly.

Ramig (1993c) also suggests that during this initial stage of parent counseling, the clinician should consider discussing the many myths that are commonly associated with stuttering and take the responsibility to correct these distorted views. Possibly the most common myth is that parents, by omission or commission, are the likely cause of their child's stuttering. As many authors have pointed out (Conture, 1990; Peters & Guitar, 1991; Rustin, 1987; Van Riper, 1982), parents often accept guilt for the problem, assuming they had a major role in the etiology. At the very least, there is often a level of frustration with a situation that requires formal intervention for a handicapping condition (Luterman, 1991). As Ramig (1993c) suggests, the reduction of possible feelings of guilt by the parents should be viewed as a major contribution of clinicians. Group meetings of parents provide an invaluable forum for dealing with these frustrations, as in this way parents begin to realize that they are not alone. The more experienced parents can provide support and share concerns and therapeutic concepts that are especially helpful (Berkowitz, Cook, & Haughey, 1994; Ramig, 1993c). Detailed descriptions of child and parent group dynamics may be found in Conture (1990, pp. 113–118).

Examples of other myths include beliefs that children stutter in order to gain attention, that once a child begins to stutter he is destined to a life of stuttering, that stuttering is always caused by some underlying psychological or emotional problem, and that stuttering can be transmitted from one family member to another by imitation or simply by hearing others (Ramig, 1993c).

Although it is not necessarily considered a myth, many clinicians tend to believe that as a group, parents of stuttering children behave differently than those of normally speaking children. As Ratner (1993) points out, however, there is no evidence for this view or for the opinion that the parental interaction style is related to the severity of a fluency disorder. Furthermore, no correlations were noted between stuttering severity at initial assessment and parental conversational behaviors of speech rate, frequency of questions, and interruptions. In addition, Weiss and Zebrowski (Weiss, 1993; Weiss & Zebrowski, 1992) found that parents of stutterers do not produce significantly more requests than parents of nonstutterers.

Facilitating Communicative Interaction

Ramig (1993c) suggests that this second stage helps the parent to develop interpersonal styles that will be conducive to fluency enhancement. The overall communication and interpersonal characteristics of the child, as well as the child-parent interaction style, should be continuously evaluated. These characteristics include linguistic as well as paralinguistic variables, many of which have been studied in recent years in an attempt to determine their effect on children's fluency (see Kelly, 1994, for a summary). Such studies have investigated the rate of the speech (Conture & Caruso, 1987; Kelly, 1994; Meyers & Freeman, 1985); parent responses to the child's fluency breaks, both verbal and nonverbal (LaSalle & Conture, 1991); the amount and type of interruptions of the child's speech by the parents (Meyers & Freeman, 1985); turn-taking behaviors and response-time latency (Kelly, 1994); the complexity of the questions posed to the child (Stocker & Usprich, 1976); and the tendency for the parent to provide verbal and nonverbal corrections to the child as he is speaking (Gregory & Hill, 1980). As these features are identified, the parent can be shown how to alter some interactions. For example, the mother can be shown how to slow her speech, provide more time for turn-taking, interrupt the child's speech less, and positively reinforce the child for using his fluency-enhancing techniques.

Conture and Caruso (1987) and Ramig (1993c) advocate the use of "Mr. Rogers" speech (referring to the soft-spoken television figure) as a prototype for slower, smoother speech and longer turn-taking pause times. Silverman (1996) suggests having the parents view videotapes of themselves and their child while the clinician points out both the undesirable and desirable ways they are responding to their child's fluency breaks. For example, the parents may be speaking rapidly and frequently interrupting or indicating by their body language (e.g., breaking eye contact) that they are not interested in what their child is saying. Recall, for example, the study by Winslow and Guitar (1994) mentioned in Chapter 2. They found that the fluency of a 5-year-old child increased when conversational demands were lessened by the implementation of turn-taking rules, while stuttering increased when these rules were withdrawn. During an obvious or severe stuttering moment, parents may unconsciously freeze or show anxiety or concern. They may have a pattern of asking their child difficult or abstract questions that require complex responses. On the other hand, of course, the parents may also be doing many appropriate things, including modeling slow, easy speech and responding with an unafraid attitude to stuttering behavior. Videotapes of clinician-child interactions also can be used to demonstrate desirable parent behavior.

Clearly the clinician plays a primary role in modeling better speaking behaviors, both inside and outside the treatment sessions. Ramig (1993c) suggests that it may be important to alter sources of family stress that appear to contribute to fluency breakdowns. Events such as arguments or conflict, financial problems, sibling rivalry, and responses to various illnesses may have an influence on the child's fluency. Of course, in some instances referral to other professionals is appropriate.

Parents as Observers and Participants

Ramig's third stage of involvement gets the parents actively involved in the treatment process. The participation of both parents is assumed to be the ideal situation, although there is minimal research on the role of the father in this process. Ramig (1993c) indicates that even if only one parent is able to take part, the result is still likely to be beneficial for the child. Initially the parent's role is to observe the interaction of the child and clinician as the clinician models changes in the above-mentioned interpersonal communication variables. The clinician may also demonstrate strategies for expanding the child's fluency or modifying moments of stuttering. As treatment progresses, the parents gradually begin to take part in the sessions by joining in with the clinician and the child. Gradually, the parents are included in treatment activities and eventually instructed to interact with the child on their own.

TREATMENT STRATEGIES AND TECHNIQUES

Although most current authors writing about treatment for young children recommend reasonably direct treatment, there is some question as to whether practicing clinicians feel the same way. Based on several recent surveys of professional clinicians (see Chapter 1), some practicing clinicians continue to be hesitant—or at least highly cautious—about working directly with young children who stutter. Whether the clinician chooses to work indirectly or directly with the younger child, however, the essence of treatment consists of both facilitating the child's capacities to produce easily fluent speech and reducing the demands placed on the child that result in fluency disruption. As Starkweather (1999) suggests, "We can prevent the complexity of stuttering from developing, or if it has developed, we can undo it, untie the knots of frustration and struggle. And the younger the child is, the easier the knots are to untie" (p. 233). Certainly the clinician will have many related goals, such as decreasing the child's response to fluency-disrupting stimuli and increasing his assertiveness and risk-taking ability.

It is also worth pointing out that many of the strategies and techniques used with older clients can be applied, in some cases with only minor alteration, particularly with older school-age children. Of the two major strategies, fluency modification approaches are most often used. However, stuttering modification techniques may also be appropriate. Particularly with younger clients, the techniques used with these two general strategies become quite similar. That is, both strategies emphasize easy, somewhat slowed movements, with light articulatory contacts and good airflow and voicing. In addition, the ultimate goal of both approaches is spontaneous fluency.

USING THE DEMANDS AND CAPACITIES MODEL

Conceptualizing treatment from a demands-and-capacities or component-model framework, as described in Chapters 2 and 5, can provide the clinician as well as parents, teachers, and other professionals with a comprehensive and clear direction of treatment. We will approach treatment for young children from this framework. That is, we will discuss things the clinician can do to increase the child's capacity to produce smooth language and speech. We can assist the child in achieving a measure of control over a speech production system that is in the process of maturation. In many instances, working on the capacities side of the equation is all that is necessary for young children who have only recently begun to exhibit breaks in their fluency. For some children, relatively minor changes in the communication environment in the form of listener reactions and modeling may be all that is necessary. For other children, a more direct modification of fluency or stuttering will occur. These children are more likely to have a family history of fluency disorders or one or more other problems that make communicating or learning more demanding. In such cases, treatment may take somewhat longer. Conture (1990) suggests that most children will take approximately 20 weeks (with a range of 10 to 30) of weekly therapy before they are ready for dismissal. He also advises, however, that the clinician should be careful not to force treatment into a parent's busy schedule. The clinician should be prepared to give both the parents and the child an intermission from weekly treatment sessions and be available for consultation with the parents during such intervals.

A realistic goal of treatment with most young children is a high level of spontaneous or normal fluency (Conture, 1990; Healey & Scott, 1995; Peters & Guitar, 1991). The future for fluency is bright for such children who receive early intervention. Although this is often the outcome of treatment for young children who are in the early stages of stuttering, a quote from Healey and Scott (1995) provides a larger view of the syndrome with which we are dealing:

> We are reluctant to base treatment effectiveness exclusively on pre- and posttreatment fluency data. This seems to be a rather narrow definition of "success." Some children in our program have demonstrated increased levels of fluency but were unable to achieve a positive attitude about themselves as fluent speakers. (p. 153)

As with adults, focusing on the child's fluency may provide the clinician with a restricted view of the syndrome and a narrow definition of progress. To be sure, high levels of fluent speech may be achieved by focusing only on the surface features of the child's behavior. However, there is little question that, even for young children, both affective and cognitive changes do and should take place during effective treatment. Of course, the young child who is beginning to stutter may not have had the time to develop the self-concept of a handicapped speaker, and thus the clinician may not need to formally intervene to modify these intrinsic changes. The clinician will find, however, children who have stuttered for only a few weeks or months who demonstrate clearly emotional reactions (e.g., frustration, anger, shame, avoidance) to their inability to speak. In any case, the monitoring of changes in these intrinsic features will provide the clinician with a broader view of progress and long-term success.

Gottwald and Starkweather (1995) provide an astute clinical suggestion that coincides nicely with the title of this text. Their comment emphasizes the importance of clinical decision-making with young children. They recommend that the clinician devote the first 10 minutes of each treatment session to reassessing the child and his current needs. This strategy is also a reasonable one to use with older clients. Obviously, the clinician will enter each session with a long-range plan and specific treatment techniques at the ready. However, by first observing the client in a natural environment and noting the type and quality of his fluency characteristics, including speech rate and secondary behaviors, the clinician is more apt to make better decisions that are

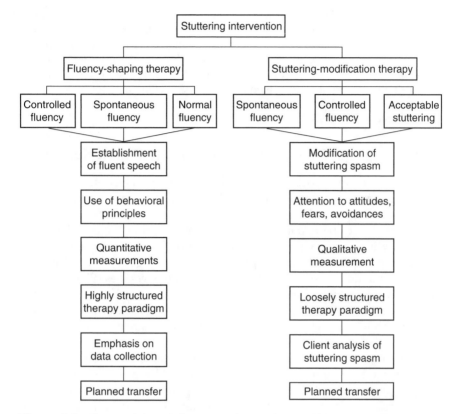

Figure 9-1. Characteristics of fluency- and stuttering-modification procedures. From Ramig and Bennett (1995), p. 140. Copyright © American Speech-Language-Hearing Association. Reprinted by permission.

focused on the immediate needs of the child rather than trying to fit the child into preselected activities.

As discussed earlier, the two major approaches to fluency treatment come together with young children. The similarities and differences of these two approaches are shown nicely in Figure 9.1, developed by Ramig and Bennett (1995).

Regardless of which overall treatment strategy is chosen, it is the clinician who is the "catalyst" for change (Silverman, 1992), providing the child with better models for speaking and the child and others with valuable information that will give them more control over their situation. The clinician can provide the child with skills for changing his speech as well as enhancing his own self-esteem and feelings about who he is.

Peters and Guitar provide the clinician with a good philosophical approach for providing treatment to the young stuttering child.

We believe that if we can provide the beginning stutterer with a sufficient number of positive and fluent speaking experiences during treatment, this fluency will generalize to more speaking situations. . . . This increased fluency will also reduce the opportunities the child has to respond to any remaining disfluencies with tension, frustration, or possibly escape and starting behaviors. The combined effect will be to allow time for the child's physiological system to mature and for normal fluency patterns to become stabilized. (1991, p. 274)

Enhancing the Child's Ability to Produce Fluent Speech

Fluency-enhancing procedures provide the child with techniques for both initiating and enhancing his fluency. The clinician cannot always assume that because the child's speech is nonstuttered, it is necessarily fluent. Speech that is to be expanded and reinforced should have high-quality fluency, which is characterized by smooth and effortless production.

Techniques for creating and promoting fluency go by several names. These techniques have been called *fluency-initiating gestures* (FIGs), *fluency-enhancing techniques, fluency-facilitating movements,* and *easy speech.* Regardless of the names for these techniques, they consist of procedures to help the child more efficiently manage the breath stream, produce gradual and relaxed use of the vocal folds, use a slower rate of articulatory movement, make gradual and smooth transitions from one sound to another, produce light articulatory contacts, and keep an open vocal tract in order to counteract constrictions resulting from tension. Many of these behaviors are already characteristic of parental or child-directed speech (slow rate, more leisurely turn-taking, shorter utterances, and more frequent use of paraphrase) (Ratner, 1993). Puppets, games, or cartoon pictures can be used to facilitate these behaviors. Conture (1990) suggests the use of cursive writing as an analogy that a child will easily understand. The child is shown how to smoothly make the transitional writing movements between letters at the same time that he is saying the sounds of the word. Not only is the clinician able to demonstrate the value of easy and flowing (versus hard and erratic) movement during serial motor tasks, it also gives her an opportunity to show the child that his speech is something *he* is *producing* rather than something that is happening to him.

It is interesting to note that although young children usually respond with greater fluency to slower and less complex speech produced by the parent or the clinician, the reasons for this effect are not well understood. To say to a parent, "Slowing down may help your child to be somewhat more fluent" is correct, but we do not understand why this holds true (Ratner, 1993, p. 244). Ratner submits there may be some higher-order conversational or interactional factor in operation. It may be that the pragmatic aspects of communication come into play more than the actual complexity of language. For example, Weiss and Zebrowski (1992) found that responsive utterances were significantly more likely to be produced fluently than assertive utterances. In addition, slowing down speech and using less complex sentence structure is likely to facilitate turn-taking.

Going beyond the specific techniques used, Ramig and Bennett (1995) provide a list of suggestions for the clinician, parents, and teachers when using a fluency-modification approach with younger school-age children. The clinician and everyone else (including parents and teachers) involved in the intervention process should:

1. Use basic and understandable terms when explaining and demonstrating what you want the child to do. These terms (e.g., "turtle speech" or "rabbit speech") should be used consistently when identifying target behaviors and reinforcing the child's actions. Regardless of the methods used, children need to have terms and concepts that enable them to think about their speech and language (Cooper & Cooper, 1991a).
2. Model, rather than instruct, the child about how to perform specific target behaviors.
3. Model slow and easy speech when interacting with the child in a variety of treatment and extra-treatment settings.
4. Model slow and easy body movements when interacting with the child, again in a variety of treatment and extra-treatment settings. These movements can be coordinated with easy, slow, and smooth speech movements. Such activities are especially good to use at the outset and completion of the treatment sessions.
5. Reinforce the child's accomplishments and feelings of self-worth in the context of as many experiences as possible.

Gottwald and Starkweather (1995) provide a succinct description of a combination of approaches, including the goals of fluency enhancement, reduction of demands, and desensitization of the child to normal fluency breaks:

> Depending on the child's specific needs, the clinician may use a reduced speech rate, many silent periods and pause times, and the language stimulation techniques of self-talk and parallel talk, but at a slow rate. Also, the clinician may reduce the number of language demands made on the child, including limiting questions requiring complex answers and reducing implied expectations for ongoing oral communication. Finally, the clinician will use normal disfluencies, such as whole word and phrase repetitions. (p. 122)

Fluency modification approaches are especially useful if the clinician is using an indirect approach. The basic goals are described by a variety of sources (Conture, 1990; Guitar, 1998; Luper & Mulder, 1964; Peters & Guitar, 1991; Van Riper, 1973).

For clinicians who are using a diagnostic-treatment model such as Riley's component approach, the clinician would quite naturally facilitate those components that have been associated with fluency failure for a particular child. Children with attending disorders would be treated in a similar fashion as nonstuttering children in need of such help. Likewise, assisting children in the improvement of their speech motor control may be a basic part of treatment for some children who stutter. Combining procedures that have much in common, Daly, Riley, and Riley (2000) recently developed a series of exercises that combine speech motor training and fluency shaping techniques. If a child appears to be unusually sensitive with high expectations (for fluency as well as other activities), the Rileys suggest helping the child to cognitively reframe those expectations that are unrealistic and contributing to anxiety and tension. They suggest creating absurd situations where the child could not possibly perform perfectly and responding with laughter with the recognition that it is impossible to perform the task "just right." As the child is given the opportunity to choose among completely unrealistic and more realistic possibilities, he begins to develop the freedom of choice, the ability to laugh at himself, and the ability to let go of unrealistic expectations. The Rileys suggest that many children who are overly sensitive feel powerless, a reaction that may be triggered by the notion that they feel they are not feeling heard. The clinician can assist children in verbalizing their feelings and analyze, with the parents and the child, stimuli that appear to trigger these reactions.

Helping the Child to Respond to Stuttering

For many children it may be enough for the clinician to make use of some or most of the above-mentioned techniques for modifying fluency. In other instances the clinician may decide to go to the next level and provide the child with techniques for helping him move through a stuttering event. With some young children, Van Riper (1973) does not recommend teaching the child to directly modify his stuttering moments. Rather, by using fluency-facilitating activities the clinician assists the child in reaching a basal level of fluency in the treatment setting. Fluency-disrupting activities are then gradually introduced (e.g., listener loss, time pressure, and greater linguistic demands). As the child's fluency becomes unstable—but prior to the point at which a child will produce fluency breaks—the clinician minimizes the disrupting activities. As a result of these procedures, the child will gradually become able to increase his tolerance and will become "toughened" to various forms of demands including communicative stress.

In order for the child to learn ways of changing the form of his stuttering, it is essential to identify both the desirable and the undesirable characteristics of his fluency breaks. One key for the child in making this distinction is for the clinician to use descriptive terms that the child can understand. Such terms should help the child differentiate the concepts of *hard, easy, smooth, gentle, stopping,* and *turtle* or *elephant* (slow) *speech* compared to *hard* or *rabbit* (fast) *speech*. The concepts are usually learned more readily if combined with illustrative body movements. The clinician and the child can, for example, alternately tighten and relax various parts of their bodies (including the speech mechanisms), helping the child to differentiate between tightness and relaxation and giving the child a sense of control over his "speech helpers." The clinician can make the experience of speaking enjoyable while giving the child a sense of power over his speech, concepts that are emphasized by virtually all writers on the topic of treatment for young children.

Particularly if a child has begun to develop some frustration about talking, a sequence of solo, tangential, and interactive play may be useful. This can be accomplished by the clinician producing nonspeech sounds as the clinician and the child play separately with their own sets of toys (solo play). The clinician models nonspeech sounds associated with the toys (sounds of animals, trucks, and airplanes) and eventually produces one-word utterances to describe the action. No emphasis is placed on the child to communicate. The clinician then begins to create minimal interactions with the toys interacting every so often (tangential play) and briefly commenting on the child's toys. Finally, as the child begins to follow the clinician's model, the clinician becomes more interactive and the activities become more cooperative, allowing for playing of games and activities that emphasize having fun and enjoying speech. This sequence of activities was originally presented by Van Riper (1973), and various interpretations are also presented by Conture (1990), Guitar (1998), Peters & Guitar (1991), and Shapiro (1999). As Conture (1990) suggests, games provide the opportunity to move into cooperative play and turn-taking during verbalization. The clinician can then begin to direct the level of communicative demand and model a variety of other activities.

Some clinicians are undoubtedly concerned about using the "s-word," *stuttering*. It is not uncommon for parents to avoid using the word stuttering in front of their children. Most writers (including myself) believe that referring to what the child is doing as stuttering is not a major issue during the treatment of young children. As Murphy (1999) suggests in his discussion of shame as it relates to stuttering, it is good for everyone to talk open and forthrightly about stuttering. It is true that if we assign positive or negative value to the word, it tends to become more powerful. However, using the word *stuttering* in a normal conversational manner is not, in and of itself, likely to make the situation worse. Whether the word *stuttering* is used or avoided, it is probably better to use behavioral terms that are more descriptive and meaningful to the child. Words such as *bumpy* and *easy speech* are less likely to be associated with negative values. As we discussed with fluency modification techniques, Ramig and Bennett (1995) also provide a list of suggestions for the clinician, parents, and teachers when using a stuttering modification approach with younger children. They indicate that the clinician should:

1. Explain the nature of the speech production system to the child and the parents, thereby providing him with greater understanding and the means of controlling his own system.
2. Illustrate the physical behaviors associated with his formulative and motoric fluency breaks, using terms that he can understand.
3. Show the child how to vary his speaking behaviors, adjusting his levels of tension and struggle. Making use of modeling and negative practice, the clinician and the child can explore ways of altering his fluency breaks. The child can gradually change the behaviors affiliated with tension and fragmentation and move toward easier, forward-moving fluency breaks. The child's speech does not have to become completely fluent, but simply easier and smoother. For example, Gregory (1989) suggests that after a child experiences a difficult and tense moment of stuttering, the clinician should direct him to produce the word again, this time reducing the tension by half. Conture's (1990) analogy of a garden hose with the possible levels of constriction that prevent the flow of water is a good way to make the child's speech production system less mysterious for him. The clinician and the child can explore procedures for "opening the clogs in the hose" and creating a more open flow of sounds. The incorporation of fluency-initiating gestures at this point is a good example of how the two general strategies can be intertwined during treatment with young children.
4. With the child leading the way, the clinician can discuss strategies for responding to people and situations that arise in the child's world. Together, the clinician and the child (as well as parents and teachers) can role-play responses to teasing, participation in social and class activities, relaxation in preparation for stressful situations, changing negative into positive self-talk, using visualizations and positive affirmations, and responding to time pressures.
5. Help the child and his parents to prepare for the possibility of relapse by considering responses to possible increases in fear, avoidance behavior, struggle behavior, and fluency breaks. The clinician, the child, and his parents can discuss self-assessment procedures as well as prescribe possible responses.

6. Develop a schedule for the maintenance and use of both stuttering-modification and fluency-maintaining skills in real-world contexts.

A central theme in stuttering-modification procedures with children is the contrasting of hard and easy speech. As described by Williams (1971), this distinction is the basis for giving the child the ability to take control of his speech system. The child learns that he is not helpless; rather, he has a choice about how to stutter and how to speak. There is much that he can do to change his speaking pattern. The clinician can take the lead and demonstrate both fluent and nonfluent speech. It is not necessary to demonstrate extreme forms of stuttering, only a degree of mild tension and fragmentation in order to make the point. The child can then be instructed to identify the moments of hard and easy speech produced by the clinician. This can also be done with audio- or videotapes of other speakers and eventually with the client himself. As the child is able to consistently identify moments of hard and easy speech, the clinician can show the child how to gradually change moments of one into the other. Struggle behavior, including blocking of airflow at various levels of the vocal tract, can be created purposely. The clinician and the child can vary the degree of construction. These actions can then be analyzed and altered in order to create greater airflow and smoother movements with easier transitions from one sound and syllable to another. It can be especially instructive for the child to take the role of the "teacher" and direct the clinician (or the parents) as she makes these adjustments in her vocal tract during a variety of activities and speaking situations.

For older children who are at the stage of treatment where they are beginning to identify and modify moments of stuttering, parents can also be shown how to highlight the child's moments of hard speech in a sensitive way and to reward smooth and easy speech as it is produced. However, the clinician cannot assume that parents will be able to do this without considerable observation and practice. Some parents will continue to be afraid of putting hard speech into their own mouths or to discuss these events even a little. As Conture (1990) indicates, some parents tend to reprimand, correct, nag, or badger the child regarding his speech, and they must be taught instead to assist in a gentle and appropriate manner.

Anything that will assist the child to produce speech with an open and flowing vocal tract will greatly facilitate fluency and help to alter the form of his stuttering. Conture's (1990) lily pad analogy, in which the child is instructed to "lightly touch" each sound or word as he lightly "talks across the lily pads" is a good example. The creation of greater airflow, as Conture (1990) explains in his garden hose analogy, and the use of software that provides feedback enabling the child to visualize appropriate respiration, airflow, phonation, and smooth speech production

(Gobel, 1989) can be beneficial also. Van Riper's (1973) modifications of his pullout techniques, Williams's (1971) technique of reminding the child to "move on" during stuttering moments, and Conture's (1990) similar recommendations to the child to "change and move forward" are all useful adaptations of stuttering modification procedures. The child, by using such suggestions, can gradually learn to release the struggled speech behavior and make the necessary transitional gestures that will enable him to move to the next sound segment. As always, it is best to model these suggestions rather than tell the child what to do.

Cognitive and Affective Considerations

As we've discussed, many authors believe that even with young children, it is important to attend to the feelings and attitudes associated with the onset of stuttering behavior. Even if a child is not showing negative reactions to his stuttering at a young age, relatively small adjustments in the parents' response to stuttering may prevent the future development of such feelings. In some instances, modeling of speech by the clinician and the parent that is easy and less complex from a motor and linguistic standpoint may be sufficient to bring about greater levels of fluency. As fluency improves, many children begin to show a decrease in their anxiety and fear associated with the stuttering experience. Other children, however, have levels of frustration and fear that are important components of the treatment process. These emotions need to be considered and dealt with, not only by the child who is stuttering but also by his parents.

Logan and Yaruss (1999) provide a comprehensive approach for helping clinicians and parents respond to the cognitive and affective features of stuttering in young children. They describe modeling and listening activities that suggest ways for parents to respond to their child and his stuttering that facilitate not only fluency, but also an improved response to the emotional and attitudinal features of the stuttering experience. Examples of modeling behaviors by the parents include practice (by role-playing with the clinician) of a calm, objective, and interested response to the child's stuttering. With the clinician leading the way, parents can become desensitized to stuttering behavior in general and their child's pattern of stuttering in particular. As parents become aware of their true feelings about their child's stuttering, they are better able to stay in the moment and openly discuss possible responses to their child's speech. With experience, parents can evaluate and monitor their nonverbal response to stuttering. The parents' mind-set about what stuttering is and what it is not will begin to change for the better. They will be able to model easy, open, and relaxed fluency breaks in their own speech. They will be able to show their child that it is possible to discuss stuttering and speaking in general in an open and matter-of-fact manner rather than taking an all-or-none view about fluency and stuttering. Parents can become better listeners and learn to affirm their child regardless of whether or not stuttering is occurring. They can reassure and encourage their child regardless of their child's level of fluency. Parent support groups (either via meetings or a telephone network) are extremely useful in helping parents to understand that they are not alone and that their feelings about their child's stuttering are both natural and acceptable. As we have said, although there are many options for parents who want to help their child, often only a few of these responses will be necessary. As Logan and Yarss report, as a result of therapeutic change, children also show improved reactions to other forms of adversity and stress, a response we have also noted with adults.

Another import feature of some programs designed for younger and older children who stutter is the development of problem-solving skills (Gregory, 1986; Riley & Riley, 2000). With the clinician as a model, the client is shown how to reevaluate his usual way of thinking about himself and his problems, including, of course, his stuttering. For example, beyond rewarding the child for using a particular technique, the clinician can ask how he liked doing the activity. We won't know that the child's reaction will be as he attempts new ways of talking and thinking. His consideration of how he experiments with his speech and with himself is important. This may remind the reader of our discussions of a "paradigm" shift in Chapter 1 and the premises of Rational Emotional Behavioral Therapy and Personal Construct Theory from earlier chapters. As applied to the stuttering experience, the goal is to enable the speaker to reevaluate his response to his situation and how he is making the process of speaking so difficult (e.g., how he is holding his breath, not allowing voicing to begin, or placing his articulators in an inappropriate position to say the next sound or syllable) and to plan better ways of responding. Such problem solving can apply to a wide variety of behaviors and decisions the speaker is making that involve his speech in educational, vocational, and social situations. Problem-solving activities can also involve the client's use of negative or positive self-talk as well as investigation the accuracy of the speaker's perceptions of listener reactions. A good deal of progress in treatment—especially for older children, adolescents, and adults—may be thought of a change from magical thinking about stuttering to a broader and more logical view about behavior and choices.

By making speaking fun and enjoyable and helping the child to create a sense of power about speaking, the clinician improves the chance of his long-term success. Such cognitive and affective changes, along with procedures for desensitizing and toughening the child to teach him to tolerate fluency disrupters in his environment, are essential aspects of treatment. Fortunately for many children, such activities are not complicated or long-term.

A review of current treatment approaches for the preschool children who stutter results in a variety of common themes that the clinician can draw from in planning treatment strategy. While there are exceptions, clinicians using virtually all programs include activities designed to achieve the following goals:

➤ Enhancing the child's enjoyment of speaking.
➤ Involving the parents in the treatment process.
➤ Improving the child's self-confidence as a speaker and self-worth as a person.
➤ Moving from simple to more linguistically complex utterances during the initial stages of treatment.
➤ Providing the child with many rewards for his success.
➤ Showing the child how to produce an easy form of speech with good air flow, an open vocal tract, and light articulatory contacts.
➤ To the degree possible, modifying any fluency disrupting aspects in the child's environment (time pressure, overtalking, linguistic complexity).
➤ Desensitizing the child to fluency disrupting factors in his environment.

 CLINICAL DECISION-MAKING

How is the clinician to know whether or not to ask the child about his concerns about his speech? As described in Chapter 3, children are not as likely as adults to describe their frustrations and fear related to the experience of stuttering but rather show it in other ways (pitch rise, cessation of air flow or voicing; substitution of the schwa vowel; or avoidance of sound, words and speaking situations). A couple of years ago a friend of mine, who is an accomplished clinician, told me of a telephone call she received from another speech-language pathologist who worked with children who stutter. The caller explained that she had worked for several months with a young child who stuttered and had been able to teach him several techniques for achieving fluency. However, despite the child's ability to understand and use the fluency-enhancing techniques, he continued to be anxious about speaking and stuttered on many occasions both in and out of the clinical setting. Her question to my friend was whether or not it might be a good idea to "do emotions" with this child. Chances are that to some degree at least, all children who stutter are bothered by the experience. If the child is not highly reactive to the stuttering experience, the clinician may not need to spend much "doing emotions." In most cases, however, spending time on the affective and cognitive aspects of the stuttering experience is an essential part of the treatment process from the outset and will be well worth the effort.

➤ Making certain that the child enjoys the therapy activities.
➤ Using fluency-facilitating activities such as slowed speech, choral reading, and unison speech.

There are also, of course, many important differences to be found in the suggestions of different authors. Clinicians using operant and fluency-shaping approaches generally obtain considerably more data and specify specific criteria for moving a child from one step of a program to another. Although the emphasis in most fluency-shaping strategies is to reward and (less frequently) punish stuttering, a close examination (or clinical observation) of these programs shows that there is typically a good deal of reassuring and encouraging taking place on the part of the clinician. In addition, the clinician is usually helping the child to identify and objectify the features of stuttered and fluent speech. The child is being shown how he can take charge of his speech system. Clinicians using stuttering modification approaches usually have a less structured interaction between the clinician and child and less emphasis on data gathering. Some clinicians of both general approaches are very direct in terms of rewarding fluency and punishing moments of stuttering, while others provide suggestion and indirect modeling for changing disrupted speech to smooth speech. Regardless of these differences, all authors believe that intervention is likely to be highly successful, particularly with the young preschool child. Undoubtedly, the enthusiasm and optimism of the clinician as she implements a logical approach for providing the child with a way to cope with his stuttering all play a critical part in treatment success. The basics of a successful treatment approach for young children seems to be related to the ability of the clinician to show the child that he is able to take control of his speaking mechanism and change the way he is speaking. As he comes to enjoy speaking and his confidence in his ability to speak in a variety of circumstances increases, it is likely that he will experience continued fluency.

STUTTERING COEXISTING WITH OTHER COMMUNICATION DISORDERS

It has been noted by several investigators that many children with fluency disorders tend to have other communication problems as well. Most often noted is the relatively high co-occurrence of articulation and phonological problems (Blood & Seider, 1981; Conture, 1990; Daly, 1981; Louko, Edwards, & Conture, 1990; Paden, Yairi, & Ambrose, 1999; Schwartz & Conture, 1988; St. Louis & Hinzman, 1986; Riley & Riley, 1979; Thompson, 1983; Yairi et al., 1996; Williams & Silverman, 1968). Reviews of this literature have resulted in estimates suggesting that something on the order of approximately one third of all children who stutter can be expected to also demonstrate articulation or phonological difficulties (Bloodstein, 1987; Conture, 1990). As we described in Chapter 5, the Riley's found that 33% of the 54 children in their original sample (1979) had moderate or severe articulation disorders. The results from the more recent sample of 50 children yielded moderate or severe articulation or phonological disorders in 50% of the children (Riley & Riley, 2000). In contrast to nonstuttering school-age control subjects, who typically demonstrate a difficulty in accurately producing speech sounds of 2% to 6.4% (Hull, Mieke, Timmons, & Willeford, 1971), well over half of children being seen for fluency intervention also have articulation disorders (Daly, 1981).

The co-occurrence of fluency disorders and language impairment is less well documented but has also been noted (Blood & Seider, 1981; Louko, Edwards, & Conture, 1990; Merits-Patterson & Reed, 1981; St. Louis & Hinzman, 1986; St. Louis, Murray, & Ashworth, 1991). Furthermore, the presence of coexisting disorders may not always be apparent at the outset of treatment. For example, a language impairment may only become evident after fluency has improved (Merits-Patterson & Reed, 1981). Although other voice or hearing problems have not been noted to occur with greater-than-typical frequency (Conture, 1990), these should be evaluated prior to the beginning of treatment.

Two Effects of Coexisting Problems

There are two basic issues the clinician must consider because of the possibility of coexisting communication problems. First, it has been observed by some clinical researchers that on occasion, children who are being treated for language disorders become more disfluent as a consequence of treatment (Conture, 1990; Merits-Patterson & Reed, 1981; Meyers, Ghatak, & Woodford, 1990). Conture (1990) suggests that if a child is receiving treatment for severe articulation problems or unusual phonological problems, the possibility of stuttering onset may be increased. Treatment for articulation or language impairments also may precipitate fluency breaks if children are placed in treatment too early. That is, premature treatment may require the child to improve his articulation before he is capable of producing sounds correctly with relative ease and without excessive scanning or effort. As a result, treatment demands may exceed the child's still-limited capacities for producing speech fluently. Conture (1990) notes that this may be most likely to occur for children who are approximately five to six years of age.

> We are inclined to speculate that increases in the length and complexity of verbally expressed languages increases the opportunities for instances of disfluency to emerge and is probably a natural byproduct of improved but still unstable expressive language skills. (p. 105)

Another therapeutic issue for children who are being treated for fluency and other impairments is the demonstrated "trading" relationships among the fluency, language, and phonological capabilities of the child. Such interaction has frequently been suggested between fluency disorders and both language and phonological capacities (Crystal, 1987; Masterson, & Kamhi, 1992; Rather, 1995, 1997; Ratner & Sih, 1987; Stocker & Gerstman, 1983; Stocker & Usprich, 1976; Watkins et al., 1999). This relationship has been particularly well documented for expressive syntax and fluency (Gaines, Runyan, & Meyers, 1991; Gordon, 1991; Gordon, Luper, & Peterson, 1986; Ratner & Sih, 1987; Stocker, 1980). The affiliation of a child's expressive and receptive capabilities is a major influence on clinical decision-making for young children who stutter. That is, the clinician should introduce fluency skills at carefully graded levels of linguistic demand (Ratner, 1995; Stocker, 1980). According to Ratner,

> Imitation and modeling tasks designed to address syntactic or morphological deficits, shown to be most efficient clinically in inducing changes in expressive language performance[,] . . . may evoke fluency failure. Similarly, fluency practice, if structured in such a way that it does not address the demand it poses on a child's expressive language capacity, may not produce desired changes in fluency. (1995, p. 183)

As discussed in Chapter 2, such trade-off relationships and their resulting effect on a child's ability to produce fluent speech provide clinical support for a capacities-and-demands model (Adams, 1990; Starkweather & Gottwald, 1990). That is, at least for some young stuttering children, any task that requires a child to formulate complex ideas with greater levels of language demand may result in decreased fluency. In fact, that is what Weiss and Zebrowski (1992) found with eight child-parent pairs. When these young stuttering children (average age 6 years, 11 months) were asked to respond to questions requiring greater linguistic sophistication, there was a greater occurrence of fluency breaks. That is, higher levels of language demand (Stocker & Usprich, 1976) resulted in significantly more disfluencies than lower-level parent requests. In addition, disfluent utterances were significantly longer and more complex than those produced fluently.

Although clinical decisions are made more complex with the presence of multiple problems, the answer to the question of whether to include in treatment a child who happens to have a fluency problem as well as other concomitant disorders is usually "yes." Articulation and language problems require long-term treatment, and the clinician is unlikely to be able to wait until these problems are resolved before initiating treatment for fluency problems. Given the success that is likely for early intervention of fluency disorders, waiting may only complicate the problem. Many authorities support the view of working on the combination of communication problems the child may have (Conture, Louko, & Edwards, 1993; Gregory & Hill, 1980; Guitar, 1998; Runyan and Runyan, 1993; Wall & Myers, 1995). Guitar (1998) indicates that he has not found that treating other speech or language problems exacerbates the child's stuttering. He also provides some particularly good examples of how the clinician may adapt clinical activities to a child with multiple problems.

Conture (1990) provides some guidelines concerning whether such a child should be seen for fluency intervention. He suggests that children with multiple problems should begin treatment as soon as possible if:

1. The child is producing two or more sound prolongations for every 10 instances of stuttering.
2. The child breaks eye contact with the listener more than half the time during conversation.
3. The child exhibits concomitant speech sound articulation problems, and especially if he produces phonological processes that are indicative of delays or deviations in phonological development.

Depending on the other associated problems, the clinician will have to decide whether the problems should be addressed sequentially or concurrently. Conture, Louko, and Edwards (1993) advocate a concurrent approach for children with both fluency and phonological problems, making use of a fluency-shaping protocol along with indirect phonological intervention. These authors do advise the clinician to avoid any overt correction of the child's speech. It is agreed by most authorities that children should not receive any direct feedback concerning the accuracy of their articulation, which would prevent possible communicative or emotional stress from impacting on the child's capacities. Obviously, each child will be different, with unique capacities and responses to communication demands. Ratner (1993) indicates that subtle forms of feedback in the form of imitation, recasts, and selective emphasis on language structures that children are finding difficult may facilitate overall communication development. The clinician should feel free to model fluency-enhancing gestures in her own speech. Certainly, the child's response to linguistic as well as emotional demands must be carefully considered, both within and outside the treatment environment.

Ratner (1995) suggests that the blending of treatments (e.g., phonology and fluency) during a treatment session may work well for some children whose fluency system does not appear to be stressed by the requirements of feedback monitoring. However, if working on one aspect of speech or language production places stress on the child's ability to produce fluent speech, it may be better to sequence treatment, achieving a stable level in one area before tackling the other. Whether or not to sequence treatment is a good example of the kind of clinical decision the experienced clinician must be entrusted to make. If fluency problems stem from problems of expressive language formulation, the clinician may choose to emphasize language intervention skills prior to fluency treatment. Obviously, as Ratner (1995) points out, an inappropriate justification for targeting language prior to—or in place of—fluency is the lack of confidence a clinician may have for conducting fluency therapy. Given the evidence concerning clinician attitudes about people who stutter and about treatment with this population of clients (see Chapter 1), this is a valid concern.

Finally, Ratner (1995) suggests some principles that clinicians can use for making clinical decisions for children with fluency and other concomitant problems:

1. The clinician should recognize that demands for phonological and grammatical processing compete with resources that permit fluent speech production.
2. The clinician should organize treatment hierarchically, proceeding from language and articulation activities that the child has established and stabilized to tasks that involve greater demands.
3. Even though it may slow progress in articulatory and linguistic growth, the clinician should structure intervention for children who stutter with minimum overt feedback.
4. The clinician, based on the child's individual capacities and responses to communicative demands, should determine whether a child's multiple impairments should be treated concurrently, sequentially, or cyclically. Furthermore, this strategy should be subject to change in the event that progress in one domain comes at the expense of regression in another.

Although children with multiple communication problems may require a greater amount of decision making by the clinician, all children—and indeed all clients—would probably benefit from the application of a similar policy. Intervention for all clients is likely to be most efficient when a careful analysis of the speaker's capacities and responses to demands are factored into the treatment strategy. Clients can—and should—be pushed to the upper ranges of their ability in order to help them to change the many features of their fluency disorder. The clinician working with young fluency-disordered children should be able to help the child to learn to *easily* produce difficult sounds or new grammatical structures without introducing the idea that they need be concerned or frightened or should struggle with their speech. It is possible to model a smooth and flowing manner of speech production while also giving the child a real sense of command over himself.

TRANSFER AND TERMINATION ISSUES

Prior to the child's dismissal from formal treatment, the clinician will want to determine how well the child has been able to transfer his new capabilities and techniques to the world outside the treatment setting. If the parents have been involved and if the child's response in extratreatment settings has been stressed from the outset, such transference is more likely to take place. Fortunately, as Conture (1991) points out, for many children the skills learned in the treatment setting transfer quite easily. Peters and Guitar (1990) and Guitar (1998) note that progress with younger children can be judged by such things as the improved use of techniques, decreased reliance on cueing by the clinician, increased control of fluency, taking risks, and decreased avoidance of speaking and speaking situations. As treatment progresses, there is a gradual shifting of the responsibility for increasing fluency from the clinician to the child and his parents. Group meetings are particularly helpful in this regard. The support and encouragement provided by parent groups does much to facilitate this change in responsibility.

Recommended criteria that the clinician may consider for the termination of formal treatment are provided by Gottwald and Starkweather (1995). Parents and teachers should feel confident about their ability to manage the child's improving fluency. These adults will need to assess and make independent decisions concerning how to alter fluency-disrupting stimuli such as time pressure and linguistic demands across a variety of social and educational settings. Parents need to be able to create an environment that corresponds to the child's capacity to maintain fluency. In addition, the young child should be normally fluent for his age. Some mild fluency breaks, particularly whole-word and phrase repetitions produced without effort, are unexceptional for three- to four-year-old children. Even fluency breaks produced with mild levels of tension may be acceptable if the clinician anticipates that the child will make continued improvement. Termination is also facilitated by a gradual phase-out of treatment that provides the clinician with the opportunity to monitor the child's progress. Ideally such monitoring should take place through age seven or eight, when basic skills underlying fluency are thought to be internalized. Finally, parents and teachers should be informed about the characteristics of relapse, made aware of the signs of incipient stuttering, and encouraged to contact the clinician if such indicators occur.

THE POSSIBILITY OF RELAPSE WITH CHILDREN

Unlike the situation for older speakers, the maintenance of the gains made during formal intervention is not usually a major problem with younger children. The available data indicates that once formal treatment has been successfully completed, the chance of regression is much less likely with children than it is with adolescents and adults who have been stuttering for much longer (Hancock, Craig, McCready, McCaul, Costello, Campbell, & Gilmore, 1998; Gottwald & Starkweather, 1995; Peters & Guitar, 1991; Starkweather, 1999; Starkweather, Gottwald, & Halfond, 1990). On the other hand, a comprehensive treatment program will include, at the very least, periodic checks for approximately two years following the end of formal treatment.

In a summary of the families seen from 1981 through 1990 at the Temple University Stuttering Prevention Center in Philadelphia, Gottwald and Starkweather (1995) indicate that

> Forty-eight of these families received individualized intervention services, ranging from parent counseling only to family counseling and direct therapy for the child. At the time these results were reported, three children and their families were still in therapy, and seven families had withdrawn from the program for a variety of reasons. The remaining 45 youngsters and their families completed the program. All 45 children were speaking normally at the time of discharge. Follow-up telephone calls to each of the families 2 years following program completion revealed that fluency had been maintained according to parent report. (p. 124)

Starkweather (1995) estimates that the relapse rate following successful treatment for young children is approximately 2%.

Partial or even complete relapse can occur, of course, and one procedure that may prevent such regression may be the use of a "buddy system." This may be especially helpful for the child who is having difficult with motivation, carryover, or maintenance. When entering into new and difficult speaking situations outside the treatment setting, the presence of someone who understands the dynamics of the situation can have a powerful supporting effect. If the clinician or parent is not there, the presence of a speech buddy may be extremely beneficial. This strategy may be particularly useful with pre-adolescent or adolescent clients who tend to spend the vast majority of their time with people other than parents or clinicians.

Hancock et al. (1998) conducted a two-to-six year follow-up of 62 children who had received one of three stuttering treatments (intensive smooth speech, parent-home smooth speech, and intensive electromyography feedback). These children, age 11–18 years, were older than those followed by Gottwald and Starkweather (1995). Children were assessed overtly during a clinic conversation with the clinician, while speaking on the clinic telephone talking to a family member or friend, and talking at home. The authors found that most of the children had maintained the gains they had achieved one year post-treatment. About half of the children had less than 1% syllables stuttered across the three speaking contexts, and nearly 70% of the children achieved less than 2% syllables stuttered two to six years following treatment. From a parent's perspective, eight of the parents (13%) believed that their child has relapsed to pre-treatment levels and 33 parents 53% felt that their child's speech had deteriorated but not to pretreatment levels.

SUGGESTIONS FOR THE CLASSROOM TEACHER

For school-age children, classroom teachers can also play a major role in facilitating therapeutic change (Ramig & Bennett, 1995). In some instances, the child's classroom teacher will have as much influence as the child's parents. In order for teachers to assume such a role, it is essential for them to have an appreciation of both the nature and treatment of stuttering. Of course, the character of the clinician-teacher relationship will depend somewhat on the model used for service delivery in the school. One possibility is a consultative model where the clinician works through the teacher and parents to help the child. A collaborative-consultative model has the clinician working with the child on an individual basis but also collaborating with the teacher and parents in planning appropriate activities in the child's daily world. A pullout model, where the children are taken out of the classroom and seen individually or in small groups by the clinician, is probably the strategy that is least apt to create professional interaction as well as long-term change for the child (Gregory, 1995).

A most efficient first step for involving classroom teachers is to present a workshop for teachers and related school personnel. Highly effective presentations can result from a basic discussion of one of the several informative videotapes available through such groups as the Stuttering Foundation of America or the National Stuttering Project (see Appendices B and C). Pamphlets, which are also available from these groups, can be distributed and questions concerning fluency and fluency disorders addressed. Nearly everyone is interested in stuttering, and it is usually relatively easy to draw an audience for these presentations.

Suggestions for the classroom teacher can be found in several sources (Cooper, 1979a; Dell, 1970; Van Riper, 1973, pp. 446–450). It is far better for the teacher to be proactive regarding a stuttering child in the classroom. Clearly this is better than waiting for a child who stutters to appear in class and then seeking advice for how to best respond to the situation. Perhaps more important, with information provided by the clinician concerning the nature of both the surface and intrinsic features of stuttering, the teacher will be much more likely to recognize a child with a fluency disorder. As the classroom teacher understands the dynamics of the syndrome, especially patterns of avoidance, postponement, and escape behavior, he will be in a much better position to help. One of the best things that speech-language pathologists in school settings can do is to provide this information via inservices, newsletters, or e-mail messages. Reardon (2000) presented a helpful checklist for helping classroom teachers in identifying students who stutter and for following their progress as they receive treatment (Figure 9-2). The reader is also referred to a recently published workbook (Chmela and Reardon, 2000) designed for speech-language pathologists working in a school setting. (See suggested readings at the conclusion of this chapter.)

As the goals and techniques of treatment are explained to the child's teacher, he is likely to become involved in treatment. As with parents, it is often better to show, rather than tell, your colleagues what takes place during your treatment sessions with the child. Such live or taped

Teacher Checklist—Fluency

Student: _____ Birthdate: _____ C.A.: _____ Grade: _____

School: _____ Teacher: _____ Section: _____ Date: _____

Speech/Language Pathologist: _____

The child above has been referred for or is receiving services regarding fluency skills. Please help me gain a better overall view of this student's speech skills by completing the following information.

Informational Checklists:

1. This student: (check all that apply)

    _____ doesn't mind talking in class.

    _____ seems to avoid speaking in class. (Does not volunteer, if called up, may frequently not reply.)

    _____ speaks with little or no outward signs of frustration.

    _____ is difficult to understand in class.

    _____ demonstrates frustration when speaking (please describe): _____

    _____ performs average or above average academically.

2. This student is disfluent or stutters when he/she: (Check all that apply)

    _____ begins the first word of a sentence.

    _____ speaks to the class.

    _____ speaks during an entire sentence.

    _____ gets upset.

    _____ uses little words.

    _____ shares ideas or tells a story.

    _____ uses main words.

    _____ answers questions.

Figure 9-2a. A checklist to assist classroom teachers in identifying students who stutter and for following their progress as they receive treatment (Reardon, 2000).

_____ talks with peers.

_____ carries on a conversation.

_____ gives messages.

_____ reads aloud.

_____ talks to adults.

_____ other _____

3. Check any of the following behaviors you have noticed in this child's speech:

_____ revisions (starting and stopping and starting over again)

_____ frequent interjections (um, like, you know)

_____ word repetitions (we-we-we)

_____ phrase repetitions (and then, and then)

_____ part-word repetitions (ta-ta-take)

_____ sound repetitions (t-t-t-take)

_____ prolongations (n-------obody)

_____ block (noticeable tension/no sound comes out)

_____ unusual face or body movements (visible tension, head nods, eye movements)

_____ other _____

In the Classroom:

1. I do/do not have concerns about this child's speech because . . .

2. I observe the most disfluency when . . .

3. When this child has difficulty speaking he/she reacts by . . .

4. When this child has difficulty speaking, I respond by . . .

Figure 9-2b.

Your Perceptions:

1. I have/have not had prior experience with a child who stutters.

2. I feel stuttering is caused by . . .

3. Some questions I have about stuttering are:

4. Some questions I have about helping this child be successful in the classroom would be:

5. The amount of knowledge I currently have regarding the disorder of stuttering is. . .

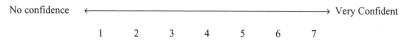

Nothing ⟵―――――――――――――――――――――⟶ A Lot

        1   2   3   4   5   6   7

6. My confidence level regarding dealing with stuttering in the classroom would be . . .

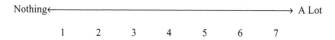

No confidence   ⟵―――――――――――――――――――⟶ Very Confident

        1   2   3   4   5   6   7

7. My comfort level when communicating with this child is . . .

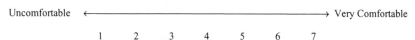

Uncomfortable   ⟵―――――――――――――――――――⟶ Very Comfortable

        1   2   3   4   5   6   7

Your Observations:

This child with PEERS . . .

1. Please describe this child's relationships with others of the same age.

2. Has this student been teased or mimicked because of his/her speech?

3. When this child has difficulty speaking, the other children react by . . .

4. Following a reaction by a peer, this child . . .

This child in GENERAL . . .

Figure 9-2c.

1. Have other students or this student's parent(s) ever mentioned his/her fluency problems? If yes, what was discussed?

2. Has this student ever talked to you about his/her speech problem. If yes, what was discussed?

3. What other information might be pertinent regarding this child's speech and language skills?

4. Do you have any other concerns regarding this child's <u>speech and language</u>, <u>academic</u>, or <u>social</u> skills?

Thank you for taking time to share this helpful information.

Please return this form to _____ by _____

                     Speech-Language Pathologist   Date

Note: Because follow-up is so important, I would like to observe this child in at least three different speaking situations. Please list some times that this student:

    Goes to lunch _____

    Has the most opportunity to share in the classroom _____

    Attends gym class _____

Figure 9-2d.

demonstrations are especially important if the child is taken from the classroom for intervention. As the classroom teacher recognizes that a child is choosing to participate in class in spite of some stuttering, the teacher will be able to reward that response (either during or following the event, and either verbally or nonverbally). When a child successfully uses a fluency-modification technique in the classroom, the teacher will be more likely to recognize it and know how to respond. When a child uses a fluency-facilitating technique and alters his usual tense and fragmented speech into a more open and forward-moving pattern, the teacher can reward the accomplishment. Until the teacher is able to interpret these seemingly small events as victories, they will go unrecognized and unrewarded. As the teacher takes part in treatment with the child, the choice of how to respond to the child in the classroom, playground, or the school lunch room will become apparent. With understanding and interaction, the teacher will be much more likely to discuss the problem with the child and be another important source of support and encouragement in the child's daily school environment.

The clinician should also alert classroom teachers that one possible outcome of successful treatment is increased participation, increased speaking, and—possibly—an increase in the occurrence of fluency breaks. As the child becomes successful at decreasing his avoidance behaviors and increasing speech assertiveness and risk-taking, one possible result may be greater participation in the classroom. Prior to treatment, the child may have been an "ideal" student, sitting quietly. Following successful treatment he may start to talk to his friends and, on occasion, stutter more as a result of his increased involvement in classroom activities.

Perhaps one of the major concepts the clinician can impart to the classroom teacher is the notion that unless she is totally insensitive, she is not likely to harm the child who stutters. The clinician can provide a great service to teachers by informing them of this fact. Yes, certainly it would be possible for an insensitive teacher to make things somewhat worse for the child who stutters. Clearly such people do exist, as reflected by reports of that sort in the National Stuttering Association publication, *Letting Go*. More often than not, however, classroom teachers are well intentioned and need to be allowed to respond naturally without fear of somehow damaging "this fragile child who stutters." As with parents, when the teacher understands the basic characteristics of stuttering behavior and avoidance responses, it becomes obvious that it is okay to discuss stuttering openly without hurting the child. The two primary messages that a clinician should impart to both the child and his parents is that "It's OK to stutter" and "You can learn to stutter in an easier way."

Many suggestions provided to parents can be applied, with slight modification, to the classroom teacher as well. For example, although there may be some exceptions, children who stutter should generally not be permitted to escape from school assignments and responsibilities. Just as the other children are required to take their turn, the child who happens to stutter must also take his turn in reciting, reading, and answering questions. To allow a child to escape these responsibilities may foster more harassment from his peers than the fact that he occasionally stutters. Some children who are fluent would, if they could, choose not to have to face the trials of class participation and public speaking. These decisions, of course, vary with the child and the circumstances, and it would be inappropriate to say that a child must always be required to take part in every speaking situation. However, the exceptions should be rare. Even children who stutter severely are able to take part in class presentations or plays. When the teacher understands that children who stutter are unlikely to stutter when playing a role—speaking with a dialect, singing, or speaking in unison with other children—the teacher is more likely to ask the child to participate. At the very least, the child could have a nonspeaking part or play a character that makes mechanical or animal sounds.

As the teacher begins to appreciate the effect of time pressure on fluency, she may decide, on occasion, to call on the child unexpectedly or early in the class, when he is less likely to stutter. The child can then relax a bit and attend to the rest of the class. By understanding the dynamics of fluency-enhancing or -disrupting stimuli for a particular child, the teacher may choose to call on him when the anticipated response is a short—perhaps one-word—answer. Of course, the teacher can reward the child for not avoiding the opportunity to participate. With the assistance of the clinician, the teacher can talk privately with the child before or after class so there can be an understanding about what will or did occur. Stuttering can be a serious topic, but the teacher can become desensitized and show the child that it is possible to openly and easily discuss the problem.

Like parents, teachers can be shown the powerful effects of listener loss on the child's fluency. The ability of the teacher to remain calm, even during a moment of severe stuttering, communicates much to the child. Nonverbal indicators of anxiety and avoidance, such as becoming tense or rigid, turning away, or breaking eye contact, can be monitored and changed with some practice. Voluntary stuttering during role-playing activities with the clinician or other teachers and desensitization activities using videotapes also can be especially helpful. Generally, but again with some few exceptions, the teacher should not help the child say a word when he is experiencing an extended long block. There may be some occasions when there is no other choice but to help the child, but this should be infrequent.

Certainly the teacher should not let other children interrupt a child while he is stuttering. Similarly, it is never beneficial for the teacher to suggest to the child that he stop and think about what he is going to say. Such comments simply indicate that the listener is naïve about the true nature of stuttering. A better response is for the teacher to restate to the class what the child has said. That is, even though the child may have struggled through his comments, the teacher can increase the value of what the child said by paraphrasing his words. Such a restating of the child's words gives them increased importance and allows the other children in the class to appreciate the content of the child's response. It may take some practice to do this gracefully, but providing such a response is clearly much better than reacting with silence and pretending that no stuttering has occurred or perhaps unintentionally conveying the impression that what the child has said is unimportant. An open and forthright response by the teacher also carries a strong statement of unconditional acceptance of the child despite his manner of speaking.

Perhaps most importantly, the classroom teacher can become an advocate for the child. If classroom teachers react negatively to a child who stutters, it is most likely due to a lack of understanding. By showing understanding, being available to the child, and rewarding what she recognizes as progress in the direction of behavioral and attitude change, the teacher, like the parent, can be a powerful force for decreasing the handicapping impact of stuttering and for preventing the maintenance and further development of the syndrome.

On those occasions when the clinician is working with a child privately or in a clinical setting outside of the child's school, making contact with the school is an important part in helping the child to transfer his ability to modify his stuttering in this important setting. The following letter (Figure 9-3) can serve as a model for informing the teachers of how to respond to a child currently undergoing treatment.

THE PROBLEM OF TEASING

Although not always an issue, teasing by other children can sometimes be a significant problem. Using a questionnaire developed to determine the nature of teasing and bullying experienced by children, Langevin, Bortnick, Hammer, and Wiebe (1998) found that 28 children (age 7 to 15 years) experienced this negative treatment more often than other children. Although the children were also teased and bullied about other things, they were especially sensitive about their stuttering. If other children choose to tease a child for whatever reason, stuttering is usually one obvious and sensitive target.

Teasing is one of the ways that the emotion of shame becomes attached to stuttering (Murphy, 1999). Shame is one of the major affective features of the stuttering experience (Bloodstein, 1995; Murphy, 1999) and dramatically influences a one's overall self-interpretation. A major aspect of shame is how we believe we are viewed by others. A common result is the desire to avoid or hide from others and a high degree of social inhibition. Somewhat less destructive is the feeling of guilt which is more often associated with a particular behavior or act. Guilt is less apt to cause concern about one's whole self and as not generally seen as having the destructive power of shame. In some instances, shame and guilt many become linked, leading to a sense of failure and defectiveness (Tangney, 1996). Shame typically originates in the reactions of others in a child's environment, including parents, classmates, and teachers. Murphy (1999) contends that shame may also result from treatment that emphasizes unobtainable fluency particularly if undue pressure is placed on the parents or the child for self-management.

Obviously, teasing in the classroom should be off-limits. However, there will be situations where the teacher will not be able to prevent this behavior by other children, and in some cases it will occur to some degree. Certainly the teacher or parent may discuss the injustice of such

To The Teachers of Fred at South Park Elementary School

Date _____

Dear _____:

Fred has been attending the Speech and Hearing Center for several months in order to modify his stuttering. He has been doing well as he learns how to monitor and modify specific features of his speech, both in the clinic setting and at home with his family and friends. As he begins a new school year, it is important that his teachers have an understanding of the techniques he is using so that his efforts to smooth his speech and take part in speaking activities are rewarded. Here are some suggestions for helping Fred continue to make progress.

- Encourage Fred's participation in all speaking activities. Avoidance of speaking situations and specific words and sounds are a significant part of the problems created by stuttering.

- Success is sometimes indicated by decreased moments of stuttering. However, success is also indicated by Fred's ability to openly change his typical stuttering moments into easy and smooth stuttering. Have him show you what this looks and sounds like.

- When Fred finds himself approaching a moment of stuttering, he will begin to slow his speech a little and stretch out the initial sounds and syllables of the word he is going to say. Although his speech at this point may not always sound perfectly normal, his best response at this time is to stretch through the word with thi "easy form of stuttering." Your recognition and positive response to his ability to do this is very helpful.

- You can find additional information about any child who stutters whom you may have in your classes by contacting the Stuttering Foundation of America, 3100 Walnut Grove Road, Suite 603, Memphis, TN, 38111-0749, phone 1-800-992-9393. In addition, there is a helpful website called the Stuttering Home Page located at Minnesota State University at Mankato:

  Stuttering Home Page: http://www.mankato.msus.edu/~stutter/

  This site has a lot of good information for adults and children and their parents who stutter as well as many links to other sites.

  I would be happy to come to your school to speak with you and other teachers concerning these and other suggestions for Fred as well as other children who happen to stutter.

  Thank you for your help. Please feel free to contact me if you have any questions about any of the recommendations described on this page.

Figure 9-3. A sample letter to be used for informing classroom teachers about how to respond to a child currently undergoing treatment.

behavior with those involved. Of course, this may not help and in fact may increase the problem in some cases. Educating the children in the class about stuttering may be helpful and having an adult who has undergone successful treatment speak to the class may be a good option. Volunteers for discussions about stuttering may be located at nearby clinics or local chapters of self-help groups. Of course, this is helpful to these people also since they are often seeking public speaking opportunities.

Silverman (1996) suggests that the classroom teacher can help the child to bring the problem out into the open by having him discuss information about stuttering and perhaps describing the accomplishments of the many highly successful and famous people who have stuttered. How to best proceed will depend on the dynamics of the situation, including the child's personality characteristics and response to various suggestions.

As described in Chapter 5, *Teasing and Bullying* is one of the components of Riley's Revised Component Model for diagnosing and treating children who stutter. As indicated, their most recent data indicate that 31% of children indicated that they had experienced such treatment by their peers. They also report that adults often associate their first remembrance of stuttering with the experience of being laughed at or teased. The Riley's state that the goals of responding to this situation when it is present, are to educate the offending children to be more tolerant of differences and to obtain the help from adults to create options for the child. Becoming more assertive in response to teasing is one option. Another possibility is to enable the child who is being teased because of stuttering to support others who are teased for other reasons. Essentially, the clinician is helping the child to become involved in solving the problem and develop a sense of power concerning this—as well as other—forms of conflict.

Role-playing with the children who are involved in teasing the child is often helpful. If those involved in the situation refuse to cooperate, the clinician can role-play with the client in order to help desensitize him to the ridicule of others. By role-playing, the child can have the opportunity to ventilate his frustration and anger. For example, the clinician and the child can take turns giving and receiving specific taunts and insulting comments. Each can gradually become desensitized to the expected comments and discuss alternative responses. The child can practice a series of verbal and nonverbal responses to teasing. Depending on the particular child, a humorous response may be considered as an alternative reaction. The child may be able to defuse or redirect the sting of the comments by acknowledging the obvious and directing the comments of others back to them. For example, the child may say: "Yes, as a matter of fact, I do stutter. But what you said was stupid and mean." In addition, depending on the circumstances and possibly the size of the children involved, the child may want to add, "And tomorrow I might no longer stutter but you may still be stupid and mean." Alternately, in response to other children imitating a child's moment of stuttering, he may say something like: "Look, if you're going to stutter you ought to learn how to do it correctly. Prolong the first sound like this and add a little more tension. If you get really good at it and you're brave enough, try it with me at school tomorrow."

Role-playing with voluntary stuttering has also been suggested as a way to desensitize a child to stuttering (Dell, 1979; Sheehan, 1975). As with adults who stutter, purposeful stuttering allows the speaker to vary and play with many different forms of stuttering and opens the door for the speaker to have fun with the stuttering experience and to begin to achieve a sense of control over his speech system. All this assumes, of course, that the clinician has already been desensitized while producing such stuttering and is open to the possibilities of experimenting with her speech in this manner. Another useful procedure involves the concept of the child's "advertising" his classmates. This form of self-disclosure will be more likely to be successful, as the child makes progress in treatment by becoming knowledgeable about himself and his stuttering, becomes desensitized to the stuttering experience, achieves a measure of fluency, and—with the help of a supportive clinician and parents—is able to become more assertive and take such risks. Although there are many ways for the child to casually disclose the fact that he sometimes stutters and is attending treatment, one particularly useful suggestion is to have the child prepare a class report on some aspect of stuttering. By practicing with the clinician, parents, small groups of classmates, eventually the presentation can be made to the entire class.

The clinician can help the child and the parents to access the Stuttering Home Page on the Internet (Appendix B), particularly the sections designed for younger speakers and the topics having to do with teasing. Young clients will begin to problem solve and come up with their own responses to this too-common problem. Exploring the information at this and other websites can be an good treatment activity and home assignment for children and their parents, especially early in treatment. The wealth of information to be found can go a long way toward increasing understanding about many aspects of the nature of stuttering and serve to make the problem less of a mystery. Clinicians should be aware, however, that there are sites on the Internet that be of no help at all and provide inaccurate, even unethical, recommendations.

EXAMPLES OF FLUENCY PROGRAMS

Although representative, the following list is far from exhaustive, for there are many excellent programs being conducted by experienced and highly qualified clinicians. Although these "prepared" programs may provide an excellent beginning for the new clinician, it is worth noting

Ham's (1999) advice that the accomplished clinician needs to be aware of many approaches. Children as well as adults will respond in unique ways to different therapeutic approaches. Furthermore, as we discussed in earlier chapters, the influence of any approach will always be somewhat different because of the characteristics of the clinician who is using the approach. As Starkweather states,

> The technique that works so dramatically for one child does not necessarily work dramatically, or at all, for other children. Stuttering is so variable and so highly individualized that, few would disagree, no one method works for all children. (1999, p. 235)

The purpose of this listing is to indicate the general principles that are employed in treating children. Further descriptions of these and other programs for children (as well as adults) may also be found in Bloodstein (1993, pp. 157–165), Guitar (1998), and Ramig and Bennett (1995). The following examples are presented in alphabetical order by the first author.

The Successful Stuttering Management Program (SSMP)

Developed by Breitenfeldt and Lorenz (1989), this is a comprehensive stuttering-modification approach designed for older adolescents and adults. Although the program is designed as an intensive treatment, many of the procedures can be used in a less intensive environment. The program includes both assessment and intervention phases that are well organized and easy to follow. The notebook that accompanies this program contains session-by-session outlines (including assignments) that focus on affective, cognitive, and behavioral features of stuttering experiences. Suggestions for transfer and maintenance activities are included.

Personalized Fluency Control Therapy (PFC)

Developed by Cooper and Cooper (1985b), this program provides the clinician with procedures for directly modifying the child's stuttering using fluency-initiating gestures. Each gesture or technique is associated with a character in order to help the children conceptualize the nature of fluency and specific modification techniques. Changes in the child's affective, cognitive, and behavioral features are an integral part of the program.

Extended Length of Utterance (ELU)

Developed by Costello (1983), this is also a fluency-shaping program that makes use of operant principles and programmed instruction. The program controls for linguistic complexity begin with monosyllabic words and continue through 20 steps to conversational speech. Depending on the child, fluency enhancing behaviors of slow speech and gentle onset are used along with a gradually increasing length and linguistic complexity of response. According to Costello, most young speakers have not yet developed a negative attitude about stuttering, so that attitude modification is done in relatively few cases. Tokens are awarded for fluent speech, and stuttering is highlighted by with drawing of tokens or feedback about the stuttering events.

CAFET for Kids

Developed by Goebel (1989), this program involves eclectic fluency and is patterned after the CAFET program for adults. The program makes use of a computer-assisted self-monitoring system (CAFET) that allows the child to regulate and change the usual fluency-enhancing targets such as a full inspiratory breath coupled with a slow exhalation of air. The computer program also provides for visual reinforcement as children achieve treatment goals.

Speak More Fluently, Stutter More Fluently

Developed by Gregory (1991), this program uses fluency-shaping procedures with school-age children. The program emphasizes relaxed speech production with additional modification of any remaining stuttering behaviors. The fluency-shaping procedures stressed include the use of smooth, slower-than-normal transitions on the first two sounds of a word or utterance and an easy initiation of phonation with smooth articulatory movement during the utterance. Emphasis is also placed on the child's maintaining normal rate, intensity, and inflection. The program incorporates learning principles and a variable lesson plan format, which can be used to individualize the treatment for each child.

Easy Does It

This program was developed by Heinze and Johnson (1985) as a fluency-shaping program for preschool children through grade two. The program consists of five phases: (a) experiencing fluency, (b) establishing fluency, (c) desensitizing to fluency disrupters, (d) transferring fluency, and (e) maintaining fluency. During each stage, parents are provided with activities for use in the home.

The Fluency Development System for Young Children (TFDS)

Developed by Meyers and Woodford (1992), this is a cognitive, fluency-shaping approach. The program includes procedures for assessment and intervention that are comprehensive but easy to follow. Child-centered activities follow "fluency rules" that emphasize slow versus fast speech, smooth versus bumpy speech, and turn-taking. Children become desensitized to time pressure and difficult speaking situations. In addition, there is a parent education and counseling scheme, which includes 13 behavioral exercises.

The Stuttering Intervention Program (SIP)

The SIP is a program developed by Pindzola (1987) for young children age three through nine (grade three). The program consists of assessment procedures, parent counseling, and intervention procedures. Also included is a protocol for differentiating incipient stuttering and normal fluency breaks. She stresses (a) both reinforcement of fluency and punishment of stuttering (in the form of feedback and repair of the stuttered moment); (b) fluency enhancing targets of stretched, soft, and smooth speech (primarily on the first syllable of a sentence or following a pause); and (c) a gradually increasing hierarchy of language complexity. This fluency-shaping program includes formatted individualized educational plans and informational handouts for both parents and teachers.

The Fluency Rules Program (FRP)

Developed by Runyan and Runyan (1986; 1993), this is a fluency-shaping program that has been designed for use in a school environment. The program incorporates seven rules for fluent speech production. The two "universal rules" of (1) "speaking slowly and saying a word once" and (2) "one word at a time" may be sufficient for achieving fluency for some children. Modeling and paced speaking are used to achieve a slower speech rate. Children receive signals from the clinician (e.g., raised index finger) for a part- or whole-word repetition. For children who do not achieve fluency using the two universal rules, additional (primary) rules of (3) "speech breathing" and (4) "gentle onset of voicing" are used. Finally, three (secondary) rules are used for some children to achieve fluency: (5) light articulatory contacts (to prevent blocking and struggle), (6) keep articulators moving (to prevent prolongations), and (7) use only the speech helpers for speaking (to eliminate secondary movements). The linguistic demands of the speaking tasks are considered. Self-monitoring procedures are strongly emphasized as the child transfers his fluency roles to other environments. The Runyans believe that treatment activities must be fun for children and that the clinician's enthusiasm and sense of humor are central elements for success.

Gradual Increase in Length and Complexity of Utterance (GILCU)

Developed by Bruce Ryan and Barbara Van Kirk (1974), GILCU is a programmed, behavioral, fluency-shaping model. It was one of the earliest programs in behavioral treatment to be widely used. The program makes use of operant-conditioning principles using verbal reward for fluency and verbal punishment for stuttering. The program is best used with the younger child who has not developed many cognitive and attitudinal features. The program takes the child through the three phases of establishment, transfer, and maintenance, with gradually increasing length and complexity of child utterances (GILCU) as the child proceeds from reading, monologue, and conversation. When necessary, fluency is established using delayed auditory feedback, with the child being instructed to speak in a monotone, slur his articulation, and prolong sounds. Transfer activities take the child from treatment to a variety of extratreatment settings. Follow-up evaluations take place at posttreatment intervals of two weeks and monthly intervals of one, 3, 6, and 12 months. If a child exceeds a specific threshold of fluency breaks during these evaluations, he is cycled back through the program.

Systematic Fluency Training for Young Children

This program was created by Shine (1980; 1988) for young children between the ages of three and nine. It is a highly structured program involving operant conditioning and programmed instruction that includes both assessment and intervention strategies. Using a fluency-shaping approach that begins with whispered (or prolonged) speech, the child is taught the usual fluency enhancing targets (e.g., light articulatory contacts, slow rate, and easy onset of phonation). The program has the child move through seven phases, beginning with picture identification using monosyllabic words, a storybook, picture matching, and transfer and maintenance of spontaneous speech. Parental involvement is emphasized.

CONCLUSION

Treatment is often successful with young preschool children who stutter, and the difficulties of transfer, maintenance, and relapse usually take considerably less time and effort than with older speakers. Regardless of the child's age, success often depends on the willingness of one or more parents to become involved in the treatment process. In many cases, one or more teachers can also be particularly helpful in transferring both

√ CLINICAL DECISION-MAKING

Throughout this text we have presented examples of decisions that clinicians are frequently asked to make along with possible responses. Of course, it is difficult to know what may be the best response to many clinical situations and often there is no way to know what response may facilitate client growth until we make a choice and see what happens. With this in mind, consider the following situations and describe one or more possible decisions or responses you might make under these circumstances.

➤ A client who has just begun treatment comes to a therapy session and states "I feel really great. I haven't stuttered at all today!"
➤ A client tells you that the treatment you demonstrated and practiced in therapy last week "doesn't work at school."
➤ A client explains to you that he has difficulty saying the word fluently when using cancellation techniques.
➤ The parents of a 12-year-old child who stutters want their child to receive treatment, but the child refuses to attend individual or group treatment sessions.
➤ A classroom teacher is unable to get a seventh grade child who stutters to ask questions in her class.
➤ A client says that his favorite method of handling his stuttering is to avoid words.
➤ An adult client tells you that despite seeing you at the clinic for several months, he is unable to tell anyone at his office that he is attending therapy.
➤ A client who is beginning to learn the technique of cancellation informs you that during everyday speaking situations outside of the clinic situation, he is unable to stand the time pressure of going back and smoothly stuttering on the word again.
➤ When practicing modification techniques with you at a mall, the client "loses it" and is unable to continue.
➤ The parents of a young client inform you that their child is being teased by a child in the neighborhood.
➤ The parents of an eight-year-old child are resistant to take part in the treatment session with their child.
➤ The clinician concludes that it may be helpful for her to model some risk-taking behavior for a client. What are examples of such modeling behavior for a child, adolescent, and adult?
➤ The parents of a young child you are seeing for treatment become confused by the amount of information about the nature of stuttering that you have provided and that they have obtained through the Internet.
➤ The wife of a client asks you why you are asking her husband to voluntarily stutter.
➤ A client asks you "How long will it take for me to stop stuttering?"

fluency-enhancing techniques and attitudes about communication. The clinician will play a significant role in educating and counseling the client's parents in order to lessen the guilt and misinformation that may have grown up around the problem. As parents gain greater understanding and control of the developmental aspects of stuttering, they will more likely become a powerful force in facilitating their child's fluency. By considering both the child's capacities for speech production and the demands that may be placed on him, the parents and the clinician can enhance his ability to achieve fluency in a variety of speaking situations both inside and outside the treatment setting. The clinician can also provide valuable information that will increase the ability of the classroom teacher to identify fluency problems and assist the child in participating in daily classroom activities.

Treatment is viewed by many authors as a process of improving a child's capacities for producing fluent speech and reducing environmental responses to fluency-disrupting stimuli (or desensitizing the speaker to stimuli that cannot be reduced or eliminated. Regardless of the overall treatment strategy chosen by the clinician, all programs emphasize such factors as enhancing the child's enjoyment of speaking, empowering the child to understand and use his "speech helpers," using fluency-facilitating techniques to achieve and expand fluency and to improve the child's self-confidence as a speaker and a person. Most authorities see no major problem in helping the child with coexisting communication problems while also intervening with fluency. Teasing is a common problem for young children who stutter. Fortunately, there are a variety of useful responses to this situation, including desensitization of the child to the situation and modeling—often via role-playing—of helpful responses.

STUDY QUESTIONS

➤ What characteristics of younger children who stutter are likely to influence both diagnostic and treatment decisions?
➤ What were the accepted views about direct intervention for young children who stuttered in the middle of the 20th century? How has this view changed in the last 20–30 years?
➤ Considering the most recent information on the onset and development of stuttering as described in Chapter 3, what are your thoughts concerning the value of concepts such as (a) primary and secondary stuttering and (b) indirect and direct treatment for young children?

➤ What do you feel are the most basic premises to keep in mind when working with a young child in the early stages of stuttering?

➤ Describe a three-stage progression of involving parents in the treatment process with their young child.

➤ What are the fluency-enhancing techniques you would consider using with a young child who stutters?

➤ With a friend, model techniques that will assist a young child who stutters in varying and modifying their stuttering behavior in the direction of easier stuttering.

➤ Describe to a friend the techniques you would consider using to help a child who stutters to change his attitude about the experience of stuttering.

➤ What decisions will you need to make when you evaluate and decide to treat a child who stutters and also exhibits one or more other communication problems?

➤ Prepare an outline of an in-service for a group of 30 classroom teachers. What are the main points you want to make about the nature of stuttering, the nature of therapy, how they may help to identify a child who stutters in their class, and how they can assist in the treatment process? What pamphlets, videos, and Internet addresses would make available to your audience?

RECOMMENDED READINGS

Chmela, K. A., & Reardon, N. A. (2000). *The school-age child who stutters: Practical ideas for working with feelings and beliefs about stuttering.* Publication No. 5. Stuttering Foundation of America.

Dell, C. (1970). *Treating the school age stutterer: A guide for clinicians.* Publication No. 14. Memphis, TN: Speech Foundation of America.

Guitar, B. (1998). *Stuttering: An integrated approach to its nature and treatment.* Baltimore: Williams & Wilkins. (See Chapters 12 & 13.)

Letting Go. The National Stuttering Project, Anaheim Hills, CA. (See Appendix B for address and related information.)

Logan, K, J., & Yaruss, J. S. (1999). Helping parents address attitudinal and emotional factors with young children who stutter. *Contemporary Issues in Communication Science and Disorders, 26,* 69–81.

Murphy, B. (1999). A preliminary look at shame, guilt, and stuttering. Chapter 11 (131143) in N. B. Ratner and E. C. Healey (Eds.), *Stuttering research and practice: Bridging the gap.* Mahwah, NJ: Lawrence Erlbaum.

Proceedings of the NIDCD Workshop on treatment efficacy research in stuttering. September 21–22, 1992. *Journal of Fluency Disorders.* (1993). 18, 2 & 3.

CHAPTER

10

INDICATORS OF PROGRESS DURING TREATMENT

> *There are, of course, observable aspects of this disorder, but do we want to say that efficacious therapies are those that deal only with the observable aspects? If anything, it should be the other way around. . . . The unobservable events seem more important than the observable ones.*
> C. Woodruff Starkweather (1999). *The effectiveness of stuttering therapy: An issue for science? Chapter 16 (231–244) in N. B. Ratner and E. C. Healey (Eds.),* Stuttering research and practice: Bridging the gap. *Mahwah, NJ: Lawrence Erlbaum.*

INTRODUCTION

Peck, in a discussion of the psychotherapeutic process, indicates that "the majority of patients, even in the hands of the most skilled and loving therapists, will terminate their therapy at some point far short of completely fulfilling their potential" (1978, p. 180). Early termination is also the nature of intervention for fluency disorders. Not all clients make as much progress as we would like, but almost any client who is ready and motivated enough to face his communication problem head-on is likely to make some progress during treatment. As the client meets with a competent clinician, he will begin to learn something about himself and his communication problem. As he is guided through the features of his stuttering, he is likely to become desensitized to the problem. He will develop a more accurate and broader view of his communication disorder, and he will gradually begin making better decisions that are less influenced by the fact that he happens to be a person who stutters. Gradually, as these and other changes occur, his disability and handicap will lessen.

Therapeutic progress is much more than the changes that take place during the time the client is immersed in formal treatment. An important aspect of the client's long-term progress is the continuum of *formal versus informal treatment*. Formal treatment may be thought of as that time when the client is receiving and paying for the services of a professional clinician. Informal treatment may be regarded as the much longer time following formal treatment, when the client is on his own. During informal treatment, there is minimal or no contact with the professional clinician. In many important ways, this latter stage of treatment is the most critical part of the overall treatment process. It is the client who is doing the changing, and the process of change cannot cease at the conclusion of formal treatment. The months and years that follow formal treatment will provide the true measure of treatment efficacy. Can the client, once he is on his own, make consistent use of the strategies and techniques acquired during formal treatment? Will he take the time to expand his ability to monitor and modify his fluency? Will he gather the energy to cultivate the cognitive and affective changes that are necessary to reduce the handicap of the syndrome, or will relapse—to a greater or lesser degree—dictate additional periods of formal intervention?

This chapter will discuss indicators of progress and ways of considering the major variables that appear to influence progress during formal treatment. Progress will be described in terms of the most obvious surface feature of the syndrome, the frequency and nature of stuttering. However, other directions of change will be proposed, changes that are more likely to indicate the successful long-term modification of the syndrome. The variables discussed in this chapter will set the stage for the final chapter, where success following formal treatment is considered.

DEFINING PROGRESS

Identifying progress during treatment is more complicated than it may first appear. Progress can be more difficult to define than it is to assess the nature of the syndrome at the outset of treatment. Certainly, clinicians will interpret progress differently, depending on the overall treatment strategy and associated techniques that are used. An indicator of progress for a client taking part in a treatment program emphasizing fluency enhancement will not necessarily be thought of as progress for another client who is taking part in a program where stuttering modification is the major goal. Determining progress during treatment is an intricate issue, as suggested by the fact that treatment efficacy is only recently being addressed in an orderly manner. (For a review on treatment efficacy research in stuttering, see Volume 18, numbers 2 and 3, of the *Journal of Fluency Disorders,* 1993). In discussing this issue with children, Conture and Guitar (1993) suggested that treatment can be considered successful if the child begins to communicate easily whenever and to whomever he chooses. This also seems to be a reasonable approach to take with adults.

The Variability of Change

Just as fluency itself can be highly variable, progress during treatment is inconsistent. In addition, fluctuations in some features of the syndrome are better indicators of change than others. Changes in some features (e.g., the percent of words stuttered) may indicate short-term progress, while changes in other features (e.g., decreased avoidance of words) may provide a better indication of long-term treatment effects. Furthermore, the rate at which these features will change is influenced, not only by the particular treatment strategy but by the treatment setting, the schedule, and the clinician.

As indicated in Chapter 1, the clinician plays a crucial role in motivating and guiding the client. It is likely, however, that another influential variable is the client himself, for personal change and growth are highly individualized. Not all clients will make the same degree of progress during formal treatment. There are, of course, clinicians who describe impressive levels of success for their treatment program. Usually, closer examination of these reports often indicates that the selection process for inclusion in the program was highly restrictive (e.g., only clients who are highly motivated, could afford the time and cost, or were responsive to the diagnostic tasks were included in treatment). In other instances, the criteria for success are overly simplistic: for example, an overt measure of the percentage of syllables stuttered within the clinic environment.

Regardless of the particular treatment strategy, clinicians who have written about treatment efficacy for adult clients seem to accept what could be called the *one third rule.* That is, regardless of the overall treatment strategy, and everything else being equal in terms of client motivation and intelligence, clinician experience, and the timing of intervention, one third of clients will make good progress; one third, moderate progress; and one third—often because they prematurely drop out of treatment—little or no progress.

Of those speakers who make good progress, there will be some that do extremely well and conclude formal treatment exhibiting little or no stuttering behavior. Perhaps even more telling, if these speakers should experience a break in their fluency, they are not likely to panic. They are able to analyze what it is they are doing and modify their breaks into smooth and comfortable forms of stuttering. They are assertive, choosing to enter into new and demanding speaking situations. When these clients are faced with a difficult communication situation, they are able to adjust to a smooth speech mode and achieve fluency-shaping targets that enable them to move through feared words and sounds. Finally, after formal treatment concludes, they are able to maintain these behaviors and attitudes about their fluency disorder.

Other clients, while not showing such marked change, will make good progress. They will regress somewhat from their levels of fluency they achieved at the conclusion of formal treatment. They will continue to stutter but with less frequency and struggle than they did prior to treatment, and they will slowly become less afraid of the stuttering experience. The fact that they are people who stutter incrementally plays a much smaller part in their lives. To be sure, they stutter on some occasions, but they also maintain their ability to make significant changes in the form of their stuttering. They gradually learn to avoid less and are progressively less likely to be at the mercy of a possible stuttering event.

Of course, there is the final third of all clients: those who make little or no progress. Often these are individuals who attend treatment for a relatively short time. As they begin to realize the full nature of their stuttering and the effort and time it will take to change the many features of their problem, their motivation begins to fade. Attendance becomes inconsistent and eventually ceases. In some cases, positive changes have occurred, but it is enough for now, and the cost of additional change is not deemed to be worth the effort. Perhaps we should decline to see such clients until they demonstrate acceptable levels of motivation at the outset. Or maybe as we give them a little knowledge and some new insights, we are setting the stage for later progress. It often seems that regardless of the longer view of change, we should attempt to do what we can for them when we have the opportunity.

In a review of 13 clinicians and their associates, Martin (1981) came to a similar conclusion about progress. He determined that one third of the clients achieved and maintained satisfactory fluency, one third achieved fluency during therapy but regressed over time, and one third either failed to complete treatment programs or were unavailable for follow-up assessment. He stressed that a major problem preventing a complete interpretation of the data was the fact that many clients left treatment prior to completion of the therapy program. Prins (1970) found comparable results, noting that 67% of 94 male clients taking part in an intensive residential program completed questionnaires indicating "much or complete" improvement. Interestingly, 65% of the subjects indicated that little or no posttreatment regression had occurred in terms of *morale*. In addition, Prins noted that once they occurred, interpersonal changes were more durable than the level of fluency or decreased avoidance of words.

Chronic Perseverative Stuttering

There is one other distinct category of clients that can be included in a discussion of therapeutic progress. These people would most likely fall into the second or third of the three groups discussed in the previous section. Cooper (1986a, 1987) argues that there is a significant group of stuttering individuals for whom fluent speech is an unrealistic goal. Any clinician who has worked for several years in the area of fluency disorders will recognize this pattern of behavior. Cooper describes this group as manifesting Chronic Perseverative Stuttering (CPS). These speakers are adolescents or adults who have stuttered for several years (at least 10) and for whom stuttering will always be a problem. Cooper indicates that these clients typically respond to treatment with increased fluency, only to experience profound levels of relapse shortly after completing formal treatment. Their predominant self-perception is that of a stutterer. They demonstrate some degree of obsessive striving for normal speech as well as a deep fear of fluency loss, even though such loss may occur infrequently.

Cooper suggests that if clinicians are unwilling to recognize that fluent speech is *not* a realistic possibility for these speakers, they are likely to create and perpetuate unwarranted feelings of guilt on behalf of their clients. He argues that an acknowledgment of this syndrome by clinicians results in a profound relief for clients who see themselves as Chronic Perseverative Stutterers. Whether this view would predispose a client to failure is debatable. Accepting the fact that some people who stutter will always have a chronic problem is simply being realistic. It is, however, important to point out that, although these speakers will always have a degree of obvious stuttering present in their speech, they may be able to alter their stuttering to the degree that they can communicate more effectively.

Paper-and-Pencil Measures

Determining progress during and following treatment is most often accomplished by client observation in a variety of settings and by administering paper-and-pencil measures of change. These are the same measures used at the outset of treatment during the diagnostic session

(Chapter 4 and Appendix A). Baseline measures obtained with these procedures can, of course, be used to indicate change during treatment. Just as the diagnostic process is a multidimensional one, so is the estimation of progress during the treatment process. Of course, as with assessment, procedures for determining progress should be appropriate for the age of the client and the attitude, cognitive, or behavioral aspects of the syndrome one wishes to assess. In some instances, other characteristics—such as the time it takes to administer the measure or the availability of the measure—become important.

As the period of formal treatment comes to a conclusion, it becomes increasingly important to determine the client's performance and response in extra-treatment speaking situations. Some assessment measures, although useful for obtaining initial diagnostic information, are specifically devised to determine progress during and following treatment. That is, they are designed to assess both intrinsic and surface features in a variety of extratreatment settings. As with diagnostic procedures, there are a wide variety of protocols for determining progress and selecting criteria for termination (from formal treatment) criteria. In Chapter 4 we presented several diagnostic measures that have been used to determine change as a function of treatment. The following section provides some examples of such research.

The Locus of Control of Behavior (LCB)

Craig, Franklin, and Andrews (1984) administered the LCB scale to a group of 45 adults who stuttered and who had received treatment in the fluency modification program at the Prince Henry Hospital in Australia. Stuttering subjects averaged scores of 32.0, while a nonstuttering control group averaged 27.0, a difference that was found to be statistically significant. Following treatment, 32 of the subjects maintained fluency levels 10 months posttreatment, and 13 subjects showed relapse (more than 2% syllables stuttered). Twenty-eight of the 32 subjects who maintained fluency also showed increased internality on the LCB scale during treatment. Of the 13 subjects who relapsed, 11 either had no change or became more external during the three-week program. These results were replicated by Craig and Andrews (1985).

Madison, Budd, and Itzkowitz (1986) studied locus of control (LOC) with 7- to 16-year-old children and found that those subjects who had a more internal locus of control *prior* to treatment tended to achieve more fluent speech during treatment. They did not, however, find a significant relationship between pretreatment LOC values and fluency levels at two follow-up measures taken two and six months posttreatment.

The results were less encouraging for the ability of the LCB to predict long-term change in a more recent study by De Nil and Kroll (1995).

These authors studied 21 adult subjects who had been enrolled in a three-week intensive behavioral treatment fluency-shaping program (the Precision Fluency Shaping Program [PFSP] of Webster, 1975). Thirteen subjects were contacted two years following treatment. While the follow-up measures indicated that the fluency gains achieved during treatment were maintained by most clients, no predictive relationship was found between LCB scores and the client's percent words stuttered. There was a significant decrease in LCB scores from pre- to posttreatment, indicating increased internality. The use of a stepwise regression analysis procedure indicated that LCB scores were found to be predictive of the speakers' self-evaluation of fluency level. However, the results did not support previously reported findings that the amount of change in locus of control toward more internality during treatment predicted success two years after treatment.

De Nil and Kroll's (1995) findings supported the findings of Andrews and Craig (1988) that total LCB scores *alone* were of limited help in predicting treatment outcome. Moreover, as pointed out by De Nil and Kroll as well as Ladouceur, Caron, and Caron (1989), the predictive value of locus of control is likely to be significantly affected by the nature of the treatment program. If for the client to assume control of his speech is a major focus of treatment (regardless of the individual's fluency level), LCB measures are more likely to change in their direction of internality. In addition, an intensive three-week period of treatment may not allow adequate time for the internalization of control.

Self-Efficacy Scaling

Blood (1995) noted a clear improvement in SESAS scores during and following a successful cognitive-behavioral treatment program for three high school clients. Treatment consisted of 25 hours of intensive work on changing speech (a modified version of the Shames and Florance, 1980, fluency-shaping program), 50 hours of relapse prevention, and two (6-month and 12-month) follow-up phases. All three clients showed gradual improvements in overall (approach and performance) scores which averaged 56.3% performance (baseline), 77.6% (post-speech change), 87.3% (post-relapse management), 89.7% (6-month follow-up), and 86.7% (12-month follow-up).

Hillis (1993) pointed out that the pragmatic nature of the SESAS approach may be interpreted as an indication of the scale's content validity. In addition, the construct validity of the SESAS approach is supported by a 28-point difference (effect size = 3.50 nonstuttering standard deviations; $p < .05$) found on the 100-point SESAS approach between 20 subjects who stuttered and the 20 who did not. The construct validity of the SESAS performance scale is supported by a 42-point difference between means (effect size = 11 nonstuttering standard deviations, $p <$ .05) on the 100-point scale between the 20 subjects who stuttered and the 20 who did not.

In order to decrease the uncontrolled variance resulting from the different levels of fluency selected by clients, Hillis (1993) modified the instructions for the performance section of the SESAS. Rather than using the original (Ornstein & Manning, 1985) instructions of having the client determine a "level of fluency" based on his stage of treatment when scoring this section, Hillis asked the client to define fluent speech as "speech [that] would be so fluent in a given situation that, in the client's opinion, a listener would not recognize that the client had a history of stuttering" (1993, p. 28).

Hillis (1993) also provided data on a variety of measures including the SESAS for an adult male stuttering client (See Figure 10-1). Despite two relapses when the client's pauses per minute and stuttered syllables per minute increased (to less than pretreatment levels), there was continued progress in that the client was judged to be speaking in a natural and fluent manner by himself, the clinician, and an independent observer. Because this was not the case in speaking situations outside the clinic, this fluency was termed "clinical fluency." At the end of treatment the client was maintaining a high level of fluency, both in the treatment environment and in selected extra-treatment situations. Nevertheless, Hillis points out that the SESAS approach score remained less than 70 and SESAS performance score less than 80 at the end of treatment—something less than normalized scores. Hillis notes that even successfully treated clients rarely score much above 80 on the modified SESAS performance scale. This is still within the range of normal speakers reported by Ornstein and Manning (1985) of 74–100, but well less than one standard deviation (8.0) of 86.2. Thus it is likely that clients can demonstrate high levels of fluent behavior but nevertheless be lagging behind in terms of cognitive change (SESAS approach) and speech performance in extra-treatment performance (SESAS performance).

The following figures indicate the changes for an adult female (SSI score of very severe) over a period of six years for the 17-item Locus of Control of Behavior Scale (Figure 10-2), and Approach (Figure 10-3) and Performance (Figure 10-4) portions of the Self-Efficacy Scale for Adult Stutterers (SESAS). This person was seen once a week for individual and group therapy. Figure 10-2 indicates extremely high LCB scores at the outset of treatment (the highest we have over recorded) with scores progressively decreasing (indicating the desired greater internality). With absences from treatment, scores would often increase in the direction of greater externality. After some two years of treatment, scores began to reach the range expected for nonstuttering speakers.

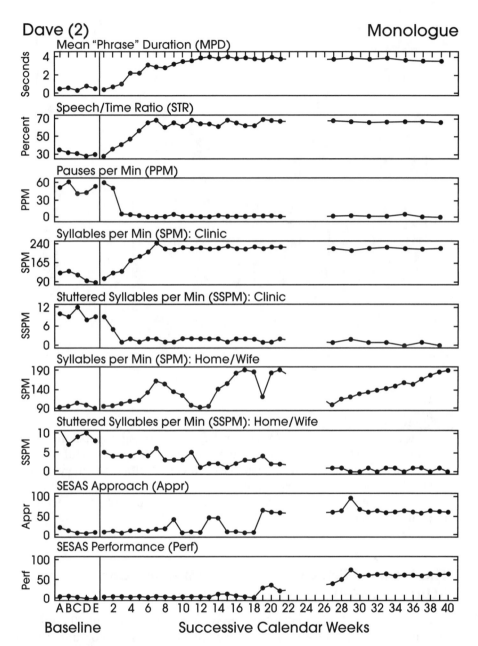

Figure 10-1. Baseline and treatment effects for an adult man on nine measurement parameters across a baseline period and 45 calendar weeks of treatment. (PPM—Pauses per Minute, MPD—Mean Phrase Duration in Seconds, STR—Speech-Time Ration, SPM—Syllables per Minute, SSPM—Stuttered Syllables per Minute, APPR-SESAS Approach, PERF-SESAS Performance). (Hillis, 1993).

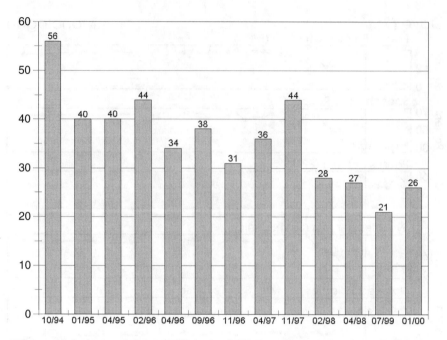

Figure 10-2. Locus of Control of Behavior (LCB) scores for an adult female with severe stuttering over six years of treatment.

Figure 10-3 indicates gradually increasing SESAS-Approach scores, and Figure 10-4 shows SESAS-Performance scores lagging behind as noted by Hillis (1993). It took some five years for this speaker with very severe stuttering to begin to achieve a level of fluency where she believed listeners would not be aware that she had a history of stuttering. Near the end of the fifth year of treatment, periods of spontaneous and natural fluency began to be observed.

The Modified Erickson Scale of Communication Attitudes (S-24)

Guitar and Bass (1978) conducted a frequently-cited study of 20 adults who underwent a three-week intensive fluency-shaping program. The study is often referred to for two reasons: (1) it provided support for the idea that the failure to change communication attitudes (as measured by the S-24) may be predictive of relapse within 12 to 18 months, and (2) it questioned the desirability of an entirely operant view of therapy. Young (1981) used a combination of regression analysis and causal modeling to

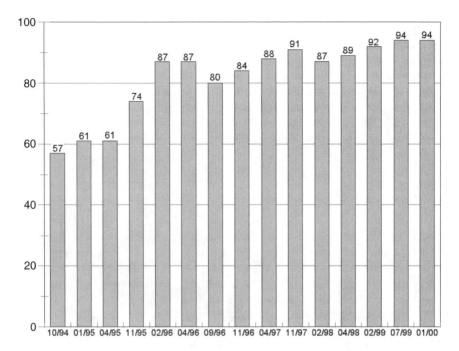

Figure 10-3. Approach scores for the Self-Efficacy Scale for Adult Stutterers for an adult female with severe stuttering over six years of treatment.

reconsider the results of the Guitar and Bass study. He found that pre-treatment S-24 scores were unrelated to either pre-or post-treatment %SS or to post-treatment S-24 scores. Although the causal modeling technique did indicate that post-treatment S-24 scores were moderately predictive of post-treatment %SS, Young questioned how much communication attitudes might change during a three-week treatment program that was not intended to focus on attitude change. He concluded that to the degree that the S-24 is capable of measuring such attitudes, the results of Guitar and Bass did support the notion that treatment programs (including behavior modification) should consider such changes. Finally, the results of a study by Andrews and Craig (1988) also found a relationship between attitude change as indicated by the S-24 and long-term change.

Paper-and-pencil measures provide helpful information for the clinician's decision-making during treatment, but these measures are not without their problems. Some can be tedious to complete, and there tend to be sequencing effects associated with multiple administrations of the measures. Clients tire of completing the forms, may fail to take the task seriously, and become test-wise about the intent of the measure, filling it

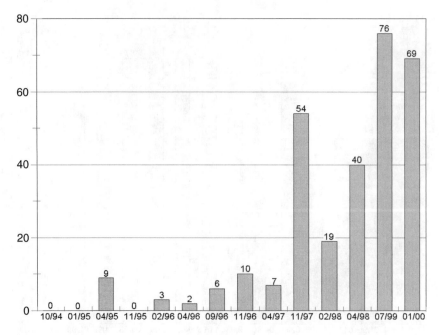

Figure 10-4. Performance scores for the Self-Efficacy Scale for Adult Stutterers for an adult female with severe stuttering over six years of treatment.

out the way they believe they "should" respond rather than indicating what they truly think or feel.

ASKING THE CLIENT

Although paper-and-pencil measures provide practical ways of estimating change and progress, it is also important to keep in mind that when the clinician wants an indication of progress, there is also the possibility of asking the client. Asking a question as simple as, "How's your speech and what are you doing about it?" can yield a wealth of information to which the clinician can respond in the treatment setting.

Obviously, a professional clinician relies on a variety of data obtained during treatment as well as findings gleaned from descriptive and experimental research. Sometimes the patterns in the data are clear, but sometimes they are not, and often the numbers conflict. In experimental investigations, individual performance is often obscured by group statistics and methods of data reduction. Furthermore, the experimental or treatment group of subjects is typically composed of a group of individuals who are far from homogeneous. Each subject exhibits a unique response to the treatment strategies and the clinician. We rarely have all the data we would like for making clinical decisions, but we do have clinical experience, and we can try different approaches depending on the needs and response of the client.

THE MULTIDIMENSIONAL NATURE OF THERAPEUTIC CHANGE

Van Riper (1973, pp. 178–199) provided a comprehensive overview of ways to consider progress during treatment. His fundamental point is that any view of progress should be comprehensive and ought to make

---

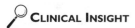 **CLINICAL INSIGHT**

One of the events that motivated the writing of this text was a presentation I attended at the annual meeting of the American Speech-Language-Hearing Association a few years ago. The six presenters who took the stage were experienced in the area of fluency disorders. These experts were charged with discussing selection criteria for matching clients to particular treatment approaches. After listening throughout the one and one-half hour session, I left with a sense of frustration. I suspected that, with the possible exception of one presenter, these speakers had managed to alienate a large portion of the approximately 100 clinicians in attendance concerning the treatment of fluency disorders. What was imparted was a frustration with the data concerning the efficacy of different treatment strategies. The emphasis was data: the lack of data, inaccurate data, and conflicting data. There was no recognition of the success that can and does take place during treatment. There was certainly little appreciation, either for the people doing the stuttering or the clinicians administering the treatment. The presenters were not giving clinicians credit for being able to identify progress. Even more so, there was no appreciation for the integrity of clinicians' decision-making abilities. Moreover, they certainly were not imparting much enthusiasm. It was a fine example of experimenters who were focusing on group results and not being able to see the people for the data.

One of the presenters who shared the frustration of this view made the suggestion that the most useful data is right in front of us during treatment. "If you want data," he suggested, "try asking the client. He might have some good information for you about what is helpful and what is not."

use of a multifactor approach. That is, several surface behaviors as well as many of the intrinsic features of the problem must be taken into account. Otherwise, success will be either overstated or unrecognized. As Sheehan suggested, the more trivial the criteria for improvement the greater the likelihood of success (1980).

As in the original assessment process, there are at least two major levels of change: change in the surface behaviors and change in the intrinsic features of the problem. The changes in the surface behavior of the client often occur relatively early in the formal treatment process. In some cases, these changes even begin to occur prior to treatment. Changes in the intrinsic features, such as attitude and cognitive aspects, lag behind (Emerick, 1988; Manning, 1991). The intrinsic changes that are reflected in the quality of the client's self-management and decision making are critical for long-term success. There are reports suggesting what seems intuitively correct, that the improvement of the surface behaviors will be more likely to be permanent if changes in the intrinsic features of the problem also occur (Emerick, 1988; Guitar, 1976; Guitar & Bass, 1978; Maxwell, 1982).

It has been shown by several investigators that change, at least in some of the surface behaviors of stuttering, can begin prior to the formal initiation of treatment (Andrews & Harvey, 1981; Bordeau & Jeffrey, 1973; Gregory, 1972; Ingham, Andrews, & Winkler, 1972; Ost, Gotestam, & Melin, 1976; Peins, McGough & Lee, 1972; Webster, 1979). For example, Andrews and Harvey (1981) measured 132 adult stutterers approximately eight months prior to the initiation of treatment and again immediately before treatment. The subjects showed significant improvements in the percentage of syllables stuttered (18.2% to 14.4%) and the rate of speech in syllables per minute (91.5 and 129.8). These changes became evident after the first three months on the waiting list. Changes in attitude, however, were much smaller. There was no significant change in the subjects' speech communication attitude, as measured by the S-24 scale (Andrews & Cutler, 1974). Furthermore, no significant change was found in two of the three measures (perceived avoidance and severity of stuttering) indicated by the Stutterers Self Rating of Reactions to Speaking Situations (Johnson, Darley, & Spriesterbach, 1963). If, as suggested in Chapter 4, clients are apt to seek treatment when their problem is most severe, this regression toward the mean is not surprising. Furthermore, the very act of finding professional help and asking for assistance is an indication of change. The client's recognition that it is now time to work on the problem is a significant initial step in the direction of change. Seeking help indicates a degree of assertiveness that was not present before. Whatever the reasons, the problem has become important enough to take action. Even though formal intervention has not yet taken place, being included on a waiting list is a tangible step in a new direction and can provide a measure of support for the speaker.

The majority of investigations on treatment efficacy utilize reduction in frequency of stuttering as the dependent variable: for example, percentage of stuttered syllables or words (Andrews, Craig, & Feyer, 1983; Ingham, 1980; Ryan, 1980; Shames & Florance, 1980). That is, the frequency of this surface feature of the problem is the primary criterion for improvement—and to some degree this makes sense. A decrease in the frequency of stuttering obviously indicates change, and sometimes such change indicates progress. There are, however, others who argue that the intrinsic aspects of the problem, the attitude and cognitive features, are at least as important (and possibly more so) for determining long-term progress (Cooper & Cooper, 1985b; Rubin, 1986; Sheehan, 1970; Starkweather, 1999; Van Riper, 1973). In addition, studies on the quality of fluent speech (also referred to as *speech naturalness*) following both stuttering-modification as well as fluency-modification strategies indicate that the absence of stuttering, in and of itself, is not necessarily an indicator of successful treatment (Onslow & Ingham, 1987).

Many features associated with the stuttering syndrome will begin to change as a function of treatment. The time and the rate of change will depend on many variables, such as the overall treatment strategy, specific treatment techniques, the nature of the fluency disorder, the age of the speaker, the severity of the problem, the needs of the client, and the intensity and the duration of treatment. As several authors have noted, to the degree that the fluency disorder is further complicated by problems such as excessive anxiety, psychological or social issues, or articulation or language disabilities, individually tailored therapy techniques become mandatory (Gregory, 1984; Riley & Riley, 1983, 1984; 2000; St. Louis, 1986b; Van Riper, 1973).

VARIABLES INFLUENCING PROGRESS

We would like to think that the treatment administered to a client is influenced, in large part, by the theoretical background received by the clinician during his academic and clinical training. Based on a series of articles commenting on how practicing clinicians select treatment approaches, this may not be the case (Apel, 1999; Kamhi, 1999; Fey and Johnson, 1998). Clinicians, it seems, frequently choose strategies and techniques that they believe will work. The treatment strategy and techniques of choice are also influenced, or at least ought to be, by information gathered by the clinician during the reading of articles in professional journals and attendance at professional meetings. As pointed out in Chapter 6, the strategy is also likely to be influenced by the professional environment where the clinician is employed. In any case, there are several important variables that will influence the quality and quantity of progress during treatment.

The Treatment Strategy

The clinician's interpretation of progress will certainly be determined by the specific goals associated with a treatment strategy. As suggested in Chapter 6, clinicians who are using programs that emphasize stuttering modification will look for somewhat different signs of progress than those employing a program of fluency modification or enhancement. If a fluency-modification approach is used, a reduction of stuttering moments is considered a basic indicator of progress. However, if the modification of stuttered moments is a goal of treatment, a decrease in stuttered moments is necessarily desirable and may, in fact, prevent the speaker from having the opportunity to identify and modify stuttered events. Furthermore, if a decrease in avoidance behavior is a primary goal of treatment, an *increase* in stuttered moments may be highly desirable and may result from an increase in speaker assertiveness and decreased avoidance of speaking situations or words.

The Nature of the Fluency Disorder

Many researchers, and probably the majority of clinicians, look to the frequency of stuttering as a primary, and sometimes the only, measure of change or progress. For some clients this measure may be a more valid indicator than for others. That is, for clients who clutter or exhibit a combination of stuttering and cluttering characteristics, the frequency of fluency breaks may provide a reasonably clear indication of progress. For these speakers, the surface behavior may be less obscured or influenced by the intrinsic features of the communication disorder. Measures such as the percentage of syllables or words that are stuttered are more likely to provide a direct indication about the severity of the problem. These speakers are either less interested in using or less able to employ techniques such as avoidance and postponement to conceal the problem. The decision-making aspects of the syndrome, while they are present, are not as likely to be a major component as they are with the more typical stuttering speaker.

The frequency of stuttering may also provide a more direct and therefore more valid indication of change for other subgroups of stutterers who are also less adept at concealing fluency breaks. Younger children, especially those who are in the early stages of developmental stuttering, usually have not yet developed sophisticated methods of hiding or avoiding their stuttering. The percentage of stuttered moments may also provide a relatively unencumbered picture of the stuttering syndrome for stutterers with psychogenic and neurogenic etiology. Moreover, there is also some indication that the surface behavior in the form of stuttering frequency may more clearly reflect progress for the mentally handicapped individual who stutters. Despite the fact that mentally handicapped speakers who stutter typically demonstrate high levels of stuttering frequency (Cooper, 1986b), these speakers often appear generally unconcerned about fluency (Bonfanti & Culatta, 1977; Cabanas, 1954). Compared to the person with normal intelligence who stutters, they tend to show fewer avoidance and postponement behaviors, as well as relatively less anxiety, associated with stuttering moments. In this sense, the intrinsic features of such speakers resemble cluttering more than stuttering. However, for the typical developmental stutterer, the frequency of stuttering is only one of many features of the syndrome, and by itself it fails to provide a complete picture of the speaker's status.

The Age of the Client

The major focus for much of this chapter has been on young adults who stutter. Of course, there are similar indicators of progress among all people who stutter. However, there are at least three age groups that are distinct enough in their response to treatment that they should be considered further: young children, adolescents, and older speakers.

As discussed earlier, young children often have good success during both direct and indirect intervention for fluency disorders. They are relatively easy to work with, and the behavioral, attitudinal, and cognitive aspects of the syndrome tend to be responsive to intervention. Success with these speakers can be measured in increased spontaneity and enjoyment of speech production, increased rate of speech, and, of course, decreases in tension and fragmentation.

As we have previously mentioned in Chapter 8, adolescents present an entirely different set of circumstances. Van Riper (1982) stated that adolescents are some of the clinician's most difficult cases. Motivation for change is relatively rare in adolescents. More recently, Daly, Simon, and Burnett-Stolnack (1995) explained that it is often extremely difficult to get adolescents to even take part in treatment. "Many adolescents drop out of therapy, miss sessions, or attend begrudgingly. [They may] downplay the effects of their stuttering on their communication and social interactions. . . . Student rationalizations for poor attendance or for not practicing are common" (1995, p. 163).

As Daly describes, adolescents are apt to be highly sensitive and easily give up during the treatment. Many teenage clients find great difficulty confronting their problem and strongly resist being singled out for anything that carries the potential social stigma of treatment. The importance of peer affiliation is a much more powerful force than the problems originating from their disorder. To complicate matters even further, adolescents often challenge the clinician's qualifications, clinical experience, and overall expertise (Daly, Simon, & Burnett-Stolnack, 1995).

In my own case, as a moderately severe high school stutterer, I firmly resisted the inconvenience and effort I knew would be necessary to work on my speech. After being referred by more than one classroom teacher for treatment, I promptly walked into the office of the two (male) clinicians and fluently announced that I had had enough therapy and wanted no part of it at this time. The Daly, Simon, & Burnett-Stolnack (1995) quote just above described me well.

For this population of clients, progress may be measured by the consistency of attendance at treatment sessions, the level of interaction with the clinician, interest shown in the topics and techniques, requests for pamphlets on stuttering, or participation in group treatment. Assuming that adolescents are willing to take part, another major indicator of progress, given the high degree of peer pressure to conform and not stand out, is a decrease in avoidance behavior.

Progress can also be noted if the client is able to keep the presence of stuttering in his speech from becoming increasingly more handicapping in his educational and social lives. Even if the clinician is unable to achieve great change in the way of modification, she can begin to demystify the problem, explain the cause-and-effect relationships of the syndrome, and let the client and his parents know that—when they are ready—help is available from professionals who specialize in the area of fluency disorders. Thus it may be possible to sow some grains of knowledge and understanding that another clinician can someday harvest.

The third group of speakers are older stutterers who have been coping with their lack of fluency for decades. Clients over the age of 50 are rarely seen in treatment and rarely included in research reports (Manning & Shirkey, 1981). This is unfortunate, for to fully understand a fluency disorder, it would appear to be essential to follow the development of the syndrome throughout the life cycle. Models of stuttering cannot be completed until the developmental changes that take place during the middle and late adult years are understood. A review of the literature, however, indicates that this subgroup of stuttering adults has received almost no investigation. Assuming a prevalence of at least .7% and the most recent census data (*World Almanac and Book of Facts*, 1995), there should be nearly 1 million stutterers over the age of 50 in the United States alone.

It is known that few people over the age of 50 are seen for treatment (Manning, Dailey, & Wallace, 1984; Manning & Monte, 1981). The physiological, including articulatory and phonatory, abilities and psychological changes, including heightened introspection and personal growth, that occur during middle and late adulthood suggest the possibility of increased fluency (Manning & Shirkey, 1981). Travis told his students that death and old age were sure cures for stuttering, and that he never knew of an old man who stuttered (1978).

Anecdotal reports have indicated that stuttering is less of a problem for older individuals. The few data available indicate some support for this argument. Manning, Dailey, and Wallace (1984) obtained attitude and personality information from 29 adults ages 52 to 82 years old who were members of two national self-help groups, the National Stuttering Project, and the National Council of Stutterers. Scores on six paper-and-pencil assessment measures indicated that the older stuttering individuals scored minimally better than the typical scores for young adults who were about to enter treatment. Scores on the Perceptions of Stuttering Inventory (PSI) (Woolf, 1967) averaged 20.3 (standard deviation of 12.0) for the older subjects, in contrast to pretreatment scores for young adults who stutter of 21.1 (Manning & Cooper, 1969) and 27.2 (Ornstein & Manning, 1985). Responses to the S24 Scale (Andrews & Cutler, 1974; Erickson, 1969) for the older speakers averaged 16.0, in contrast to mean pretreatment scores of 19.4 (Howie, 1981), 20.0 (Guitar & Bass, 1978), and 15.6 (Ornstein & Manning, 1985). Scores on the Self-Efficacy Scale for Adult Stutterers (SESAS) (Ornstein & Manning, 1985) averaged 70.5% for approach items and 60.5% on the performance items, in contrast to 66.2% and 55.8% for young adult stutterers (Ornstein & Manning, 1985). In addition, the older participants ranked the approach tasks significantly higher than the performance tasks, just as the younger subjects had done ($p < .05$) (Ornstein & Manning, 1985). Finally, responses to a 25-item bipolar-adjective scale (Woods & Williams, 1976) indicated no significant differences between the 29 stuttering and 13 nonstuttering older subjects.

When asked to indicate whether the handicap associated with stuttering had lessened over the years, the large majority of the subjects agreed that this had been the case. Using a seven-point, equally appearing interval scale to rank their perceived severity as young adults and at the present time, subjects scored their current severity as significantly less ($p < .005$). Furthermore, in response to open-ended queries concerning past and current perceived severity, subjects responded with statements such as, "Stuttering is less of a problem now [since] there is not so much competition"; "I accept myself more now than when I was younger"; "I've become more insightful about personal problems as I grow older"; and "Stuttering has less of an all-consuming hold on me than when I was younger." Because of the way the subjects were selected, this group of older stutterers best represents those older individuals who are actively involved in self-help groups. Nevertheless, the availability of data suggests that although older speakers who stutter may be considered to be equally severely compromised as their younger counterparts, they consider themselves less handicapped by the problem.

The Intensity of Treatment

Intensive treatment is often desirable for many behavioral problems. When people are ready to change, the clinician must be ready to respond, and she must strike when the fire is hot. Often if the client becomes totally immersed in the treatment process, he is more likely to experience rapid changes in the behaviors and attitudes that have persisted for many years (Gregory, 1983; Ingham, 1984; Shames & Florance, 1980; Webster, 1975, 1986). Azrin, Nunn, and Frantz (1979) and Webster (1975) have advocated short-term, intensive approaches, on grounds that it takes a big push to get off dead center and to begin moving in a new direction.

Intensive treatment often presents logistical problems. Many people are not able to leave their work for weeks at a time or cannot commute to and from the treatment site. Potential clients can't always afford the cost of intensive treatment. Moreover, while intensive programs can result in rapid behavioral change, treatment is sometimes followed by dramatic relapses (Kuhr & Rustin, 1985; Prins, 1970). An intensive program, especially if it involves having the client live apart from his typical environment, may yield rapid change in behavioral as well as cognitive aspects of the syndrome. However, for some people, the transition back to the typical world can be traumatic, especially if it is not well thought out and approached in a systematic manner. The old discriminative stimuli and expectancies, on the part of the speaker as well as the listener, are still operating. Relapse is often the case, even for those who practice diligently. Perhaps the suggestion by Cooper (1979a) provides the ideal situation. He advises intensive treatment to modify the surface behaviors, followed by less intensive treatment to allow for change in the intrinsic features of the syndrome and to also allow for maintenance activities.

In any case, if the time is right and the client is ready, significant progress can take place. Moreover, when the changes occur, the clinician must recognize the nature of the breakthroughs. She must recognize the victories when they occur, even though often they are small ones. If the clinician is unable to identify success—the small victories that signal progress—they will go unrecognized and unrewarded. The following section describes the nature of such victories by describing several directions of progress.

INDICATORS OF PROGRESS

Increasing the Client's Self-Monitoring Ability

A basic indicator of progress is the speaker's ability to tune into what he is doing when he stutters and what he is capable of doing in order to enable himself to speak fluently. Even if he is not yet able to *modify* his production, he may be able to accurately *monitor* what he is doing to make speaking so difficult. Accurate self-monitoring of any behavior or thought process is a preparatory step toward taking responsibility and transforming the event.

A good place to begin monitoring is to identify listener reactions. What are the subtle and not so subtle responses to stuttering in terms of body language and verbal responses? Role-playing can be particularly helpful as both client and clinician portray responses observed in extra-treatment situations. Another target of monitoring activities can be the attitudes and behaviors of other clients. Using audio- and videotape segments of treatment sessions. Early in treatment, clients tend to have more success confronting and analyzing stuttering behaviors in others than in themselves. The clinician can provide realistic examples of stuttering behaviors for the client to identify. These can take the form of generic stuttering or replicate behaviors unique to the client. Of course, there will be many subtle aspects of the speaker's stuttering that may take some time and effort for the clinician to distinguish. Real-time analysis, whereby the client identifies stuttering events as they are happening, is usually too demanding at the outset of treatment. This is especially true if the client indicates high levels of fear and avoidance. Audio- or videotapes of the speaker are often essential prior to on-line analysis.

Progress can also be noted in the ability of the client to identify progressively more subtle moments of stuttering. Moments of stuttering can be broken down into their component parts. That is, the speaker may have repeated the initial syllable of the word but also constricted the vocal tract at the level of the glottis, shifted his eyes to the side, and inserted the starter sound "ah" in order to postpone an upcoming feared word. It is essential that both the clinician and client be able to accurately identify the most subtle features of the client's fluency breaks before they can begin to systematically modify these aspects of the syndrome.

Eventually the client will be able to monitor his own speech production via both auditory and, perhaps more importantly, proprioceptive feedback. Auditory feedback provides some indication of the nature and quality of fluent speech, but proprioceptive feedback provides a more direct indication of the status of the vocal tract and both the accuracy and ease of articulatory movement. Proprioceptive feedback provides a better way to monitor the quality of fluency: the degree to which the speech is produced in an open, flowing, and effortless manner. It is a major step in treatment as the client becomes able—using, for example, delayed auditory feedback and articulatory and proprioceptive training—to heighten his ability to monitor proprioceptively.

The value of accurate self-monitoring is illustrated by two investigations that considered the effectiveness of treatment. Martin and Haroldson (1982) studied 20 adults who stuttered who were administered time-outs contingent on their stuttering moments during a behavioral-modification treatment program. All subjects showed significant reductions during treatment, but those who experienced *self-administered* time-outs showed significantly less extinction and significantly greater generalization than those who experienced only experimenter time-outs. Ingham (1982) investigated two adults who had failed to make progress in previous treatment. The subjects took part in a treatment program stressing the self-evaluation of performance. The subjects evaluated their own video recordings for percent stuttering and words spoken per minute. If they achieved prescribed targets for these behaviors, they were able to decrease making the recordings and evaluations. Both overt and covert assessments of their speaking behavior indicated that self-evaluation training was associated with substantially reduced stuttering for up to six months posttreatment.

Self-monitoring will continue to be a critical element of long-term success. Van Riper reported that his own stuttering increased in frequency (although not, he felt in severity) after an initial heart attack at age 65. He described "little sluggish prolongations" (1978) that mostly disappeared after his recovery. Following his retirement he again noticed an increase in the frequency and, occasionally, the severity of his stuttering. He found he was experiencing more frequent and longer tremors as well as some laryngeal blocks. Because these fluency breaks were surprising, he speculated that these changes were probably due to his lack of monitoring of his speech. He speculated that the hard work of closely monitoring his speech and "stuttering fluently" was no longer worth the effort.

During the initial stages of treatment, the client's monitoring is focused on the overt stuttering behavior. Although the focus early in treatment is on monitoring rather than the modification of stuttering events, as the speaker improves his ability to catch his behavior nearer to the initiation of the stuttering event, some instinctive and positive changes in the stuttering often take place. That is, the speaker will not only recognize what he is doing to make speaking difficult, he will begin to make some changes in his behavior. He may provide himself with some airflow, or he may slightly decrease a constriction in his vocal tract that will assist him in smoothing his speech. These changes are small and transient victories to be sure, but the clinician should look for them and reward these subtle changes in the form of stuttering. As Conture (1990) indicates, the client's consistent identification at the beginning or the middle of stuttering events sometimes become associated with his ability to change his stuttering behavior.

As treatment progresses, such self-monitoring activities continue to be pivotal for long-term progress outside the treatment environment. In addition, self-evaluation also comes to mean the monitoring of the cognitive aspects of change, such as the self-talk the client provides to himself prior to and following successful, as well as less-than-successful, speaking situations.

Increasing the Client's Ability to Produce "Open Speech"

Victories can be observed during every treatment session by the clinician and the client if close attention is paid to the *form* of the fluency breaks. Early in treatment the fluency breaks are typically characterized by a greater degree of vocal tract constriction and effort. As the speaker begins to understand the nature of his speech production system and becomes able to modify moments of stuttering, progress can be observed in the form of greater airflow, increased smoothness, and blending of the sounds and words. Perhaps most importantly, he begins to produce speech with less vocal and articulatory effort. As he becomes able to monitor his production, especially via proprioceptive feedback, he will be able to appreciate the difference between the tension and constriction of his old way of speaking and the new flowing and effortless production using an open vocal tract. The speaker as well as the listener can hear the increased openness and ease of such speech movements. At each such occurrence of enhanced airflow and smoothness of articulatory movement, there is the opportunity for the clinician to reward the progress. The client's speech may not be completely fluent, but the changes are obvious and satisfying. The result is a much easier form of stuttering. As Conture (1990) suggests, a shortening in the duration of stuttering (even though the frequency may not change) is a sign of progress. The client is stuttering, to be sure, but it is speech that is produced with less effort and is much easier to listen to. Certainly this new form of speech is not the old helpless, reflexive stuttering. It is a clear indication of progress.

Decreasing the Frequency and Duration of Motoric Fluency Breaks

Decreasing the frequency of motoric fluency breaks is an obvious goal of treatment and a commonly used indicator of progress. As the speech becomes more open and flowing, both the frequency and especially the duration of stuttering moments should show some obvious change. It may be that the frequency of brief stuttering events may even increase somewhat if the speaker is successful in changing his patterns of avoidance and word substitution. However, if the duration and associated tension—in terms of both the degree and the sites of physical tension—decreases, real progress is being accomplished. Again, this progress will be more likely to be recognized by the speaker if self-monitoring is maintained.

Bloodstein (1987) suggests that successful treatment should result in speech that sounds not only natural but also spontaneous, and that subjects should be free of the need to monitor their speech. St. Louis and

Westbrook (1987) suggest that clients should be free from stuttering before being dismissed from treatment. Whether it is realistic to expect adults who have stuttered for most of their lives to be completely fluent before being dismissed from formal treatment is questionable. While it is possible that this level of nonmonitored fluency may be a realistic goal for some clients, it is not often the case for the typical adult developmental stutterer. Obviously, there should be relatively few stuttering moments as formal treatment is concluded, but there are still likely to be occasions where some form of stuttering takes place. It may take the form of either overt stuttering or, even more likely, unstable stuttering that is just under the surface. There may also continue to be some degree of avoidance and word substitution. These responses to the possibility of stuttering are extremely powerful and overlearned. They will not simply go away in response to a few months or even years of treatment. In addition, there are likely to be several attitudinal and cognitive aspects of the syndrome still operating.

A decrease in the number of stuttering moments is a sign of progress to be sure. More important than immediate changes in frequency, however, are changes in the form of the stuttering moments. Early in the change process, changes toward easier and open stuttering reflect the ability of the speaker to both monitor and self-manage his speech. He is gradually beginning to take charge of previously uncontrollable behavior. Underlying the successes of these surface changes is the management of the cognitive and affective aspects of the syndrome. As the speaker becomes able to take charge of his speech during these events, which previously were associated with fear and helplessness, he comes to see that there are alternatives other than struggling with the old, maladaptive behaviors and ways of thinking about the experience. As the techniques of fluency modification become practiced in gradually more stressful speaking situations, the success expands and self-efficacy will gradually increase. If these techniques are practiced by the client between formal treatment sessions, they tend to become automatic in the presence of stress. However, it takes *overpractice* to achieve such automaticity. Authorities in the area of motor learning suggest that even basic motor skills do not begin to become habituated until they are performed 2500 to 3000 times. As we mentioned in Chapter 1 when discussing the value of clinicians practicing their craft, experience gained by the client as he appreciates his success and understands the nature of his failures will lead to invaluable learning. The motivation, dedication, and persistence necessary for continued change sets the stage for that knowledge.

Any moderately complex behavior requires much repetition in order for mastering skills, especially when there are elements of time pressure and fear. A final example involves learning another activity that also possesses elements of balance, possible loss of control, and even anxiety or fear—much like Brad's story of rock climbing in Chapter 8. Although the following description is about learning to paddle a kayak in white water, with very few changes, it could easily be about learning to rely on therapeutic techniques outside of the clinic. Clinicians can use a variety of such speech or non-speech examples in order to demonstrate their understanding of the demands faced by clients as they practice their therapy techniques.

As a result of much practice and persistence, persons who stutter can succeed both in and out of treatment. The speaker gains ability and confidence, and he is more likely to successfully repair his mistakes in the stream of speech. He begins to realize that he is not helpless. He comes to understand that it is possible for him to be able to count on and successfully use well-practiced responses to previously

---

CLINICAL INSIGHT

One of our teenage clients who was beginning to realize how much he was going to have to practice his treatment techniques brought this story back to the group therapy session when he returned from a skiing trip to Colorado. He had been watching people learning to negotiate a hill with a series of mogals and wondered out loud to a nearby instructor how long it would take to master such a difficult section. The instructor responded by saying, "Well, if you practiced every day for about six hours and you did that for about six months you would be pretty good. But you still wouldn't master it." Only after hearing that did the client fully appreciate how much he was going to have to practice so that he would become "pretty good" at using his therapy techniques.

Another story about the degree of practice and overlearning that must take place in order to master difficult and complex activities was related by Daly (1999). He described how every spring he and his friends charter a sailboat and spend a week on the Chesapeake Bay. One year one of his friends wasn't able to come along and another person took his place. The new fellow happened to be a professional oboe player. Each morning he would come up on deck and practice his oboe. His playing was enjoyable for everyone but eventually one of the crew members asked him why he continued to practice even though he was on a vacation. He responded by saying, "If I didn't practice for one day, I would know it. If I didn't practice for two days, the oboe section would know it. And if I didn't practice for three days, the entire orchestra would know it."

🔍 **CLINICAL INSIGHT**

Kayaking in white water requires a high level of balance and confidence. It is easy to lose control, finding yourself under the surface of the water and in a threatening situation. In the beginning stages of learning to kayak, anxiety and fear are often present. Complicating the situation is the fact that the novice tends to be rigid and inflexible, especially as the stress associated with a series of difficult rapids approaches. The likelihood of a mistake is high. However, with continued practice, the paddler's skill increases. Progress is seen as the paddler's strokes become integrated and blended together. A crucial step takes place when the person learns to repair a mistake by rolling back to the surface.

Learning to roll a kayak takes considerable practice. It is best to begin in the safe confines of a pool or lake. The paddlers practice first with the assistance of an instructor, and then by themselves. The instructor explains the rationale and details of the rolling technique, and, together, the instructor and the paddler go over the sequence of events that must take place if the roll is to be successful. The techniques are done deliberately and slowly, in a preplanned manner by setting up in the ideal roll position. With the assistance of the instructor, the paddler learns to roll to both the left and the right, to roll with the kayak filled with water, and to roll without a paddle using only the arms and an associated hip snap. Eventually, the paddler learns to roll without first setting up in a roll position in order to approximate the unexpected situations found on the river. Finally, it is time to move from the safety of the flat water to the unpredictable tumult of the river.

Depending on such factors as water temperature, turbulence, and obstacles that appear in the boater's path, the first attempts of the paddler to roll in a moving stream are not likely to be successful. The likelihood of success decreases dramatically when the stresses of time pressure, distraction, and especially fear enter the picture. The paddler's initial reaction to being upside down for the first time in white water is apt to be similar to the first experience of being upside down in flat water: one of fear, or even panic. The techniques that worked so well in the safety of the pool are quickly forgotten and the first reaction of the paddler is to exit the boat and swim to the surface. It is not until the paddler is able to overlearn the techniques that they can be counted on. The techniques must be practiced to the point that they are automatic and the paddler does not have to think about them. If the paddler takes time to think, what he will think about is how scared he is.

As the paddler learns to react to the situations on the river in this manner, positive things begin to occur. Confidence builds and paddling skills

---

🔍 **CLINICAL INSIGHT** (CONTINUED)

increase geometrically. The person becomes more flexible and begins to adopt a style of working with, rather than against, the power of the water. If a mistake is made, the person will repair it by getting back to the surface and achieving control. The person will begin to experiment and play with different new techniques, intentionally entering difficult sections of the river. The paddler gradually becomes less rigid, paddling with greater flexibility. Because he is more flexible, the paddler and the boat are able to absorb the impacts that previously had such a profound influence on their progress. The paddler gradually gains confidence in his ability to correct errors and thus, is less concerned about making them. Fewer mistakes are made. After a time, the person begins looking around for more challenging rapids to paddle and new rivers to navigate.

---

feared situations, to manipulate and play with possibilities within the turmoil of the stuttering moment. Moreover, he is free to move ahead and achieve new success in increasingly more difficult speaking situations.

For the adult who as been stuttering for many years, practice with therapy techniques must take place for many months and years before the techniques will become functional. Furthermore, it may be that continued practice and learning over time results in "remodeling" of the central nervous system as described in Chapter 2. Those individuals who have relatively few factors predisposing them for nonfluent speech production and are also fortunate enough to be able to practice treatment techniques to the point where they are mastered, may be those speakers who are able to achieve spontaneous or automatic fluency.

Increasing the Frequency of Formulative Fluency Breaks

Nearly all clinicians would agree that progress during treatment is reflected by decreases in the occurrence of motoric fluency breaks. However, as Goldman-Eisler (1961) and Starkweather (1987) have indicated, fluency breaks are an important aspect of normal speech formulation. Adults who stutter, while they obviously produce more motoric fluency breaks, also demonstrate significantly fewer formulative fluency breaks (Manning & Monte, 1981). If speech is to be normalized for people who stutter, one important aspect of that process, aside from a decrease in motoric breaks, may well be an increase to near-normal levels of formulative fluency breaks (Manning & Monte, 1981).

As the speaker in treatment experiences fewer motoric fluency breaks, there are fewer pauses and fewer opportunities for him to consider alternative ways of expressing what he wants to say. In order to have an opportunity to formulate his ideas, he may need to include some formulative breaks in order to express himself. As with normal speakers, the breaks provide the chance to organize and reorganize his thoughts. Many speakers who stutter will be unwilling to voluntarily stop to use a formulative fluency break because they fear that beginning speech again may precipitate another moment of stuttering. Accordingly, if treatment has been successful, the speaker will be more likely to make use of formulative breaks, being less concerned about his ability to continue once he has organized his thoughts. He does not have to be concerned about pauses, especially pauses that allow the formulation of thought. Because many clients have not had the opportunity to practice using formulative breaks for formulating speech, during the later stages of treatment it may be helpful for them to practice sequencing or branching activities. It is an opportunity to speak "without putting on the brakes" and to free-associate. Once a reasonably high degree of fluency is achieved, the client needs to practice speaking in a less inhibited manner, slowly freeing himself from scanning ahead for feared words and pretasting feared sounds.

Even for those speakers who demonstrate a nearly total absence of stuttering moments in all speaking situations, investigators have shown that many are not necessarily perceived as normal (Ingham & Onslow, 1985; Onslow & Ingham, 1987; Runyan, Hames, & Proseck, 1982; Sacco, Metz, & Schiavetti, 1992). One reason for the unnaturalness of such post-treatment speech may be the lack of normal, effortless, formulative breaks. Manning and Monte (1981) suggested the possible prognostic value of promoting an *increase* in the number of formulative fluency breaks as one way to determine the stability of fluency. Given the presence of formulative breaks even in accomplished adult speakers, a lack of these breaks suggests something other than normal fluency. Although there are no data yet available to support this suggestion, it may be that the increase of formulative fluency breaks to near-normal levels may be one of the surface behaviors that could be used to predict relapse.

Increasing the Naturalness of Fluent Speech

As described earlier, there are many aspects of change that indicate success during formal treatment. One of these is the clinical research on speech naturalness that beginning in the late 1970s. The impetus for studying the speech naturalness of individuals treated for stuttering came from observations that many people who had undergone successful treatment using fluency-modification strategies continued to sound less than satisfactory. That is, although the frequency of stuttering had decreased dramatically, listeners found that many speakers continued to sound unnatural. Their speech was effortful, uncomfortable to listen to, and contained auditory or visual features that prevented the listener from fully attending to the content of the message. Despite an otherwise successful treatment experience, many speakers found that they were still regarded by themselves and others as having a problem (Schiavetti and Metz, 1997).

Development of a Naturalness Rating Scale

In an early attempt to investigate this effect, Ingham and Packman (1978) studied the normalcy of speech following treatment by comparing nine adolescents and adults who had undergone treatment with a prolonged speech procedure. These subjects were compared with nine normally fluent speakers matched for age and sex. The stuttering clients, seven males and two females, ranged in age from 13 to 24 years old. Listeners rated whether one-minute speech samples were either natural or unnatural. The authors found that the listeners' ratings of naturalness of the post-treatment clients were not significantly different from those of the normal speakers.

In 1984, Martin, Haroldson, and Triden began the development of a reliable scale for rating speech naturalness. The scale consisted of a nine-point Likert scale with 1 equivalent to highly natural-sounding speech and 9 equivalent to highly unnatural-sounding speech. This scale has been used in virtually all subsequent investigations of speech naturalness.

1	2	4	5	6	7	8	9
Highly Natural							Highly Unnatural

The original investigations by Martin, et al. did not provide listeners with a definition of naturalness and asked the listeners to "make your rating on how natural or unnatural the speech sounds to you" (p. 54). Subsequent studies have typically used identical or slightly altered instructions.

Martin, et al. had 30 listeners use the scale to assess the speech naturalness of 10 adults who stuttered (ages 20–53) speaking without delayed auditory feedback, 10 adults who stuttered (ages 20–51) speaking under delayed auditory feedback, and a group of 10 normal speaking adults (ages 21–45). They found that both groups of speakers who stuttered (those with and without delayed auditory feedback) sounded significantly less natural than the nonstuttering samples. The mean naturalness ratings for the speakers who stuttered (without delayed auditory feedback) was 6.52. The stuttering speakers under delayed auditory feedback received a naturalness rating of 5.84. The speech of the nonstuttering speakers (without delayed auditory feedback) received a score of 2.12. Based on interrater agreement and rater consistency, Martin, et al. concluded that observers are able to quantify speech naturalness.

Following the introduction of this scaling technique there was increased interest by a variety of researchers on this topic. Using the same nine-point scale, Ingham, Gow, and Costello (1985) studied the speech naturalness of 15 fluent speakers and 15 treated stutterers who had completed the initial phases of a prolonged speech treatment program. Listeners judged the stutterers' speech to be significantly more unnatural than the nonstutterers' speech. The listeners were also asked to identify whether or not the samples came from "normal speakers." Interestingly, listeners judged an equal amount of samples from both the stutterers and the nonstutterers to be from "normal speakers."

In a two-part investigation, Ingham and Onslow (1985) used the Martin, et al. nine-point scale for assessing the speech naturalness of clients during a treatment program. They conducted a two-part investigation in which they first described the speech naturalness of clients enrolled in a prolonged speech treatment program. The clients were adolescent speakers (3 males and 21 females) ranging from 10 to 14 years of age. One-minute speech samples taken at different phases of the treatment program (instatement, transfer, and maintenance phase) were presented to a practicing clinician. The clinician used the nine-point scale to rate naturalness. The speakers were all found to improve their speech naturalness, but not at the same rate.

Three of the subjects who took part in the first part of the study participated in a second study. These three speakers were chosen for a follow-up study based on their speech naturalness scores during the final stages of the instatement phase of treatment. All three subjects had a speech naturalness score of 4 or higher. Each of these subjects spoke spontaneously while maintaining a targeted speaking rate. Every 15 seconds, a clinician made a naturalness rating of between 1 and 9. The ratings were displayed so that the speaker could see them. The subjects were told that they would be given their naturalness rating score at the end of a five-minute period. The results indicated that feedback to the speakers about their ratings resulted in an improvement in the speech naturalness ratings.

Onslow, Adams, and Ingham (1992) considered the reliability of the nine-point scale in a clinical situation. Their intent was (1) to determine the reliability of listeners' repeated ratings of one subject's speech, (2) to compare the reliability of sophisticated and unsophisticated judges' speech naturalness, and (3) to evaluate the influence of the duration of the speech sample. Speech samples were obtained from 10 adults and adolescents who were receiving treatment in a prolonged speech program. The listeners were 30 sophisticated and 30 unsophisticated judges. Subgroups of listeners rated speech samples of 15, 30, or 60 seconds in duration. The results indicated that the judges were inconsistent in their ratings, suggesting that procedures for rating naturalness need to be developed. There were no important differences between sophisticated and unsophisticated raters. Ratings made for 30 and 60 seconds resulted in the highest agreement and intraclass correlations.

The Effect of Feedback

Ingham, Martin, Haroldson, Onslow, and Leney (1985) considered the effect of feedback on the improvement of speech naturalness. In this case, the subjects were six males who stuttered between the ages of 16 and 55. The speakers had either never received treatment or had not received treatment for the past two years. The subjects varied widely in their frequency of stuttering and history of treatment. Each subject spoke spontaneously while being monitored by two clinicians. One clinician counted stuttered and nonstuttered syllables, while the other clinician evaluated the speaker using the none-point naturalness scale. Every 30 seconds, the clinician displayed the naturalness rating for the subject to see. Each subject was instructed to keep the naturalness ratings low and to sound as natural as possible. The speakers were not told, however, how to accomplish this task. The results indicated that five of the six subjects showed some improvement in their speech naturalness scores while also increasing fluency.

Ingham, Ingham, Onslow, and Finn (1989) were interested in how naturalness felt and sounded to the speaker, and thus considered the effects of instructions to clients to rate and change their own speech naturalness. Three males between the age of 22 and 30, who were currently in a stuttering treatment program, volunteered for this study. Two experimenters listened to each subject as he spoke for five minutes during a series of two- to four-hour sessions. One experimenter counted stuttered and nonstuttered syllables, while the other experimenter made naturalness ratings of between 1 and 9 every 30 seconds. The clients also rated their own speech naturalness.

The results indicated that when the clients were asked to make their speech sound more unnatural, both the subjects' and judges' ratings were similar. When the clients were asked to improve their speech naturalness ratings, they judged their speech to be more natural, but the judges did not note the same improvements. Differences in the clients' and judges' speech naturalness ratings suggested that clients are able to recognize features of their naturalness better than listeners. The authors suspected that the two groups of listeners were using different criteria for making the judgment of speech naturalness. The clients indicated that they listened for unusual prolongations or prosody in their speech to help them rate their naturalness.

Finn and Ingham (1994) also studied stutterers' self-ratings of naturalness. They found, as did Ingham, et al. (1989), that adult stuttering speakers produce rather reliable self-ratings of speech naturalness, particularly when they listened to previously recorded speech samples. The speakers were also able to consistently differentiate between how natural their speech felt and sounded.

Runyan, Bell, and Proseck (1990) considered whether there was a difference between the speech naturalness of nonstutterers and clients who had been successfully treated in six different treatment programs. They investigated whether the identification of stuttering was related to speech naturalness. Finally, they considered if pretreatment severity (mild, moderate, or severe) was related to posttreatment naturalness scores.

Tape-recorded samples of speech from treated clients (280 samples) and normal speakers were used. The recorded samples were the same as those described by Runyan and Adams (1978). The clinicians who supplied the speech samples also supplied the pretreatment severity ratings of these subjects. The different clients had participated in a variety of different treatment programs (Van Riperian, metronome-conditioned speech retraining, delayed auditory feedback, operant conditioning, precision fluency shaping, or holistic treatment). Ten graduate students in speech-language pathology who had received training in fluency and fluency disorders served as judges. These listeners identified whether each speech sample was from a client or nonstutterer. Once this was decided, they again listened to the sample and rated each speaker's naturalness using Martin, Haroldson, & Triden's (1984) nine-point scale. Listener responses were examined and speech samples were divided into two groups: easily identified and treated, or difficult-to-identify, clients.

The results indicated that significant differences were found between speech naturalness ratings of treated clients and fluent speakers. Listeners judged the treated clients' speech as being more unnatural than that of normal speakers. Moreover, (the difficult-to-identify clients were rated as sounding significantly more natural than the easily identified clients ($p < .003$). The difficult-to-identify clients' mean speech naturalness score (2.38) was not significantly different from the normal speakers' mean score (2.79). Finally, the authors found that posttreatment naturalness ratings of all clients were similar despite differences in pretreatment severity ratings. Posttreatment scores were 4.26 for subjects judged to be mild, 3.82 for subjects judged to be moderate, and 3.68 for subjects judged to be severe.

Onslow, Hayes, Hutchings, and Newman (1992) also considered the effect of pretreatment severity on both pre- and posttreatment naturalness ratings. Thirty-six subjects between 9 and 50 years of age (mean of 21 years) were studied. Fifteen listeners rated the naturalness of a 30-second speech sample from each subject. The results indicated that the most severe clients prior to treatment had naturalness scores that were more than two values higher (less natural) than the least severe clients. These results differed from those of Runyan, Bell, and Prosek (1990), who found similar posttreatment speech naturalness rating of all speakers, regardless of pretreatment severity.

Acoustic Features of Speech Naturalness

Metz, Schiavetti, and Sacco (1990) examined the speech of nonstutterers and treated clients for acoustic features related to naturalness. Twenty clients (15 males and 5 females) were seen following treatment. These were adolescent subjects ranging in age from 9 to 20 years old with a mean age of 14.5 years. Using the Stuttering Severity Instrument (SSI) (Riley, 1972) prior to treatment, 7 subjects were rated as moderately severe, 11 were rated as severe, and 2 were determined to be very severe. Twenty nonstuttering subjects were matched with the stuttering speakers for the factors of sex and age (within one year). Subjects read a passage and described a picture.

Results indicated that the clients to stuttered were perceived as sounding more unnatural than the speakers who did not. This was true for both the read and spontaneous speech samples. Voice onset time (VOT) and sentence duration were found to be significantly related to—and predictive of—speech naturalness, with the VOT values being most predictive of naturalness during spontaneous speech. Sentence duration was the primary predictor of naturalness during reading.

The Effect of Speaking Task

Nearly all investigations of speech naturalness have used monologue speech or some combination of monologue and oral reading. Some were not specific concerning the speech task. Onslow, Adams, and Ingham (1992) first studied the effect of speaking task by comparing the influence of monologue and conversational speech. Subjects were seven males ranging in age from 14 to 36 years (average age of 21) who had received treatment. The subjects were matched in age (within six months) with seven nonstuttering male speakers.

All subjects were recorded during conversation and monologue on three different occasions. Ninety-six speech samples were selected for analysis by listeners. Using the nine-point scale developed by Martin et al.

(1984), a group of 29 undergraduate university students assigned naturalness scores. The results showed no significant differences in the naturalness scores of conversation or monologue for either the speakers who stuttered or those that did not. The results confirmed the external validity of previous studies that were based only on monologue speech or failed to make the speech task clear.

Audio and Video Samples

All of the studies discussed thus far used audio recordings of speech samples. There are, of course, many visual components of stuttering that are related to judgments of speech naturalness in the everyday world. In a first attempt to distinguish possible visual components, Martin and Haroldson (1992) studied six male and four female speakers who stuttered (ages 20–62) and six male and four female fluent speakers (ages 21–64). Twenty-four undergraduate college students made speech naturalness ratings of one-minute speech samples. Using the nine-point scale, subjects rated both audio and audiovisual speech samples. Another group of 30 undergraduate students rated stuttering *severity* of the stuttered speech samples. Stuttering severity was also rated using a nine-point scale, with 1 representing very mild stuttering and 9 representing very severe stuttering.

The results indicated that the naturalness judgments of nonstuttering speakers were not significantly different for audio and audiovisual samples (2.30 and 2.27, respectively). However, for the subjects who stuttered, audiovisual samples were consistently judged as being more unnatural than audio only samples (6.81 and 6.04, respectively). The rating of stuttering severity influenced the naturalness ratings. These results may have been influenced by the fact that the speech samples of the stuttering subjects in this study were not stutter free with stuttered words averaging 17.4%.

Kalinowski, Nobel, Armson, and Stuart (1994) determined the pre- and posttreatment speech naturalness of five adult speakers with relatively few syllables stuttered (0–4%) clients and five adult speakers with more syllables stuttered (23% or greater). Sixty-four naive listeners (32 male and 32 female college students) rated these adult male speakers using the Martin et al. nine-point scale. The listeners rated both pre- and posttreatment one-minute videotape recordings of conversational speech. All subjects had taken part in the Precision Fluency Shaping Program (Webster, 1975) and, at the completion of formal treatment, were either nearly or completely stutter-free. However, despite the posttreatment reduction in the frequency of stuttering for mild as well as severe subjects, both groups of speakers were rated as being significantly more unnatural sounding (higher scores on the naturalness scale) following treatment. In addition, the five subjects with severe pretreatment stuttering were rated with significantly less natural than those with mild stuttering. These findings coincide with those of Franken, Boves, Peters, and Webster (1992), who found that the naturalness scores of 32 clients with severe stuttering who underwent fluency shaping treatment remained unchanged from pretreatment to posttreatment. That is, while it is to be expected that severe stuttering is likely to result in listener judgments of highly unnatural speech, increased fluency that is produced in an effortful and carefully controlled manner will also be judged as unnatural. These findings coincide with Starkweather's (1992) suggestion that even with increased fluency, some therapy procedures often tend to diminish the quality of a person's speech.

In summary, the naturalness of speech is becoming recognized as an important consideration in determining the success of treatment. The scale developed by Martin, Haroldson, and Triden's appears to be reliable for either oral reading or spontaneous speech. Some (but not all) clients improve their speech naturalness as a result of treatment and do so at their own rate. Speakers who differ on naturalness ratings at the outset of treatment may be rated much the same after treatment, although pre- and posttreatment severity ratings influence judgments of naturalness. Moreover, feedback appears to enhance the speaker's ability to improve naturalness, although listeners and clients may have different criteria for determining naturalness. Listeners tend to evaluate an audio recording of a speaker as being more natural than when both audio and visual signals are presented. Lastly, voice onset time and sentence duration have been suggested as important acoustic features of speech naturalness.

Although several studies have included adolescents (Ingham & Onslow, 1985; Ingham & Packman, 1978; Metz, Schiavetti, & Sacco, 1990; Onslow, Adams, & Ingham, 1992; Onslow, Hayes, Hutchins, & Newman, 1992), there are no naturalness data concerning children who stutter. In addition, there may be other acoustic features that could be considered beyond voice onset time and sentence duration, such as formant transition measures (particularly the second formant), that have been found to be useful in predicting the status of other (nonstuttering) speakers.

In their review of the issues inherent in measuring speech naturalness, Schiaveti and Metz (1997) provide an extensive list of future questions that can be addressed. It may be that a comparison of internal (listeners decide) and external (predetermined) standards would result in the adoption of external standards that would add consistency to the criteria used to make such judgments. Defining naturalness for listeners would allow for training and result in greater consistency across studies and very likely provide more useful clinical and research measurements. In addition, it would also be useful to understand the criteria for judging speech naturalness that are used by experienced (professional) and inexperienced (naïve) listeners. They also suggest the possible use of alternative scaling procedures, such as sensory modality matching, absolute magnitude estimation, or "natural measurement," which have been used to validate several social opinion variables that are similar to judgments of speech naturalness (p. 409). There is a need to understand how physiological and acoustic characteristics of speech make speaking sound and feel natural. What, for example, are the visual characteristics of unnaturalness? Finally, they suggest that answers to these questions may better explain posttreatment speech patterns and help predict relapse: Are there parameters of unnaturalness that are not tolerated by some clients and invite relapse?

The research on speech naturalness indicates that the goal of treatment is considerably more complex than assisting clients to decrease the frequency of stuttering. Some moments of stuttering are not likely to detract from a speaker's naturalness and spontaneity, particularly if these breaks are smooth and relatively effortless. Clinicians who understand the importance of these smooth breaks are most likely to appreciate this change. However, the research suggests that even naïve listeners may prefer speech with fluency breaks in contrast to unnatural-sounding and highly controlled speech devoid of all fluency disruptions.

There is a wide range of performance that is possible, but fluency without ease of listening represents something short of a complete therapeutic success. If the client's nonstuttered speech is something less than fluent—if it sounds unnatural or if the fluency is tenuous—this may also be one of the surface behaviors with some value in forecasting relapse. If a person's fluent but unnatural speech continues to elicit negative response from listeners, it may be that clients will soon grow tired of the practice necessary to maintain their new and unnatural speech and return to their original and familiar form of stuttering. Adams and Runyan (1981) state that the client who is ready for dismissal should have speech that is objectively and perceptively indistinguishable from that of normal speakers. The client's speech should not only be free of stuttering but should be produced at an acceptable rate, sound natural, and be free of perceptible signs of *tenuous* fluency. Some speakers, after several years of experience, may be able to achieve spontaneous fluency. However, as suggested earlier in this chapter, these are lofty and perhaps unrealistic goals for many adults who stutter (although not necessarily for younger children). Nonetheless, such changes in speech naturalness should certainly be viewed as important signs of progress.

Metalinguistic Changes

The language a person uses to describe his situation provides important clues about who he is and where he is going. The way a person depicts his situation or problem often indicates important signs of progress during treatment. Moreover, as described in Chapter 7 in our discussion of cognitive restructuring approaches to counseling and treatment, by changing the way we describe a problem, we can often change the problem itself. The client's language will reflect his level of "stuckness" and degree to which he is able to assume responsibility for his choices and his world.

As people progress through effective treatment, they begin to think and talk differently about themselves and their speech. The intrinsic features of affective and cognitive change are reflected in the words the client uses to describe himself, his speech, and his interactions with others. How the client talks about himself and his speech provides a window for viewing these intrinsic features.

Early in treatment the client typically feels helpless. He believes he is unable to do much to change his speech or himself. There is a high degree of mystery associated with stuttering. He may say such things as "When *it* happens I feel helpless," or "When I'm in a block I feel lost and I don't know what to do." As treatment progresses, clients slowly begin to develop the "language of fluency" (Blodgett & Cooper, 1988; Cooper & Cooper, 1985), as well as use more appropriate self-talk (Daly, 1986; Emerick, 1988; Maxwell, 1982). As the client begins to successfully change his previously uncontrollable behavior, he will begin to change the way he observes himself and his speech. Moreover, he will begin to describe his behavior and actions in more objective, specific, and realistic ways. The client will begin to interpret stuttering as something that he is *doing* rather than something that is happening to him. He will begin to say such things as:

> When I stutter, sometimes I stop the airflow at the vocal folds. I was able to change the way I repeated that syllable into a smoother and easier way of stuttering. Even though that was a difficult telephone call, I was able to make the call and successfully achieve most of my fluency targets.

These metalinguistic changes provide the clinician with important evidence of change and indicate that the client is beginning to take charge of the problem. Such utterances may be used as a way to monitor cognitive change, or—in some cases—the clinician can take a more active role and point out to the client how he is describing himself and his problem. It may be possible for the client to begin talking about his problem in a different way in order to, in turn, facilitate new and better ways of thinking about himself and his speech (Daly, 1986; Emerick, 1988; Maxwell, 1982). The client's language will reflect some degree of liberation from their problem. That is, coinciding with the fact that the speaker shows a greater degree of fluency, they are more liberated in terms of their choices and have a greater involvement in life. One adult female client related how she approached a feared speaking situation she had previously avoided. Afterwards she related to her clinician that "I stuttered as much as I always have but this time I didn't feel ashamed." As discussed in Chapter 6, facilitating these cognitive changes is similar to the cognitive-restructuring activities, as advocated by several others in the field of fluency disorders (Curlee, 1984; Fransella, 1972; Hayhow & Levy, 1989; Johnson, 1946; Kuhr & Rustin, 1985; Williams, 1979; Williams, 1995).

Increasing Open Decision-Making

Coinciding with the client's gradual reinterpretation of himself and his speech is his increasing ability to make choices that are based on information other than the possibility of stuttering. The client begins to open his focus beyond the influence of stuttering and consider other, more expansive, possibilities and options. With this wider focus comes the adjustment to new responsibilities and challenges. Furthermore, once a new way of viewing life becomes available to the client, he has the obligation—if he is to be true to himself—to act on this new information. If his hard-won progress is to continue, he must make new choices and accept new challenges. There will be many opportunities for open decision-making during daily work and social activities. Years of avoidance and less-than-complete interpersonal involvement will gradually change. However, it is important for the clinician as well as the client to recognize that what is changing is not only the surface behavior of the client's speech but a way of living. One of our clients recently described how her increased confidence in her ability to use stuttering modification techniques has transferred to other aspects of her life such as competition for job positions, performance during music recitals, and social interaction in general.

Decreased Avoidance

As avoidance decreases, the frequency of fluency breaks may increase. Early in treatment, less avoidance and greater participation in speaking activities may yield a slight increase in the frequency of stuttering. There may even be an increase in the duration and tension of stuttering events. Although these changes may not be pleasant to the client, if a stuttering-modification strategy is being used, they can be viewed as progress within the context of the overall treatment process. The good news is that decreased avoidance translates directly into decreased handicap. Taking part in (speaking) activities and making better choices may not be the first step for each client, but it is always a critical step. Furthermore, a decrease in avoidance behavior permits the client to go directly at the problem and the associated fear. It is not simply the stuttering that composes the problem, but uncontrolled and helpless stuttering. As experienced clinicians have pointed out for decades, much of the handicapping effect of stuttering is the result of maladaptive efforts to avoid any type of overt stuttering. A temporary increase in the frequency and duration of stuttering may be viewed as a small and often necessary price to pay for increased approach behavior and assertiveness.

Increased (Speech) Assertiveness

With a decrease in avoidance behavior, there is likely to be a corresponding increase in overall assertiveness. In reality, being more assertive about one's speaking behavior is likely to translate into increased assertiveness in general. There may be changes in roles and relationships as the person no longer plays the primary role of a stutterer (Sheehan, 1970). It is a distinctive indicator of progress when the speaker begins to decrease his reflexive self-censorship and beings to consider many speaking situations he once considered unimaginable. This is not to say that he will now take part in these situations with ease or idyllic fluency, but choosing to take part nonetheless and to consider new opportunities is a significant measure of progress.

Increased Risk-Taking

Closely associated to an increase in speech assertiveness is an increase in risk-taking. Just as an athlete, in order to improve his skills, reaches to the edge of his ability (or sometimes, for a moment, just beyond), the speaker is extending the envelope of his experience and performance. Each time the client extends himself into positions of responsibility for organizing social or work-related activities, he is expanding his world. He is risking failure, of course, and sometimes degrees of failure will occur. Taking on these challenges is more indicative of progress for some clients than others. However, for many clients, this expansion of risk-taking activities provides evidence of the cognitive changes that are part of long-term success.

Improved Self-Concept, Improved Self-Esteem, and Role Changes

Self-concept and self-esteem have been referred to many times in the literature on fluency disorders. According to Peck (1978), self-esteem is the cornerstone of psychological change. Although persons who stutter have not been found to have a unique self-concept or to be lacking in self-esteem, this concept has frequently been mentioned as an aspect of treatment programs (Van Riper, 1973, pp. 364–367).

Self-esteem is not something that can be given to you. Nonetheless, the stage can be set by loving parents and friends as well as by a competent clinician. As the clinician provides a secure and stable therapeutic environment, growth will be likely to occur. When the client experiences success in the self-management of surface and intrinsic aspects of his fluency disorder, self-esteem and the self-concept begin to shift in a positive

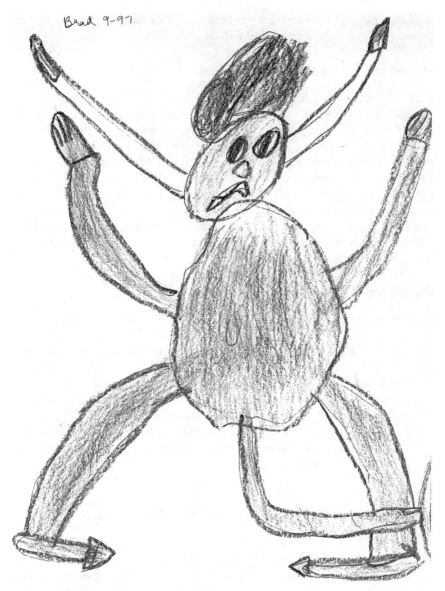

Brad 9-97

Figure 10-5. Brad's picture of the "stuttering monster."

direction. This is certainly the case with children who are still in the process of developing their self concept. Of course, this is a major reason why intervention for fluency problems is much more likely to result in long-term success with this group of clients. The drawings by Brad, age 10, provide a clear description of how he sees his stuttering block (Figure 10-5) and his view of the treatment experience (Figure 10-6). Carol, age 6,

Brad Age 10

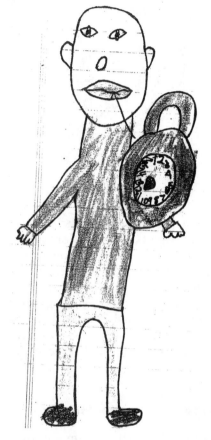

my lips are locked
up. I'm stuttering.
The lock has a
combination to open
it. And the combination
is to use tools and
practice.

Figure 10-6. Brad's picture of treatment for stuttering.

is able to indicate her feelings about herself before and after three months of successful therapy, including how to deal with teasing (Figure 10-7). Adults are also able to make big changes that are reflected in a changed view of themselves during and following treatment. They are able to redefine themselves and create an altered paradigm of their lives. Such changes can be quantified by self-reports during individual and group treatment sessions as well as by measures such as the locus of control (Kuhr & Rustin, 1985).

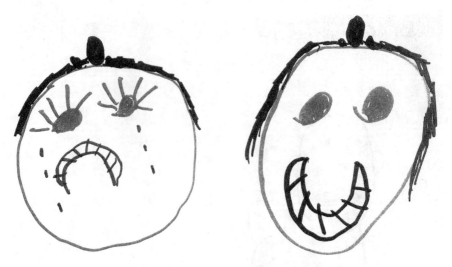

Figure 10-7. Carol's self-drawing before and after three months of treatment.

Success also can be observed through the reports of others in the speaker's environment, such as teachers, parents, a spouse, or friends, who indicate to the client or the clinician the changes both in fluency and participation in activities. For example, Conture (1990) indicates that early signs of improvement often take the form of others' reporting that they are noticing an improvement in speech or related behavior. These reports may appear spontaneously or may be elicited from those in the client's environment who are able to provide candid feedback. This feedback should be taken seriously and regarded as a valid indicator of change.

Increased Distancing and Objectivity Through Humor

With the client's development of greater objectivity, self-monitoring, and modification abilities, he learns to generate the ability to back up and distance himself from his problem. Such cognitive change may be reflected in the presence of humor. As discussed in Chapter 1, in most cases the clinician must lead the way in identifying and appreciating the humorous aspects of the situation, providing the "new eyes" for viewing this old problem. However, once the process has been initiated, surprising results often occur. A different view often occurs during group treatment sessions, where one humorous story by a client often leads to a change in perspective by others. The question "What humorous thing occurred this week because of your stuttering?" may elicit incredulous looks from new members of the group. Experienced members, however, often provide wonderfully humorous stories that—more often than not—allow the new members of the group to summon equally amusing stories from their past. With the distance afforded by the passage of time, the client is able to release the damaging effects of the experience and see the incident with new eyes. The entire group can share the experience and participate in a new interpretation of an old predicament. Along with the examples found in Chapter 1, here are two additional examples of the many stories we have heard over the years.

The various types of listener reactions, from mildly inappropriate to obviously patronizing, can be painful to endure at the moment they occur, but they lose some of their bite when distance and objectivity are applied to the wound. Taking a humorous perspective can be a healthy way to deal with these events. The ability of the clients to adjust such situations with humor can provide the clinician with a way to gauge progress in terms of objectivity, distancing, and mastery.

CLINICAL INSIGHT

Related to changes in self-concept is the possibility of viewing stuttering less as a problem and more as a gift. A few years ago during a professional meeting in San Antonio, my wife and I were having dinner with a group of about 10 people. As I looked at everyone around the table, I thought about how much I enjoyed being with these people. I mentioned to them that had I never stuttered I would never have met a single one of them and would not be with them at this wonderful place. Three other people at the table who also had a history of stuttering agreed that our being together was a wonderful example of how our stuttering could truly be thought of as a gift. Diverse people in stuttering support groups come together and develop life-long friendships that never would have occurred otherwise. Often, people who stutter develop a sensitivity and understanding for others and their problems that may not have occurred. Working to achieve fluent speech often results in an understanding of what a grand experience it is to produce smooth and easy speech, something that most everyone takes for granted. Of course, no one would choose stuttering as a personal characteristic or think of it as a gift at the outset. But, in fact, it can become one depending on how we interpret our situation.

CRITERIA FOR THE TERMINATION OF FORMAL TREATMENT

There are few guidelines concerning the termination of formal treatment. For children the decision may be clearer. Once the child is able to maintain easy, fluent speech in a variety of situations at home and in school for several months, the decision to conclude treatment is reasonable.

For adults the issue is more complex. After all, the adult who stutters has had extensive practice, and the behavioral and cognitive aspects are resistant to change. If the process of change for adults is viewed as a continuum of formal-informal treatment, it will never be quite complete. Van Riper (1973) provided guidelines for terminating treatment. He suggested, for example, that if the client becomes bored and unexcited about treatment or even about maintaining fluency, it may be time to terminate formal treatment. Certainly it is better to anticipate the end of treatment and to schedule a final exit meeting or two rather than have the client simply cease attending. Such lack of closure leaves the clinician feeling at a loss about the final outcome.

Discussing the criteria for termination from the outset of treatment is one solution to this dilemma. It is probably never too soon for the clinician to begin asking the client to address the issue of termination. Often

---

🔍 CLINICAL INSIGHT

James, a middle-aged man, had attended therapy for only a short time but was already considerably desensitized to his stuttering. One day during group therapy, he related how, during his college years, he had eventually worked up the courage to call a young woman he had noticed in one of his classes for a date. He rarely used the telephone and never had telephoned a woman's dormitory before. [Note: Although it may be difficult for today's readers to appreciate this, in those days there was only a single telephone located in the hallway of each floor of the woman's dorm.] The coed James wanted to call was named Harriet, and rather than risk saying an entire sentence such as "May I speak to Harriet?" he decided to simply say "Harriet?" to whoever happened to answer the telephone. He dialed the dormitory and the telephone began ringing. After a few moments, a woman came to the phone and answered it. James froze, and the very best he could do was produce a series of breathy sounds as he kept repeating the initial "H" of Harriet's name. After this went on for several seconds, he heard the coed partially cover the phone and announce to the other women in the hall, "It's him again!"

the client will respond with, "You're the expert, you tell me." Of course, the clinician is the expert about fluency disorders in a generic sense, but the client must become an expert about his own situation and therapy goals. Requesting him to operationally define when he will be able to be on his own is a valid issue from the outset of treatment.

🔍 CLINICAL INSIGHT

Walt had recently graduated from college and had enrolled himself in an intensive treatment program at a local university. As part of a group therapy assignment, he and others members of the group were assigned to walk across campus to the streets of the college town and keep a record of their behavior as well as listener reactions as they asked for directions from strangers. Walt and his partner decided they would ask for the location of the police station. Still in the early stages of treatment and clearly disfluent, his task was a daunting one. He attempted to find the listener who posed the least possible threat. Entering the first street adjacent to the campus, he spied the best of all possible targets. Coming around the corner and approaching him on the street was a grandmother. As he approached her, he positioned himself so that even if he stuttered, she would have no alternative but to stop. She was the prototypical grandmother. She wore a cloth coat and a hat with a veil. She was carrying a shopping bag in each hand along with an umbrella. As Walt began to ask his question, she stopped. She looked up at him and placed both shopping backs on the sidewalk. Walt continued stuttering his way through his required question asking about the location of the police station. As he completed his sentence, she responded. Yes, she did know the location of the police station. She spoke very slowly, a fact that was enhanced by her lipstick-red mouth and the veil attached to the front of her hat. "See the . . . big . . . red . . . light?" she asked as she turned and pointed to the stop light one block behind her. She continued, even slower now, "When you get to that big . . . red . . . light . . . turn . . . (and she paused even longer here as she took the elbow of his right arm) . . . left." At that same moment, to emphasize her instructions, she spun him around to his left. Somewhat wide-eyed and mortified for the moment, he pondered these events as he made his way back to the group meeting. As he shared his experience with the other group members, everyone, including Walt, appreciated the humorous telling of his story. There was genuine empathy and laughter all around as each member of the group shared similar experiences with well-meaning but overly patronizing listeners.

If the clinician and the client agree that termination is appropriate, it makes sense to schedule a meeting to review the progress. The clinician can make it clear that she is available for consultation and that group treatment on an informal basis is also possible. Referral to a support group such as a local chapter of the National Stuttering Association can serve to keep the client's momentum going and assist in keeping him desensitized and assertive concerning his fluency.

Although clients sometimes leave treatment before we deem it desirable, it is also possible to err in the direction of keeping the client in treatment for too long. Continued treatment beyond what is necessary or helpful may serve to reinforce the client's dependency. In addition, there is a law of diminishing returns whereby at a certain point, the cost—financial or otherwise—is no longer worth the effect. Ideally, during an exit meeting, both the client and the clinician can recognize and agree that, for now at least, they have each done their best.

On occasion, termination from formal treatment may be temporary. If the client has reached a plateau and little progress is noted for several weeks, such leveling-off may suggest that the client—not to mention the clinician—needs a break. A break from treatment may be indicated if the client becomes bored or other issues such as financial constraints or the logistics of attending treatment become preeminent. Just as in the case of attending graduate school or beginning a period of arduous athletic training, pushing ahead at full speed is not always the best strategy. Sometimes it is best to back away for a while. A break may provide the opportunity to reassess priorities and evaluate and regain motivation. Perhaps the clinician needs to assist the client in backing away from the treatment process. It may be that a vacation from treatment is the best investment for future growth. Temporary dismissal from treatment may not be an easy decision, for there is the chance that we will lose the clients and progress will cease. Nonetheless, forgoing treatment for a time can be an essential step in the overall process.

CONCLUSION

Clinicians must be able to recognize success when it occurs, often in the form of small victories. Certainly change during treatment is far from linear, with many plateaus, successes, and failures. Some change may even occur prior to initiating formal treatment, as clients regress toward the mean following acceptance into a program. Although some adult clients achieve spontaneous fluency, many others do not, particularly those who drop out of treatment prior to dismissal. There is no combination of assessment measures that allows the clinician to predict which clients will be successful. The probability of success varies across many factors, including age, motivation, and intensity of treatment. Progress may be noted in either a decrease or an increase in the frequency of stuttering, an increase in formulative breaks, and especially the presence of shorter and less effortful stuttering events. Progress is also seen in more open decision-making in the form of decreased avoidance, greater speech assertiveness and risk-taking, and greater objectivity about the stuttering experience.

It is never too early in treatment to begin considering criteria for termination: What will it take for this client to be on his own and to manage his speech without the assistance of the clinician? Planning for termination and possible relapse will bring closure to formal treatment. A return to treatment as needed may be a good option, and such a decision should not be viewed as failure, but rather an opportunity for continued growth.

STUDY QUESTIONS

➤ How do you conceptualize change for clients who stutter? What do you consider to be the principle characteristics of change when treating children and adults who stutter?

➤ How would you go about quantifying the attitudinal, behavioral, and cognitive changes of (a) children and (b) adults who stutter?

➤ Using at least a three-minute sample of spontaneous speech, rate at least five "normal" adult speakers using the nine-point naturalness rating scale described in this chapter. Also do this for at least three adolescents or adults who are at the end of the treatment process.

➤ What are some of the key variables that appear to influence the ability of speakers to produce speech that is natural?

➤ What are you basic criteria for the termination of formal treatment for an adolescent or adult who has been coming to you for treatment?

RECOMMENDED READINGS

DiClemente, C. C. (1993). Changing addictive behaviors: A process perspective. *Current Directions in Psychological Science, 2*(4), 101–106.

Hillis, J. W. (1993). Ongoing assessment in the management of stuttering: A clinical perspective. *American Journal of Speech-Language Pathology, 2*(1), 24–37.

Prochaska, J. O., DiClemente, C. C., & Norcross, J. C. (1992). In search of how people change: Applications to addictive behaviors. *American Psychologist, 47*(9), 1102–1114.

Sheehan, J. G. (1980). Problems in the evaluation of progress and outcome. In W. H. Perkins (Ed.), *Strategies in stuttering therapy for seminars in speech, language and hearing* (pp. 389–401). New York: Thieme-Stratton.

CHAPTER

DETERMINING PROGRESS FOLLOWING TREATMENT

> *Speaking to people is not just a way of making a living for me; it's an affirmation of the ability that we all share to face an adversary or challenge without fear. And I enjoy it every bit as much as I enjoyed competing in basketball. . . . As I've traveled across the country telling my story and trying to get people to draw on their own inner strength and to fight to realize their dreams, I've received as many compliments, as much praise, as I ever received in basketball. While it's seldom publicized and not as dramatic as being chosen to play in an NBA All-Star game or having my jersey retired, it's every bit as rewarding as anything I experienced on the basketball court. (p. 198)*
>
> Bob Love (2000). The Bob Love Story.
> *Chicago, IL: Contemporary Books.*

INTRODUCTION

Is it realistic to think of adults recovering as a result of treatment for fluency disorders? Alternatively, is it more reasonable to think of treatment as an evolving process of recovery, as is the case with other complex human problems? Although investigators of treatment efficacy and relapse indicate that substantial changes take place during treatment for the majority of clients, a review of this literature suggests that, with sporadic exceptions, relatively few people who stutter into adulthood become completely normal speakers. Even following what could be considered by all accounts a successful treatment experience, there are likely to be some residual effects of having stuttered for years or even decades. Nearly all autobiographical accounts written by people who have undergone successful treatment, contain descriptions of the long-term effects of being a person who stutters (e.g., Chmela, 1998; Daly, 1998; Johnson, 1930; Krall, 1998; Manning, 1991b, 1998; Murry & Edwards, 1980; Quesal, 1998; Ramig, 1998; St. Louis, 1998). These effects need to be countered with continued vigilance and the practice of techniques that allow the achievement of smooth and flowing speech in a variety of speaking situations.

As we have stated many times throughout this book, stuttering is a complex combination of attitude, behavioral, and cognitive features bound together with degrees of anxiety and fear. Because of its complex nature, stuttering is resistant to long-term change, particularly for adults. Unless a speaker is able to lose his memory of having stuttered for many years (e.g., Johnson & Johnson, 2000) he is not likely to see himself as a fluent speaker. On the other hand, there are speakers who have stuttered for decades who are able to become extremely fluent and who rarely think of themselves as people who stutter.

In a number of ways, altering the stuttering syndrome is similar to other areas of clinical intervention where relapse is a common phenomenon, such as marital problems, drug addiction, alcoholism, weight reduction, and smoking cessation (Lefcourt, 1976). For example, one-year success rates for intensive smoking-cessation programs range from 20% to 40%; they range from 10% to 20% for nonintensive interventions (DiClemente, 1993). On a somewhat more optimistic note, a review of the relapse literature by Craig (1998) indicated that relapse for individuals with addictive disorders have decreased from 70% by 12 months post-intervention in the 1960s and 1970s to 12-month rates of 40%–60% in the 1990s. This improvement is thought to have occurred as a result of anti-relapse programs including follow-up programs, enhancement of self-efficacy, and attendance at self-help support groups.

After formal treatment is concluded, the client is on his own. It is then that the crucial process of informal treatment begins. This phase of the treatment process has most often been termed *maintenance* and typically lasts much longer than formal treatment. In many important ways, for the adult who stutters this stage of treatment continues for the rest of the speaker's life. During maintenance the person who stutters must be able to fully accept the responsibility of self-management, a function he should gradually begin to assume as early as possible during the stages of formal treatment.

OUR LIMITED VIEW OF CHANGE

One of the major considerations following the period of formal treatment is the possibility of relapse. This is especially true during the first few months and years following the termination of formal intervention. Relapse is most obvious in terms of the surface features of the problem as indicated by the speaker's fluency level. However, more importantly, relapse also takes place in the direction of the pretreatment attitude and cognitive features of the syndrome. Just as the assessment of stuttering is multidimensional, the evaluation of maintenance must be multidimensional as well. Concentration on a single feature (especially the frequency of stuttering) tends to exclude the important affective and cognitive features of the problem, features that those who stutter perceive as critical (Prins, 1970). In any case, maintenance of the many changes that take place during formal treatment is difficult when the client is on his own, doing battle alone against a long history of stuttering and the well learned survival techniques that he has used for years. Therefore, a major portion of this chapter is devoted to understanding relapse and the strategies for dealing with this common problem.

As discussed in the first chapter, student clinicians rarely have the opportunity to observe more than a single semester of all the changes that occur as a result of treatment. At best, clinicians are usually able to see a only small window of progress, and often this is indicated only by frequency counts of stuttered events. Significant life-style changes or not quantified or even noted. To some degree, this can also the case for professional clinicians. Although the professional clinician will likely follow a client throughout the duration of formal treatment, there is often little or no interaction with the client during the long process of informal treatment. Some clients do maintain contact with the clinic, but mostly—as Van Riper (1973) points out—these are clients who need additional help. The majority of clients go off on their own, leaving the clinician with no idea about their progress over the many years of informal treatment. Boberg (1981; 1986) was one of the first clinical researchers to recognize this problem and suggested that comprehensive clinical programs should have a system for assisting the client in the maintenance of clinical gains as well as refresher programs emphasizing client self-management of cognitive and attitudinal changes.

MAINTENANCE AND TRANSFER

Of the three stages of treatment—establishment of fluency, transference of new abilities to extra-treatment speaking situations, and maintenance of the new abilities following formal treatment—maintenance has come to be regarded as the most challenging aspect of the treatment process (Boberg, 1981). Maintenance is burdensome for the client, for he is working against many forces that are pulling in the direction of pretreatment performance and cognition.

Furthermore, maintenance is enigmatic for the clinician, for it is typically difficult to maintain contact with the client. Even when contact is continued, there are many practical—and even some ethical—problems that make it difficult to obtain accurate data concerning posttreatment performance. Maintenance of the changes achieved during informal treatment will be more likely to occur if, during the period of formal treatment, the clinician has enabled the client to focus on the *transfer* of cognitive, affective, and behavioral changes to a variety of extra-treatment settings. Gregory states, "The essence of effective therapy is transfer" (1995, p. 199). As mentioned earlier, transfer refers to the generalization of gains made in the treatment environment to extra-treatment situations. Rather than wait until partial or complete fluency is achieved in treatment before beginning these transfer activities, most clients can benefit from such activities from the outset of treatment. During the first treatment sessions, the speaker can begin the process of desensitizing to a large variety of environmental stimuli that have had a powerful handicapping effect. The clinician can assist in extending the victories of identification and self-monitoring to real-world speaking situations. Activities, objects, and individuals that are brought to the treatment setting can serve as powerful discriminative stimuli that will cue the client for achieving a similar performance outside the treatment environment. Even something as basic as a tape recorder can function as a discriminative stimulus in extra-treatment speaking situations (Howie, Woods, & Andrews, 1982).

As discussed in earlier chapters, the lack of homogeneity among clients is a major variable that contributes to the inconsistent effects of treatment. This lack of client as well as environmental homogeneity may also provide a good explanation for the difficulty of successful client maintenance following treatment. For example, Boberg (1986) suggested that differences in long-term progress are as likely to be due to personality factors and the ability of the clients as they are to the treatment program or even the clinician. During informal treatment, there is little or no direct influence by the clinician concerning the fluency-disrupting stimuli in the client's world. The client is on his own as he responds to the stimuli and attempts to alter his old roles and the expectancies of those in his environment. Clearly his success, or lack thereof, will have a critical impact on long-term effects of intervention.

THE NATURE OF RELAPSE

By discussing the nature of relapse with the client and preparing him for the possibility of regression, is the clinician creating a self-fulfilling prophecy? If the topic of regression is never mentioned, is relapse less apt to occur, or does the clinician have an obligation to prepare the client for something that, in some form at least, is likely to happen? Certainly, the literature indicates that for adult clients, the possibility of relapse is real. The clinician's understanding of the nature of this experience and preparing the client to respond to relapse is one of the clinician's responsibilities.

The Possibility of Relapse

Many authors have recognized relapse as a common event following treatment for adults who stutter (Bloodstein, 1987; Craig, 1998; Kuhr & Rustin, 1985; Martin, 1981; Perkins, 1979; Silverman, 1981; Van Riper, 1973). Prins (1970) found that about 40% of clients taking part in an intensive residential program experienced some regression following treatment. Although Prins noted that clients believed that maximum regression occurred within six months after the termination of formal treatment, other writers have suggested that clients should be followed for at least two to five years following formal treatment (Bloodstein, 1995; Conture & Guitar, 1992; Young, 1975). Martin (1981) reviewed the literature and estimated relapse at approximately 30%. Craig and Hancock (1995) found that 71.7% of 152 adults surveyed experienced relapse but that the majority found that they subsequently regained fluency. They also found that relapse tended to be cyclical, occurring up to three times in a year.

Cooper (1977) views relapse as part of the human condition. Silverman (1981) suggests that relapse is likely to occur with a 40% to 90% probability. Van Riper states, "Relapses and remissions are the rule, not the exception, for the adult stutterer if long-term follow-up investigations are conducted" (1973, p. 178). St. Louis and Westbrook report that "relapse is a ubiquitous and familiar problem in stuttering therapy" (1987, p. 252). Perkins states that "maintenance of fluency is the perennial weak link in the therapeutic chain" (1979, p. 119) of stuttering treatment. Finally, as Bloodstein (1995) maintains, although we are adept at making people who stutter fluent, we know little about how to keep them that way.

Thus for most clients, some type of follow-up is necessary. The learning curve is long, and as Van Riper was fond of saying, the old habits are always the strongest. Clients should at least have the option of continuing treatment in some form for as long as they need it. This, of course, is not likely to happen if coming back to the center is viewed, by the clinician or the client, as an indication of failure. If changing the syndrome of stuttering in adults is viewed as a long-term process—which in the majority of cases it surely is—then the client returning for follow-up sessions is not a sign of failure. Rather, it is a natural and acceptable part of the process of change. Additional treatment, more than anything else, simply means that those involved are intelligent enough to recognize that they are likely to benefit from further effort and growth. Fortunately, many clients do not require a return to intensive individual treatment. Often, group treatment sessions or support group meetings once or twice a month will enable many clients to get back on track and continue making progress.

Relatively little is known about relapse in children or adolescents. Craig et al. (1996) followed 97 children (aged 9–14) for one year posttreatment and found that 3 of 10 children experienced relapse (2% SS). In a subsequent study Hancock and Craig (1998) followed 77 of these same children in order to identify possible predictors of relapse (2% SS). A regression analysis indicated that only pretreatment % SS and immediate posttreatment trait anxiety were significant predictors (accounting for 14.4% and 8% of the variance, respectively). That is, children who stuttered to a greater degree prior to treatment were more likely to relapse. Surprisingly, the children who indicated higher immediate posttreatment measures of trait anxiety (within the normal range) were *less likely* to relapse. The authors concluded that perhaps the normal but heightened anxiety resulted in the children being more willing to work on their fluency skills. A variety of other variables (age and sex of the children, number of years stuttered, family history of stuttering) had little predictive value. Although we are unaware of any investigations of the phenomena, we have encountered many college-age students who, although they report what appeared to be highly successful treatment in the early elementary grades, experience an increase in stuttering behavior as they approach their early 20s.

Defining Relapse

Defining relapse following formal treatment is nearly as difficult as determining the severity of the stuttering at the outset. As Craig (1998) points out, a medical definition that defines relapse using an all-or-none criterion (the presence or absence of a disease) clearly does not work well for stuttering. An all-or-none criterion may be used for some addictive behaviors (such as setting a threshold of total abstinence for the use of alcohol or cigarettes). However, it's clear that most people who stutter will have residual attitudes and behaviors following treatment, and zero stuttering is not likely to always be the case.

Most investigators who have studied relapse in stuttering have used the presence of overt stuttering as the one—and often the only—measure of relapse. Some investigators have considered the percentage of syllables stuttered (% SS) and have used a relapse criteria of 2% SS (Craig, Franklin, & Andrews, 1984; Craig & Hancock,1984; Evesham & Fransella, 1985) or 4% SS (Boberg, 1981). Blood (1995) and Ladouceur, Caron and Caron (1989) used 3% SS to define treatment success.

Of course, the frequency of stuttering is usually far from the only and often not the initial indicator of regression. As Van Riper stated,

"Stuttering does not mean relapse. Another moment of fear is no catastrophe" (1973, p. 209). Changes in the attitudinal and cognitive aspects of the problem, often in the form of negative self-talk, are likely to take the lead in the progression of relapse. As an example, Craig and Hancock (1995) found that adults with significantly raised levels of trait anxiety were three times more likely to experience relapse. When elements of avoidance and fear begin to multiply and increasingly influence the speaker's decision making, overt stuttering will not be far behind. Recognizing the great variability of stuttering frequency and the variability of fluency across different speaking situations, Craig and Calver (1991) defined relapse as "stuttering to a degree which was not acceptable to yourself for at least a period of one week" (p. 283), a definition that is probably more realistic and functional than many others.

Relapses may take many forms and may range from brief periods that are mildly irritating to long episodes that are extremely handicapping. The clinician may be able to determine that the client has reached the threshold of a relapse based on observable affective, behavioral, and cognitive aspects of the syndrome. However, the presence and degree of relapse are probably best determined by the client himself. When the client gets to the point where he believes he is no longer confident of managing his speech on his own or that his decisions are increasingly based on the possibility of stuttering, relapse has reached a clinical level. If he is making choices because of the *possibility* of a stuttering event, the problem has again become significant. At that point, it is both reasonable and desirable to seek additional professional help.

POSSIBLE CAUSES OF RELAPSE

While describing the shadow side of implementing change, Egan (1998) briefly discusses the idea of "entropy," the tendency of things to break down or fall apart. Applied to humans who are attempting to change, this may be thought of as the tendency to give up actions that have been initiated. Of course, we have all experienced this. We lose some weight, we get in a little better shape and then we fall back a bit . . . or maybe a lot. As we begin a process of change, the actions we are taking seem reasonable, even exciting. However, with the hard work of the daily routine, enthusiasm fades and lack of time and other priorities soon interfere. As Egan describes, we are distracted or become discouraged and flounder. Citing Brownell et al. (1986) he makes the important distinction between the clinician preparing a client for the mistakes they may make and "giving them permission" to make mistakes and implying that they are inescapable. Perhaps even more important, he suggests that there is a critical distinction between a "lapse" and a "relapse" and that a small slip does not need to result in a relapse.

Silverman (1981) suggested a number of possible reasons for relapse. Clients who are especially likely to relapse are those who, following treatment, believe themselves to be cured. Believing they have experienced a cure, they are less likely to continue the rigorous process of self-management. Other clients may regress as they come to lose confidence in the treatment program. This is more apt to occur if they have experienced relapse following previous treatment experiences. As Silverman points out, people tend to expect events to replicate themselves.

Another possible reason for relapse may be that the clinician and the client have thresholds for fluency breaks that are too liberal. In this case, small fluency breaks are accepted and left unmodified. Relapse is also more likely to occur if clients are released from treatment too soon, although how soon is "too soon" may be difficult to assess. It may be worthwhile seeing the client through one relapse while the support of the clinician is immediately available. The presence of stuttering can provide an escape from responsibilities or work. This probably does not occur enough to explain relapse in most people, but, no doubt, it is one force that can nudge the client back into his old pattern of avoidance. We all make use of excuses to avoid performing unpleasant tasks. For any client, but perhaps especially for adolescents, an emotional crisis resulting in loss of self-esteem may negatively influence fluency (Daly, Simon, & Burnett-Stolnack, 1995). As Daly, et al. indicate, adolescent clients are likely to see many negative events—be they social-, academic-, or treatment-related—as catastrophic.

Neurophysiological Loading

Several authors who have gathered and studied data concerning etiology, spontaneous recovery, and relapse for subjects with fluency disorders suggest that some of these speakers possess an underlying physiological or neurophysiological condition (Boberg, 1986; Moore & Haynes, 1980; Perkins, Kent, & Curlee, 1990; Zimmerman, 1980, 1981). This may be especially likely for clients with "genetic loading," who have a family history of stuttering. Boberg (1986) suggests that just as recovery from stuttering may be related to a family history of stuttering (Sheehan & Martyn, 1966), there also may be a greater chance of relapse for such speakers (Cooper, 1972; Neavers, 1970).

If these findings are accurate, there are some important implications for the treatment process. That is, the treatment techniques acquired by the client may be thought of as providing skills necessary to *compensate* for an innate deficiency (Boberg, 1986). These findings also imply that the maintenance of these skills is best viewed as a lifelong process. This would be the case even if the speaker were not seen as having a deficiency. If, as Starkweather and Gottwald (1990) and Conture (1990) suggest, the demands placed on the speaker consistently exceed the person's capacities to produce speech, fluency breaks will be apt to occur. The treatment techniques then would provide a response to the discrepancy between the demands placed on the speaker and his individual capacities. In any case, the person must maintain appropriate self-management abilities to compensate for this situation.

Continued Effort Is Required

Changing the surface and intrinsic features of the stuttering syndrome takes considerable effort. This effort is apparent throughout the often arduous process of formal treatment. However, for some people, the continuing effort and vigilance that are required for long-term change are not perceived as worth the effort. As Cooper (1977) has pointed out, it takes a good deal of psychic energy to initiate and maintain all the necessary changes in the stuttering syndrome. As with most things, this does become easier with practice and success. However, if, as a result of treatment, the problem itself becomes less handicapping to the client, the continued effort may not be worth the effect. The problem will no longer be a major one for the person, and he may decide to devote his finite time and energies to issues in his life that he considers more important. Whether clinicians like it or not, this is the scenario that often occurs. Progress can continue in the direction of enhanced fluency and improved self-management, but the curve of success is never linear and does not always travel in an upward direction.

Client Adjustment to a New Role

Joseph Sheehan often suggested that for treatment to be successful, the client must eventually make the adjustment of viewing himself as something beyond an individual who stutters. As proposed by theories such as Personal Construct Theory, in many important ways the speaker must evolve as a person and form a new paradigm, a new view of himself and his possibilities (Boberg, Howie, & Woods, 1979; Dalton, 1987, 1994; Emerick, 1988; Evesham & Fransella, 1985; Fransella, 1972; Fransella & Dalton, 1990; Hayhow & Levy, 1989). Kuhr and Rustin (1985) noted, for example, that following treatment, those clients who were most satisfied with their fluency also made changes in their lifestyle, which Kuhr and Rustin associated with the maintenance of fluency. Unfortunately, it takes some time to change decades of expectancies in the face of many old and powerful stimuli. As Fransella (1972) suggests, the speaker knows how events will transpire with him in the role of a person who stutters; he is less able to predict events if he speaks fluently. As Dalton (1987) explains, at some level, the speaker makes a "choice" to stutter, not because he prefers to do so in the usual sense, but because it is what is familiar and consistent with how he understands his world. This choice is not abnormal:

It is a perfectly understandable outcome of many years of living in the stuttering experience.

Near the end of successful treatment, some clients may express some anxiety, and even vague feelings of guilt, concerning their new fluency. Kuhr and Rustin (1985) found evidence of minor depression in several fluent speakers during maintenance following formal treatment. Clients may state that they are not as comfortable as they thought they would be with their fluency. They may even have the vague feeling that they are deceiving others. They do not feel like themselves. Their new fluency and all the responsibility for self-management that comes along with it have changed the self they had grown used to. In addition, although the speaker may be fluent and feel that his fluency is earned, there may be the feeling of waiting for the other shoe to fall. He may be afraid of losing his fluency, thinking, "Yes, I'm fluent now. But what happens if I lose it?"

While the new fluency may be nice, it will not always feel comfortable, at least immediately. As Williams (1995) explains from the perspective of Personal Construct Theory, even when fluent, the speaker is attempting gain evidence of support for their new construct of themselves and their world. The person is now acting in ways that are not congruent with their long-held view of themselves. It will take some time before the client, as well as others in the environment, can adjust to the speaker's new way of communicating and interacting with others. Of course, the client's fluency may not be something that others in their lives are used to, either. If treatment has been successful, many aspects of the syndrome have changed, and not just the speaker's fluency. Enormous changes have occurred on many levels and it will take some time for everyone, speakers and listeners alike, to adjust to the many implications of these changes. On the other hand, as these cognitive and affective changes occur, there will be new options for thinking and behaving that the person would never have imagined.

Listener Adjustment to a New Speaker

The speaker is not the only one adjusting to a new role. Because successful treatment for stuttering impacts the listener as well, it may be necessary for others in the client's daily environment to change their usual response to this person. If other people in the client's life fail to understand and recognize the nature of changes that have occurred, they will be less likely to reinforce these changes. Should this be the case, long-term progress is less likely to occur.

If treatment is genuinely successful, there are some important changes in the client's thinking about himself and others. As discussed in Chapter 6, for some clients, changes in speech assertiveness and risk-taking are likely to influence ways of interacting and communicating with others. Not only must the client adjust to a new role beyond that of a person who stutters, others may have to shift their position in order to establish a new equilibrium in the relationships. The other people in the client's life must recognize that they may also need to readjust their roles. Of course, these other people may not want to change. Following treatment, there will be forces brought about by others in their expectations that the client will continue playing his old role. Kuhr and Rustin provide an example of just such a response. They described a wife who felt uncomfortable when her husband returned home with fluent speech, following successful in-patient treatment. His wife's reaction was a negative one: She accused the clinician, saying, "You took him away and made him fluent" (1985, p. 234).

On the other hand there are examples of good adjustments by others in the client's life that contribute much to the continued pattern of growth. In the following example, the client is a middle-aged woman who has stuttered severely and only recently began to make even the most routine telephone calls.

Clinician: You say you are beginning to make some of your own telephone calls now?

Client: Oh yes, sometimes I would answer calls when I was at home but I would never place calls. If there was I call that I felt I had to make I would ask my husband to do it.

Clinician: Are you finding that making the calls is becoming less anxiety-producing?

Client: Yes, at least some of them. The other thing that I've begun to do is make some of my husband's calls. You know . . . for things related to his business and our personal travel, airlines reservations and things like that.

Clinician: Wow, that's great. How does he like that?

Client: He thinks it great too. He's busy with his new job and he really appreciates it.

Related to these old expectancies of others is the pressure that is often placed on the speaker to exhibit fluency following treatment. This pressure may be particularly true if the speaker has attended an intensive program away from his home and family. Upon returning home, there may be expectancy and pressure to demonstrate much-improved or even perfect fluency. The occurrence of stuttering will likely be viewed as an immediate sign of failure: "How awful, after all this time, effort, and money and he still stutters!" Although many clients can show much-improved fluency, the fear of even a single fluency break can be immense. One good response to the pressure of others to be fluent when they say such things as, "Your speech is wonderful now that you've had therapy. You don't stutter at all any more, do you," might be to say something such as, "Wwwwell, I'm do-do-doing my best!" (Van Riper, personal communication, October, 1971).

Speaking in a Nonhabitual Manner

It has been argued by several writers and clinicians that treatment programs that bring about increased fluency by encouraging the person to speak in a nonhabitual manner tend to have only a temporary impact on a speaker's fluency (Bloodstein, 1949, 1950; Boberg, 1986; Van Riper, 1973, 1990). A review of the research on the measurement of speech naturalness for stuttering speakers by Schiavetti and Metz (1997) suggested that some speakers who achieved stutter-free speech sounded as unnatural after treatment as they had prior to treatment. Altering an individual's habitual rate and manner of articulation is obviously possible for relatively short periods of time, and without question, such altered ways of speaking can result in rapid increases in fluency. However, such changes in habitual speech production are difficult to change in the long term. It takes concentration and a great deal of effort to maintain what are clearly nonhabitual respiratory, phonatory, and articulatory patterns.

Without question, some speakers are able to maintain these altered ways of producing speech. For others, however, the use of these altered patterns eventually wears off. Kalinowski, Nobel, Armson, and Stuart (1994) obtained reading passages from five adults with mild stuttering and five adults with severe stuttering. The subjects were randomly selected from clients who had undergone an intensive fluency-shaping program. Reading passages of one minute each from both pre- and posttreatment recordings were rated by sixty-four listeners for speech naturalness. Despite the fact the pretreatment samples contained several instances of stuttering and the posttreatment audio samples were largely free from stuttering events, the listeners indicated that posttreatment recordings resulted in a significant decrease in speech naturalness for both mildly and severely stuttering clients. The authors suggested that perhaps one reason why many individuals who stutter may fail to conscientiously use target behaviors following their discharge from treatment is because of the unsatisfactory therapeutic effects of unnatural-sounding speech.

Starke (1994) points out that the use of artificial speech often results in prosodic distortion. Although the altered ways of producing speech may promote fluency in a traditional sense, they may also result in messages being misperceived. Because of the altered prosody, there is a distinct possibility of a distortion in the speaker's communicative intentions and the relationship between the speaker and the listener, an effect Starke terms "message incompatibility conflict" (1994). Although the speaker may no longer be stuttering in his typical manner, the pragmatics of human communication may suffer unless the listener is able to understand that speech modification techniques are being used.

Finally, there are preliminary data suggesting that listener response to stuttering modification techniques also elicit less than favorable reactions by nonprofessional listeners. Manning, Burlison, and Thaxton (1999) had groups of naïve listeners use a bipolar scale, a handicap scale, and open-ended questions to evaluate an adult male who simulated mild stuttering (SSI=17) or utilized stuttering modification techniques (cancellations or pullouts). Listeners plainly preferred the condition where the speaker was stuttering over the condition when the speaker was using stuttering modification techniques. The results suggested that everyday listeners may be likely to react less favorably to a speaker (with mild levels of stuttering) who is modifying his stuttered speech than when the same speaker is simply stuttering.

Failure to Follow Maintenance Procedures

Boberg (1986) suggests that in many ways, the requirements of practicing self-management techniques (regardless of whether the techniques involve stuttering modification or fluency modification) can be a highly punishing experience. As we have indicated, the use of nearly all modification techniques carries with it a loss of spontaneity and an emphasis on how the speech is produced rather than what is being said. As Boberg (1986) suggests, being accountable for using the speech modification techniques may be more internally punishing for many speakers than hoping for the periods of normal speech that occur. Boberg suggests that most people who stutter who have experienced treatment will continue to practice these techniques "only if the perceived positive consequences of practice outweigh the perceived negative consequences" (1986, p. 498).

The Cyclical Nature of Fluency

In earlier chapters we discussed how the cyclical nature of fluency in children and adults contributes to the difficulty of diagnosing stuttering and predicting future levels of fluency. This characteristic of fluency also continues following treatment. Kamhi (1982) points out that some people who stutter must expend considerably more effort than others to achieve and maintain fluency due to the natural variability of their speech-production systems. For some speakers, such variability as well as relapses are more common and perhaps more severe. Kamhi suggests that knowing the stimuli that are likely to produce stress, the speaker can learn to predict and work through these occurrences. The higher the level of fluency desired, the more work is usually required to maintain that level.

OVERT AND COVERT MEASURES OF LONG-TERM CHANGE

One of the difficulties in determining how clients are performing following treatment involves the method of assessment. That is, if speakers are aware of the assessment, will they respond differently than they might otherwise? Howie, Woods, and Andrews (1982) compared the effect of overt and covert measures, both prior to and following treatment. Twenty-two adult males who stuttered were assessed before—and 15 were contacted after—intensive fluency treatment. Howie, et al. found no difference between overt and covert measures in terms of percent syllables stuttered (% SS) before treatment. However, following treatment, there were significantly more stuttering events noted following treatment when the speakers were measured covertly. Both overt and covert samples consisted of two (one monologue and one face-to-face conversation with a stranger) three-minute samples of speech, which were audiotaped. All but 3 of the 15 subjects assessed posttreatment stuttered more during covert assessment than during overt assessment.

There is some evidence that such differences in percent syllables stuttered between overt and covert measures become less pronounced with increased time posttreatment (Ingham, 1975; Howie, Tanner, & Andrews, 1981). Andrews and Craig (1982) suggest that after approximately 18 months posttreatment, covert assessment may no longer be necessary.

PREDICTING SUCCESS FOLLOWING TREATMENT

To date, researchers have had little success predicting the long-term success of treatment. It is difficult to know what features to monitor as predictors. It is also difficult to know which features of the syndrome should be used as criterion measures. The results of Andrews and Craig (1988) provide support for a multidimensional approach for predicting long-term success. Using a combination of three factors, they found that 97% of the subjects who maintained high skill mastery (0% syllables stuttered), normal speech attitudes as indicated by such measures as the Modified Erickson Scale of Communication Attitudes (S-24) (Andrews & Cutler, 1974), and an internal locus of control as indicated by the Locus of Control of Behavior Scale (LCB) (Craig, Franklin, & Andrews, 1984) were able to maintain success. Perhaps more telling is the fact that none of the subjects who failed to achieve any of these goals was able to maintain their posttreatment fluency level. In a related study, Madison, Budd, and Itzkowitz (1986) found that pretreatment locus of control (LOC) measures corresponded to the degree of change in stuttering following treatment for a group of 7- to 16-year-old children. That is, those children who had a more internal LOC prior to intervention tended to achieve more fluent speech during treatment. However, no significant relationship was found between pretreatment LOC scores and fluency levels during evaluations conducted at both two and six months following treatment.

Another attempt to predict long-term success was conducted by DeNil and Kroll (1994). They considered to what extent adult stutterers' scores on the Locus of Control of Behavior Scale (Craig, Franklin, & Andrews, 1984) are predictive of their ability to maintain speech fluency both immediately following intensive treatment and approximately two years later. Twenty-one subjects participated in a three-week intensive treatment program based on the Precision Fluency Shaping Program (Webster, 1975). Thirteen subjects who were contacted again two years later participated in a follow-up evaluation, which consisted of the administration of several scales, the reading of a brief passage, and a conversation with a research assistant. All subjects were seen by an assistant who was unknown to the subjects and unaware of their previous performance. Furthermore, the assessment took place in a new and unfamiliar location. While subjects showed a significant long-term improvement in fluency, no predictive relationship was found between scores on the LCB scale and level of fluency, as measured in percent words stuttered, either posttreatment or follow-up. However, LCB scores were found to be predictive of the subjects' fluency self-evaluation measured posttreatment and at follow-up. The study suggests that while the LCB may contribute to the prediction of the long-term treatment outcome, particularly as perceived by the client, other client and process variables will need to be considered.

Using a measure such as the locus of control is intuitively appealing. Early in treatment, clients typically express the feeling that stuttering is something that happens to them. When they stutter, they feel helpless and have no control (Van Riper, 1982). In one way or another, all treatment programs place a major emphasis on the client's self-management of his speech behavior and his cognitive interpretation of his circumstances (Adams, 1983; Kuhr & Rustin, 1985). As treatment progresses, speakers must gradually internalize cognitive and behavioral changes. If they do not, these speakers are more likely to relapse once formal treatment is completed (Boberg, Howie, & Woods, 1979). Other researchers (Craig, Franklin, & Andrews, 1984; Andrews & Craig, 1985) have demonstrated that changes in clients' LCB scores toward more internal control during treatment are related to the long-term treatment outcome. On the other hand, Ladouceur, Caron, and Caron (1989) found no relationship between LCB scores and fluency improvement in nine adults. Surprisingly, they found that some clients became more externally oriented during treatment while also acquiring increased fluency. Although

Ladouceur, et al. suggested that the changes in fluency, internal control, at least as gauged by the LCB, and behavior may have to do with the treatment strategy used.

Using a correlation approach, Craig (1988) considered the relationship between % SS 10 to 18 months following treatment (an intensive fluency-shaping approach) and a large variety of pretreatment variables including subject demographics (age, sex, and social status), stuttering severity (% SS and syllables per minute speech rate as measured in syllables per minute (SPM), health perceptions, self-reported avoidance and reaction to stuttering, neuroticism and extroversion, locus of control, formal practice, attendance at self-help meetings. He found no strong associations between demographic, severity, psychological, or self-help variables and follow-up fluency. In addition, there were small to moderate correlations between follow-up % SS and pretreatment severity, % SS ($r = 0.424$) and SPM ($r = 0.515$). That is, those with greater stuttering and slower speech rates were more likely to stutter more at follow-up. Finally, there was no single predictor variable that that showed a strong correlation across the subjects.

Craig (1998) summarizes the suggestions for preventing relapse and achieving long-term success following treatment. At the center of the issue is the concept of self-control. Constant effort and continued practice will most likely be the basic requirements for continued change. Craig suggests that success involves such things as practice of treatment activities and objectives that are achievable; using positive (self-)reinforcement; practicing self-monitoring skills; scheduling follow-up treatment; and emphasis of self-responsibility. It seems that understanding and overcoming probable relapses is complex and—just as stuttering itself—requires a multidimensional approach.

THE IMPORTANCE OF SUPPORT GROUPS

One of the more important influences on the long-term maintenance of treatment gains may be the client's involvement in self-help groups (Appendix B). Whether these groups are referred to as self-help, support, or advocacy groups, they all can provide sources of information and motivation for those who stutter as well as their families and friends. For the speaker who has isolated himself as a result of his stuttering, support groups are particularly valuable (see Crowe, 1997b). Possibly for the first time in his life, the person will find that he is among many others who share a common problem. He finds that the unique part of him that has, for so long, set him apart from others now provides a way to connect and bond with many people. Although an empathetic clinician and successful treatment may promote dramatic decreases in isolation for a client, there is probably nothing as effective as a good support group for increasing a person's social involvement.

The meetings of the local chapters of support groups also furnish important opportunities to practice techniques and stabilize cognitive changes following formal treatment. The encouragement of the other members is apt to enhance increases in motivation and assertiveness. Group membership can also provide an important social function for some of the members, fostering interaction in an accepting, penalty-free environment. It is a place where members can continue the process of coming to terms with the problem. Appendix B provides the addresses, telephone, fax, and Internet connections for a variety of such groups.

The development of self-help groups is closely related to the development and growth of consumerism (Hunt, 1987; Ramig, 1993b). For a variety of cultural and economic reasons, many members of society and people with disabilities in particular, are hesitant about seeking professional help. In cases where individuals feel that they have failed to benefit from intervention, there is sometimes a confrontational attitude toward professionals. Coming together with other people who have similar problems can be an empowering and exciting experience. Empathy and support from your fellow travelers is all but assured. Importantly, this form of help can be obtained at relatively little cost. For all these reasons, Egan (1998) indicates that self-help groups are one of the most popular sources of help for people with a variety of problems and this is certainly the case for those who stutter.

As Hunt (1987) describes (citing Katz & Bender, 1976), support groups are volunteers who come together for mutual assistance with common problems, handicaps, or chronic complaints. They provide face-to-face contact among members and stress members' personal responsibility. The groups provide a variety of members' needs including the facilitation of personal change, fostering of personal responsibility by members, provision of information and advice, discussion of alternative treatments, fund-raising, and political activities relating to the goals of the group. Most often, however, the majority of the activities relate to providing members with support and information.

Hunt (1987) reported that the greatest virtue of support groups was providing the members with a sense of relief from the feeling of isolation and establishing contact with others who understand their distress and frustration. A survey conducted by Krass-Lehrman and Reeves (1989) of 600 National Stuttering Project (NSP) members (141 questionnaires returned) indicated that the *least* important focus of the groups was to provide an adjunct to formal treatment. Ramig (1993b), in a survey of 62 support group participants, found that 49 indicated that their fluency had improved "at least somewhat" as a direct result of their involvement in such groups. Interestingly, there was also some indication that group members had to attend something approaching twenty meetings for this to be the case. More importantly, 55 of the 62 respondents indicated that support group involvement resulted in "at least somewhat positive" or "very positive" impact on their daily life.

In order to appreciate the nature of such groups, we will provide a brief history of two of them. The first one, The British Stammering Association (BSA), was founded in 1968. As is often the case, the initial development of such groups results from the efforts of one person (in this case, Robin Harrison) who is willing to dedicate many years of administrative, public relation, and fund-raising activities in order to get the group off the ground. A review of the BSA membership by Hunt (1987) indicated that a small proportion of the total population of people with fluency disorders belonged to the group. The age range for the membership is generally from 25 to 40, with few teenagers. The average age of people in groups was higher than those in treatment, where few clients over the age of 50 are typically found (Manning & Shirkey, 1981). The size of most local groups was 4 to 6 members. It ranged from as small as two to a rarely exceeded upper limit of 12. The most common goal reported by individual chapters was to transfer and maintain techniques learned in formal treatment. Although group members often practiced treatment techniques during the meetings, much of the discussion centered on adjusting to the cognitive aspects of the fluency disorder, including fears, anxieties, and feelings of inferiority, powerlessness, and frustration. Hunt (1987) reports that this was especially true for groups with "more mature members" who have had success in controlling their speech.

Most of the local chapters tended to be short-lived, lasting for only one or two years. In order for a local group to continue for any length of time, strong leadership is essential. In addition, from time to time, the group needs to elicit the support of local speech-language pathologists for referrals as well as advice. Finally, as Hunt suggests, the group must discipline itself so that it will be more than a social group. It must have specific guidelines and objectives that focus on the self-management of fluency disorders.

The largest group in the United States is The National Stuttering Association (NSA). Originally founded by Michael Sugarman and Bob Goldman in 1977 and known for more than 20 years as the National Stuttering Project (NSP), the purpose of this group is to provide information and support to children and adults who stutter, their families, and professional clinicians. The guiding principle of this group is reflected in their statement, "If you stutter, you are not alone." Participation in the NSA group expanded during the leadership of John Albach and is composed of several thousand members throughout the United States and more than 50 local support groups. The NSA Board of Directors develops the organization's mission and goals and the administrative staff is responsible for daily operations. As of this writing, the current Chair of the Board of Directors is Lee Reeves and the Executive Director is Annie Bradberry. NSA's monthly publication, *Letting Go,* is sent to all members and provides information and support in the form of articles, letters, stories, and reflections written by members. The activities include the monthly newsletter, news releases and public service announcements, participation in the annual National Stuttering Awareness week (May), and the creation and distribution of many brochures, books, tapes, the local group meetings, and regional workshops. In recent years, the development of a highly informative web page with links to related services provides another helpful source of information. All these activities as well as an annual national convention of 500–600 adults and children who stutter and their families are designed to educate, advocate, and instill a sense of solidarity and confidence in the members. The specific goals of NSA are to provide an opportunity for members to share with others their fears, frustrations, and triumphs; practice therapeutic techniques in a safe and supportive environment; take part in speaking experiences they would otherwise be likely to avoid; develop positive cognitive and affective strategies for managing their fluency disorder; and assist other members in achieving these goals.

There are, as Hunt (1987) points out, some potential difficulties in the functioning of support groups. Some groups tend to see themselves as treatment groups without the therapist. Of course, there is the potential in such situations for inappropriate or counterproductive attitudes, information, and techniques to be promoted. Furthermore, Hunt (1987) suggests that many people who could benefit from participation do not belong to such groups because they refuse to define themselves as persons who stutter. Cooper (1987), Silverman (1996), and Ramig (1993b) have all pointed out that many clinicians have a skeptical view of support groups, generally because they fail to understand the positive potential of group membership. Overall, however, these groups play an important, often critical role, in providing individuals with an opportunity for support and encouragement that is essential for long-term success following treatment. As consumers of treatment services, they are also able to provide an effective voice for improved training and service delivery to professional and legislative groups.

REPORTS OF LONG-TERM SUCCESS

There are many individuals who, following formal treatment for what were moderate-to-severe stuttering, are able to achieve a high level of fluency. In some cases, such people are able to attain spontaneous fluency and may become more fluent than many nonstuttering speakers. Most likely, these are speakers who do not possess the high level of neurophysiological loading for stuttering discussed earlier. There are few, if any, other individuals in the immediate or extended family who are know to have stuttered. Following formal treatment, they have been able to more or less transfer their ability to use fluency enhancing and fluency modification techniques to their everyday world. As the following descriptions indicate, they have been able to alter the way they think about themselves and their speech.

TRANSFER AND MAINTENANCE ACTIVITIES

A basic theme in changing human behavior is that the individual must gradually take the major responsibility for identifying and modifying his

---

🔍 CLINICAL INSIGHT

Adult male, age 53: Basically, I want to share that striving for perfection impeded my improvement. I read about William Jennings Bryan (The Golden Tongued orator) and he was my goal. When I readjusted my sights to become "as fluent as my motor system would allow," then I started to make progress. Gradual progress over a three- or four-year period, with occasional relapses and real breakdowns (like when three people very close to me—one my mother—died within a two-week period). My speech suffered tremendously, but even then I knew that I was grieving and when I grew strong again, and focused attention to my speech again, that I would regain my fluency. I never doubted that. My belief system remained positive that I would speak fluently again, as fluently as my timing system or motor coordination abilities would allow. But striving for perfection was abandoned as unrealistic, and really as unnecessary for success and happiness.

Also, when I took my stuttering out from under the microscope and saw that disfluencies were only a part of me, that helped. When I saw that other qualities (like being a good friend, listener, and caring person to others) was also a part of who and what I was—then I put speech (stuttered or fluent) in a proper perspective. I worked on using light pressure on my first sounds, sure, but also on improving tennis or sailing skills, too. And becoming a better administrator and writer, etc. Putting disfluencies in perspective helped—I realized that our Creator may have more challenges in store for me other than just becoming a perfect speaker. So I decided to work not only on fluency but on other "talents" I have too. That thinking seemed to send me in a more positive direction.

own behavior and attitudes concerning his situation (DiClemente, 1993; Egan, 1998. In the case of fluency disorders, the client must become sophisticated about stuttering in general, and his own stuttering in particular. The speaker must be able to recognize his errors and assign activities for confronting and changing his mistakes. Moreover, in order for change to take place, the speaker must do the majority of his practice outside the context of the treatment setting. Formal training takes place for only a few hours each week, and changes are not likely to occur unless the individual is disciplined enough to practice on his own. To the degree that a person does well in extratreatment settings during formal treatment, he will be likely to do well in those same situations during the months and years of informal treatment.

🔍 CLINICAL INSIGHT

Adult male, age 52: I completed an intensive program of treatment in my mid-20s. That was 28 years ago at this writing. I made obvious progress during the 20-week period of formal treatment. I learned how to decrease my avoidance behaviors (a big part of my stuttering) and to change the way I was stuttering. Very slowly, I began to take charge of my speech, especially specific behaviors associated with my stuttering. I also began to make some preliminary changes in the way I thought about my speech, both my stuttering as well as my fluent speech. But these cognitive changes, what I was telling myself about myself and my speech, came along at a much slower pace. Following my dismissal from treatment, I continued to expand my new ways of speaking, of stuttering, and thinking in more and more speaking situations. I slowly continued to make progress but it certainly wasn't linear. It was many years, at least 15, before the handicap of stuttering decreased to the point where it was really insignificant.

Now, nearly three decades following my dismissal from treatment, I find that I do something that could be classified as stuttering less than 20 times a year. I continue to think of myself as someone who stutters. It is just that I don't do it very often. Of course, it is no big deal to think of yourself as someone who stutters when it no longer represents a problem. Although I still do stutter on rare occasions, I now regard the situation more with curiosity and as a challenge to myself to use fluency-enhancing or modification techniques—I try to stutter in an open and easy manner. And most important, the fact that I might stutter has absolutely no influence on the choices I make.

Throughout this chapter we have described the importance of activities for transferring and maintaining abilities and attitudes learned during treatment to outside-of-therapy situations. These activities can and should begin at the outset of treatment for both children and adults who stutter. Performance in the real world with real time pressure and competition for communication is what counts. Many of the following suggestions for continued progress apply to children as well as older clients. For younger speakers, of course, parent involvement and understanding of the treatment process is critical for supporting and reinforcing the desired progress at all levels of change.

The following is a compilation of suggestions presented by St. Louis and Westbrook (1987) and includes activities suggested by Van Riper (1958, 1973); Boberg (1983); Boberg and Kelly (1984); Boberg and Sawyer (1977); Ryan (1979, 1980); Daly (1987); Dell (1980); Shames and Florance (1980); Howie, Tanner, and Andress (1981); St. Louis (1982); Williams, (1983); Craig (1998), and the current author.

➤ Clinicians should not be naïve or surprised when a client experiences a relapse.

➤ The clinician can stress that it is natural and expected for the client's quantity and quality of his fluency to swing from greater to lesser amounts and that this does not need to be interpreted as a disastrous event. Clients can be taught to think of a relapse as a temporary "lapse" and an opportunity to re-commit to make use of cognitive and behavioral techniques of change.

➤ The clinician can make it clear to the client that continued consultation and support are available following the termination of formal treatment. Returning to treatment is not only acceptable, it is expected.

➤ Treatment intensity can vary and decrease gradually, with individual meetings gradually occurring less often. Individual treatment sessions can gradually be supplemented with group meetings.

➤ Treatment can be transformed from face-to-face meetings to contact via the telephone or postcards. Audio- or videotape recordings of self-practice sessions can be mailed to the clinician, who can mail back critiques.

➤ Videotapes made in treatment can be used on a home VCR, enabling the client to demonstrate techniques learned in treatment and to record examples of the client's ability to use the techniques in extra-treatment speaking situations.

➤ Prior to dismissal from formal treatment, the clinician and client can discuss the reasons for relapse and plan specific client responses at the first indications of relapse (e.g., design voluntary stuttering activities in order to decrease the fear and avoidance of specific sounds, words, and speaking situations).

➤ Following formal treatment, the client can continue to seek new, assertive speaking situations where the envelope of comfort can gradually be expanded. If professional or social contacts do not provide such opportunities, the client may consider taking part in groups such as Toastmasters or Dale Carnegie.

➤ The client can expand his assertive and risk-taking behaviors for both speech and nonspeech activities, expanding and cultivating other talents and interests.

➤ The client may contact local groups and organizations to talk about his interests and professional experiences. Libraries are often interested in finding such speakers.

➤ The client may consider contacting local agencies that need volunteers to read newspapers or books on tape to older people who cannot read or to the blind.

➤ The client can continue to reassess opportunities for changes in his lifestyle, including possible alteration of interpersonal, vocational, and social roles.

➤ The client can continue to improve and expand on a variety of non-speaking skills that are likely to enhance his participation in life and his interaction with others.

➤ The client can join and take an active part in a local self-help or support group, possibly assuming a leadership role.

➤ The client can continue to monitor and evaluate his positive-negative self-talk, using the stopping and positive redirection activities (see Chapter 6).

➤ The client can take part in cognitive behavioral techniques that decrease anxiety and fear of social interactions.

➤ Clients can be taught to identify potentially high-risk situations regarding lifestyle, negative moods, or threatening environments and develop methods of coping with these situations.

➤ The client can practice the use of positive affirmations on a regular basis.

➤ The client can volunteer to work in a formal treatment setting with adults and children who have fluency disorders.

➤ The client can read selections of the Stuttering Foundation of America's *Advice to those who stutter* (Publication No. 9) and practice the suggestions contained in the chapters.

CONCLUSION

Although change occurs throughout formal treatment, progress must continue long after formal intervention has been completed. Unfortunately, as is the case with many complex human problems, relapse is not unusual, particularly for adult clients. Emphasis on transfer and maintenance activities that include extra-treatment performance will help decrease the possibility of relapse. Following formal treatment, continued vigilance and effort are required for long-term success. It is helpful to understand that a small lapse does not mean that a relapse is imminent.

As a result of treatment, some clients will become fluent. Others will continue to stutter but in a smoother and effortless form, and some—for now at least—will make little change. Nearly all speakers have the potential to develop to the point where they have very little, and in some cases, essentially no handicap because of their speech.

It is also important to realize that many in the client's environment will probably need to adjust not only to his newly acquired fluency, but also to reformed relationships and altered roles. Family members and friends may need to adapt to a speaker who may be considerably more assertive than previously. Membership in one or more support groups both during and following treatment is highly recommended for maintaining both behavioral and attitudinal changes. There is an ever-increasing source of useful information available from the internet as well as materials from related groups (Appendix C). If treatment is successful, the client must gradually assume the responsibility for self-evaluating and systematically altering both the surface and intrinsic features of stuttering. He may also begin to enjoy an ever-expanding participation in many areas of life he has so energetically avoided in the past.

STUDY QUESTIONS

➤ What is your response to an adult who asks you what his chances are of relapse following treatment?
➤ How is relapse usually defined in the literature?
➤ What are some of the early indicators of relapse?
➤ What are some possible causes of relapse following treatment?
➤ What are some procedures or measures you would consider for attempting to predict relapse in your clients?
➤ What is your opinion of the assistance provided to people who stutter and their families by the self-help movement?
➤ Considering the transfer and maintenance described in this chapter, develop examples of activities that you could use to change one or more of your habitual behaviors.

RECOMMENDED READINGS

Boberg, E. (1983). Behavioral transfer and maintenance programs for adolescent and adult stutterers. pp. 41–61. In J. Fraser Gruss (Ed.) *Stuttering therapy:*

Transfer and maintenance (Publication No. 19). Memphis, TN: Stuttering Foundation of America.

Craig, A. (1998). Relapse following treatment for stuttering: A critical review and correlative data. *Journal of Fluency Disorders, 23*, 1–30.

Hood, S. B. (1998). *Advice to those who stutter* (Publication No. 9). Memphis, TN: Stuttering Foundation of America.

Manning, W. H. (1991). Making progress during and after treatment. In W. H. Perkins (Ed.), *Seminars in speech and language,* 12:349–354. New York: Thieme Medical Publishers.

EPILOGUE

Throughout this text I have tried to be true to the goals stated in the preface. However, one of those goals continues to rise above all the others. This is the need to create enthusiasm in clinicians for helping children, adolescents, and adults with fluency disorders. Enthusiasm is created and enhanced by exploration. Just as we encourage those we are trying to help to take action, the professional clinician must continually take action to seek new information and consider new strategies and techniques. With a graduate degree at the outset, the professional clinician will take part in a process of learning and change that is similar to the journey we ask our clients to take.

With an understanding of the many possibilities and choices of intervention, the experienced and wise clinician is free to focus on the needs of the person who has come to us for help. Rather than concentrating on doctrine or techniques, the professional is able to make clinical decisions based on her experience and the accurate perception of a client's need at a moment in time. This is no simple task and it will take a lifetime of practice to do it well.

Clinicians who work with people who stutter, especially those that are entering the field, need to know that magnificent changes are possible in the speech and the lives of those who come to us for help. If there is any doubt of this, read the descriptions of successful treatment that are cited in the opening paragraph of the final chapter of this text.

Not every speech-language pathologist is equipped to work in the area of fluency disorders for, as in each of the specialty areas of our parent field, it takes some unique abilities. However, for those who choose to come to the assistance of these people who because of their stuttering are struggling to communicate with others and to seek fulfillment as human beings, there are exciting and rewarding victories to be shared and marvelous colleagues who are willing to help.

REFERENCES

Ackoff, R. (1974). *Redesigning the future*. New York: Wiley.

Adams, M. R. (1977a). A clinical strategy for differentiating the normal nonfluent child and the incipient stutterers. *Journal of Fluency Disorders, 2,* 141–148.

Adams, M. R. (1977b). The young stutterer: Diagnosis, treatment and assessment of progress. *Seminars in Speech, Language and Hearing, 1,* 289–299.

Adams, M. R. (1983). Learning from negative outcomes in stuttering therapy: Getting off on the wrong foot. *Journal of Fluency Disorders, 8,* 147–153.

Adams, M. R. (1984). The differential assessment and direct treatment of stuttering, In J. Costello (Ed.), *Speech disorders in children* (pp. 260–295). San Diego, CA: College-Hill Press.

Adams, M. R. (1990). The demands and capacities model I: Theoretical elaborations. *Journal of Fluency Disorders, 15,* 135–141.

Adams, M. R. (1993). The home environment of children who stutter. *Seminars in Speech and Language, 14*(3), 185–191.

Adams, M. R., & Hayden, P. (1976). The ability of stutters and nonstutterers to initiate and terminate phonation during production of an isolated vowel. *Journal of Speech and Hearing Disorders, 19,* 290–296.

Adams, M. R., & Runyan, C. (1981). Stuttering and fluency: Exclusive events or points on a continuum? *Journal of Fluency Disorders, 6,* 197–218.

Agnello, J. G. (1975). Voice onset and voice termination features of stutterers. In L. M. Webster & L. C. Furst (Eds.), *Vocal tract dynamics and disfluency*. New York: Speech and Hearing Institute.

Ainsworth, S. (Ed.). (1992). *Counseling stutterers* (Publication No. 18, 4th ed.). pp. 171–186. Memphis, TN: Speech Foundation of America.

Albach, J., & Benson, V. (Eds.). (1994). *To say what is ours. The best of 13 years of letting GO.* (3rd Ed.). San Francisco, CA: National Stuttering Project.

Alfonso, P. J., Watson, B. C., & Baer, T. (1987). Measuring stutterers' dynamic vocal tract characteristics by x-ray microbeam pellet tracking. In H. F. M. Peters & W. Hulstijn (Eds.), *Speech motor dynamics in stuttering*. New York: Springer-Verlag.

Allen, G. (1975). Speech rhythm: Its relation to performance universals and articulatory timing. *Journal of Phonetics, 3,* 75–86.

Alport, G. W. (1937). *Personality, a psychological interpretation*. New York: Hold.

Alport, G. W. (1961). *Pattern and growth in personality*. New York: Holt, Rinehart & Winston.

Ambrose, N. G., Cox, N., & Yairi, E. (1997). The genetic basis of persistent and recovered stuttering. *Journal of Speech and Hearing Research, 40,* 567–580.

Ambrose, N. G., & Yairi, E. (1994). The development of awareness of stuttering in preschool children. *Journal of Fluency Disorders, 19,* 229–246.

Ambrose, N. G., & Yairi, E. (1995). The role of repetition units in the differential diagnosis of early childhood incipient stuttering. *American Journal of Speech-Language Pathology, 4*(3), 82–88.

Ambrose, N. G., Yairi, E., and Cox, N. (1993). Genetic factors in childhood stuttering. *Journal of Speech and Hearing Research, 36,* 701–706.

American Academy of Neurology. (1990). Assessment: The clinical usefulness of botulinum toxin-A in treating neurologic disorders. *Neurology, 40,* 1332–1336.

American Psychiatric Association. (1987). *Diagnostic and statistical manual of mental disorders* (3rd ed.-rev. [DSM-III-R]). Washington, DC: American Psychiatric Association.

American Psychiatric Association. (1994). *Diagnostic and statistical manual of mental disorders* (4th ed.-rev. [DSM-IV]). Washington, DC: American Psychiatric Association.

American Psychological Association. (1947). Recommended graduate training program in clinical psychology: Report of the committee on training in clinical psychology. *American Psychologist, 2,* 539–558.

American Speech-Language-Hearing Association. (1984). Guidelines for caseload size for speech-language services in the schools. *ASHA, 26,* 53–58.

Amman, J. O. C. (1700/1965). *A dissertation on speech* (reprint). New York: Stechert-Hafner.

Andrews, G. (1984). Epidemiology of stuttering. In R. F. Curlee & W. H. Perkins (Eds.), *Nature and treatment of stuttering: New directions* (pp. 1–12). San Diego, CA: College Hill Press.

Andrews, G., & Craig, A. (1982). Stuttering: Overt and covert assessment of the speech of treated subjects. *Journal of Speech and Hearing Disorders, 47,* 96–99.

Andrews, G., & Craig, A. R. (1985). The prediction and prevention of relapse in stuttering. The value of self-control techniques and locus of control measures. *Behavior Modification, 9,* 427–442.

Andrews, G., & Craig, A. R. (1988). Prediction of outcome after treatment for stuttering. *British Journal of Psychiatry, 153,* 236–240.

Andrews, G., Craig, A., & Feyer, A. M. (1983). *Therapist's manual for the stuttering treatment programme.* Sydney, Australia: Prince Henry Hospital, Division of Communication Disorders.

Andrews, G., Craig, A., Feyer, A., Hoddinott, S., Howie, P., & Neilson, M. (1983). Stuttering: A review of research findings and theories circa 1982. *Journal of Speech and Hearing Disorders, 48,* 226–246.

Andrews, G., & Cutler, J. (1974). Stuttering therapy: The relation between changes in symptom level and attitudes. *Journal of Speech and Hearing Disorders, 39,* 312–319.

Andrews, G., Guitar, B., & Howie. P. (1980). Meta-analysis of the effects of stuttering treatment. *Journal of Speech and Hearing Disorders, 45,* 287–307.

Andrews, G., & Harris, M. (1964). *The syndrome of stuttering* (Clinics in Developmental Medicine No. 17). London: Spastics Society Medical Education and Information Unit, in association with W. Heinemann Medical Books.

Andrews, G., & Harvey, R. (1981). Regression to the mean in pretreatment measures of stuttering. *Journal of Speech and Hearing Disorders, 46,* 204–207.

Andrews, G., & Neilson, M. (1981). *Stuttering: A state of the art seminar.* Paper to the annual meeting of the Speech-Hearing Association, Los Angeles, CA.

Andrews, G., Quinn, P. T., & Sorby, W. A. (1972). Stuttering: An investigation into cerebral dominance of speech. *Journal of Neurology, Neurosurgery, and Psychiatry, 25,* 414–418.

Andrews, G., Yates-Morris, A., Howie, P., & Martin, N. G. (1991). Genetic factors in stuttering confirmed. *Archives of General Psychiatry, 48*(11), 1034–1035.

Apel, K. (1999). Checks and balances: Keeping the science in our profession. *Language, Speech, and Hearing Services in Schools, 30,* 99–108.

Arnold, G. E. (1960). Studies in tachyphemia:I. Present concepts of etiologic factors. *Logos, 3,* 25–45.

Arnott, N. (1928). *Elements of physics.* Edinburgh, Scotland: Adams.

Aronson, A. E. (1973). *Psychogenic voice disorders: An interdisciplinary approach to detection, diagnosis, and therapy.* New York: W. B. Saunders.

Aronson, A. E. (1978). Differential diagnosis of organic and psychogenic voice disorders. In F. L. Darley and D. C. Spriesterbach (Eds.), *Diagnostic methods in speech pathology* (2nd ed., pp. 535–560). New York: Harper and Row.

Aronson, A. E. (1992). *Clinical voice disorders. An interdisciplinary approach.* New York: Thieme.

Aronson, A. E., Brown, J., Litin, E. M., & Pearson, J. S. (1968). Spastic dysphonia. I: Voice, neurological and psychiatric aspects. *Journal of Speech and Hearing Disorders, 33,* 219–231.

Attanasio, J. (1987). The dodo was Lewis Carroll you see: Reflections and speculations. *Journal of Fluency Disorders, 12,* 107–118.

Attanasio, J. (1997). Was Moses a person who stuttered? Perhaps not. *Journal of Fluency Disorders, 22,* 65–68.

Azrin, N. H., Nunn, R. G., & Frantz, S. E. (1979). Comparison of regulated breathing versus abbreviated desensitization on reported stuttering episodes. *Journal of Speech and Hearing Disorders, 44,* 331–339.

Backus, O. (1947). Intensive group therapy in speech rehabilitation. *Journal of Speech Disorders, 12,* 39–60.

Backus, O. (1957). Group structure in speech therapy. In L. E. Travis (Ed.), *Handbook of speech pathology* (pp. 1025–1064). New York: Appleton-Century-Crofts, Inc.

Baken, R. J. (1987). *Clinical measurement of speech and voice.* Boston: Little, Brown, & Co.

Bamberg, C., Hanley, J., & Hillenbrand, J. (1990). Pitch and amplitude perturbation in adult stutterers and nonstutterers. Paper presented to the annual meeting of the American Speech-Language-Hearing Association, Seattle, WA.

Bandura, A. (1977). Toward a unifying theory of behavior change. *Psychological Review, 1,* 191–215.

Bannister, D. (1966). Psychology as an exercise in paradox. *Bulletin of the British Psychological Society, 19,* 21–26.

Barbara, D. A. (Ed.). (1965). *New Directions in Stuttering: Theory and Practice.* Springfield, IL: Charles C. Thomas.

Barbara, D. A. (1982). *The psychodynamics of stuttering.* Springfield, IL: Charles C. Thomas.

Battle, D. E. (1993). Introduction. In D. E. Battle (Ed.), *Communication disorders in multicultural populations* (pp. XV–XXIV). Stoneham, MA: Andover Medical Publishers/Butterworth-Heinemann.

Baumgartner, J. M. (1999). Acquired Psychogenic Stuttering. In R. Curlee (Ed.), *Stuttering and related disorders of fluency* (2nd ed., pp. 269–288). New York: Thieme Medical Publishers, Inc.

Baumgartner, J., & Duffy, J. (1997). Psychogenic stuttering in adults with and without neurologic disease. *Journal of Medical Speech-Language Pathology, 52,* 75–95.

Beech, H., & Fransella, F. (1968). *Research and experiment in stuttering.* Oxford, England: Pergamon Press.

Bell, A. M. (1853). *Observations on defects of speech, the cure of stammering, and the principles of elocution.* London: Hamilton-Adams.

Bennett, E. M., & Chemela, K. A. (1998). The mask of shame: Treatment strategies for adults who stutter. In E. C. Healey & H. F. M. Peters (Eds.), *Proceedings of the 2nd World Congress on Fluency Disorders* (pp. 340–342). Nijmegen, The Netherlands: Nijmegen University Press.

Berenson, B. G., & Carkhuff, R. R. (1967). *Sources of gain in counseling and psychotherapy.* New York: Holt, Rinehart & Winston.

Berenson, B. G., & Mitchell, K. M. (1974). *Confrontation: For better or worse.* Amherst, MA: Human Resource Development Press.

Berkowitz, M., Cook, H., & Haughey, J. (1994). Fluency program developed for the public school setting. *Language, Speech and Hearing Services in Schools, 25,* 94–99.

Berlin, C. I., Lowe-Bell, S. S., Cullen, J. K., Jr., Thompson, C. L., & Loovis, C. F. (1973). Dichotic speech perception: An interpretation of right-ear advantage and temporal offset effects. *Journal of the Acoustical Society of America, 53,* 699–709.

Berlin, C. I., & McNeil, M. R. (1976). Dichotic Listening. In N. J. Lass (Ed.), *Contemporary issues in experimental phonetics.* New York: Academic Press.

Berry, M. F. (1938). Developmental history of stuttering children. *Journal of Pediatrics, 11,* 209–217.

Bhatnagar, S.C., & Andy, O.J. (1995). *Neuroscience for the Study of Communicative Disorders.* Baltimore, MD: Williams & Wilkins.

Black, J. W. (1951). The effect of delayed sidetone upon vocal rate and intensity. *Journal of Speech and Hearing Disorders, 16,* 56–60.

Blanton, S., & Blanton, M. G. (1936). *For stutterers.* New York: Appleton-Century.

Bloch, E. L., & Goodstein, L. D. (1971). Functional speech disorders and personality: A decade of research. *Journal of Speech and Hearing Disorders, 36,* 295–314.

Blodgett, E. G., & Cooper, E. B. (1988). Talking about it and doing it: Meta linguistic capacity and prosodic control in three to seven year olds. *Journal of Fluency Disorders, 13,* 283–290.

Blood, G. (1995). A behavioral-cognitive therapy program for adults who stutter: Computers and counseling. *Journal of Communication Disorders, 28,* 165–180.

Blood, G. (1995). POWER^2: Relapse management with adolescents who stutter. *Language, Speech, and Hearing Services in Schools, 26,* 169–179.

Blood, G. W., & Blood, I. M. (1982). A tactic for facilitating social interacting with laryngectomees. *Journal of Speech and Hearing Disorders, 47,* 416–419.

Blood, G. W., & Hood, S. B. (1978). Elementary school-age stutterers' disfluencies during oral reading and spontaneous speech. *Journal of Fluency Disorders, 3,* 155–165.

Blood, G., & Seider, R. (1981). The concomitant problems of young stutterers. *Journal of Speech and Hearing Disorders, 46,* 31–33.

Bloodstein, O. (1949). Conditions under which stuttering is reduced or absent: A review of literature. *Journal of Speech and Hearing Disorders, 14,* 295–302.

Bloodstein, O. (1950). Hypothetical conditions under which stuttering is reduced or absent. *Journal of Speech and Hearing Disorders, 15,* 142–153.

Bloodstein, O. (1958). Stuttering as anticipatory struggle reaction. In J. Eisenson (Ed.), *Stuttering: A symposium,* pp. 1–69. New York: Harper & Row.

Bloodstein, O. (1960). The development of stuttering I. Changes in nine basic features. *Journal of Speech and Hearing Disorders, 25,* 219–237.

Bloodstein, O. (1961). The development of stuttering III. Theoretical and clinical implications. *Journal of Speech and Hearing Disorders, 26,* 67–82.

Bloodstein, O. (1974). The rules of early stuttering. *Journal of Speech and Hearing Disorders, 39,* 379–394.

Bloodstein, O. (1987). *A handbook on stuttering* (4th ed.). Chicago: National Easter Seal Society.

Bloodstein, O. (1992). Response to Hamre: Part I. *Journal of Fluency Disorders, 17,* 29–32.

Bloodstein, O. (1993). *Stuttering: The search for a cause and cure.* Needham Heights, MA: Allyn & Bacon.

Bloodstein, O. (1995). *A handbook on stuttering* (5th ed.). San Diego: Singular Publishing Group.

Bloodstein, O. (1999). Opening comments to the sixth annual leadership conference of the ASHA Special Interest Division, San Diego, CA.

Bloodstein, O., & Grossman, M. (1981). Early stutterings: Some aspects of their form and distribution. *Journal of Speech and Hearing Research, 24,* 298–302.

Bloodstein, O., & Shogun, R. (1972). Some clinical notes on forced stuttering. *Journal of Speech and Hearing Disorders, 37,* 177–186.

Bloom, C. & Cooperman, D. K. (1999). *Synergistic stuttering therapy: A holistic approach.* Boston: Butterworth-Heinemann

Bluemel, C. S. (1932). Primary and secondary stammering. *Quarterly Journal of Speech, 18,* 187–200.

Bluemel, C. S. (1957). *The riddle of stuttering.* Danville, IL: Interstate.

Boberg, E. (1983). Behavioral transfer and maintenance programs for adolescent and adult stutterers. In J. Fraser Gruss (Ed.), *Stuttering therapy: Transfer and maintenance* (Publication No. 19, pp. 41–61). Memphis, TN: Stuttering Foundation of America.

Boberg, E. (Ed.). (1986). Maintenance of fluency: An Experimental program. In E. Boberg (Ed.) *Maintenance of fluency: Proceedings of the Banff Conference* (pp. 71–112). New York: Elsevier.

Boberg, E., Howie, P., & Woods, L. (1979). Maintenance of fluency: A review. *Journal of Fluency Disorders, 4,* 93–116.

Boberg, E., & Kully, D. (1984). Techniques for transferring fluency. In W. H. Perkins (Ed.), *Current therapy of communication disorders: Stuttering disorders* (pp. 178–201). New York: Thieme-Stratton.

Boberg, E., & Sawyer, L. (1977). The maintenance of fluency following intensive therapy. *Human Communication, 2,* 21–28.

Boberg, E., Yeudall, L. T., Schopflocher, D., & Bo Lassen, P. (1983). The effect of an intensive behavioral program on the distribution of EEG alpha power in stutterers during the processing of verbal and visuospatial information. *Journal of Fluency Disorders, 8,* 245–263.

Bobrick, B. (1995). *Knotted tongues.* New York: Simon and Schuster.

Bonfanti, B. H., & Culatta, R. (1977). An analysis of the fluency patterns of institutionalized retarded adults. *Journal of Fluency Disorders, 2,* 117–128.

Bordeau, L. A., & Jeffrey, C. H. (1973). Stuttering treated by desensitization. *Journal of Behavior Therapy and Experimental Psychiatry, 4,* 209–212.

Borden, G. D., Kim, D. H., & Spiegler, K. (1991). Acoustics of stop consonant-vowel relationships during fluent and stuttered utterances. *Journal of Fluency Disorders, 12*(3), 175–184.

Bosshardt, H. (1990). Subvocalization and reading rate differences between stuttering and nonstuttering children and adults. *Journal of Speech and Hearing Research, 33,* 776–785.

Bosshardt, H., & Nandyal, I. (1988). Reading rates of stutterers and nonstutterers during silent and oral reading. *Journal of Fluency Disorders, 13,* 407–420.

Botterill, W. & Cook, F. (1987). Personal construct theory and the treatment of adolescent disfluency. In L. Rustin, H. Purser & D. Rowley (Eds.), *Progress in the treatment of fluency disorders* (pp. 147–165). London: Taylor & Francis.

Brady, J.P., & Berson, J. (1975). Stuttering, dichotic listening, and cerebral dominance. *Archives of General Psychiatry, 32,* 1449–1452.

Branch, C., Milner, B., & Rasmussen, T. (1964). Intercarotid sodium amytol for lateralization of cerebral speech dominance. *Journal of Neurosurgery, 21,* 399–405.

Breitenfeldt, D. H., & Lorenz, D. R. (1989). *Successful stuttering management program.* Cheney: Eastern Washington University.

Brill, A. A. (1923). Speech disturbances in nervous and mental diseases. *Quarterly Journal of Speech, 9,* 129–135.

Brin, M. F., Stewart, C., Blitzer, A., & Diamond, B. (1994). Laryngeal botulinum toxin injections for disabling stuttering in adults. *Neurology, 44,* 2262–2266.

Brisk, D. J., Healey, E. C., & Hux, K. A. (1997). Clinicians' training and confidence associated with treating school-age children who stutter: A national survey. *Language, Speech, and Hearing Services in Schools, 28,* 164–176.

Broadbent, D.E., & Gregory, M. (1964). Accuracy of recognition for speech presented to the right and left ears. *Quarterly Journal of Experimental Psychology, 16,* 359–360.

Brodnitz, F. S. (1976). Spastic dysphonia. *Annals of Otorhinolaryngology, 85,* 210–214.

Brown, G., & Cullinan, W. L. (1981). Word-retrieval difficulty and disfluent speech in adult anomic speakers. *Journal of Speech and Hearing Research, 24,* 358–365.

Brownell, K.D., Marlatt, G. A., Lichtenstein, E. & Wilson, G. T., (1996). Understanding and preventing relapse. *American Psychologist, 41,* 765–782.

Brutten, G. J., & Dunham, S. (1989). The Communication Attitude Test: A normative study of grade school children. *Journal of Fluency Disorders, 14,* 371–377.

Brutten, G. J., & Shoemaker, D. J. (1967). *The modification of stuttering.* Englewood Cliffs, NJ: Prentice-Hall.

Bryngleson, B. (1935). Method of stuttering. *Journal of Abnormal Psychology, 30,* 194–198.

Bryngleson, B. (1938). Prognosis in stuttering. *Journal of Speech Disorders, 3,* 121–123.

Bryngleson, B., Chapman, B., & Hansen, O. (1944). *Know yourself: A guide for those who stutter.* Minneapolis: Burgess Publishing.

Bullen, A. K. (1945). A cross cultural approach to the problem of stuttering. *Child Development, 16,* 1–88.

Burks, H. (1976). *Burks behavioral rating scales.* Los Angeles: Western Psychological Services.

Burton, A. (1972). *Interpersonal psychotherapy.* Englewood Cliffs, NJ: Prentice-Hall.

Cabanas, R. (1954). Some findings in speech and voice therapy among mentally deficient children. *Folia Phoniatrica, 6,* 34–39.

Cannito. M. P. (1991). Neurobiological interpretations of spasmodic dysphonia. In D. Vogel and M. P. Cannito (Eds.), *Treating disordered speech motor control: For clinicians by clinicians* (pp. 275–317). Austin: Pro-Ed.

Cannito, M. P., Burch, A. R., Watts, C., Rappold, P. W., Hood, S. B., & Sherrard, K. (1997). Disfluency in spasmodic dysphonia: A multivariate analysis. *Journal of Speech, Language, and Hearing Research, 40,* 627–641.

Cannito, M. P., & Sherrard, K. C. (1995). *Fluency in spasmodic dysphonia I: Oral reading rate and disfluency occurrence.* Unpublished manuscript.

Carkhuff, R. R., & Berenson, B. G. (1967). *Beyond counseling and psychotherapy.* New York: Holt, Rinehart & Winston.

Carlise, J. A. (1985). *Tangled tongue: Living with a stutter.* Toronto, Canada: University of Toronto Press.

Caruso, A. J. (1988). Childhood stuttering: A review of behavioral, acoustical, and physiological research [abstract]. *ASHA, 30,* 73.

Caruso, A. J., Abbs, J. H., & Gracco, V.L. (1988). Kinematic analysis of multiple movement coordination during speech in stutterers. *Brain, 111,* 439–456.

Caruso, A., Conture, E., & Colton, R. (1988). Selected temporal parameters of coordination associated with stuttering in children. *Journal of Fluency Disorders, 12,* 67–82.

Caruso, A. J., Gracco, V. L., & Abbs, J. H. (1987). A speech motor control perspective on stuttering: Preliminary observation. In H. F. M. Peters & Hulstijn (Eds.), *Speech motor dynamics in stuttering* (pp. 245–258). Wien: Springer Verlag.

Cerf, A., & Prins, D. (1974). *Stutterers' ear preference for dichotic syllables.* Paper presented to the annual meeting of the American Speech-Language-Hearing Association, Las Vegas.

Chmela, K. A. (1998). Thoughts on recovery. In E. C. Healey & H. F. M. Peters (Eds.), *Proceedings of the 2nd World Congress on Fluency Disorders* (pp. 376–378). Nijmegen, The Netherlands: Nijmegen University Press.

Chmela, K. A., & Reardon, N. A. (2000). *The school-age child who stutters: Practical ideas for working with feelings and beliefs about stuttering* (Publication No. 5). Stuttering Foundation of America.

Clark, H. (1971). The importance of linguistics for the study of speech hesitations. In D. Horton & J. Jenkins (Eds.), *The perception of language: Proceedings of the symposium, University of Pittsburgh.* Columbus, OH: Charles E. Merrill.

Colburn, N. (1985). Clustering of disfluency in stuttering children's early utterances. *Journal of Fluency Disorders, 10,* 51–58.

Cole, L. (1986). The social responsibility of the researcher. In F. H. Bess, B. S. Clark, & H. R. Mitchell (Eds.), *Concerns for minority groups in communication disorders* (ASHA Reports No. 16, ISSN 0569-8553, pp. 93–100). Rockville, MD: American Speech-Language-Hearing Association.

Cole, L. (1989). E pluribus pluribus: Multicultural imperatives for the 1990s and beyond. *Journal of the American Speech-Language-Hearing Association, 31,* 65–71.

Collins, C. R., & Blood, G. W. (1990). Acknowledgement and severity of stuttering as factors influencing nonstutterers' perceptions of stutterers. *Journal of Speech and Hearing Disorders, 55,* 75–81.

Combs, A., & Snygg, D. (1959). *Individual behavior.* New York: Harper.

Conners, C. K. (1997). *Conners' rating scales—revised.* New York: Multi-Health Systems, Inc.

Conture, E. G. (1982). Stuttering in young children. *Journal of Developmental and Behavioral Pediatrics, 3,* 163–169.

Conture, E. G. (1990). *Stuttering* (2nd ed.). Englewood Cliffs, NJ: Prentice-Hall.

Conture, E. G. (1996). Treatment efficacy: stuttering. *Journal of Speech and Hearing Research, 39,* S18–26.

Conture, E. G. (1997). Evaluating childhood stuttering. In R. Curlee & G. Siegel (Eds.), *Nature and treatment of stuttering, new directions* (2nd ed., pp. 239–256). Needham Heights, MA: Allyn & Bacon.

Conture, E. G. (2000). *Stuttering* (3rd ed.). Needham Heights, MA: Allyn & Bacon.

Conture, E., & Caruso, A. (1987). Assessment and diagnosis of childhood disfluency. In L. Ruskin, D. Rowley, & H. Purser (Eds.), *Progress in the treatment of fluency disorders* (pp. 57–82). London, England: Taylor & Francis.

Conture, E., Colton, R., & Gleason, J. (1988). Selected temporal aspects of coordination during fluency speech of young stutterers. *Journal of Speech and Hearing Research, 31,* 640–653.

Conture, E., & Guitar, B. (1993). Evaluating efficacy of treatment of stuttering: School-age children. *Journal of Fluency Disorders, 18,* 253–287.

Conture, E., & Kelly, E. (1988). *Nonverbal behavior of young stutterers and their mothers.* Paper presented to the annual meeting of the American Speech-Language-Hearing Association, Boston, MA.

Conture, E. & Kelly, E. (1991). Young stutterers' non-speech behaviors during stuttering. *Journal of Speech and Hearing Research, 34,* 1041–1056.

Conture, E., Louko, L., & Edwards, M. L. (1993). Simultaneously treating stuttering and disordered phonology in children: Experimental therapy, preliminary findings. *American Journal of Speech-Language Pathology, 2*(3), 72–81.

Conture, E. G., McCall, G. N., & Brewer, D. (1977). Laryngeal behavior during stuttering. *Journal of Speech and Hearing Research, 20,* 661–668.

Conture, E., Rothenberg, M., & Molitor, R. (1986). Electroglottographic observations of young stutterers' fluency. *Journal of Speech and Hearing Research, 29,* 384–393.

Conture, E., & Schwartz, H. (1984). Children who stutter: diagnosis and remediation. *Communication Disorders, 9,* 1–18.

Conture, E. G., & Zebrowski, P. M. (1992). Can child speech disfluencies be mutable to the influences of speech-language pathologists, but immutable to the influence of parents? *Journal of Fluency Disorders, 17,* 121–130.

Cooper, E. B. (1968). A therapy process for the adult stutterer. *Journal of Speech and Hearing Disorders, 33,* 246–260.

Cooper, E. B. (1972). Recovery from stuttering in a junior and senior high school population. *Journal of Speech and Hearing Research, 15,* 632–638.

Cooper, E. B. (1973). The development of a stuttering chronicity prediction checklist: A preliminary report. *Journal of Speech and Hearing Disorders, 38,* 215–223.

Cooper, E. B. (1975a). *Clinician attitudes toward stutterers: A study of bigotry?* Paper presented at the annual meeting of the American Speech-Language-Hearing Association, Washington, DC.

Cooper, E. B. (1975b). *Clinician Attitudes Toward Stuttering Inventory (CATS).* Allen, TX: DLM.

Cooper, E. B. (1977). Controversies about stuttering therapy. *Journal of Fluency Disorders, 2,* 75–86.

Cooper, E. B. (1979a). Intervention procedures for the young stutterer. In H. Gregory (Ed.), *Controversies about stuttering* (pp. 63–96). Baltimore, MD: University Park Press.

Cooper, E. B. (1979b). *Understanding stuttering: Information for parents.* Chicago: National Easter Seal Society for Crippled Children and Adults.

Cooper, E. B. (1985). *Cooper personalized fluency control therapy—revised.* Allen, TX: DLM.

Cooper, E. B. (1986a). The mentally retarded stutterer. In K. O. St. Louis (Ed.), *The atypical stutterer* (pp. 123–154). San Diego, CA: Academic Press.

Cooper, E. B. (1986b). Treatment of dysfluency: Future trends. *Journal of Fluency Disorders, 11,* 317–327.

Cooper, E. B. (1987). The chronic perseverative stuttering syndrome: Incurable stuttering. *Journal of Fluency Disorders, 12,* 381–388.

Cooper, E. B. (1990). *Understanding stuttering: Information for parents.* Chicago: National Easter Seal Society.

Cooper, E. B. (1993). Red herrings, dead horses, straw men, and blind alleys: Escaping the stuttering conundrum. *Journal of Fluency Disorders, 18,* 375–387.

Cooper, E. B., Cady, B. B., & Robbins, C. J. (1970). The effect of the verbal stimulus words wrong, right and tree on the disfluency rates of stutterers and nonstutterers. *Journal of Speech and Hearing Research, 13,* 239–244.

Cooper, E. B., & Cooper, C. S. (1965). Variations in adult stutterer attitudes towards clinicians during therapy. *Journal of Communication Disorders, 2,* 141–153.

Cooper, E. B., & Cooper, C. S. (1985a). Clinician attitudes toward stuttering: A decade of change (1973–1983). *Journal of Fluency Disorders, 10,* 19–33.

Cooper, E. B., & Cooper, C. S. (1985b). The effective clinician. In E. B. Cooper and C. S. Cooper, *Personalized fluency control therapy—revised (handbook)* (pp. 21–31) Allen, TX: DLM.

Cooper, E. B., & Cooper, C. S. (1985c). *Personalized fluency control therapy—revised (handbook).* Allen, TX: DLM.

Cooper, E. B., & Cooper, C. S. (1991a). A fluency disorders prevention program for preschoolers and children in the primary grades. *American Journal of Speech-Language Pathology, 1,* 28–31.

Cooper, E. B., & Cooper, C. S. (1991b). *Multicultural considerations in the assessment and treatment of fluency disorders.* Paper presented at the American Speech-Language-Hearing Association Annual Convention, Atlanta, GA.

Cooper, E. B., & Cooper, C. S. (1992). *Clinician attitudes toward stuttering: two decades of change.* Paper presented to the annual meeting of the American Speech-Language-Hearing Association, San Antonio, TX.

Cooper, E. B., & Cooper, C. S. (1993). Fluency disorders. In D. E. Battle (Ed.), *Communication disorders in multicultural populations* (pp. 189–211). Stoneham, MA: Andover Medical Publishers/Butterworth-Heinemann.

Corcoran, J. A., & Stewart, M. (1998). Stories of stuttering: A qualitative analysis of interview narratives. *Journal of Fluency Disorders, 23,* 247–264.

Cordes, A. K. (1998). Current status of the stuttering treatment literature. In A. K. Cordes & R. J. Ingham (Eds.), *Treatment efficacy for stuttering: A search for empirical bases.* San Diego, CA: Singular Publishing.

Cordes, A. K., & Ingham, R. J. (1998). *Treatment efficacy for stuttering: A search for empirical bases.* San Diego, CA: Singular Publishing.

Coriat, I. H. (1943). Psychoanalytic concept of stammering. *Nervous Child, 2,* 167–171.

Costello, J. M. (1983). Current behavioral treatment of children. In D. Prins & R. J. Ingham (Eds.), *Treatment of stuttering in early childhood: Methods and issues* (pp. 69–112). San Diego, CA: College-Hill Press.

Cousins, N. (1979). *Anatomy of an illness.* New York: Norton.

Covey, S. (1989). *The seven habits of highly effective people.* New York: Simon & Schuster.

Cox, J. J., Seider, R. A., & Kidd, K. K. (1984). Some environmental factors and hypotheses for stuttering in families with several stutterers. *Journal of Speech and Hearing Research, 27,* 543–548.

Craig, A. (1990). An investigation into the relationship between anxiety and stuttering. *Journal of Speech and Hearing Disorders, 55,* 290–294.

Craig, A. (1998). Relapse following treatment for stuttering: A critical review and correlative data. *Journal of Fluency Disorders, 23,* 1–30.

Craig, A., & Andrews, G. (1985). The prediction and prevention of relapse in stuttering. The value of self-control techniques and locus of control measures. *Behavior Modification, 9,* 427–442.

Craig, A and Calver, P. (1991) Following up on treated stutterers: Studies on perceptions of fluency and job status. *Journal of Speech and Hearing Research, 34,* 279–284.

Craig, A., Franklin, J., & Andrews, G. (1984). A scale to measure locus of control of behavior. *British Journal of Medical Psychology, 57,* 173–180.

Craig, A. and Hancock, K. (1995). Self-reported factors related to relapse following treatment for stuttering. *Australian Journal of Human Communication Disorders, 23,* 48–60.

Craig, A. and Hancock, K. (1996). Anxiety in children and young adolescents who stutter. *Australian Journal of Human Communication Disorders, 24,* 28–38.

Craig, A., Hancock, K., Chang, E., McCready, C., Shepley, A., McCaul, A., Costello, D., Harding, S., Kehran, R., Masel, C., & Reilly, K. (1996). A controlled trial for stuttering in persons aged 9 to 14 years. *Journal of Speech and Hearing Research, 38,* 808–826.

Cross, D. E., & Luper, H. L. (1983). Relation between finger reaction time and voice reaction time in stuttering and nonstuttering children and adults. *Journal of Speech and Hearing Research, 26,* 356–361.

Cross, D. E., Shadden, B. B., & Luper, H. L. (1979). Effects of stimulus ear presentation on the voice reaction time of adult stutterers and nonstutterers. *Journal of Fluency Disorders, 4,* 45–58.

Crowe, T. A. (1997a). Counseling: Definition, history, rationale. In T. A. Crowe (Ed.), *Applications of Counseling in Speech-Language Pathology and Audiology* (pp. 3–29). Baltimore: Williams & Wilkins.

Crowe, T. A. (1997b). Emotional aspects of communicative disorders. In T. A. Crowe (Ed.), *Applications of Counseling in Speech-Language Pathology and Audiology* (pp. 30–47). Baltimore: Williams & Wilkins.

Crowe, T. A., & Cooper, E. B. (1977). Clinician attitudes toward and knowledge of stuttering. *Journal of Communication Disorders, 10,* 343–357.

Crowe, T. A., DiLollo, A. P., & Crowe, B. T., *Crowe's Protocols: A Comprehensive Guide to Stuttering Assessment.* San Antonio, TX: The Psychological Corporation.

Crystal, D. (1987). Towards a "bucket" theory of language disability: Taking account of interaction between linguistic levels. *Clinical Linguistics and Phonetics, 1,* 7–22.

Culatta, R., & Goldberg. S. A. (1995). *Stuttering therapy: An integrated approach to theory and practice.* Boston: Allyn & Bacon.

Curlee, R. (1984). Counseling with adults who stutter. In W. Perkins (Ed.), *Stuttering disorders.* New York: Thieme-Stratton.

Curlee, R. (1985). Training students to work with stutterers. In E. Boberg (Ed.), *Stuttering: Part one. Seminars in speech and language, 6*(2), 131–144. New York: Thieme-Stratton.

Curlee, R. (1993). Evaluating treatment efficacy for adults: Assessment of stuttering disability. *Journal of Fluency Disorders, 18,* 319–331.

Curlee, R. (2000). Demands-Capacities versus Demands-Performance. *Journal of Fluency Disorders* (in press).

Curlee, R. & Yairi, E. (1997). Early intervention with early childhood stuttering: A critical examination of the data. *American Journal of Speech-Language Pathology, 6,* 8–18.

Curry, F., & Gregory, H. (1969). The performance of stutterers on dichotic listening tasks thought to reflect cerebral dominance. *Journal of Speech and Hearing Research, 12,* 73–81.

Dalton, P. (1987). Some developments in personal construct therapy with adults who stutter. In C. Levy (Ed.), *Stuttering therapies: Practical approaches* (pp. 61–70). London: Croom Helm.

Dalton, P. (1994) A persona l construct approach to communication problems. In P. Dalton (Ed.), *Counseling people with communication problems* (pp. 15–27). London: Sage Publications.

Daly, D. A. (1981). Differentiation of stuttering subgroups with Van Riper's developmental tracks: A preliminary study. *Journal of the American Student Speech and Hearing Association, 9,* 89–101.

Daly, D. A. (1986). The clutterer. In K. O. St. Louis (Ed.), *The atypical stutterer* (pp. 155–192). Orlando, FL: Academic Press.

Daly, D. (1987). Use of the home VCR to facilitate transfer of fluency. *Journal of Fluency Disorders, 12,* 103–106.

Daly, D. A. (1988). *Freedom of fluency.* Tucson, AZ: LingaSystems.

Daly, D. A. (1992). Helping the clutterer: Therapy considerations. In F. Myers & K. St. Louis (Eds.), *Cluttering: A clinical perspective* (pp. 27–41). San Diego, CA: Singular Publishing Group, Inc.

Daly, D. A. (1993). Cluttering: Another fluency syndrome. In R. Curlee (Ed.), *Stuttering and related disorders of fluency* (pp. 151–175). New York: Thieme Medical Publishers.

Daly, D. A. (1994). Practical techniques that work with children and adolescents who stutter. Paper presented to the annual meeting of the American Speech-Language-Hearing Association, New Orleans.

Daly, D. A. (1998). Stuttering: Recovering or recovered. In E. C. Healey & H. F. M. Peters (Eds.), *Proceedings of the 2nd World Congress on Fluency Disorders* (pp. 379–380). Nijmegen, The Netherlands: Nijmegen University Press.

Daly, D. A. (1999). Personal Communication.

Daly, D. A., & Burnett, M. L. (1996) Cluttering: assessment, treatment planning, and case study illustration. *Journal of Fluency Disorders, 21,* 239–248.

Daly, D. A., & Burnett, M. L. (1999). Cluttering: Traditional views and new perspectives. In R. Curlee (Ed.), *Stuttering and related disorders of fluency* (2nd ed., pp. 222–254). New York: Thieme Medical Publishers, Inc.

Daly, D. A., & Kimbarow, M. L. (1978). Stuttering as operant behavior: Effects of the verbal stimuli wrong, right, and tree on the disfluency rates of school-age stutterers and nonstutterers. *Journal of Speech and Hearing Research, 21,* 589–597.

Daly, D., Riley, J., & Riley, G. (2000) *Speech motor exercises.* Austin, TX: ProEd.

Daly, D., Simon, C., & Burnett-Stolnack, M. (1995). Helping adolescents who stutter focus on fluency. *Language, Speech, and Hearing Services in Schools, 26,* 162–168.

Davis, J. M., & Farina, A. (1970). Appreciation of humor: An experimental and theoretical study. *Journal of Personality and Social Psychology, 15*(2), 175–178.

DeBuck, A. (1970). *Egyptian readingbook, exercises and Middle Egyptian tests.* Leiden, Holland: Nederlands Instituut Voor Nabije Oosten.

Dell, C. (1970). *Treating the school age stutterer: A guide for clinicians* (Publication No. 14). Memphis, TN: Speech Foundation of America.

De Nil, L. F. (1999) Stuttering: A neurophysiological perspective. Chapter 7 In N. B. Ratner & E. C. Healey (Eds.), *Stuttering research and practice: Bridging the gap* (pp. 85–102). Mahwah, NJ: Lawrence Erlbaum.

De Nil, L. F., & Abbs, J. H. (1990). Influence of rate on stutterers' articulatory movements: A microbeam study. *ASHA, 32,* 72.

De Nil, L. F., & Brutten, G. J. (1991). Speech-associated attitudes of stuttering and nonstuttering children. *Journal of Speech and Hearing Research, 34,* 60–66.

De Nil, L. F., & Kroll, R. M. (1995). The relationship between locus of control and long-term stuttering treatment outcome in adult stutterers. *Journal of Fluency Disorders, 20,* 345–364.

De Nil, L. F., Kroll, R. M., Kapur, S., & Houle, S. (2000). A positron emission tomography study of silent and oral single word reading in stuttering and non-stuttering adults. *Journal of Speech, Hearing, and Language Research* (in press).

Denny, M., & Smith, A.. (1992). Gradations in a pattern of neuro-muscular activity associated with stuttering. *Journal of Speech and Hearing Research, 35,* 1216–1229.

DeVore, J., Nandur, M., & Manning, W. (1984). Projective drawings and children who stutter. *Journal of Fluency Disorders, 9,* 217–226.

Dewar, A., Dewar, A. D., & Anthony, J. F. K. (1976). The effect of auditory feedback masking on concomitants of stammering. *British Journal of Disorders of Communication, 11,* 95–102.

DiClemente, C. C. (1993). Changing addictive behaviors: A process perspective. *Current Directions in Psychological Science, 2*(4), 101–106.

Dietrich, S. (1997). Central auditory processing in males who stutter. *Proceedings of the 2nd World Congress on Fluency Disorders* (pp. 73–76). Nijmegen, The Netherlands: Nijmegen University Press.

Doopdy, I., Kalinowski, J., Armson, J. (1993). Stereotypes of stutterers and non-stutterers in three rural communities in Newfoundland. *Journal of Fluency Disorders, 18,* 363–373.

Dorman, M.F., & Porter, R.J. (1975). Hemispheric lateralization for speech perception in stutterers. *Cortex, 11,* 181–185.

Douglass, E., & Quarrington, B. (1952). The differentiation of interiorized and exteriorized secondary stuttering. *Journal of Speech and Hearing Disorders, 17,* 377–385.

Dunlap, K. (1917). The stuttering boy. *Journal of Abnormal Psychology, 12,* 44–48.

Dunlap, K. (1932). *Habits: Their making and unmaking.* New York: Liveright.

Dykes, R., & Pindzola, R. (1995). Racial/ethnic differences in the prevalence of school-aged stutterers. Paper presented to the annual meeting of the American Speech-Language-Hearing Association, Orlando.

Egan, G. (1990). *The skilled helper: A systematic approach to effective helping* (4th ed.). Pacific Grove, CA: Brooks/Cole Publishing Co.

Egan, G. (1998) *The Skilled Helper: A problem-management approach to helping* (6th ed.). Pacific Grove, CA: Brooks/Cole Publishing Co.

Eisenson, J., & Ogilvie, M. (1963). *Speech correction in the schools* (2nd ed.). New York: Macmillan.

Ellis, A. (1977). The basic clinical theory of rational-emotive therapy. In A. Ellis & R. Grieger (Eds.), *Handbook of rational-emotive therapy* (pp. 218–250). New York: Springer.

Emerick, L. (1974). Stuttering therapy: Dimensions of interpersonal sensitivity. In L. L. Emerick & S. B. Hood (Eds.), *The client-clinician relationship: Essays on interpersonal sensitivity in the therapeutic transaction* (pp. 92–102). Springfield, IL: Charles C. Thomas.

Emerick, L. (1988). Counseling adults who stutter: A cognitive approach. *Seminars in Speech and Language* (Thieme Medical Publishers), *9*(3), 257–267.

Erickson, R. L. (1969). Assessing communication attitudes among stutterers. *Journal of Speech and Hearing Research, 12,* 711–724.

Evesham, M. (1987). Residential courses for stutterers: Combining technique and personal construct psychology. In C. Levy (Ed.), *Stuttering therapies: Practical approaches* (pp. 61–70). London: Croom Helm.

Evesham, M., & Fransella, F. (1985). Stuttering relapse: The effect of a combined speech and psychological reconstruction programme. *British Journal of Disorders of Communication, 20,* 237–248.

Fairbanks, G. (1954). Systematic research in experimental phonetics—I. A. A theory of the speech mechanism as a servomechanism. *Journal of Speech and Hearing Disorders, 19,* 133–139.

Falsenfeld, S. (1997). Epidemiology and genetics of stuttering. In R. Curlee & G. Siegel (Eds.), *Nature and treatment of stuttering, new directions* (2nd ed., pp. 3–23). Needham Heights, MA: Allyn & Bacon.

Fant, G. (1960). *The acoustic theory of speech production.* The Hague, Holland: Mouton.

Farrelly, F., & Brandsma, J. (1974). *Provocative therapy.* Cupertino, CA: Meta Publications.

Faulkner, R. O. (1962). *A concise dictionary of Middle Egyptian.* Oxford, England: University Press.

Fenichel, O. (1945). *The psychoanalytic theory of neurosis.* New York: Norton.

Fey, M., & Johnson, B. (1998). Research to practice (and back again) in speech-language intervention. *Topics in Language Disorders, 18*(2), 23–34.

Fibiger, S. (1994). Did Moses and Demosthenes stutter? *Journal of Fluency Disorders Abstracts of the First World Congress on Fluency Disorders, 19,* 173.

Filmore, C. J. (1979). On fluency. In *Individual differences in language ability and language behavior.* New York: Academic Press.

Finitzo, T., Pool, K. D., Freeman, F. J., Devous, M. D., Sr., & Watson, B. C. (1991). Cortical dysfunction in developmental stutterers. In H. F. M. Peters, W. Hulstijn,

& C. W. Starkweather (Eds.), *Speech motor control and stuttering* (pp. 251–262). Amsterdam: Elsevier.

Fish, J. M. (1995). Does problem behavior just happen? Does it matter? *Behavior and Social Issues, 5*(1), 3–12.

Fisher, R., & Ury, W. (1981). *Getting to yes: Negotiating agreement without giving in.* Boston: Houghton Mifflin.

Fitch, J. L., & Batson, E. A. (1989). Hemispheric asymmetry of alpha wave suppression in stutterers and nonstutterers. *Journal of Fluency Disorders, 9*, 51–65.

Fosnot, S. (1993). Research design for examining treatment efficacy in fluency disorders, *Journal of Fluency Disorders, 18*, 221–251.

Fowler, C. (1978). Timing control in speech production. *Dissertation Abstracts International, 38*, 3927–3928.

Fox, P. T., Ingham, R. J., Ingham, J. C., Hirsch, T. B., Downs, J. H., Martin, C., Jerabek, P., Glass, T., & Lancaster, J. L. (1996). A PET study of the neural systems of stuttering. *Nature, 382*, 158–162.

Fox, P. T., Lancaster, J. L., & Ingham, R. J. (1993). On stuttering and global ischemia—Letter to the editor. *Archives of Neurology, 50*, 1287–1288.

Franken, C. M., Boves, L., Peter, H. F. M., & Webster, R. L. (1992) Perceptual evaluation of speech before and after fluency shaping therapy. *Journal of Fluency Disorders, 17*, 223–241.

Fransella, F. (1972). *Personal change and reconstruction.* New York: Academic Press.

Fransella, F., & Dalton, P. (1990). *Personal construct counseling in action.* London: Sage.

Freud, S. (1905/1961). Jokes and their relation to the unconscious. In James Strachey (Ed.), *The complete psychological works of Sigmund Freud* (vol. 8). London: Hogarth Press.

Freud, S. (1928). Humor. *International Journal of Psychoanalysis, 9*, 1–6.

Freund, H. (1966). *Psychopathology and the problems of stuttering.* Springfield, IL: Charles C. Thomas.

Gaines, N., Runyan, C., & Meyers, S. (1991). A comparison of young stutterers' fluent versus stuttered utterances on measures of length and complexity. *Journal of Speech and Hearing Research, 34*, 37–42.

Gay, T. (1978). Effect of speaking rate on vowel formant movements. *Journal of the Acoustical Society of America, 63*, 223–230.

Gay, T., & Hirose, H. (1973). Effect of speaking rate on labial consonant production: a combined electromyographic high-speech motion picture study. *Phonetrica, 27*, 203–213.

Gay, T., Ushijima, T., Hirose, H., & Cooper, F. S. (1974). Effect of speaking rate on labial consonant-vowel articulation. *Journal of Phonetics, 2*, 47–63.

Geschwind, N., & Galaburda, A. M. (1985). Cerebral lateralization: Biological mechanisms, associations, and pathology: I. A hypothesis and a program for research. *Archives of Neurology, 42*, 429–459.

Gildston, P. (1967). Stutterers' self-acceptance and perceived self-acceptance. *Journal of Abnormal and Social Psychology, 72*, 59–64.

Gillespie, S. K., & Cooper, E. G. (1973). Prevalence of speech problems in junior and senior high schools, *Journal of Speech and Hearing Research, 16*, 739–743.

Glasner, P. J., & Rosenthal, D. (1957). Parental diagnosis of stuttering in young children. *Journal of Speech and Hearing Disorders, 22*, 288–295.

Glauber, I. P. (1958). The psychoanalysis of stuttering. In Jon Eisenson (Ed.), *Stuttering: A symposium* (pp. 71–119). New York: Harper & Brothers.

Glauber, I. P. (1982). *Stuttering: A psychoanalytic understanding.* New York: Human Sciences Press.

Goebel, M. (1989). *CAFET-for-kids.* Annandale, VA: Annandale Fluency Clinic.

Goldman-Eisler, F. (1958). The predictability of words in context and the length of pauses in speech. *Language and Speech, 1,* 226–231.

Goldman-Eisler, F. (1961). The continuity of speech utterance: Its determinants and its significance. *Language and Speech, 4,* 220–231.

Goldstein, J. H. (1976). Theoretical notes on humor. *Journal of Communication, 26,* 104–112.

Goleman, D. (1985). Switching therapists may be best. *Indianapolis News,* p. 9.

Goodstein, L. D. (1958). Functional speech disorders and personality: A survey of the research. *Journal of Speech and Hearing Research, 1,* 359–376.

Gordon, K. C., Hutchinson, J. M., & Allen, C. S. (1976). An evaluation of selected discourse characteristics in normal geriatric subjects. *Idaho State University Laboratory Research Reports, 1,* 11–21.

Gordon, P. (1991). Language task effects: A comparison of stuttering and nonstuttering children. *Journal of Fluency Disorders, 16,* 275–287.

Gordon, P., Luper, H., & Peterson, H. J. (1986). The effects of syntactic complexity on the occurrence of disfluencies in 5 year old nonstutterers. *Journal of Fluency Disorders, 11,* 151–164.

Gottwald, S. F. (1999). Family communication pattern and stuttering development: An analysis of the research literature. In N. B. Ratner & E. C. Healey (Eds.), *Stuttering research and practice: Bridging the gap* (pp. 175–192). Mahwah, NJ: Lawrence Erlbaum Associates.

Gottwald, S. R., & Starkweather, C. W. (1995). Fluency intervention for preschoolers and their families in the public schools. *Language, Speech, and Hearing Services in Schools, 26,* 117–126.

Gottwald, S. R., & Starkweather, C. W. (1999). Stuttering prevention and early intervention: A multi-process approach. In M. Onslow and A. Packman (Eds.), *The handbook of early stuttering intervention* (pp. 53–82). San Diego, CA: Singular Publishing Company.

Gregory, H. H. (1972). An assessment of the results of stuttering therapy. *Journal of Communication Disorders, 5,* 320–334.

Gregory, H. H. (1979). Controversial issues: Statement and review of the literature. In H. H. Gregory (Ed.), *Controversies about stuttering therapy* (pp. 1–62). Baltimore, MD: University Park Press.

Gregory, H. H. (1983). *The clinician's attitudes in counseling stutterers* (Publication No. 18). Memphis, TN: Stuttering Foundation of America.

Gregory, H. H. (1984). Prevention of stuttering: Management of the early stages. In R. F. Curlee & W. H. Perkins (Eds.), *Nature and treatment of stuttering: New directions.* San Diego: College-Hill Press.

Gregory, H. H. (1986). *Stuttering: Differential evaluation and therapy.* Austin, TX: ProEd.

Gregory, H. H. (1989). *Stuttering therapy: A workshop for specialists.* Unpublished manuscript, Evanston, IL: Northwestern University and the Stuttering Foundation of America.

Gregory, H. H. (1991). Therapy for elementary school-age children. *Seminars in Speech and Language, 12,* 323–335.

Gregory, H. H. (1995). Analysis and commentary. *Language, Speech, and Hearing Services in Schools, 26*(2), 196–200.

Gregory, H. H., & Hill, D. (1980). Stuttering therapy for children. In W. Perkins (Ed.), *Stuttering disorders,* (pp. 351–363). New York: Thieme-Stratton.

Guitar, B. (1976). Pretreatment factors associated with the outcome of stuttering therapy. *Journal of Speech and Hearing Research, 18,* 590–600.

Guitar, B. (1997). Therapy for children's stuttering and emotions. In R. F. Curlee & G. M. Siegel (Eds.), *Nature and Treatment of Stuttering: New Directions* (2nd ed., pp. 280–291). Boston, MA: Allyn & Bacon.

Guitar, B. (1998). *Stuttering: An integrated approach to its nature and treatment.* Baltimore: Williams & Wilkins.

Guitar, B. E., & Bass, C. (1978). Stuttering therapy: The relation between attitude change and long-term outcome. *Journal of Speech and Hearing Disorders, 43,* 392–499.

Guitar, B., & Peters, T. J. (1980). *Stuttering: An integration of contemporary therapies* (Publication No. 16). Memphis, TN: Stuttering Foundation of America.

Haefner, R. (1929). *The educational significance of left-handedness.* New York: Teachers College, Columbia University Press.

Hagerman, C. F., & Greene, P. N. (1989). Auditory comprehension of stutterers on a competing message task. *Journal of Fluency Disorders, 14,* 109–120.

Hall, J. W., & Jerger, J. (1978). Central auditory function in stutterers. *Journal of Speech and Hearing Research, 21,* 324–337.

Hall, K. D., & Yairi, E. (1992). Fundamental frequency, jitter, and shimmer in preschoolers who stutter. *Journal of Speech and Hearing Research, 35,* 1002–1008.

Hall, P. K. (1977). The occurrence of disfluencies in language-disordered school-age children. *Journal of Speech and Hearing Disorders, 42,* 364–369.

Ham, R. (1986). *Techniques of stuttering therapy.* Englewood Cliffs, NJ: Prentice-Hall.

Ham, R. E. (1990). *Therapy of stuttering, preschool through adolescence.* Englewood Cliffs, NJ: Prentice-Hall.

Ham, R. E. (1992). I know the chapter, but what's the verse? *Journal of Fluency Disorders, 17,* 39–41.

Ham, R. E. (1993). Chronic perseverative stuttering syndrome: constructive or casuistic? *American Journal of Speech-Language Pathology, 2*(3), 16–20.

Ham, R. E. (1999). *Clinical management of stuttering in older children and adults.* Gaithersburg, MD: Aspen Publishers. Ind.

Hamre, C. (1992). Stuttering prevention I: Primacy of identification. *Journal of Fluency Disorders, 17,* 3–23.

Hancock, K., & Craig, A. (1998). Predictors of stuttering relapse one year following treatment for children aged 9 to 14 years. *Journal of Fluency Disorders, 23,* 31–48.

Hancock, K, Craig, A., McCready, C., McCaul, A., Costello, D., Campbell, K., & Gilmore, G. (1998). Two- to six-year controlled-trial stuttering outcomes for children and adolescents. *Journal of Speech, Language, and Hearing Research, 41,* 1242–1252.

Hanson, B. R., Gonhoud, K. D., & Rice, P. L. (1981). Speech situation checklist. *Journal of Fluency Disorders, 6,* 351–360.

Hastorf, A. H., Windfogel, J., & Cassman, T. (1979). Acknowledgement of handicap as a tactic in social interaction. *Journal of Personality and Social Psychology, 37,* 1790–1797.

Hayden, P. A., Scott, D. A., & Addicott, J. (1977). The effects of delayed auditory feedback on the overt behaviors of stutterers. *Journal of Fluency Disorders, 2,* 235–246.

Hayhow, R., & Levy, C. (1989). *Working with stuttering.* Bicester, Oxon, England: Winslow Press.

Healey, E. C. (1982). Speaking fundamental frequency characteristics of stutterers and nonstutterers. *Journal of Communications Disorders, 15*(1), 21–29.

Healey, E. C. (Ed.). (1995, June). *Division 4 Newsletter, 5*(2). Rockville, MD: American Speech-Language-Hearing Association.

Healey, E. C., & Gutkin, B. (1984). Analysis of stutterers' voice onset times and fundamental frequency contours during fluency. *Journal of Speech and Hearing Research, 27,* 219–225.

Healey, E. C., & Scott, L. A. (1995). Strategies for treating elementary school-age children who stutter: An integrative approach. *Language, Speech, and Hearing Services in Schools, 26,* 151–161.

Henri, B. P. (1994, January). Graduate student preparation: Tomorrow's challenge. *Asha, 36,* 43–46.

Heinze, B. A., & Johnson, K. L. (1985). *Easy does it–1: Fluency activities for young children.* East Moline, IL: LinguiSystems.

Heinze, B. A., & Johnson, K. L. (1987). *Easy does it–2: Fluency activities for school-aged stutterers.* East Moline, IL: LinguiSystems.

Helm, N. A., Butler, R. B., & Canter, G. J. (1980). Neurogenic acquired stuttering. *Journal of Fluency Disorders, 5,* 269–279.

Helm, N. A., Yeo, R., Geschwind, M., Freedman, M., & Wenstein, C. (1986). Stuttering: Disappearance and reappearance with acquired brain lesions. *Neurology, 36,* 1109–1112.

Helm-Estabrooks, N. (1986). Diagnosis and management of neurogenic stuttering in adults. In K. O. St. Louis (Ed.), *The atypical stutterer* (pp. 193–217). Orlando, FL: Academic Press.

Helm-Estabrooks, N. (1993). Stuttering associated with acquired neurological disorders. In Curlee, R. (Ed.), *Stuttering and related disorders of fluency.* New York: Thieme Medical Publishers.

Helm-Estabrooks, N. (1999). Stuttering associated with acquired neurological disorders. In R. Curlee (Ed.), *Stuttering and related disorders of fluency* (2nd ed., pp. 255–268). New York: Thieme Medical Publishers, Inc.

Hillis, J. W. (1993). Ongoing assessment in the management of stuttering: A clinical perspective. *American Journal of Speech-Language Pathology, 2*(1), 24–37.

Hillis, J., & Manning, W. H. (1996, November). Extraclinical generalization of speech fluency: A social cognitive approach. Presentation to the annual meeting of the American Speech-Language-Hearing Association, Seattle.

Hillis, J., & Manning, W. (1998, November) Multidimensional assessment of self-efficacy for speech fluency. Computer laboratory presentation to the annual meeting of the American Speech-Language-Hearing Association, San Antonio, TX.

Hillman, R. E., & Gilbert, H. R. (1977). Voice onset time for voiceless stop consonants in the fluent reading of stutterers and nonstutterers. *Journal of the Acoustical Society of America, 61,* 610–611.

Hinsie, L. E., & Campbell, R., J., (1970). *Psychiatric dictionary* (4ᵗʰ ed.). New York: Oxford University Press.

Hodson, B. W. (1986). *The assessment of phonological processes—Revised.* Austin, TX: Pro-Ed.

Hood, S. B. (1974). Clients, clinicians and therapy. In L. L. Emerick & S. B. Hood (Eds.), *The client-clinician relationship: Essays on interpersonal sensitivity in the therapeutic transaction* (pp. 45–59). Springfield, IL: Charles C. Thomas.

Hood, S. B. (1998). *Advice to those who stutter* (Publication No. 9). Memphis, TN: Stuttering Foundation of America.

Howie, P. M. (1981). Concordance for stuttering in monozygotic and dizygotic twin pairs. *Journal of Speech and Hearing Research, 24,* 317–321.

Howie, P., Woods, C., & Andrews, J. (1982). Relationship between covert and overt speech measures immediately before and immediately after stuttering treatment. *Journal of Speech and Hearing Disorders, 47,* 419–422.

Howie, P. M., Tanner, S., & Andrews, G. (1981). Short and long term outcome in an intensive treatment program for adult stutterers. *Journal of Speech and Hearing Disorders, 46,* 104–109.

Hubbard, C. P., & Yairi, E. (1988). Clustering of disfluencies in the speech of stuttering and nonstuttering preschool children. *Journal of Speech and Hearing Research, 31,* 228–233.

Huggins, A. (1978). Speech timing and intelligibility. In J. Requin (Ed.), *Attention and performance VII* (pp. 218–241). Hillsdale, NJ: Lawrence Erlbaum.

Hull, F., Mieke, P., Timmons, R., & Willeford, J. (1971). The National Speech and Hearing Survey: Preliminary Results. *ASHA, 13,* 501–509.

Hunt, B. (1987). Self-help for stutterers—Experience in Britain. In L. Rustin, H. Purser, & K. D. Rowley (Eds.), *Progress in the treatment of fluency disorders* (pp. 198–212). London: Taylor & Francis.

Hunt, H. (1861/1967). *Stammering and stuttering, their nature and treatment.* New York: Hafner Publishing Company.

Ingham, R. J. (1975). A comparison of covert and overt assessment procedures in stuttering therapy outcome evaluation. *Journal of Speech and Hearing Research, 16,* 246–254.

Ingham, R. J. (1980). *Stuttering therapy manual: Hierarchy control schedule. A clinician's guide.* Sydney, Australia: Cumberland College of Health Sciences, School of Communication Disorders.

Ingham, R. J. (1982). The effects of self-evaluation and training and maintenance and generalization during stuttering treatment. *Journal of Speech and Hearing Disorders, 47,* 271–280.

Ingham, R. J. (1984). *Stuttering and behavior therapy: Current status and experimental foundations.* San Diego, CA: College-Hill Press.

Ingham, R. J. (1990). Commentary on Perkins (1990) and Moore and Perkins (1990): On the valid role of reliability in identifying "What is stuttering." *Journal of Speech and Hearing Disorders, 55,* 394–397.

Ingham, R. J. (1993). Stuttering treatment efficacy: Paradigm dependent or independent? *Journal of Fluency Disorders, 18,* 133–145.

Ingham, R. J., Andrews, G., & Winkler, R. (1972). Stuttering: A comparative evaluation of the short term effectiveness of four treatment techniques. *Journal of Communication Disorders, 5,* 91–117.

Ingham, R. J., & Cordes, A. K. (1999). On watching a discipline shoot itself in the foot: Some observations on current trends in stuttering treatment research. In N. B. Ratner & E. C. Healey (Eds.), *Stuttering research and practice: Bridging the gap.* Mahwah, NJ: Lawrence Erlbaum Associates.

Ingham, R. J., Fox, P. T., & Ingham, J. C. (1994). Brain image investigation of the speech of stutterers and nonstutterers. *ASHA, 36,* 188.

Ingham, R. J., Fox, P. T., Ingham, J. C., Zamarripa, F., Martin, C., Jerabek, P., & Cotton, J. (1996). Functional-lesion investigation of developmental stuttering with Positron Emission Tomography. *Journal of Speech and Hearing Research, 39,* 1208–1227.

Ingham, R. J., Gow, M., & Costello, J. M. (1985). Stuttering and speech natural-ness: Some additional data. *Journal of Speech and Hearing Disorders, 50,* 217–219.

Ingham, R. J., Ingham, J. C., Onslow, M., & Finn, P. (1989). Stutterers' self-ratings of speech naturalness: Assessing effects and reliability. *Journal of Speech and Hearing Research, 32,* 419–431.

Ingham, R. J., Martin, R. R., Haroldson, S. K., Onslow, M., & Leney, M. (1985). Modification of listener-judged naturalness in the speech of stutterers. *Journal of Speech and Hearing Research, 28,* 495–504.

Ingham, R. J., & Onslow, M. (1985). Measurement and modification of speech nat-uralness during stuttering therapy. *Journal of Speech and Hearing Disorders, 50,* 261–181.

Ingham, R. J., & Packman, A. C. (1978). Perceptual assessment of normalcy of speech following stuttering therapy. *Journal of Speech and Hearing Research, 21,* 63–73.

Ivy, A. E. (1983). *Intentional interviewing and counseling.* Pacific Grove, CA: Brooks/Cole.

Jacobs, M. K., & Goodman, G. (1989). Psychology and self-help groups: Prediction on a partnership. *American Psychologist, 44,* 536–545.

Jezer, Marty. (1997). *Stuttering: A Life Bound Up in Words.* New York, NY: Basic Books.

Johnson, G. G., & Johnson, M. M. (2000). Stutter free speech the hard way—via transient global amnesia. *The Speak Easy Newsletter, 20*(1) 4–6.

Johnson, W. (1930). *Because I stutter.* New York: Appleton-Century-Crofts.

Johnson, W. (1946). *People in quandaries.* New York: Harper Brothers.

Johnson, W. (1956). *Speech handicapped school children.* New York: Harper & Row.

Johnson, W. (1958). The six men and the stuttering. In J. Eisenson (Ed.), *Stuttering* (pp. xi–xxiv). New York: Harper & Brothers.

Johnson, W. (1961). Measurement of oral reading and speaking rate and disfluen-cy of adult male and female stutterers and nonstutterers. *Journal of Speech and Hearing Disorders* (Monograph Supplement 7), 1–20.

Johnson, W. (1962). *An open letter to the mother of a "stuttering" child.* Danville, IL: Interstate Printers and Publishers.

Johnson, W., & Associates. (1959). *The Onset of stuttering.* Minneapolis: University of Minnesota Press.

Johnson, W., Darley, F. L., & Spriestersbach, D. C. (1963). *Diagnostic methods in speech pathology.* New York: Harper & Row.

Johnson, W., & Leutenegger, R. R. (Eds.). (1955). *Stuttering in children and adults.* Minneapolis: University of Minnesota Press.

Jones, R. (1966). Observations on stammering after localized cerebral injury. *Journal of Neurology, Neurosurgery, and Psychiatry, 29*, 192–195.

Kalinowski, J., Nobel, S., Armson, J., & Stuart, A. (1994). Pretreatment and post-treatment speech naturalness ratings of adults with mild and severe stuttering. *American Journal of Speech-Language Pathology, 3*(2), 61–66.

Kamhi, A. G. (1982). The problem of relapse in stuttering: Some thoughts on what might cause it and how to deal with it. *Journal of Fluency Disorders, 7*, 459–467.

Kamhi, A. G. (1999). To use or not to use: Factors that influence the selection of new treatment approaches. *Language, Speech, and Hearing Services in Schools, 30*, 92–98.

Kanfer, F. H. (1975). Self-management methods. In F. H. Kanfer & A. P. Goldstein (Eds.), *Helping people change* (pp. 416–431). New York: Pergamon Press.

Kanfer, F. H., & Schefft, B. K. (1988). *Guiding therapeutic change.* Champaign, IL: Research Press.

Katz, A. H., & Bender, E. (1976). *The strength in us: Self-help groups in the modern world.* New York: Franklin Watts.

Kelly, E. M. (1994). Speech rates and turn-taking behaviors of children who stutter and their fathers. *Journal of Speech and Hearing Research, 37*, 1284–1294.

Kelly, E. M. (2000). Modeling stuttering etiology: clarifying levels of description and measurement. *Journal of Fluency Disorders, 25* (in press).

Kelly, E. M., Martin, J. S., Baker, K. I., Rivera, N. J., Bishop, J. E., Kriziske, C. B., Stettler, D. B., & Stealy, J. M. (1997). Academic and clinical preparation and practices of school speech-language pathologists with people who stutter. *Language, Speech, and Hearing Services in Schools, 28*, 195–212.

Kelly, G. A. (1955a). *The psychology of personal constructs,* Volume 1. New York: Norton.

Kelly, G. A., (1955b). *The psychology of personal constructs,* Volume 2. New York: Norton.

Kent, R. D. (1983). Facts about stuttering: Neurologic perspectives. *Journal of Speech and Hearing Disorders, 48*, 249–255.

Kent R. D. (1997). *The Speech Sciences.* San Diego, CA: Singular Publishing Group.

Kent, R. D., & Read, C. (1992). *The acoustic analysis of speech.* San Diego, CA: Singular Publishing Group.

Kertesz, A. (1989). Anatomical and physiological correlations and neuroimaging techniques in language disorders. In A. Ardila & F. Ostrosky-Solis (Eds.) *Brain organization of language and cognitive processes.* New York: Plenum Press.

Kidd, K. K. (1977). A genetic perspective on stuttering. *Journal of Fluency Disorders, 2*, 259–269.

Kidd, K. (1984). Stuttering as a genetic disorder. In R. F. Curlee & W. H. Perkins (Eds.), *Nature and treatment of stuttering: New directions* (pp. 149–169). Boston: Allyn & Bacon.

Kidd, K., Heimbuch, R., Records, M. A., Oehlert, G., & Webster, R. (1980). Familial stuttering patterns are not related to one measure of severity. *Journal of Speech and Hearing Research, 23*, 539–545.

Kidd, K. K., Kidd, J. R., & Records, M. A. (1978). The possible causes of the sex ratio in stuttering and its implications. *Journal of Fluency Disorders, 3*, 13–23.

Kidd, K. K., Reich, T., & Kessler, S. (1973). *Genetics, 74* (Part 2), s137.

Kimmel, D. C. (1974). *Adulthood and aging*. New York: John Wiley & Sons.

Kimura, D. (1961). Cerebral dominance and the perception of verbal stimuli. *Canadian Journal of Psychology, 15*, 166–171.

Kimura, D. (1964). Left-right differences in the perception of melodies. *Quarterly Journal of Experimental Psychology, 16*, 355–358.

Kirby, G., Delgadillo, J., Hillard, S., & Manning, W. (1992). *Visual imagery, relaxation, and cognitive restructuring integrated in fluency therapy*. Paper presented to the annual meeting of the American Speech-Language-Hearing Association, San Antonio, TX.

Klich, R. J., & May, G. M. (1982). Spectrographic study of vowels in stutterers' fluent speech. *Journal of Speech and Hearing Research, 25*(3), 364–370.

Kline, M., & Starkweather, C. (1979). *Receptive and expressive language performance in young stutterers* [Abstract]. *ASHA, 21*, 797.

Kloth, S. A., Kraaimaat, F. W., Janssen, P., & Brutten, G. J. (1999). Persistence and remission of incipient stuttering among high-risk children. *Journal of Fluency Disorders, 24*, 23–265.

Koszybski, A. (1941). *Science and sanity: An introduction to non-Aristotelian systems and general semantics* (2nd Ed.). New York: Int. Non-Aristotelian Library Publishing Co.

Kozhevnikov, V. A., & Chistovich, L. A. (1965). *Speech: Articulation and perception* (Joint Publications Research Service, 30, 543). Washington, DC: United States Department of Commerce.

Krall, T. (1998). My long term path toward recovery from stuttering. In E. C. Healey & H. F. M. Peters (Eds.), *Proceedings of the 2nd World Congress on Fluency Disorders* (pp. 388–389). Nijmegen, The Netherlands: Nijmegen University Press.

Kramer, M. B., Green, D., & Guitar, B. (1987). A comparison of stutterers and non-stutterers on masking level differences and synthetic sentence identification tasks. *Journal of Communication Disorders, 20*, 379–390.

Krass-Lehrman, T., & Reeves, L. (1989). Attitudes toward speech-language pathology and support groups: Results of a survey of members of the National Stuttering Project. *Texas Journal of Audiology and Speech Pathology, 15*(1), 22–25.

Kroll, R. M., De Nil, L. F., Kapur, S. & Houle, S. (1997). A positron emission tomography investigation of post-treatment brain activation in stutterers. In H. F. M. Peters & W. Hulstijn, (Eds.), *Proceedings of the Third Speech Motor Production and Fluency Disorders* (pp. 307–320). Amsterdam: Elsevier.

Kubie, L. S. (1971). The destructive potential of humor on psychotherapy. *American Journal of Psychiatry, 127*, 861–866.

Kuhlman, T. (1984). *Humor and psychotherapy*. Homewood, IL: Dow Jones-Irwin.

Kuhr, A., & Rustin, L. (1985). The maintenance of fluency after intensive in-patient therapy: Long-term follow-up. *Journal of Fluency Disorders, 10*, 229–236.

Ladouceur, R., Caron, C., & Caron, G. (1989). Stuttering severity and treatment outcome. *Journal of Behavior Therapy and Experimental Psychiatry, 20*, 49–56.

LaSalle, L. R., & Conture, E. G. (1991). Eye contact between young stutterers and their mothers. *Journal of Fluency Disorders, 16*(4), 173–199.

LaSalle, L. R., & Conture, E. G. (1995). Disfluency clusters of children who stutter: Relation of stutterings to self-repairs. *Journal of Speech and Hearing Research, 38*(5), 965–977.

Lass, N., Ruscello, D., Pannbaker, M., Schmitt, J., & Everly-Myers, D. (1989). Speech-language pathologists' perceptions of child and adult female and male stutterers. *Journal of Fluency Disorders, 14,* 127–134.

Lass, N. J., Ruscello, D. M., Schmitt, J. F., Pannbacker, M. D., Orlando, M. B., Dean, K. A., Ruziska, J. C., & Bradshaw, K. H. (1992). Teachers' perceptions of stutterers. *Language, Speech and Hearing Services in Schools, 23,* 78–81.

Lee, B. S. (1951). Artificial stutter. *Journal of Speech and Hearing Disorders, 16,* 53–55.

Lauter, J. L., Herscovitch, P., Formby, C., & Raichle, M. E. (1985). Tonotopic organization in human auditory cortex revealed by positron emission tomography. *Hearing Research, 20,* 199–205.

Lefcourt, H. M. (1976). *Locus of control: Current trends in theory and research.* Hillsdale, NJ: Erlbaum.

Lefcourt, H., & Martin, R. (1989). *Humor and life stress: Antidote to adversity.* New York: Springer-Verlag.

Lefcourt, H., Sordoni, C., & Sordoni C. (1974). Locus of control and the expression of humor. *Journal of Personality, 42,* 130–143.

Leith, W. R. (1986) Treating the stutter with atypical cultural influences. In K. O. St. Louis (Ed.), *The atypical stutterer: Principles and practices of rehabilitation* (pp. 9–34). Orlando, FL: Academic Press.

Lemert, E. M. (1953). Some Indians who stutter. *Journal of Speech and Hearing Disorders, 18,* 168–174.

Lemert, E. M. (1962). Stuttering and social structure in two Pacific societies. *Journal of Speech and Hearing Disorders, 27,* 3–10.

Lengevin, M., Bortnick, K., Hammer, T., & Wiebe, E. (1998). Teasing/bullying experienced by children who stutter: Toward development of a questionnaire. *Contemporary Issues in Communication Sciences and Disorders, 25,* 12–24.

Levine, J. (1977). Humour as a form of therapy. In A. J. Chapman & H. C. Foot (Eds.), *It's a funny thing, humour* (pp. 127–137). Oxford, England: Pergamon.

Levy, C. (1983). Group therapy with adults. In P. Dalton (Ed.), *Approaches to the treatment of stuttering* (pp. 150–171). London and Canberra, Australia: Croom Helm.

Lichtheim, M. (1973). *Ancient Egyptian literature, a book of readings: Volume 1. The Old and Middle Kingdoms.* Berkeley: University of California Press.

Liebetrau, R.M., & Daly, D.A. (1981). Auditory processing and perceptual abilities of "organic" and "functional" stutterers. *Journal of Fluency Disorders, 6,* 219–232.

Lincoln, M. A., Onslow, M., & Reed, V. (1997). Social validity of the treatment outcomes of an early intervention program for stuttering. *American Journal of Speech-Language Pathology, 6,* 77–84.

Lindaman, E. B., & Lippitt, R. O. (1979). *Choosing the future you prefer: Goal setting guide.* Washington, DC: Development Publications.

Loban, W. (1976). *Language development: Kindergarten through grade twelve.* Urbana, IL: National Council of Teachers of English.

Logan, K, J., & Yaruss, J. S. (1999). Helping parents address attitudinal and emotional factors with young children who stutter. *Contemporary Issues in Communication Science and Disorders, 26,* 69–81.

Longhurst, T. M., & Siegel, G. M. (1973). Effects of communication failure on speaker-listener behaviors. *Journal of Speech and Hearing Disorders, 16,* 128–140.

Louko, L., Edwards, M. E., & Conture, E. (1990). Phonological characteristics of young stutterers and their normally fluent peers: Preliminary observations. *Journal of Fluency Disorders, 15,* 191–210.

Love, L. R., & Jefress, L. A. (1971). Identification of brief pauses in the fluent speech of stutterers and nonstutterers. *Journal of Speech and Hearing Research, 14,* 229–240.

Love, R. E. (2000). *The Bob Love story.* Chicago, IL: Contemporary Books.

Lowe-Bell, S. S., Cullen, J. K., Jr., Berlin, C. I., Thompson, C. L., & Willett, M. E. (1970). Perceptions of simultaneous dichotic and monotic monosyllables. *Journal of Speech and Hearing Research, 13,* 812–822.

Luchsinger, R., & Arnold, G. E. (1965). *Voice-speech-language clinical communicology: Its physiology and pathology.* Belmont, CA: Wadsworth.

Ludlow, C. L. (1990). Treatment of speech and voice disorders with botulinum toxin. *The Journal of the American Medical Association, 264,* 2671–2675.

Luper, Harold L., & Mulder, R. L. (1964). *Stuttering therapy for children.* Englewood Cliffs, NJ: Prentice-Hall.

Luterman, D. (1979). *Counseling parents of hearing impaired children.* Boston: Little, Brown, & Co.

Luterman, D. M. (1991). *Counseling the communicatively disordered and their families* (2nd ed.). Austin, TX: Pro-Ed.

Madison, L. S., Budd, K. S., & Itzkowitz, J. S. (1986). Changes in stuttering in relation to children's locus of control. *Journal of Genetic Psychology, 147,* 233–240.

Malecot, A., Johnston, R., & Kizziar, P. A. (1972). Syllabic rate and utterance length in French. *Phonetica, 26,* 235–251.

Mallard, A. R., Gardner, L., & Downey, C. (1988). Clinical training in stuttering for school clinicians. *Journal of Fluency Disorders, 13,* 253–259.

Mallard, A. R., & Westrbook J. B. (1988). Variables affecting stuttering therapy in school settings. *Language, Speech, and Hearing Services in Schools, 19,* 362–370.

Manders, E., & Bastijns, P. (1988). Sudden recovery from stuttering after an epileptic attack: A case report. *Journal of Fluency Disorders, 13,* 421–425.

Manning, W. (1977). In pursuit of fluency. *Journal of Fluency Disorders, 2,* 53–56.

Manning, W. (1991a). Sports analogies in the treatment of stuttering: Taking the field with your client. *Public School Caucus, 10*(2), 1, 10–11.

Manning, W. H. (1991b). Making progress during and after treatment. In, W. H. Perkins (Ed.) *Seminars in speech and language,* (Vol. 12, pp. 349–354). New York: Thieme Medical Publishers.

Manning, W. H. (1994). The SEA-Scale: Self-efficacy scaling for adolescents who stutter. Paper presented to the annual meeting of the American Speech-Language-Hearing Association, New Orleans, LA.

Manning, W. H. (1998). Long term recovery from stuttering. In E. C. Healey & H. F. M. Peters (Eds.), *Proceedings of the 2nd World Congress on Fluency Disorders* (pp. 381–383). Nijmegen, The Netherlands: Nijmegen University Press.

Manning, W. H. (1999a). Progress under the surface and over time. In N. B. Ratner & E. C. Healey (Eds.), *Stuttering Research and Practice: Bridging the Gap* (pp. 123–129). Mahwah, NJ: Lawrence Erlbaum.

Manning, W. (1999b). Management of adult stuttering. In R. Curlee (Ed.), *Stuttering and related disorders of fluency* (pp. 160–180). New York: Thieme Medical Publishers, Inc.

Manning, W. H., & Beachy, T. S. (1994). *Humor as a variable in the treatment of fluency disorders.* Paper presented to the First World Congress on Fluency Disorders, Munich, Germany.

Manning, W., Burlison, A., & Thaxton, D. (1999). Listener response to stuttering modification techniques. *Journal of Fluency Disorders, 24,* 267–280.

Manning, W., & Cooper, E. B. (1969). Variations in attitudes of the adult stutterer toward his clinician related to progress in therapy. *Journal of Communication Disorders, 2,* 154–162.

Manning, W., Dailey, D., & Wallace, S. (1984). Attitude and personality characteristics of older stutterers. *Journal of Fluency Disorders, 9,* 207–215.

Manning, W., & Monte, K. (1981). Fluency breaks in older speakers: Implications for a model of stuttering throughout the life cycle. *Journal of Fluency Disorders, 6,* 35–48.

Manning, W., Perkins, D., Winn, S., & Cole, D. (1984). *Self-efficacy changes during treatment and maintenance for adult stutterers.* Paper presented to the annual meeting of the American Speech-Language-Hearing Association, San Francisco, CA.

Manning, W., & Shirkey, E. (1981). Fluency and the aging process. In D. S. Beasley & G. A. Davis (Eds.), *Aging: Communication Processes and Disorders* (pp. 175–189). New York: Grune & Stratton.

Manning W., & Shrum, W. (1973). The concept of control in stuttering therapy: A reappraisal. *Division for Children with Communication Disorders Bulletin, 9*(1), 32–34.

Market, K. E., Montague, J. C., Buffalo, M. D., & Drummond, S. S. (1990). Acquired stuttering: Descriptive data and treatment outcome. *Journal of Fluency Disorders, 15,* 21–34.

Martin, R. R., & Haroldson, S. (1986). Stuttering as involuntary loss of speech control: Barking up a new tree. *Journal of Speech and Hearing Disorders, 51,* 187–190.

Martin, R. R., & Lefcourt, H. (1983). Sense of humor as a moderator of the relation between stressors and moods. *Journal of Personality and Social Psychology, 45,* 1313–1324.

Martin, R. R., & Lefcourt, H. (1984). Situational humor response questionnaire: Quantitative measure of sense of humor. *Journal of Personality and Social Psychology, 47,* 145–155.

Martin, R. R., & Lindamood, L. P. (1986). Stuttering and spontaneous recovery; Implications for the speech-language pathologist. *Language, Speech, and Hearing Services in Schools, 17,* 207–218.

Martin, R. R. (1981). Introduction and perspective: Review of published research. In E. Boberg (Ed.), *Maintenance of fluency* (pp. 1–30). New York: Elsevier.

Martin, R. R., & Haroldson, S. K. (1982). Contingent self-stimulation for stuttering. *Journal of Speech and Hearing Disorders, 47,* 407–413.

Martin, R. R., & Haroldson, S. K. (1992). Stuttering and speech naturalness: Audio and audiovisual judgements. *Journal of Speech and Hearing Research, 35,* 521–528.

Martin, R. R., Haroldson, S., & Kuhl, P. (1972a). Disfluencies in child-child and child-mother speaking situations. *Journal of Speech and Hearing Research, 15,* 753–756.

Martin, R. R., Haroldson, S., & Kuhl, P. (1972b). Disfluencies of young children in two speaking situations. *Journal of Speech and Hearing Research, 15,* 831–836.

Martin, R. R., Haroldson, S. K., & Triden, K. A. (1984). Stuttering and speech naturalness. *Journal of Speech and Hearing Disorders, 49,* 53–58.

Maslow, A. (1968). *Towards a Psychology of Being* (2nd ed.). Princeton, NJ: Van Nostrand.

Masterson, J., & Kamhi, A. (1992). Linguistic trade-offs in school-age children with and without language disorders. *Journal of Speech and Hearing Research, 35,* 1064–1075.

Matkin, N., Ringle, R., & Snope, T. (1983). Master report of surveys discrepancies. In N. Rees & T. Snope (Eds.), *Proceedings of the Conference on Undergraduate, Graduate and Continuing Education* (ASHA Reports No. 13). Rockville, MD: American Speech-Language-Hearing Association.

Maxwell, D. (1982). Cognitive and behavioral self-control strategies: Applications for the clinical management of adult stutterers. *Journal of Fluency Disorders, 7,* 403–432.

McCall, G. N. (1974). Spasmodic dysphonia and the stuttering block: Commonalities or possible connections. In L. M. Webster & L. C. Furst (Eds.), *Vocal tract dynamics and dysfluency* (pp. 124–151). New York: Speech & Hearing Institute.

McCarthy, P., Culpepper, N., & Lucks, L. (1986). Variability in counseling experience and training among ESB accredited programs. *ASHA, 28,* 49–53.

McClean, M., Goldsmith, H., & Cerf, A. (1984). Lowerlip EMG and displacement during bilabial disfluencies in adult stutterers. *Journal of Speech and Hearing Research, 27,* 342–349.

McDearmon, J. R. (1968). Primary stuttering at the onset of stuttering: A reexamination of data. *Journal of Speech and Hearing Research, 11,* 631–637.

McDonald, E. T., & Frick, J. V. (1954). Store clerks' reactions to stuttering. *Journal of Speech and Hearing Disorders, 19,* 306–311.

McFarland, D. H., & Moore, W. H., Jr. (1982). Alpha asymmetries during an electromyographic biofeedback procedure for stuttering. Paper presented to the annual convention of the American Speech-Language-Hearing Association, Toronto, Canada.

McFarlane, S., & Goldberg, L. (1987). Factors influencing treatment approaches, prognosis and dismissal criteria for stuttering [Abstract]. *ASHA, 29,* 164–165.

McGhee, P. E., & Goldstein, J. H. (1977). *Handbook of humor research: Volume 1, Basic issues.* New York: Springer-Verlag.

McLelland, J. K., & Cooper, E. B. (1978). Fluency-related behaviors and attitudes of 178 young stutterers. *Journal of Fluency Disorders, 3,* 253–263.

Mehrabian, A., & Reed., H. (1969). Factors influencing judgments of psychopathology. *Psychological Reports, 24,* 323–330.

Merits-Patterson, R., & Reed, C. (1981). Disfluencies in the speech of language delayed children. *Journal of Speech and Hearing Research, 24,* 55–58.

Metz, D. E., Schiavetti, N., & Sacco, P. R. (1990). Acoustic and psychophysical dimensions of the perceived speech naturalness of nonstutterers and posttreatment stutterers. *Journal of Speech and Hearing Disorders, 55,* 516–525.

Meyers, S., Ghatak, L., & Woodford, L. (1990). Case descriptions of nonfluency and loci: Initial and follow-up conversations with three preschool children. *Journal of Fluency Disorders, 14,* 383–398.

Meyers, S., Hall, N. E., & Aram, D. M. (1990). Fluency and language recovery in a child with a left hemisphere lesion. *Journal of Fluency Disorders, 15,* 159–173.

Meyers, S., & Woodford, L. (1992). *The fluency development system for young children.* Buffalo, NY: United Educational Services.

Meyers, S. C., & Freeman, F. J. (1985). Mother and child speech rates as a variable in stuttering and disfluency. *Journal of Speech and Hearing Research, 28,* 436–444.

Miller, S., & Watson, B. C. (1992). The relationship between communication attitude, anxiety and depression in stutterers and nonstutterers. *Journal of Speech and Hearing Research, 35,* 789–798.

Mineka, S. (1985). Animal models of anxiety-based disorders: Their usefulness and limitations. In A. H. Tuma & J. Mase (Eds.), *Anxiety and the anxiety disorders.* Hillsdale, NJ: Lawrence Erlbaum Associates.

Molt, L., & Brading, T. (1994). Hemispheric patterns of auditory event-related potentials to dichotic CV syllables in stutterers and normal speakers. In C. W. Starkweather & H. F. M. Peters (Eds.) *Proceedings of the 1st World Congress on Fluency Disorders,* Munich, Germany.

Molt, L. F., & Guilford, A. M. (1979). Auditory processing and anxiety in stutterers. *Journal of Fluency Disorders, 4,* 255–267.

Moore, S. E., & Perkins, W. (1990). Validity and reliability of judgements of authentic and simulated stuttering. *Journal of Speech and Hearing Disorders, 55,* 383–391.

Moore, W. (1984). Hemispheric alpha asymmetries during an electromyographic biofeedback procedure for stuttering: A single-subject experimental design. *Journal of Fluency Disorders, 9,* 143–162.

Moore, W., & Haynes, W. (1980). Alpha hemispheric asymmetry and stuttering: Some support for a segmentation dysfunction hypothesis. *Journal of Speech and Hearing Research, 23,* 229–247.

Morgenstern, J. J. (1956). Socio-economic factors in stuttering. *Journal of Speech and Hearing Disorders, 21,* 25–33.

Morreall, J. (1982). *Taking laughter seriously.* Albany: State University of New York Press.

Mueller, H. G., & Bright, K. E. (1994). Monosyllabic procedures in central testing. In J. Katz (Ed.), *Handbook of clinical audiology,* 4th ed. Baltimore, MD: Williams & Wilkins.

Murphy, A. T., & Fitzsimons, R. M. (1960). *Stuttering and personality dynamics.* New York: Ronald Press.

Murphy, B. (1999). A preliminary look at shame, guilt, and stuttering. In N. B. Ratner & E. C. Healey (Eds.), *Stuttering research and practice: Bridging the gap* (pp. 131–143). Mahwah, NJ: Lawrence Erlbaum.

Murray, F. P., & Edwards, S. G. (1980). *A stutterer's story.* Danville, IL: Interstate Printers and Publishers.

Murray, H. L., & Reed, C. G. (1977). Language abilities of preschool stuttering children. *Journal of Fluency Disorders, 2,* 171–176.

Myers, F. L., & St. Louis, K. O. (1992). Cluttering: Issues and controversies. In F. L. Myers & K. O. St. Louis (Eds.), *Cluttering: A clinical perspective* (pp. 11–22). San Diego, CA: Singular Publishing Group, Inc.

Mysak, E. D. (1960). Servo theory and stuttering. *Journal of Speech and Hearing Disorders, 25,* 188–195.

Neaves, R. (1970). To establish a basis for prognosis in stammering. *British Journal of Disorders of Communication, 5,* 46–58.

Neeley, J. N. (1961). A study of the speech behavior of stutterers and nonstutterers under normal and delayed auditory feedback. *Journal of Speech and Hearing Disorders* (Monograph Supplement No. 7), 63–82.

Neilson, M., & Neilson, P. (1987). Speech motor control and stuttering: A computational model of adaptive sensory-motor processing. *Speech Communications, 6,* 325–333.

Newman, P. W., Harris, R. W., & Hilton, L. M. (1989). Vocal jitter and shimmer in stuttering. *Journal of Fluency Disorders, 14,* 87–95.

Nezu, A., Nezu, C., & Blissett, S. (1988). Sense of humor as a moderator of the relations between stressful events and psychological distress: A prospective analysis. *Journal of Personality and Social Psychology, 54,* 520–525.

Nippold, M., & Rudzinski, M. (1995). Parents' speech and children's stuttering: A critique of the literature. *Journal of Speech and Hearing Research, 38,* 978–989.

Oates, D. (1929). Left-handedness in relation to speech defects, intelligence, and achievement. *Forum of Education, 7,* 91–105.

Ohman, S. (1965). Coarticulation in VCV utterances: Spectrographic measurements. *Journal of the Acoustical Society of America, 39,* 151–168.

Ojemann, R. (1931). Studies in sidedness: III. Relation of handedness to speech. *Journal of Educational Psychology, 22,* 120–126.

Onslow, M. (1992). Identification of early stuttering: Issues and suggested strategies. *American Journal of Speech-Language Pathology, 1*(4), 21–27.

Onslow, M. (1999). Review of *Stuttering: An Integrated Approach to Its Nature and Treatment,* 2nd Edition, Baltimore, MD: Williams & Wilkins. *Journal of Fluency Disorder, 24,* 319–332.

Onslow, M., Adams, R., & Ingham, R. (1992). Reliability of speech naturalness ratings of stuttered speech during treatment. *Journal of Speech and Hearing Research, 35,* 994–1001.

Onslow, M., Hayes, B., Hutchins, L., & Newman, D. (1992). Speech naturalness and prolonged-speech treatments for stuttering: Further variables and data. *Journal of Speech and Hearing Research, 35,* 274–282.

Onslow, M., & Ingham, R. J. (1987). Speech quality measurement and the management of stuttering. *Journal of Speech and Hearing Disorders, 52,* 2–17.

Ornstein, A., & Manning, W. (1985). Self-efficacy scaling by adult stutterers. *Journal of Communication Disorders, 18,* 313–320.

Orton, S.T. (1927). Studies in stuttering. *Archives of Neurology and Psychiatry, 18,* 671–672.

Ost, L., Gotestam, K. G., & Melin, L. (1976). A controlled study of two behavioral methods in the treatment of stuttering. *Behavior Therapy, 7,* 587–592.

Otsuki, H. (1958). Study on stuttering: Statistical observations. *Otorhinolaryngology Clinic, 5,* 1150–1151.

Paden, E. P. (1970). *A History of the American Speech and Hearing Association 1925–1958.* Washington, DC: American Speech and Hearing Association.

Paden, E. P., Yairi, E., & Ambrose, N. G. (1999). Early childhood stuttering II: Initial status of phonological abilities. *Journal of Speech, Language, and Hearing Research, 42,* 1113–1124.

Panelli, C., McFarlane, S., & Shipley, K. (1978). Implications of evaluating and interviewing with incipient stutterers. *Journal of Fluency Disorders, 3,* 41–50.

Patterson, C. H. (1985). *The therapeutic relationship: Foundations for an eclectic psychotherapy.* Pacific Grove, CA: Brooks/Cole.

Pauls, D. L. (1990). A review of the evidence for genetic factors in stuttering ASHA Reports Series. *American Speech-Language-Hearing Association, 18,* 34–38.

Peck, M. S. (1978). *The road less traveled.* New York: Simon & Schuster.

Peins, M., McGough, W. E., & Lee, B. S. (1972). Evaluation of a tape-recorded method of stuttering therapy: Improvement in a speaking task. *Journal of Speech and Hearing Research, 15,* 364–371.

Perkins, W., Kent, R. D., & Curlee, R. F. (1990). A theory of neuropsycholinguistic function in stuttering. *Journal of Speech and Hearing Research, 34,* 734–752.

Perkins, W. H. (1973). Replacement of stuttering with normal speech: II. Clinical procedures. *Journal of Speech and Hearing Disorders, 38,* 295–303.

Perkins, W. H. (1979). From psychoanalysis to discoordination. In H. Gregory (Ed.), *Controversies about stuttering therapy,* 97–127. Baltimore, MD: University Park Press.

Perkins, W. H. (1983). The problem of definition: Commentary on stuttering. *Journal of Speech and Hearing Disorders, 48,* 246–249.

Perkins, W. H. (1990). What is stuttering? *Journal of Speech and Hearing Disorders, 55,* 370–382.

Peters, T. J., & Guitar, B. (1991). *Stuttering, an integrated approach to its nature and treatment.* Baltimore, MD: Williams & Wilkins.

Pickett, J. M. (1980). *The sounds of speech communication.* Baltimore, MD: University Park Press.

Pindzola, R. (1987). *Stuttering intervention program.* Austin, TX: Pro-Ed.

Pinsky, S. D., & McAdam, D. W. (1980). Electroencephalographic and dichotic indicies of cerebral laterality in stutterers. *Brain & Language, 11,* 374–397. Pool, K. D., Devous, M. D., Sr., Freeman, F. J., Watson, B. C., & Finitzo, T. (1991). Regional cerebral blood flow in developmental stutterers. *Archives of Neurology, 48,* 509–512.

Postma, A., & Kolk, H. (1992). Error monitoring in people who stutter: Evidence against auditory feedback defect theories. *Journal of Speech and Hearing Research, 35,* 1024–1032.

Postma, A., & Kolk, H. (1993). The covert repair hypothesis: Prearticulatory repair processes in normal and stuttered disfluencies. *Journal of Speech and Hearing Research, 36,* 472–487.

Postma, A., Kolk, H. H. J., & Povel, D. J. (1990). Speech planning and execution in stutterers. *Journal of Fluency Disorders, 15,* 49–59.

Poulos, M. G., & Webster, W. G. (1991). Family history as a basis for subgrouping people who stutter. *Journal of Speech and Hearing Research, 34,* 5–10.

Preus, A. (1972). Stuttering in Down's syndrome. *Scandinavian Journal of Education Research, 15,* 89–104.

Prins, D. (1970). Improvement and regression in stutterers following short-term intensive therapy. *Journal of Speech and Hearing Disorders, 35,* 123–135.

Prins, D. (1997). Modifying stuttering—The stutterer's reactive behavior: perspectives on past, present, and future. In R. Curlee & G. Siegel (Eds.), *Nature and treatment of stuttering, New directions* (2nd ed., pp. 335–355). Needham Heights, MA: Allyn & Bacon.

Prins, D., & Hubbard, C. (1988). Response contingent stimuli and stuttering: Issues and implications. *Journal of Speech and Hearing Research, 31,* 696–709.

Prochaska, J. O. & DiClemente, C.C. (1992). Stages of change in the modification of problem behaviors. In Herson, M., Eisler, R., & Miller, P. (Eds.), *Progress in behavior modification* (pp. 184–218). Sycamore, IL: Sycamore Publishing Company.

Prochaska, J. O., DiClemente, C. C., & Norcross, J. C. (1992). In search of how people change: Applications to addictive behaviors. *American Psychologist, 47*(9), 1102–1114.

Quarrington, B., Seligman, J., & Kosower, E. (1969). Goal setting behavior of parents of beginning stutterers and parents of nonstuttering children. *Journal of Speech and Hearing Research, 12,* 435–42.

Quesal, R. W. (1998). Knowledge, understanding, and acceptance. In E. C. Healey & H. F. M. Peters (Eds.), *Proceedings of the 2nd World Congress on Fluency Disorders* (pp. 384–387). Nijmegen, The Netherlands: Nijmegen University Press.

Ramig, P. R. (1993a). High reported spontaneous recovery rates: Fact or fiction? *Language, Speech, and Hearing in Schools, 24,* 156–160.

Ramig, P. R. (1993b). The impact of self-help groups on persons who stutter: A call for research. *Journal of Fluency Disorders, 18,* 351–361.

Ramig, P. R. (1993c). Parent-clinician-child partnership in the therapeutic process of the preschool and elementary-aged child who stutters. *Seminars in Speech and Language, 14,* 226–236.

Ramig, P. R. (1998). My long-term recovery from stuttering. In E. C. Healey & H. F. M. Peters (Eds.), *Proceedings of the 2nd World Congress on Fluency Disorders* (pp. 390–391). Nijmegen, The Netherlands: Nijmegen University Press.

Ramig, P., & Bennett, E. (1995). Working with 7- to 12-year-old children who stutter: Ideas for intervention in the public schools. *Language, Speech, and Hearing Services in Schools, 26,* 138–150.

Rao, P R. (1991) Neurogenic stuttering as a manifestation of stroke and a mask of dysnomia. *Clinics in Communication Disorders, 1,*(1), 31–37.

Ratner, N. (1993). Parents, children, and stuttering. *Seminars in Speech and Language, 14*(3), 238–247.

Ratner, N. (1997). Stuttering: A psycholinguistic perspective. In R. Curlee & Siegel (Eds.), *Nature and treatment of stuttering: New directions* (pp. 99–127) (2nd ed.). Boston: Allyn & Bacon.

Ratner, N. (2000). Performance or capacity, the model still requires definitions and boundaries it doesn't have. *Journal of Fluency Disorders,* (in press).

Ratner, N., & Sih, C. (1987). The effects of gradual increases in sentence length and complexity on children's dysfluency. *Journal of Speech and Hearing Disorders, 52,* 278–287.

Ratner, N. B. (1995). Treating the child who stutters with concomitant language or phonological impairment. *Language, Speech, and Hearing in Schools, 26,* 180–186.

Ratner, N. B., & Healey, E. C. (1999) Bridging the gap between stuttering research and practice: An overview. In N. B. Ratner & E. C. Healey (Eds.), *Stuttering research and practice: Bridging the gap* (pp. 1–12). Mahwah, NJ: Lawrence Erlbaum Associates.

Reardon, N. A. (2000). Working with teachers. Presentation to the Stuttering Foundation of America Conference, *Stuttering therapy: Practical ideas for the school clinician.* Charleston, SC, June 10, 2000.

Reich, A., Till, J. A., & Goldsmith, H. (1981). Laryngeal and manual reaction times of stuttering and nonstuttering adults. *Journal of Speech and Hearing Research, 24*(2), 192–196.

Riley, G. (1981). *Stuttering prediction instrument for young children* (rev. ed.). Austin, TX: Pro-Ed.

Riley, G., & Riley, J. (1979). A component model for diagnosing and treating children who stutter. *Journal of Fluency Disorders, 4,* 279–293.

Riley, G., & Riley, J. (1983). Evaluation as a basis for intervention. In D. Peins & R. Ingham (Eds.), *Treatment of stuttering in early childhood* (pp. 128–152). San Diego, CA: College-Hill.

Riley, G., & Riley, J. (1984). A component model for treating stuttering in children. In M. Prins (Ed.), *Contemporary approaches in stuttering therapy.* Boston: Little, Brown.

Riley, G., & Riley, J. (1985). *Oral motor assessment and treatment: Improving syllable production.* Austin, TX: ProED.

Riley, G., & Riley, J. (2000). A revised component model for diagnosing and treating children who stutter. *Contemporary Issues in Communication Sciences and Disorders, 27* (in press).

Riley, G. A. (1994). Stuttering severity instrument for children and adults—third edition. (SSI-3). Austin, TX: Pro-Ed.

Riley, G. D. (1972). A stuttering severity instrument for children and adults. *Journal of Speech and Hearing Disorders, 37,* 314–321.

Robb, M., Blomgren, M., & Chen, Y. (1998). Formant frequency fluctuation in stuttering and nonstuttering adults. *Journal of Fluency Disorders, 23,* 73–84.

Robinson, V. M. (1991). *Humor and the health professions.* Throrfare, NJ: Slack.

Rogers, C. R. (1951). *Client-centered therapy.* Boston: Houghton Mifflin.

Rogers, C. R. (1961). *On becoming a person.* Boston: Houghton Mifflin.

Rogers, C. R. (Ed.). (1967). *The therapeutic relationship and its impact.* Madison: University of Wisconsin Press.

Rogers, C. R. (1980). *A way of being.* Boston: Houghton Mifflin.

Rogers, C. R. (1986). *Person-Centered Review, 1,* 125–140.

Rosenbek, J., Messert, B., Collins, M., & Wertz, T. (1978). Stuttering following brain damage. *Brain and Language, 6,* 82–86.

Rosenheim, E. (1974). Humor in psychotherapy: An interactive experience. *American Journal of Psychotherapy, 28,* 584–591.

Roth, C. R., Aronson, A. E., & Davis, L. J., Jr. (1989). Clinical studies in psychogenic stuttering of adult onset. *Journal of Speech and Hearing Disorders, 54,* 634–646.

Rousey, C. G., Arjunan, K. N., & Rousey, C. L. (1986). Successful treatment of stuttering following closed head injury. *Journal of Fluency Disorders, 11,* 257–261.

Rubin, H. (1986). Postscript: Cognitive therapy. In G. H. Shames & H. Rubin (Eds.), *Stuttering then and now* (pp. 474–486). Columbus, OH: Merrill.

Rubin, H., & Culatta, R. (1971). A point of view about fluency. *ASHA, 13,* 93–116.

Rudolf, S. R., Manning, W. H., & Sewell, W. R. (1983). The use of self-efficacy scaling in training student clinicians: Implications for working with stutterers. *Journal of Fluency Disorders, 8,* 55–75.

Runyan, C. M., & Adams, M.R. (1978). Perceptual study of the speech of "successfully therapeutized stutterers." *Journal of Fluency Disorders, 3,* 25–29.

Runyan, C. M., Bell, J. N., & Prosek, R.A. (1990). Speech naturalness ratings of treated stutterers. *Journal of Speech and Hearing Disorders, 55,* 434–438.

Runyan, C. M., Hames, P. E., & Proseck, R. A. (1982). A perceptual comparison between paired stimulus and single stimulus methods of presentation of the fluent utterances of stutterers. *Journal of Fluency Disorders, 7,* 71–77.

Runyan, C. M., & Runyan, S. (1993). Therapy for school-age stutterers: An update on the fluency rules program. In R. Curlee (Ed.), *Stuttering and related disorders of fluency* (pp. 101–114). New York: Thieme Medical Publishers, Inc.

Runyan, C. M., & Runyan, S. E. (1986). A fluency rules therapy program for young children in the public schools. *Language, Speech, and Hearing Services in Schools, 17,* 276–284.

Rusk, T. (1989). *So you want to change: Helping people help themselves.* Presentation given at the Twelfth Annual Conference for Trainers, Consultants, and other HRD Professionals, sponsored by University Associates (San Diego), San Francisco, CA.

Rustin, L. (1987). The treatment of childhood dysfluency through active parental involvement. In L. Rustin, H. Purser, & H. Rowley (Eds.), *Progress in the treatment of fluency disorders* (pp. 166–180). London: Taylor & Francis.

Rustin, L., & Cook, F. (1995). Parental involvement in the treatment of stuttering. *Language, Speech, and Hearing Services in Schools, 26,* 127–137.

Ryan, B. (1979). Stuttering therapy in a framework of operant conditioning and programmed learning. In H. Gregory (Ed.), *Controversies about stuttering therapy* (pp. 129–174). Baltimore, MD: University Park Press.

Ryan, B. (1980). *Programmed therapy for stuttering children and adults* (3rd ed.). Springfield, IL: Charles C. Thomas.

Ryan, B., & Van Kirk, B. (1974). The establishment, transfer, and maintenance of fluent speech in 50 stutterers using delayed auditory feedback and operant procedures. *Journal of Speech and Hearing Disorders, 39,* 3–10.

Sacco, P. R., Metz, D. E., & Schiavetti, N. (1992). *Speech naturalness of nonstutterers and treated stutterers: Acoustical correlates.* Paper presented to the annual meeting of the American Speech-Language-Hearing Association, San Antonio, TX.

Sagan, C. (1996). *The demon-haunted world: Science as a candle in the dark.* New York: Random House.

Salamy, J. N., & Sessions, R. B. (1980). Spastic dysphonia. *Journal of Fluency Disorders, 5,* 281–290.

Saltuklaroglu, T., & Kully, D. (1998). Further validation of the self-efficacy scale for adult stutterers. University of Alberta (unpublished manuscript).

Satcher, D. (1986). Research needs for minority populations. In F. H. Bess, B. S. Clark, & H. R. Mitchel (Eds.), *Concerns for minority groups in communication disorders* (pp. 89–92). (ASHA Reports, No. 16, ISSN 0569-8553). Rockville, MD: American Speech-Language-Hearing Association.

Schaeffer, M. L., & Shearer, W. M. (1968). A survey of mentally retarded stutterers. *Mental Retardation, 6,* 44–45.

Schiavetti, N., & Metz, D. E. (1997). Stuttering and the measurement of speech naturalness. In R. Curlee & G. Siegel (Eds.), *Nature and treatment of stuttering, new directions* (2nd ed., pp. 298–412). Needham Heights, MA: Allyn & Bacon.

Schiff, J. L. (1975). *Cathexis reader: Transactional analysis treatment of psychosis.* New York: Harper & Row.

Schimel, J. (1978). The function of wit and humor in psychoanalysis. *Journal of the American Academy of Psychoanalysis, 6*(3), 369–379.

Schwartz, H. D. (1999). *A primer of stuttering therapy.* Needham Heights, MA: Allyn and Bacon.

Schwartz, H., & Conture, E. (1988). Subgroupings of young stutterers: Preliminary behavioral observations. *Journal of Speech and Hearing Research, 31,* 62–71.

Schwartz, H. D., Zebrowski, P. M., & Conture, E. G. (1990). Behaviors at the outset of stuttering. *Journal of Fluency Disorders, 15,* 77–86.

Scripture, E. W. (1931). *Stuttering, lisping, and correction of the speech of the deaf.* New York: Macmillan.

Shames, G. H., & Florance, C. L. (1980). *Stutter free speech: A goal for therapy.* Columbus, OH: Merrill.

Shapiro, D. A. (1999). *Stuttering intervention: A collaborative journey to fluency freedom.* Austin, TX: Pro-Ed.

Shaywitz, B. A., Pugh, K. R., Constable, R. T., Shaywitz, S. E., Bronen, R. A., Fulbright, R. K., Shankweiler, D. P., Katz, L., Fletcher, J. M., Skudlarski, P., & Gore, J. C. (1994). Localization of semantic processing using functional magnetic resonance imaging. *Human Brain Mapping, 2,* 149–158.

Sheehan, J. (1958). Projective studies of stuttering. *Journal of Speech and Hearing Disorders, 23,* 18–25.

Sheehan, J. (1970). *Stuttering: Research and therapy.* New York: Harper & Row.

Sheehan, J. (1975). Conflict theory and avoidance-reduction therapy. In J. Eisenson (Ed.), *Stuttering, a second symposium* (pp. 97–198). New York: Harper & Row.

Sheehan, J., & Martyn, M. (1966). Spontaneous recovery from stuttering. *Journal of Speech and Hearing Research, 9,* 121–135.

Sheehan, J. G. (1980). Problems in the evaluation of progress and outcome. In W. H. Perkins (Ed.), *Seminars in speech, language and hearing* (pp. 389–401). New York: Thieme-Stratton.

Sheehan, J. G., & Costley, M. S. (1977). A reexamination of the role of heredity in stuttering. *Journal of Speech and Hearing Disorders, 42,* 47–59.

Sheehy, G. (1974). *Passages: Predictable crises of adult life.* New York: Bantam Books.

Shields, D. (1989). *Dead languages.* New York: Knopf.

Shine, R. E. (1980). Direct management of the beginning stutterer. *Seminars in Speech, Language and Hearing, 1,* 339–350.

Shine, R. E. (1988). *Systematic fluency training for young children* (3rd ed.). Austin, TX: ProEd.

Siegel, G. (1970). Punishment, stuttering and disfluency. *Journal of Speech and Hearing Disorders, 13,* 677–714.

Siegel, G. (2000). "Demands and capacities" or "demands and performance." *Journal of Fluency Disorders, 25* (in press).

Silverman, E. (1973). Clustering: A characteristic of preschoolers' speech disfluency. *Journal of Speech and Hearing Research, 16,* 578–583.

Silverman, E. (1974). Disfluency behavior of elementary-school stutterers and nonstutterers. *Language, Speech, and Hearing Services in Schools, 5,* 32–37.

Silverman, E., & Zimmer, C. (1982). Demographic characteristics and treatment experiences of women and men who stutter. *Journal of Fluency Disorders, 7,* 273–285.

Silverman, F. H. (1975). How "typical" is a stutterer's stuttering in a clinical environment? *Perceptual and Motor Skills, 40,* 458.

Silverman, F. H. (1976). Long-term impact of a miniature metronome on stuttering: An interim report. *Perceptual and Motor Skills, 43,* 398.

Silverman, F. H. (1981). Relapse following stuttering therapy. In N. J. Lass (Ed.), *Speech and language, advances in basic research and practice* (Vol. 5, pp. 56–78). New York: Academic Press.

Silverman, F. H. (1988a). Impact of a T-shirt message on stutterer stereotypes. *Journal of Fluency Disorders, 13,* 279–281.

Silverman, F. H. (1988b). The monster study. *Journal of Fluency Disorders, 13,* 225–231.

Silverman, F. H. (1996). *Stuttering and other fluency disorders.* Englewood Cliffs, NJ: Prentice Hall.

Silverman, F. H., & Hummer, K. (1989). Spastic dysphonia: A fluency disorder? *Journal of Fluency Disorders, 14,* 285–291.

Slater, S. C. (1992, August). 1992 Omnibus Survey: Portrait of the professions. *ASHA, 34,* 61–65.

Smith, A. (1989). Neural drive to muscles in stuttering. *Journal of Speech and Hearing Research, 32,* 252–264.

Smith, A. (1990). Toward a comprehensive theory of stuttering: A commentary. *Journal of Speech and Hearing Disorders, 55,* 398–401.

Smith, A. (1999). Stuttering: A unified approach to a multifactorial, dynamic disorder. In N. B. Ratner and E. C. Healey (Eds.), *Stuttering research and practice: Bridging the gap* (pp. 27–44). Mahwah, NJ: Lawrence Erlbaum.

Smith, A., Denny, M, Shaffer, L, Kelly, E. and Hirano, M. (1996). Activity of intrinsic laryngeal muscles in fluent and disfluent speech. *Journal of Speech and Hearing Research, 39,* 329–348.

Smith, A., Denny, M., & Wood, J. (1991). Instability in speech muscle systems in stuttering. In H. F. M. Peters, W. Hulstijn, & W. Starkweather (Eds.), *Speech motor control and stuttering* (pp. 231–242). New York: Elsevier.

Smith A., & Kelly, E. (1997) Stuttering: A dynamic, multifactoral model. In R. F. Curlee & G. M. Siegel (Eds.), *The nature and treatment of stuttering: New directions* (2nd Ed., pp. 204–217). Needham Heighs, MA: Allyn & Bacon.

Snidecor, J. C. (1947). Why the Indian does not stutter. *Quarterly Journal of Speech, 33,* 493–495.

Sommers, R. K., Brady, W., & Moore, W. H., Jr. (1975). Dichotic ear preferences of stuttering children and adults. *Perceptual and Motor Skills, 41,* 931–938.

Sommers, R. K., & Caruso, A. J. (1995). *American Journal of Speech-Language Pathology, 4*(3), 22–28.

Spielberger, C. D., Edwards, C. D., Luschene, R. E., Montuori, J., & Platzek, D. (1972). *STAIC preliminary manual.* New York: Consulting Psychologists Press, Inc.

Springer, S.P., & Deutsch, G. (1989). *Left brain, right brain.* New York: W. H. Freeman and Company.

St. Louis, K. O. (1982). *Transfer and maintenance of fluency in stuttering clients.* Short course presented to the annual meeting of the American Speech-Language-Hearing Association, Toronto, Ontario.

St. Louis, K. O. (1986a). *The atypical stutterer: Principles and practices of rehabilitation.* Orlando, FL: Academic Press.

St. Louis, K. O. (1986b). The problem of the atypical stutterer: An introduction. In K. O. St. Louis (Ed.), *The atypical stutterer: principles and practices of rehabilitation* (pp. 1–8). New York: Academic Press.

St. Louis, K. (1996). Are "stutterer," disfluent," dysfluent," and "PWS" labels confusing? Insensitive. Paper presented at the Annual Meeting of the American Speech-Language-Hearing Association, Seattle, WA.

St. Louis, K. (1998). A typical (?) stutterer's story. In E. C. Healey & H. F. M. Peters (Eds.), *Proceedings of the 2nd World Congress on Fluency Disorders* (pp. 392–393). Nijmegen, The Netherlands: Nijmegen University Press.

St. Louis, K. O., & Durrenberger, C. H. (1992). *Clinician preferences for managing various communication disorders.* Paper presented at the American Speech-Language-Hearing Association Convention, San Antonio, TX.

St. Louis, K. O., & Hinzman, A. R. (1986). Studies of cluttering: Perceptions of cluttering by speech-language pathologists and educators, *Journal of Fluency Disorders, 11,* 131–149.

St. Louis, K. O., & Lass, N. J. (1981). A survey of communicative disorders students' attitudes toward stuttering. *Journal of Fluency Disorders, 6,* 49–80.

St. Louis, K., Hanley, J., & Hood, S. (1999). Terminology Pertaining to Fluency and Fluency Disorders. Technical paper prepared for Special Interest Division 4, American Speech Language and Hearing Association (1997). *ASHA,* Suppl. No. 19, Mar/April.

St. Louis, K., Murray, C., & Ashworth, M. (1991). Coexisting communication disorders in a random sample of school-aged stutterers. *Journal of Fluency Disorders, 16,* 13–23.

St. Louis, K., & Myers, F. (1995). Clinical management of cluttering. *Language, Speech, and Hearing in Schools, 26,* 187–195.

St. Louis, K. O., & Rustin, L. (1992). Professional awareness of cluttering. In F. M. Myers & K. O. St. Louis (Eds.), *Cluttering: A clinical perspective* (pp. 23–35). San Diego, CA: Singular Publishing Group, Inc.

St. Louis, K. O., & Westbrook, J. B. (1987). The effectiveness of treatment for stuttering. In L. Rustin, H. Purser, & D. Rowley (Eds.), *Progress in the treatment of fluency disorders* (pp. 235–257). London: Taylor & Francis.

Stager, S. V., & Ludlow, C. (1994). Responses of stutterers and vocal tremor patients to treatment with botulinum toxin. In J. Jankovic & M. Hallatt (Eds.), *Therapy with botulinum toxin* (pp. 481–490). New York: Marcel Dekker, Inc.

Starke, A. (1995). Why do stutterers reject artificial speech? The message incompatibility conflict. *Proceedings of the 1994 Meeting of the International Fluency Association* (V. II, pp. 445–452). University Press Nijmegen, Netherlands.

Starkweather, C. W. (1987). *Fluency and stuttering.* Englewood Cliffs, NJ: Prentice-Hall.

Starkweather, C. W. (1992). Response and reaction to Hamre, "Stuttering Prevention I." *Journal of Fluency Disorders, 17,* 43–55.

Starkweather, C. W. (July 8, 1995). Personal communication.

Starkweather, C.W. (1997). Therapy for younger children. In R. F. Curlee and G. M. Siegel (Eds.), *Nature and treatment of stuttering* (2nd ed., pp. 257–279). Boston: Allyn and Bacon.

Starkweather, C.W. (1999).The effectiveness of stuttering therapy: An issue for science? In N. B. Ratner and E. C. Healey (Eds.), *Stuttering research and practice: Bridging the gap* (pp. 231–244). Mahwah, NJ: Lawrence Erlbaum.

Starkweather, C. W., & Givens-Ackerman, J. (1997). *Stuttering.* Austin, TX: Pro-Ed.

Starkweather, C. W. & Givens-Ackerman, J. (2000). Personal communication.

Starkweather, C. W., & Gottwald, S. R. (1990). The demands and capacities model II: Clinical implications. *Journal of Fluency Disorders, 15,* 143–157.

Starkweather, C. W., & Gottwald, S. R. (2000). The demands and capacities model: Response to Siegel. *Journal of Fluency Disorders, 25* (in press).

Starkweather, C. W., Gottwald, S. R., & Halfond, M. H. (1990). *Stuttering prevention: A clinical method.* Englewood Cliffs, NJ: Prentice-Hall.

Starkweather, C. W., Hirschmann, P., & Tannenbaum, R. (1976). Latency of vocalization: Stutterers v. nonstutterers. *Journal of Speech and Hearing Research, 19,* 481–492.

Starkweather, C. W., St. Louis, K. O., Blood, G., Peters, T., & Westbrook, J. (1994). American Speech-Language-Hearing Association (1995, March). Guidelines for Practice in Stuttering Treatment. *ASHA, 37* (Suppl. 14, p. 26).

Stetson, R. H. (1951). *Motor phonetics* (2nd ed.). Amsterdam: North-Holland.

Stocker, B. (1980). *The Stocker Probe technique for diagnosis and treatment of stuttering in young children.* Tulsa, OK: Modern Education Corporation.

Stocker, B., & Gerstman, L. (1983). A comparison of the probe technique and conventional therapy for young stutterers. *Journal of Fluency Disorders, 8,* 331–339.

Stocker, B., & Usprich, C. (1976). Stuttering in young children and level of demand. *Journal of Fluency Disorders, 1,* 116–131.

Strub, R. L., Black, F. W., & Naeser, M. A. (1987). Anomalous dominance in sibling stutterers: Evidence from CT scan asymmetries, dichotic listening, neurophysiological testing, and handedness. *Brain and Language, 30,* 338–350.

Studdert-Kennedy, M., & Shankweiler, D. (1970). Hemispheric specialization for speech perception. *Journal of the Acoustical Society of America, 48,* 579–594.

Sugarman, M. (1980). It's O.K. to stutter: A personal account. *Journal of Fluency Disorders, 5,* 149–157.

Sussman, H.M. (1971). The laterality effect in lingual-auditory tracking. *Journal of the Acoustical Society of America, 49,* 1874–1880.

Sussman, H. M., & MacNeilage, P. F. (1975). Hemispheric specialization for speech production and perception in stutterers. *Neuropsychologia, 13,* 19–26.

Sussman, H. M., MacNeilage, P. F., & Lumbley, J. (1974). Sensorimotor dominance and the right-ear advantage in mandibular-auditory tracking. *Journal of the Acoustical Society of America, 56,* 214–216.

Sussman, H. M., MacNeilage, P. F., & Lumbley, J. (1975). Pursuit auditory tracking of dichotically presented tonal amplitudes. *Journal of Speech and Hearing Research, 18,* 74–81.

Thompson, J. (1983). *Assessment of fluency in school-age children* (resource guide). Danville, IL: Interstate Printers and Publishers.

Thompson, J. (1984). Update: School-age stutterers. *Journal of Fluency Disorders, 9,* 199–206.

Throneberg, R. N., & Yairi, E. (1994). Temporal dynamics of repetitions during the early stages of childhood stuttering: An acoustic study. *Journal of Speech and Hearing Research, 37,* 1067–1075.

Tiffany, W. R. (1980). The effects of syllable structure on diadochokinetic and reading rates. *Journal of Speech and Hearing Research, 23,* 894–908.

Tiger, R. J., Irvine, T. L., & Reiss, R. P. (1980). Cluttering as a complex of learning disabilities. *Language, Speech, and Hearing Services in the Schools, 11,* 3–14.

Toscher, M. M., & Rupp, R. R. (1978). A study of the central auditory processes in stutterers using the Synthetic Sentence Identification (SSI) test battery. *Journal of Speech and Hearing Research, 21,* 779–792.

Travis, L. E. (1931). *Speech Pathology.* New York: Appleton-Century-Crofts.

Travis, L. E. (1957). The unspeakable feelings of people with special reference to stuttering. In L. E. Travis (Ed.), *Handbook of speech pathology* (pp. 916–946). New York: Appleton-Century-Crofts.

Travis, L. E. (1971). The unspeakable feelings of people with special reference to stuttering. In L. E. Travis (Ed.), *Handbook of speech pathology and audiology* (pp. 1001–1003). New York: Appleton-Century-Crofts.

Travis, L. E. (July 10, 1978). Personal communication.

Travis, L. E., & Knott, J. R. (1936). Brain potentials for normal speakers and stutterers. *Journal of Psychology, 2,* 137–150.

Travis, L. E., & Knott, J. R. (1937). Bilaterally recorded brain potentials from normal speakers and stutterers. *Journal of Speech Disorders, 2,* 239–241.

Travis, L.E., & Malamud, W. (1937). Brain potentials from normal subjects, stutterers, and schizophrenic patients. *American Journal of Psychiatry, 93,* 929–936.

Trotter, W. D., & Silverman, F. H. (1973). Experiments with the stutteraid. *Perceptual and Motor Skills, 36,* 1129–1130.

Truax, C. B., & Carkhuff, R. R. (1966). *Toward effective counseling and psychotherapy.* Chicago: Aldine Press.

Tuckman, B. (1965). Developmental sequence in small groups. *Psychological Bulletin, 63,* 384–399.

Tudor, M. (1939). *An experimental study of the effect of evaluative labeling on speech fluency.* Master's thesis, University of Iowa.

Umeda, N. (1975). Vowel duration in American English. *Journal of the Acoustical Society of America, 58,* 434–445.

Valiant, G. E. (1977). *Adaptation to life.* Boston: Little, Brown & Co.

Van Borsel, J., Van Lierde, K., Van Cauwenberge, P., Guldemont, I., & Van Orshoven, M., (1998). Severe acquired stuttering following injury of the left supplementary motor region: A case report. *Journal of Fluency Disorders, 23,* 49–58.

Van Riper, C. (1937). The preparatory set in stuttering. *Journal of Speech Disorders, 2,* 149–154.

Van Riper, C. (1939). *Speech correction: Principles and methods* (11th ed.). Englewood Cliffs, NJ: Prentice-Hall.

Van Riper, C. (1971). *The nature of stuttering.* Englewood Cliffs, NJ: Prentice-Hall.

Van Riper, C. (1973). *The treatment of stuttering* (2nd ed.). Englewood Cliffs, NJ: Prentice-Hall.

Van Riper, C. (1974). A handful of nuts. *Western Michigan Journal of Speech Therapy, 11*(2), 1–3.

Van Riper, C. (1975). The stutterer's clinician. In Jon Eisenson (Ed.), *Stuttering, a second symposium* (pp. 453–492). New York: Harper & Row.

Van Riper, C. (1977). *Adult Stuttering Therapy.* A series of eight video tapes produced at Western Michigan University, Kalamazoo, MI. Distributed by The Stuttering Foundation of America.

Van Riper, C. (July 1, 1978). Personal communication.

Van Riper, C. (1979). *A career in speech pathology.* Englewood Cliffs, NJ: Prentice-Hall.

Van Riper, C. (1982). *The nature of stuttering* (2nd ed.). Englewood Cliffs, NJ: Prentice-Hall.

Van Riper, C. (1984). Henry Freund: 1896–1982. *Journal of Fluency Disorders, 9,* 93–102.

Van Riper, C. (1990). Final thoughts about stuttering, *Journal of Fluency Disorders, 15,* 317–318.

Van Riper, C. (1992a). Foreword. In F. Florence & K. St. Louis (Eds.), *Cluttering: A clinical perspective* (pp. xii–xix). Leicester, England: Wurr Publications.

Van Riper, C. (1992b). Some ancient history. *Journal of Fluency Disorders, 17,* 25–28.

Viswanath, N. S., Rosenfield, D. B., & Nudelman, H. B. (1992). Stutterers and cerebral blood flow: Letter to the editor. *Archives of Neurology, 49,* 346–347.

Wada, J., & Rasmussen, T. (1960). Intracarotid injection of sodium amytal for the lateralization of cerebral speech dominance. *Journal of Neurosurgery, 17,* 266–282.

Waldrop, J., & Exter, T. (1990). What the 1990 census will show. *American Demographics, 12,* 20–30.

Walker, C., & Black, J. (1950). *The intrinsic intensity of oral phrases* (Joint Project Report No. 2). Pensacola, FL: United States Naval School of Aviation Medicine, Naval Air Station.

Wall, M. J. (1980). A comparison of syntax in young stutterers and nonstutterers. *Journal of Fluency Disorders, 5,* 345–352.

Wall, M. J., & Myers, F. L. (1995). *Clinical management of childhood stuttering* (2nd ed.). Austin, TX: Pro-Ed.

Walle, G. (1975). *The prevention of stuttering, part 1* (film). Memphis, TN: Stuttering Foundation of America.

Watkins, R. V., Yairi, E., & Ambrose, N. G. (1999). Early childhood stuttering III: Initial status of expressive language abilities. *Journal of Speech, Language, and Hearing Research, 42,* 1025–1135.

Watson, B. C., & Freeman, F. J. (1997). Brain imaging contributions. In R. F. Curlee & G. M. Siegel (Eds.), *Nature and Treatment of Stuttering: New Directions.* Needham Heights, MA: Allyn & Bacon.

Watson, B. C., Freeman, F. J., Devous, M. D., Chapman, S. B., Finitzo, T., & Pool, K. D. (1994). Linguistic performance and regional cerebral blood flow in persons who stutter. *Journal of Speech and Hearing Research, 37,* 1221–1228.

Watson, B. C., Pool, K. D., Devous, M. D., Freeman, F. J., & Finitzo, T. (1992). Brain blood flow related to acoustic laryngeal reaction time in adult developmental stutterers. *Journal of Speech and Hearing Research, 35,* 555–561.

Watson, J. B. (1988). A comparison of stutterers' and nonstutterers' affective, cognitive, and behavioral self-reports. *Journal of Speech and Hearing Research, 31,* 377–385.

Webster, E. (1966). Parent counseling by speech pathologists and audiologists. *Journal of Speech and Hearing Disorders, 31,* 331–345.

Webster, E. (1968). Procedures for group counseling in speech, pathology and audiology. *Journal of Speech and Hearing Disorders, 31,* 331–345.

Webster, R. L. (1974). A behavioral analysis of stuttering: Treatment and theory. In *Treatment methods in psychopathology.* New York: Wiley.

Webster, R. L. (1975). *Clinicians' program guide: The precision fluency shaping program.* Roanoke, VA: Communication Development Corp.

Webster, R. L. (1979). Empirical considerations regarding stuttering therapy. In H. H. Gregory (Ed.), *Controversies about stuttering therapy* (pp. 209–239). Baltimore, MD: University Park Press.

Webster, R. L. (1986). Postscript: Stuttering therapy from a technological point of view. In G. H. Shames & H. Rubin (Ed.), *Stuttering then and now* (pp. 407–414). Columbus, OH: Merrill.

Weisel, A., & Specktor, G. (1998). Attitudes toward own communication and toward stutterers. *Journal of Fluency Disorders, 23,* 157–172.

Weiss, A. L. (1993). The pragmatic context of children's disfluency. *Seminars in Speech and Language, 14*(3) 215–224.

Weiss, A. L., & Zebrowski, P. M. (1992). Disfluencies in the conversation of young children who stutter: Some answers about questions. *Journal of Speech and Hearing Research, 35,* 1230–1238.

Weiss, D. A. (1964). *Cluttering.* Englewood Cliffs, NJ: Prentice-Hall.

Weiss, D. A. (1967). Similarities and differences between stuttering and cluttering. *Folia Phoniatrica, 19,* 98–104.

West, R., & Ansberry, M. (1968). *The rehabilitation of speech* (4th ed.). New York: Harper & Row.

Wexler, K. (1982). Developmental disfluency in 2-, 4-, and 6-year-old boys in neutral and stress situations. *Journal of Speech and Hearing Research, 25,* 229–234.

White, E. B. (1954/1960) Some remarks on humor. The second tree from the corner. In J. J. Enck, E. T. Forter, & A. Whitley (Eds.), *The comic in theory and practice* (pp. 102–108). New York: Appleton-Century-Crofts.

Williams, D. (1979). A perspective on approaches to stuttering therapy. In H. Gregory (Ed.), *Controversies about stuttering therapy* (pp. 241–268). Baltimore, MD: University Park Press.

Williams, D. (1983). Working with children in the school environment. In J. Fraser Gruss (Ed.), *Stuttering therapy: Transfer and maintenance* (Publication No. 19). Memphis, TN: Stuttering Foundation of America.

Williams, D. (1985). Talking with children who stutter. In J. Fraser (Ed.), *Counseling stutterers* (pp. 35–45). Memphis, TN: Stuttering Foundation of America.

Williams, D., & Silverman, F. (1968). Note concerning articulation of school-age stutterers. *Perceptual and Motor Skills, 27,* 713–714.

Williams, D. E. (1971). Stuttering therapy for children. In L. E. Travis (Ed.), *Handbook of speech pathology* (pp. 1073–1093). New York: Appleton-Century-Crofts.

Williams, D. E., Silverman, F. H., & Kools, J. A. (1968). Disfluency behavior of elementary school stutterers and nonstutterers: The adaptation effect. *Journal of Speech and Hearing Research, 11,* 622–630.

Williams, D. F., Wener, D. L. Cluttering and stuttering exhibited in a young professional: Post hoc case study (clinical impressions). *Journal of Fluency Disorders, 21,* 1–9.

Williams, R. (1995). Personal construct theory in use with people who stutter. In M. Fawcus (Ed.), *Stuttering: From theory to practice.* London: Whurr Publishers.

Wingate, M. (1959). Calling attention to stuttering. *Journal of Speech and Hearing Research, 2,* 326–335.

Wingate, M. (1964). A standard definition of stuttering. *Journal of Speech and Hearing Disorders, 29,* 484–489.

Wingate, M. (1968). Research trends in stuttering. *Voice,* (Journal of the California Speech and Hearing Association), *17,* 2–6.

Wingate, M. E. (1969). Sound and pattern in "artificial" fluency. *Journal of Speech and Hearing Research, 12,* 677–686.

Wingate, M. E. (1971). The fear of stuttering. *Journal of the American Speech-Language-Hearing Association, 13,* 3–5.

Wingate, M. E. (1988). *The structure of stuttering, a psycholinguistic analysis.* New York: Springer-Verlag.

Winslow, M. & Guitar, B. (1994). The effects of structured turn-taking on disfluencies: A case study. *Language, Speech, and Hearing Services in Schools, 25,* 251–257.

Wolfe, V. I., Ratusnik, D. L., & Feldman, A. (1979). Acoustic and perceptual comparison of chronic and incipient spastic dysphonia. *Laryngoscope, 89,* 1478–1486.

Wood, F., Stump, D., McKeehan, A., Sheldon, S., & Proctor, J. (1980). Patterns of regional cerebral blood flow during attempted reading aloud by stutterers both on and off Haloperidol medication: Evidence for inadequate left frontal activation during stuttering. *Brain and Language, 9,* 141–144.

Wood, F. B., Flowers, D. L., & Naylor, C. E. (1991). Cerebral laterality in functional neuroimaging. In F. L. Kitterle (Ed.), *Cerebral laterality: Theory and research.* Hillsdale, NJ: Lawrence Erlbaum Associates.

Woods, C. L., & Williams, D. E. (1976). Traits attributed to stuttering and normally fluent males. *Journal of Speech and Hearing Research, 19,* 267–278.

Woolf, G. (1967). The assessment of stuttering as struggle, avoidance and expectancy. *British Journal of Disorders of Communication, 2,* 158–171.

World Almanac and Book of Facts. (1995). Mahwah, NJ: Funk and Wagnalls Corp.

World Health Organization. (1977). *Manual of the international statistical classification of diseases, injuries, and causes of death* (Vol. 1). Geneva: World Health Organization.

World Health Organization. (1980). *International classification of impairments, disabilities, and handicaps: A Manual of classification of classification relating to the consequences of disease.* Geneva, Switzerland: World Health Organization.

Wu, J. C., Maguire, G., Riley, G., Fallon, J., LaCasse, L., Chin, S., Klein, E., Tang, C., Cadwell, S., & Lottenberg, S. (1995). A positron emission tomography deoxyglucose study of developmental stuttering. *NeuroReport, 6,* 501–505.

Wyatt, G. L. (1969). *Language learning and communication disorders in children.* New York: Free Press.

Yairi, E. (1981). Disfluencies of normally speaking two-year-old children. *Journal of Speech and Hearing Research, 24,* 490–495.

Yairi, E. (1982). Longitudinal studies of disfluencies in two-year-old children. *Journal of Speech and Hearing Research, 25,* 155–160.

Yairi, E. (1983). The onset of stuttering in two- and three-year-old children. *Journal of Speech and Hearing Disorders, 48,* 171–177.

Yairi, E. (1993). Epidemiologic and other considerations in treatment efficacy research with preschool-age children who stutter. *Journal of Fluency Disorders, 18*(2–3), 197–219.

Yairi, E. (1997). Home environment and parent-child interaction in childhood stuttering. Curlee & G. Siegel (Eds.), *Nature and treatment of stuttering, New directions* (2nd ed., pp. 24–48). Needham Heights, MA: Allyn & Bacon.

Yairi, E., & Ambrose, N. G. (1992a). A longitudinal study of stuttering in children: A preliminary report. *Journal of Speech and Hearing Research, 35,* 755–760.

Yairi, E., & Ambrose, N. G. (1992b). Onset of stuttering in preschool children: Selected factors. *Journal of Speech and Hearing Research, 35,* 782–788.

Yairi, E., & Ambrose, N. G. (1999). Early childhood stuttering I: Persistency and recovery rates. *Journal of Speech, Language, and Hearing Research, 42,* 1097–1112.

Yairi, E., Ambrose, N. G., & Niermann, R. (1993). The early months of stuttering: A developmental study. *Journal of Speech and Hearing Research, 36,* 521–528.

Yairi, E., Ambrose, N. G., Paden, E. P., & Throneburg, R. N. (1996). Predictive factors of persistence and recovery: Pathways of childhood stuttering. *Journal of Communication Disorders, 29,* 51–77.

Yairi, E., & Carrico, D. (1992). Pediatricians' attitudes and practices concerning early childhood stuttering. *American Journal of Speech-Language Pathology, 1,* 54–62.

Yairi, E., & Clifton, N. F. (1972). Disfluent speech behavior of preschool children, high school seniors and geriatric persons. *Journal of Speech and Hearing Research, 15,* 714–719.

Yairi, E., & Hall, K. D. (1993). Temporal relations within repetitions of preschool children near the onset of stuttering: A preliminary report. *Journal of Communication Disorders, 26,* 231–244.

Yairi, E., & Lewis, B. (1984). Disfluencies at the onset of stuttering. *Journal of Speech and Hearing Research, 27,* 155–159.

Yairi, E., & Williams, D. (1971). Reports of parental attitudes by stuttering and nonstuttering children. *Journal of Speech and Hearing Research, 14,* 596–604.

Yaruss, J. S. (1997a). Clinical measurement of stuttering behaviors. *Contemporary Issues in Communication Science and Disorders, 24,* 33–44.

Yaruss, J. S. (1977b). Improving assessment of children's oral motor development in clinical settings. In W. Hulstijn, H. F. M. Peters, & P. H. H. M. Van Lieshout (Eds.), *Speech production: Motor control, brain research, and fluency disorders* (pp. 565–571). Amsterdam: Elsevier Science.

Yaruss, J. S. (1998). Describing the consequences of disorders: Stuttering and the international classification of impairments, disabilities, and handicaps. *Journal of Speech, Language, and Hearing Research, 41,* 249–257.

Yaruss, J. S. (2000). The role of performance in the demands and capacities model. *Journal of Fluency Disorders, 25* (in press).

Yaruss, J. S., & Conture, E. G. (1995). Motor and child speaking rates and utterance lengths in adjacent fluent utterances. *Journal of Fluency Disorders, 20,* 257–278.

Yates, A. J. (1963). Delayed auditory feedback. *Psychological Bulletin, 60,* 213–232.

Young, M. A. (1975). Onset, prevalence, and recovery from stuttering. *Journal of Speech and Hearing Disorders, 40,* 49–58.

Young, M. A. (1981). A reanalysis of "Stuttering therapy: The relation between attitude change and long-term outcome." *Journal of Speech and Hearing Disorders, 46,* 221–222.

Zebrowski, P. M. (1997). Assisting young children who stutter and their families: Defining the role of the speech-language pathologist. *American Journal of Speech-Language Pathology, 6*(2), 19–28.

Zebrowski, P. M., Conture, E. G., & Cudahy, E. A. (1985). Acoustic analysis of young stutterers' fluency: Preliminary observations. *Journal of Fluency Disorders, 10,* 173–192.

Zemlin, W. R. (1988). *Speech and hearing science: Anatomy and physiology* (3rd ed.). Englewood Cliffs, NJ: Prentice-Hall.

Zenner, A., Ritterman, S., Bowden, S., & Gronhovd, D. (1978). Measurement and comparison of anxiety levels of parents of stuttering, articulatory defective and normal-speaking children. *Journal of Fluency Disorders, 3,* 273–284.

Zimmerman, G. (1980). Stuttering: A disorder of movement. *Journal of Speech and Hearing Research, 23,* 122–136.

Zimmerman, G. (1981). Stuttering: In need of a unifying conceptual framework. *Journal of Speech and Hearing Research, 24,* 25–31.

Zinker, J. (1977). *Creative process in Gestalt therapy.* New York: Random House.

Zinsser, W. (1988). *Learning to write.* New York: Harper and Row.

APPENDIX

ANNOTATIVE LISTING OF ASSESSMENT PROCEDURES

1. Adams, M.R. (1977a). A clinical strategy for differentiating the normal nonfluent child and the incipient stutterer. *Journal of Fluency Disorders, 2,* 141–148.

This measure is designed for preschool children. The clinician first obtains a 300–500 word sample of conversational speech. The following five behaviors are used to identify nonnormal speech: (1) more than 10 fluency breaks per 100 words, (2) occurrences of part-word repetitions and prolongations, (3) part-word repetitions of four or more units, (4) cessation of airflow/voicing, and (5) schwa vowel substitutions. The analysis can be somewhat time-consuming, and the clinician must be certain that one or more representative samples of the child's speech can be obtained.

2. Ammons, R., & Johnson, W. (1944). Iowa Scale of attitudes toward stuttering. In Studies in the psychology of stuttering. *Journal of Speech Disorders, 9,* 39–49.

This five-point rating scale consists of 45 statements about stutterers and what they should or should not do or feel in various speaking situations. The stutterer's intolerance (avoidance) may indicate the need for counseling therapy or modification of attitudes through hierarchial practice.

3. Andre, S., & Guitar, G. (1979). The A-19 Scale for children who stutter. See Guitar, B., & Grimes, S. (1979). *Developing a scale to assess communication attitudes in children who stutter.* Paper presented to the annual meeting of American Speech-Language-Hearing Association. See also Peters, T., & Guitar, B. (1991). *Stuttering, an integrated approach to its nature and treatment* (p. 179). Baltimore, MD: Williams & Williams.

This 19-item scale was designed to assess communication attitudes in children who stutter. The child responds by saying "yes/no" to each of the questions (e.g., Do you like to talk on the phone?). As with the S-scale mentioned above (Erickson, 1969), the scale is obtained by comparing the subject's responses to the way a stutterer would respond. Nonstuttering children typically respond as a stutterer would to an average of 8.17 items. Stuttering children respond as a stutterer to an average of 9.07 items ($SD = 2.44$).

4. Andrews, G., & Cutler, J. (1974). S-24 Scale. Stuttering therapy: The relations between changes in symptom level and attitudes. *Journal of Speech and Hearing Disorders, 39,* 312–319.

This popular measure is a shortened version of the 39-item Erickson S-Scale (1969). Using regression analysis, the authors developed a more efficient 24-item version of the original scale, which may be used for repeated measures (e.g., during treatment). This scale contains 24 true-false items that the speaker completes. It is designed for use with older teenagers and adults and contains items such as "I usually feel that I am making a favorable impression when I talk." Nonstuttering adults typically respond as a stutterer would to an average of 9.14 of the items ($SD = 5.38$). Stuttering adults respond as a stutterer to an average of 19.22 of the items ($SD = 4.24$). The S-24 is quickly and easily administered.

5. Brutten, G. J., & Dunham, S. L. (1989). The Communication Attitude Test: A normative study of grade school children. *Journal of Fluency Disorders, 14,* 371–377.

This 35-item questionnaire, revised in 1997 and called the CAT-R, is designed to assess the speech-associated beliefs of children. The children who stutter circle true or false about negative or positive attitudes toward speech. Sample items include: "I like the way I talk. Talking is easy for me. I am afraid the words won't come out when I talk." Scoring is done by assigning a 0 to all responses that reflect a positive attitude toward speech and a 1 for responses that reflect a negative attitude. Brutten and DeNill (1991) studied 63 stuttering children from Belgium

(7–14 years of age) who scored an average of 15.95 (*SD* = 7.28), compared with 134 control subjects, who averaged 8.57 (*SD* = 5.22).

6. Brutton, E., & Shoemaker, D. (1974). Fear Survey Schedule. In *The Southern Illinois Behavior Checklist*. Carbondale, IL: Southern Illinois University.

This is an adaptation of the Fear Survey Schedule developed by J. Wolpe and P. Lang, Educational and Industrial Service, San Diego, CA.

This schedule is designed for both children (80 items) and adults (51 items). The subject responds by circling a point on a 1 (no fear) to 5 (great fear) scale indicating the amount of fear associated with a variety of things (sharp objects, being criticized, death, being misunderstood, meeting with someone in authority). Average scores for nonstuttering children were 162.5, but no scores were given for stuttering children. Average scores for nonstuttering adults were 70.45, and average scores for stuttering adults were 108.08.

7. Brutten, E., & Shoemaker, D. (1974). Speech Situation Checklist. In *The Southern Illinois Checklist*. Carbondale, IL: Southern Illinois University.

This checklist is designed for both children (55 items) and adults (51 items). The checklist was developed to assess speech-related anxiety and speech disruptions. The subject is asked to respond to typical speaking situations (talking on a telephone, giving your name, making introductions, or asking for help with homework) by using an interval scale from 1 (no anxiety; no disruptions) to 5 (much anxiety; many disruptions). Average scores for nonstuttering children were 96.90 (anxiety level) and 86.92 (disruption level). Average scores for stuttering adults were 100.74 (anxiety level) and 105.40 (disruption level). Average scores for stuttering adults were 100.74 (anxiety level) and 105.40 (disruption level).

8. Cooper, E. B. (1973). Cooper Chronicity Prediction Checklist for school-age stutterers: A research inventory for clinicians. *Journal of Speech and Hearing Disorders, 38,* 215–223. Also in E. Cooper. Personalized fluency control therapy. DLM Teaching Resources, 1 DLM Park, Allen, Texas 75002.

This inventory utilizes questions and clinical observations regarding case history, child attitudes, parental attitudes, and behavioral symptomology to predict the likelihood of a child "outgrowing" stuttering. The clinician completes the checklist after sampling the child's speech and interviewing the parent(s). There are a total of 27 questions covering "historical," "attitudinal," and "behavioral" indicators of chronicity. The clinician scores each question by indicating, "yes," "no," "not available," or "unknown." "Yes" responses may indicate that stuttering is likely to become a chronic problem. A total score of 0–6 suggests possible recovery; 7–15 indicates continued vigilance, and 16–27 is predictive of chronicity. Longitudinal data needs to be obtained and weighing of items needs to be done before this potentially useful inventory will yield helpful assessment information.

9. Cooper, Eugene. (1985). Client and clinician perceptions of stuttering severity ratings. In *Personalized fluency control therapy* (p. 127). DLM Teaching Resources, 1 DLM Park, Allen, Texas 75002.

The client is asked for a self-rating of global severity, which may then be compared to the clinician's perception of the client's severity. The clinician rates four aspects of severity: frequency, duration, tension, and concomitant behaviors.

10. Cooper, Eugene. (1985). Concomitant Stuttering Behavior Checklist. In *Personalized fluency control therapy* (p. 125). DLM Teaching Resources, 1 DLM Park, Allen, Texas 75002.

Clinical observations are recorded on this assessment form. Thirty-two behaviors that may accompany moments of stuttering are observed in five categories: posturing, respiratory, facial, syntactic/semantic, and vocal behaviors. These may be monitored during reevaluations.

11. Cooper, Eugene. (1985) Parent Attitudes toward Stuttering Checklist. In *Personalized fluency control therapy* (p. 105). DLM Teaching Resources, 1 DLM Park, Allen, Texas 75002.

Parental attitudes and feelings may be identified with this 25-item checklist. Areas of parental concern or misperceptions may then be targeted in counseling sessions.

12. Cooper, Eugene. (1985) Situation Avoidance Behavior Checklist. In *Personalized fluency control therapy* (p. 124). DLM Teaching Resources, 1 DLM Park, Allen, Texas 75002.

Fifty common speech situations are listed to ascertain those that are avoided. The score is the total number of situations avoided and may be useful in monitoring progress during treatment or to establish a hierarchy of tasks during treatment.

13. Cooper, Eugene. (1985). Stuttering Attitudes Checklist. In *Personalized fluency control therapy*. DLM Teaching Resources, 1 DLM Park, Allen, Texas 75002.

Twenty-five statements are used to assess a client's own feelings and attitudes toward stuttering. This pencil-and-paper checklist is claimed useful with children and adults, although modifications will be necessary for young or poor readers. The total score may be useful for pre-, during, and posttreatment assessments. Individual statements may indicate topics for counseling and discussion of feelings.

14. Cooper, Eugene. (1985) Stuttering Frequency and Duration Estimate Record. In *Personalized fluency control therapy* (pp. 121–123). DLM Teaching, 1 DLM Park, Allen, Texas 75002.

The severity of stuttering, based on only frequency (percentage) and duration, is assessed with this instrument. Severity is assessed under the conditions of answering questions that elicit a one- to two-word response, recitation of the alphabet, and reading of a 200-syllable passage.

15. Craig, A. R., Franklin, J. A., & Andrews, G. (1984). [Locus of Control of Behavior (LCB) Scale.] A scale to measure locus of control behavior. *British Journal of Medical Psychology, 57*, 173–180.

This 17-item, Likert-type scale was constructed to measure the degree to which a person perceives events as being a consequence of his own behavior and subsequently takes responsibility for maintaining new (desired) behavior. Designed for adults, the scale has been shown to have good internal reliability and is not influenced by sex, age, or social desirability of subject responses. The scale appears to differentiate between individuals with and without chronic behavioral conditions. Items 1, 5, 7, 8, 13, and 16 are reverse-scored. Higher scores on the LCB Scale reflect greater self-perception of external control (chronic stutterers averaged 31.01), while lower scores indicate greater internal control (control subjects averaged means of 27.9 and 28.3). The scale may help predict those stutterers who will relapse after treatment and those who have the ability to maintain change in behavior they previously believed to be uncontrollable.

16. Crowe, T. A., DiLollo, A. P., & Crowe, B. T. (2000). *Crowe's protocols: A comprehensive guide to stuttering intervention.* San Antonio, TX: The Psychological Corporation.

This protocol provides the most comprehensive assessment options yet devised for children and adults who stutter. The protocols include forms and scales (3- point and 7-point) for obtaining case history and cultural information as well as client self-assessment. Other components include assessment of affective, behavioral, cognitive, speech status, stimulability and measures of severity. Several sections and forms are designed to provide information for counseling during treatment. Forms are designed to be completed by the client or by the clinician through respondent interview. An abbreviated protocol is also provided.

17. Daly, D. A. (1992–1993). Daly's Checklist for Possible Cluttering. *Clinical Connection*, p. 6.

This checklist consists of 33 descriptive statements on a four-point scale (1 = not at all, 2 = just a little, 3 = pretty much, 4 = very much). Adults, children, or both answer by reflecting how well the statements describe them. Preliminary evidence suggests that a score of 60 or above indicates the diagnosis of cluttering. A score between 30 and 60 may be indicative of a clutterer-stutterer. Daly also suggests that the following items may be particularly critical: 2, 3, 7, 9, 10, 12, 14, 20, 25, and 33.

18. DeVore, J., Nandur, M., & Manning, W. (1984). Projective drawings and children who stutter. *Journal of Fluency Disorders, 9,* 217–226.

These authors provide preliminary information indicating significant differences between the drawings of children (ages 5 to 10 years) who stuttered and those who did not. Children who did not stutter drew significantly larger drawings that were placed nearer to the center of the page. Significant changes were found for the drawings of the children who stuttered after treatment. That is, the clients drew larger figures and began to place them more toward the center of the page as treatment progressed. No significant differences were found between the groups of children after the stutterers received treatment. These preliminary results suggest that projective drawings may provide a means of assisting personality dynamics of young stutterers and personality change that might otherwise go undetected and unrewarded.

19. Erickson, R. (1969). [Scale of Communication Attitudes (S-Scale)]. *Journal of Speech and Hearing Research, 12,* 711–724.

Designed for older adolescents and adults, this scale consists of 39 statements ("I find it easy to talk with almost anyone"; or "Some words are harder than others for me to say."). The subject responds by indicating true or false. Stutterers tend to answer an average of 30 items, while nonstutterers typically answer no more than four items in this fashion.

20. Erickson, R. (1969). [Severity Scale and Adjective Checklist]. In Assessing communication attitudes among stutterers. *Journal of Speech and Hearing Research, 12,* 711–724.

Eighty adjectives that are descriptive of various feelings and types of behaviors potentially experienced during interpersonal communication are included in the Adjective Checklist (ACL).

21. Goldberg, Stanley A. (1981). The Child Fluency Assessment Instrument; The Adolescent Fluency Assessment Instrument; The Adult Fluency Assessment Instrument. In *Behavioral cognitive stuttering therapy*, C. C. Publication, Inc., P.O. Box 23699, Tigard, OR 97223.

These three assessment instruments are extensive systems for appraising the many facets of stuttering. Included are case history questions, frequency counts, situational rating scales, self-perception questionnaires, and—in the child and adolescent version—questions for assessing parental attitudes.

22. Gough, H. G., & Heilbrun, A. B. Adjective Checklist. *The Adjective Checklist.* Palo Alto, CA: Consulting Psychologists Press.

This all-purpose checklist of favorable adjectives has been used with stuttering to monitor attitudinal shifts as a function of therapy. The checklist consists of 24 scales covering areas such as self-confidence, personal adjustment, and achievement.

23. Hanson, B. R., Gonhoud, K. D., & Rice, P. L. (1981). Speech Situation Checklist. *Journal of Fluency Disorders, 6,* 351–360.

These authors used discriminative analysis to select the most discriminating items in the original SSC (Brutton & Shoemaker, 1974). The resulting 21 items provide a screening device for identifying stutterers who experience a high level of speech-related anxiety.

24. Johnson, W., Darley, F., & Spriestersbach, D. (1952). Stutterer's Self Ratings of Reactions to Speech Situations (SSR). In *Diagnostic manual in speech correction.* New York: Harper & Row.

The measure provides a comprehensive view of the client's reactions to 40 extratreatment speaking situations. The client uses a 1–5 scale to indicate a self-measurement in each of four categories: Frequency (how often he encounters the situation), Avoidance (how likely he would be to avoid the situation), Reaction (how much he would like or dislike speaking in this situation), and Stuttering (the estimated severity of stuttering in each situation). Total scores are computed by averaging the scaled totals for each of the four categories.

25. Johnson, W., Darley, F., & Spriestersbach, D. (1963). [Iowa Scale of Attitudes Toward Stuttering.] In *Diagnostic methods in speech pathology.* New York: Harper & Row.

This 45-item scale is designed to assess the attitudes toward stuttering of older children and adult stutterers and their listeners. The subject responds to each item (e.g., "A stutterer should not try out for the debating team.") by circling one of five points on an ordinal scale ranging from "strongly agree" to "strongly disagree." The lower the score, the better the attitude of the respondent. Average group scores on the data obtained by these authors ranged from a 1.36 (clinicians) to 11.73 (controls). Scores for a group of 63 stutterers averaged 1.53.

26. Johnson, W., Darley, F., & Spriestersbach, D. (1963). Iowa Scale for rating the severity of stuttering. In *Diagnostic methods in speech pathology.* New York: Harper & Row.

This scale provides the clinician with descriptive categories of stuttering behavior ranging from (1) very mild–stuttering on less than 1% of words, very little tension, disfluencies generally less than one second in duration, patterns of disfluency simple, and no associated body movements, to (7) very severe–stuttering on more than 25% of words, very conspicuous tension, disfluencies average more than four seconds in duration, very conspicuous distorting of sounds, facial grimaces, and conspicuous associated movements.

27. Lanyon, R. (1967). Stuttering Severity Scale (SS). *Journal of Speech and Hearing Research, 10,* 836–843.

This paper-and-pencil scale is designed to evaluate the overt behaviors and attitudes of older teens and adults who stutter. The 64 items ("I worry about the fact that I'm a stutterer. When I talk I often become short of breath.") are answered as true or false. The scores on the 64 items are converted to ratings on a 1 (mild) to 7 (severe) scale.

28. Lewis, D., & Sherman, D. (1951–1952). Sherman-Lewis Scale. *Journal of Speech and Hearing Disorders, 16,* 320–326, and *Journal of Speech and Hearing Disorders, 17,* 316–320.

For clients displaying overt struggle behaviors, this five-point scale rates the frequency of overt struggle, degree of tension present, duration of blocks, pattern of blocking, and distracting movements of the body. Using a nine-point equal-interval scale (1 = least severe; 9 = most severe), the speech-language pathologist listens to a sample of conversational speech and directly assigns a value. Intra- and interjudge reliability scores were good using this approach. A correlation of +.98 was obtained between groups of undergraduate students, and a correlation of +.97 was obtained between women and men.

29. Luper, Harold L. and Mulder, R. L. (1964). Stuttering Diagnostic and Evaluative Checklist. In *Stuttering therapy for children* (pp. 207–211). Englewood Cliffs, NJ: Prentice-Hall.

This checklist includes features of stuttering: case history descriptions, disfluency symptoms (regarding repetitions, prolongations, hard attacks, and interjections), consistency and adaptation, secondary mannerisms, and concealment devices.

30. Manning, W. (1994). *The SEA-Scale: Self-efficacy scaling for adolescents who stutter.* Paper presented to the annual meeting of the American Speech-Language-Hearing Association, New Orleans, LA.

Based on the work of Bandura (1977), this technique is designed to measure the confidence that an adolescent stutterer can (1) enter into speaking situations typically found outside of treatment and (2) achieve a predetermined level of fluency in the speaking situation. Using a decimal scale the subject assigns a whole number value (1 to 10) to each situation, and these scores are then averaged across all one-hundred speaking situations in order to obtain a total score for the approach and performance items. The scale is composed of 13 subscales (after Watson, 1988). The overall alpha level for all 100 items was 0.98, with subscale alphas ranging from 0.74 to 0.94. Forty adolescents who stuttered scored significantly ($p < .001$) lower (mean = 7.21; SD = 1.8) than a matched group of nonstuttering control subjects (mean = 8.65; SD = 1.2). The technique is likely to be most helpful in assessing extratreatment performance during and following treatment.

31. Martin, R. R., Haroldson, S. K., & Woessner, G. L. (1988). Perceptual scaling of stuttering severity. *Journal of Fluency Disorders, 13*, 27–47.

After observers judged stuttering severity on a seven-point scale with equal-appearing intervals, observers judged "on line" the severity of stutterers' speech under normal circumstances and under delayed auditory feedback.

32. McDonough, A., & Quesal, R. W. (1988). Locus of control orientation of stutterers and nonstutterers. *Journal of Fluency Disorders, 13*, 97–106.

This task is used to determine whether an adult or adolescent client believes in an internal or external locus of control for speech. It consists of eight questions or statements that are answered "yes" or "no."

33. Ornstein, A., & Manning, W. (1985). Self-efficacy scaling by adult stutterers. *Journal of Communication Disorders, 18*, 313–320.

Based on the work of Bandura (1977), this technique is designed to measure the confidence that an adult stutterer can (1) enter into speaking situations typically found outside treatment and (2) achieve a predetermined level of fluency in the speaking situation. Using a decile (10–100) scale, the subject assigns a value to each situation and these scores are then averaged across the 50 speaking situations in order to obtain a total score for both approach and performance sections. The technique is likely to be most helpful in assessing extra-treatment performance during and following treatment. (See also Hillis, 1993.)

34. Pindzola, R. H., & White, D. T. (1986). A protocol for differentiating the incipient stutterer. *Language Speech and Hearing Services in Schools,* *17* (1), 2–15.

This protocol assesses behaviors such as type, size, frequency, and duration of the disfluencies, level of effort, rhythm, use of avoidance tactics, visual (secondary) mannerisms, and historical and psychological indicators. A unique feature of this protocol is a normal-versus-abnormal rating grid for interpreting each behavior.

35. Riley, G. A. (1994). *Stuttering Severity Instrument for Children and Adults*—Third Edition. (SSI-3). Austin, TX: Pro-Ed.

Originally developed in 1972 (Riley, G., A Stuttering Severity Instrument for Children and Adults (1972). *Journal of Speech and Hearing Disorders, 37,* 314–322), this is the third edition of this instrument designed to provide scale values for stuttering severity for both children and adults. Speakers who can read are asked to (1) describe their job or school and (2) read a short passage. Nonreaders are given a cartoon picture task to which they respond. Scoring is accomplished across three areas. The frequency of the fluency breaks tabulated and the percentage of stuttering is converted to a task score (range, 4–18). The duration of the three longest stuttering moments (fleeting to more than 60 seconds) is tabulated and converted to a task score (range, 1–7). Last, physical concomitant across four categories are scaled on a 0-to-5 scale (0 = none, 5 = severe and painful looking) and totaled (range, 0–20). The total overall score ranges from 0 to 45 points.

36. Riley, G. (1981). *Stuttering Prediction Instrument for Young Children.* C. C. Publications, Inc., P.O. Box 23699, Tigard, OR 97223. Rev. ed., Austin, TX: Pro-Ed.

Designed to predict chronicity of stuttering in young children (ages 3–8), this instrument is divided into five sections: (1) history, (2) parent's reactions, (3) part-word repetitions, (4) prolongations, and (5) frequency. After interviewing the parents, the conversational speech of the child is elicited using pictures and tape recordings. The speech samples are then analyzed for the behaviors and scored by assigning numerical values to the child's behavior. The total possible score is 40. The average score of 22.2 (standard deviation of 7.01) was obtained by children who continued to stutter, whereas those children who did not become chronic stutterers had an average score of 6.17 (standard deviation of 3.13).

37. Riley, G., & Riley, J. (1986). [Oral Motor Assessment Scale (OMAS).] *Oral motor assessment and treatment.* Tigard, OR: C. C. Publications.

This scale provides norms for assessing the accuracy of target speech sounds, the even flow of articulatory sequences of syllables, and rate of production. This scale is designed to provide a comprehensive and quantitative measure of a child's neuromotor development.

38. Riley, G. and Riley, J. (1989). Physician's screening procedure for children who may stutter. *Journal of Fluency Disorders, 14,* 57–67.

This screening is designed to assist clinicians in making diagnostic decisions in preschool children. It is devised as a data-based screening protocol and can be used by physicians and speech-language pathologists for assessing degree of abnormality of a child's disfluency and reactions to it.

39. Ryan, B. (1980). Stuttering interview (SI, Form A). In *Programmed therapy for stuttering children and adults.* Springfield, IL: Charles C. Thomas.

The format for this 20-item interview ranges from "automatic" (saying the alphabet) to "conversational" speech. Intended for young children, speech is elicited by using a variety of materials (pictures, puppets, reading material). Scoring is accomplished by relating the frequency scores and types of fluency breaks to a scale. Scale values range from 0 (normal) to 3 (severe).

40. Ryan, B. (1974). [Stuttering Interview (SI, Form B)]. In *Programmed therapy for stuttering children and adults.* Springfield, IL: Charles C. Thomas.

Scoring for this 14-item interview is similar to that of Form A described in (38). This form is designed to be used with upper elementary and high school students as well as adults.

41. Sherman, D. (1952). Clinical and experimental use of the Iowa Scale of Severity of Stuttering. *Journal of Speech Hearing Disorders, 17,* 316–320.

This scale has a range from 0 to 7 (with 0 indicating "no stuttering"). Each point is associated with stuttering frequency and duration, amount of muscle tension, and facial grimaces and general body movement. This scale is used for rating the severity of stuttering and utilizing information about behaviors that occur during moments of stuttering.

42. Shine, Richard E. (1980). Assessment form: Systematic fluency training for young children. In *Systematic fluency training for children.* C. C. Publications, Inc., P.O. Box 23699, Tigard, OR 97223.

This assessment form covers history of the stuttering problem, rate of stuttering (during assorted speaking tasks), severity rating, a speech sample, and a checklist of affected physiological speaking processes.

43. Shumak, I. C. (1955). A speech situation rating sheet for stutterers. In Johnson, W. & Leutenegger, R. R. (Eds.) *Stuttering in children and adults* (pp. 341–347). Minneapolis: University of Minnesota Press.

Forty common speech situations are rated on four aspects of adjustment: avoidance, reaction, stuttering, and frequency. Pre-, during, and posttreatment administrations of this scale may monitor attitudinal improvements. The scale also may assist in hierarchy ranking of speaking situations for practice.

44. Silverman, F. H. (1980). Stuttering Problem Profile (SPP). *Journal of Speech and Hearing Disorders, 45,* 119–123.

The SSP was created with the idea of assisting the clinician and the client in identifying treatment goals for adults who stutter. The profile consist of 86 first-person statements ("I am usually willing to stutter openly. I now rarely anticipate stuttering."). The profile is not scored, but rather the stutterer indicates those statements that he would like to be able to make at the termination of treatment but could not honestly be made at the outset. The list may be added to in order to make the statements more relevant to the client's interests and goals.

45. Stocker, B. (1980). *The Stocker Probe.* Tulsa, OK: Modern Education Corporation.

This procedure is designed to differentiate the chronic young stutterer from the child whose stuttering is temporary. The procedure is based on the assumption that the more novel the message, the greater the communication demand is on the speaker. Two common objects are used and the clinician asks the child a total of 10 questions across five "levels of demand." The levels of demand range from Level I (The clinician hands the child a ball and asks "Is it hard or is it soft?") to Level V (The clinician says, "Make up a story about the ball."). At any level of demand, the frequency of disfluencies are associated with clinical levels of severity: 1–10 (mild), 11–20 (moderate), 21–30 (severe), and 31 (very severe).

46. Van Riper, C. (1982). [Profile of Stuttering Severity.] In *The nature of stuttering* (p. 201). Englewood Cliffs, NJ: Prentice-Hall.

This profile provides a quick assessment of severity across four behavior areas: frequency, duration, tension/struggle, and postponement/ avoidance. The clinician uses a 1–7 scale for each behavior, with a scale value of 1 representing less than 1% of stuttered words and no postponement avoidance behavior. A scale value of 7 represents stuttering on 25% or more words, excessive tension and struggle in the trunk of the body, duration of breaks lasting five seconds or more, and postponement/ avoidance occurring more than 70% of the time. This is one of the few behavioral scales that includes the important factor of avoidance behavior and can be used with both children and adults.

47. Watson, J. B. (1987). Profiles of stutterers' and nonstutterers' affective, cognitive, and behavioral communication attitudes. *Journal of Fluency Disorders, 12,* 389–405.

This self-report inventory for adults obtains ratings of different types of speaking situations, using five response scales reflecting behavioral, affective, and cognitive aspects of attitudes. Examination of profile characteristics revealed two significant discriminators, classification as a stutterer or nonstutterer, and an overall speech rating. Nondiscriminatory characteristics include sex, age, education, therapy experiences, stuttering severity self-rating, onset of stuttering, total therapy time, current therapeutic status, and familial history.

48. Williams, D. (1978). Stutterers' Self-Ratings of Reactions of Speech Situations. In F. Darley & D. Spriestersbach, *Diagnostic methods in speech pathology* (2nd ed.), New York: Harper & Row.

This self-rating scale was created to determine specific speaking situations that a speaker was having difficulty adjusting to outside the treatment setting as well as the possible need for continued counseling. It is appropriate for use with adolescents (14 years and above) and adults. The stutterer rates his reaction to 40 speaking situations (e.g., ordering in a restaurant, saying hello to a friend, or telephoning to make an appointment) using a 1 to 5 scale. Four categories of reactions are scored for each question: avoidance, reaction, stuttering, and frequency. For example, a scale value of 1 indicated that the speaker would never avoid the situation, and a scale value of 5 indicated that the speaker would avoid the situation whenever possible. The scale values for all situation are averaged over all 40 speaking situations for each of the four reaction categories.

49. Williams, D., Darley, F., & Spriestersbach, D. (1978). Measures of Disfluency of Speaking and Oral Reading (Form 5). In F. Darley & D. Spriestersbach, *Diagnostic methods in speech pathology*, (2nd ed.), New York: Harper & Row.

Designed for the older adolescent and adult, this measure consists of two speaking tasks (job description and description of the pictures from the Thematic Apperception Test and two oral reading tasks). The examiner calculates a disfluency index and types of disfluencies as a percentage of breaks per 100 words. These disfluency types considered are: interjections, part-word repetitions, word repetitions, phrase repetitions, revisions, incomplete phrases, broken words, prolonged sounds, dysrhythmic phonation in words, and tension-pauses.

50. Woods, C., & Williams, D. (1976). Bi-Polar Adjective Scale. In "Traits attributed to stuttering and normally fluent males." *Journal of Speech and Hearing Research, 19*, 267–278.

This scale consists of 25 paired adjectives (open-guarded, tense-relaxed, daring-hesitant) organized in a 7-point semantic differential format. It may be used by clinicians or others (including the stutterer) in an attempt to describe the perceived personality characteristics of children or adults. Rather than a measure for differentiating stutterers from nonstutterers, it may be best applied as an indication of cognitive and attitude change for the client during treatment.

51. Woolf, G. (1967). Perception of Stuttering Inventory (PSI). In "The assessment of stuttering as struggle, avoidance and expectancy." *British Journal of Disorders of Communication, 2*, 158–171.

This inventory is intended to determine the avoidance, struggle, and expectancy of older adolescent and adult stutterers. The subject responds to 60 behavioral and attitude characteristics by indicating whether they are characteristic themselves. Those items that are not typical of their behavior are left unmarked. Examples of inventory items include: "Avoiding talking to people in authority" (avoidance), "Having extra and unnecessary facial movement" (struggle), and "Adding an extra sound in order to get started" (expectancy).

APPENDIX

RESOURCES AND SUPPORT GROUPS IN FLUENCY DISORDERS

American Speech-Language-Hearing Association (ASHA)
10801 Rockville Pike
Rockville, MD 20852
Phone: 301-897-5700
Fax: 301-471-0457
Web: http://www.asha.org

Specialty Commission on Fluency Disorders
P.O. Box 4475
Morgantown, WV 26504-4475

The Birch Tree Foundation
3615 Hamilton Street
Philadelphia, PA 19104
Phone: 215-222-4559
Fax: 215-222-4564
E-mail: givins@earthlink.net
Web: http://birch-tree.org

The British Stammering Association (BSA)
15 Old Ford Road
London, England E2 9PJ
Phone: 0181-983 1003
Fax: 0181-983 3591
Web: http://www.stammer.demon.co.uk

Canadian Association for People Who Stutter (CAPS)
2269 Lakeshore Boulevard, West
Etobikoke, Ontario, Canada M8V 3X6
Phone: 416-252-0842
Fax: 416-252-0720
Web: http://chat.carleton.ca/~dblock/caps.html

Friends: The Association of Young People Who Stutter
1220 Rosita Road
Pacifica, CA 94044-4223
Phone: 650-355-0215
E-mail: LCaggiano@aol.com
Web: http://friendswhostutter.org

International Fluency Association (IFA)
Box 870242
Tuscaloosa, AL 35487-0242
Phone: 205-348-7131
Fax: 205-348-1845
E-mail: ECOOPER@UA1VM.UA.EDU

National Council on Stuttering
558 Russell Road   9242 Gross Point Road, #305
DeKalb, IL 60115   Skokie, IL 60077-1338
Phone: 815-756-6986   708-677-8280

National Stuttering Association (NSA)
(formally the National Stuttering Project or NSP)
5100 E. La Palma Avenue
Suite 208
Anaheim Hills, CA 92807
Phone: 800-364-1677
Fax: 714-693-7554
E-mail: NSPMAIL@AOL.COM
Web: http://www.nsastutter.org

Speak Easy International
233 Concord Drive
Paramus, NJ 07652
Phone: 201-262-0895

Stuttering Foundation of America (SFA)
3100 Walnut Grove Road
Suite 603
Memphis, TN 38111-0749
Phone: 800-992-9392 / 901-452-7343
Fax: 901-452-3931
E-mail: STUTTERSFA@AOL.COM
Web: http://www.stuttersfa.org

Stuttering Resource Foundation
Ellen Rind, Director
123 Oxford Road
New Rochelle, NY 10804
Phone: 800-232-4772 / 914-632-3925
Fax: 914-235-0615
E-mail: ESR1@IONA.BITNET
Web: http://www.stuttersfa.org

International Stuttering Association (ISA)
c/o Mel Hoffman
811 Nisqually Drive
Sunnyvale, CA 94087
Phone: 408-245-5654
Fax: 408-730-8154
E-mail: JAAN_PILL@SBE.SCARBOROUGH.ON.CA

ELECTRONIC NETWORK SYSTEMS

The following is not a complete list of Internet addresses for information about stuttering. Some addresses may change or be unavailable for a time. Many of these sources can provide valuable information, but caution should be used, especially when investigating services and treatment options.

The Stuttering Home Page. Begun in 1994, this was the first major resource on the World Wide Web about stuttering. It is an information-rich site and also links to many resources and websites that have been placed online by various treatment programs. This will most likely be one of the most efficient places to begin your search for information and links on the web.

http://www.stutteringhomepage.com

PARENTS-W@F-BODY.ORG A mailing list for parents concerned about stuttering behaviors in children. Professionals, students, and others interested are also welcome to join. To subscribe send the following message to majordomo@f-body.org, **subscribe parents-w** or send a request to the list owner, Larry Burd, at larry_burd@compuserve.com.

SID4@VM.TEMPLE.EDU is a mailing list for members of the ASHA Special Interest Division 4, on stuttering and other fluency disorders. Any ASHA member is welcome to join Division 4 which will then make them eligible to join the closed mailing list. To subscribe, send e-mail to: listserv@vm.temple.edu with the message **subscribe sid4 firstname lastname.**

STUT-HLP@ECNET.NET is an open list, designed as a virtual support group for people who stutter and their families. To subscribe, send an E-mail to lisproc2@ecnet.net and type **subscribe Stutt-hlp firstname lastname** in the body of the message. The list owner is Robert Quesal.

STUTT-L@LISTSERV.TEMPLE.EDU is an open list originally designed for researchers, clinicians, and theorists interested in stuttering. It also has many people who stutter who participate. To subscribe, address E-mail to listserv@listserv.temple.edu and type **subscribe Stutt-L firstname lastname** in the body of the message. The list owner is Woody Starkweather.

STUTT-X@ASUVM.INRE.ASU.EDU is an open list designed for the discussion about research of communication disorders, fluency disorders in particular. To subscribe, send an e-mail to listserv@asuvm.inre.asu.edu and type **subscribe Stutt-X firstname lastname** in the body of the message. The list owner is Donald Mower.

WORDFREE@VM.TEMPLE.EDU is a closed mailing list for young persons who stutter. Anyone who stutters and is old enough to use e-mail on a computer but younger than age 20 is welcome. To join, address e-mail to listserv@vm.temple.edu and type **subscribe wordfree firstname lastname** in the body of the message. The list owner is Woody Starkweather.

Web sites from around the world. Many of these sites contain valuable information about stuttering support organizations, including newsletters, conference papers, and articles, as well as information about the organization.

Australia—Speak Easy: http://www.vicnet.net.au/ausspeak

Australia—Pacesetters: http://www.ideal.net.au/wicksp/

Canada—Speakeasy: http://www.vibrate.net/speakeasy/

Canada—Association des jeunes begues du Quebec: http://www.ajbq.qc.ca/

Canada—British Columbia Association of People Who Stutter: http://www.haserv.com/bcaps/

European League of Stuttering Associations: http://www.europe.is/elsa

Iceland—Malbjorg: http://www.geocities.com/HotSprings/5492/index.html

Israel—Israeli Stuttering Support Group: http://www.anglefire.com/il/bravid/Hstutt.html

South Africa—Speakeasy: http://www.ix.co.za./speakeash/

United Kingdom—British Stammering Association: http://www.stammer.demon.co.uk/

United States—Friends:Association of Young People Who Stutter: http://www.friendswhostutter.org/

United States—National Stuttering Association: http://www.nspstutter.org

United States—Stuttering Foundation of America: http://www.stuttersfa.org

United States—International Fluency Association: http://www.ruhr-uni-bochum.de/psy-deknat/projekte/verbindungen/bossardt/index.html

United States—International Stuttering Association: http://www.xs4all.nl/edorlow/isa.html

United States—Passing Twice: http://www.geocities.com/WestHollywood/3223/

United States—SLPsWhoStutter: http://www.egroups.com/subscribe/SLPsWhoStutter/

APPENDIX

USEFUL BOOKLETS AND VIDEOTAPES FOR PARENTS, TEACHERS, AND SPOUSES

FOR GENERAL USE

Understanding Stuttering, Cooper, E. G. (1990.) Information for Parents, Chicago, IL: National Easter Seal Society. This booklet describes the nature and possible causes of stuttering. Also discussed are diagnostic signs of stuttering, suggestions for parents of stuttering children, and the nature of treatment programs. (28 pages.)

Help! This child is stuttering. Selmar, J. W. (1991.) Austin, TX: Pro-Ed, Inc. Written for parents and teachers of school-age children who stutter, this booklet provides suggestions concerning selecting a speech-language pathologist and the nature of a treatment programs. (41 pages.)

A Guide for Parents of Children Who Stutter. National Stuttering Project. Designed as a brief guide for parents of stuttering children according to three experts in the field. (15 pages.)

Stuttering Foundation Publications

These booklets are edited by Malcolm Fraser, founder of SFA, or his daughter Jane. They are inexpensive ($1.00–$2.00) and contain concise information for clinicians, parents, teachers, and interested others.

Advice to those who stutter, Publication #9. (2nd ed.). Practical advice by 28 men and women speech-language pathologists who have been stutterers. (155 pages.)

If your child stutters: A Guide for Parents, Publication #11. (Third Revised Edition.) Suggestions for parents when helping the young stuttering or disfluent child. (56 pages.)

Self-Therapy for the Stutterer, Publication #12. (7th Edition.) Written for adults who are unable to obtain formal treatment, the booklet describes self-therapy activities. (192 pages.)

Do You Stutter: A Guide for Teens, Publication #21. Written by seven speech-language pathologists who give practical advice to teens on coping with stuttering. (80 pages.)

Stuttering and Your Child: Questions and Answers, Publication #22. Written for parents, teachers, and day care personnel for helping young children who stutter. (64 pages.)

FOR PROFESSIONAL USE

Stuttering Words, Publication #2. A glossary of terms associated with fluency and fluency disorders. (64 pages.)

Therapy for Stutterers, Publication #10. Outlines a program of treatment for clinicians who are working with adult or older adolescents. (120 pages.)

Treating the School Age Stutterer, A Guide for Clinicians, Publication #14. Written by Carl Dell, Ph.D., this booklet describes a large variety of clinical procedures for young stutterers. (112 pages.)

Stuttering: An Integration of Contemporary Therapies, Publication #16. Describes combining the treatment strategies of stuttering modification and fluency modification for stutterers of all ages. (80 pages.)

Counseling Stutterers, Publication #18. This booklet discusses the counseling aspects of treatment for adults and parents of children undergoing treatment. (80 pages.)

Stuttering Therapy: Transfer and Maintenance, Publication #19. Discusses the importance of transfer and maintenance procedures during and following the final stages of formal treatment. (112 pages.)

Stuttering Therapy: Prevention and Intervention with Children, Publication #20. A discussion of prevention and early intervention strategies and techniques with young children. (152 pages.)

Brief Informational Pamphlets from the Stuttering Foundation of America

If you Think Your Child is Stuttering
Turning On to Therapy
The Child Who Stutterers at School: Notes to the Teacher
How to React When Speaking with Someone Who Stutters

Videotapes

Childhood Stuttering: A Videotape for Parents. Conture, E., Guitar, B., & Williams, D. (1994). Stuttering Foundation of America. A 30-minute tape that describes the nature of stuttering in children and helpful ways for parents to respond.

Prevention of Stuttering Part I: Identifying the Danger Signs. This 33-minute video demonstrates the early signs of stuttering behavior in young children.

Speaking of Courage (1992). A one-hour video of three children who describe their stories of living with stuttering. The video stresses the importance of understanding by parents, family members, and professionals for both the detection and support of a child who stutters. In the United States: Suncoast Media, Inc. 12551 Indian Rocks Road, #15, Largo, Florida 34644, Tel: 813-596-1112, 1-800-899-1008, Fax: 813-596-3939.

Voices to Remember (1992). A one-hour video of four adults as seen through the eyes of an 11-year old child. The video discusses the effects of stuttering on the educational, social, and professional lives of four adults. The effects of treatment and support group groups are stressed. In the United States: Suncoast Media, Inc. 12551 Indian Rocks Road, #15, Largo, Florida 34644, Tel: 813-596-1112, 1-800-899-1008, Fax: 813-596-3939.

Therapy in Action: The School-Age Child Who Stutters. Conture, E., Guitar, B., Fraser, J. in collaboration with Campbell, J., Gregory, H., Ramig, P., & Zebrowski, P. (1997). Stuttering Foundation of America. A 38-minute tape describing the examples of stuttering and intervention techniques for young school-age children.

APPENDIX

GUIDELINES FOR PRACTICE IN STUTTERING TREATMENT

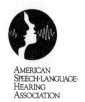

AMERICAN
SPEECH-LANGUAGE-
HEARING
ASSOCIATION

Guidelines for Practice in Stuttering Treatment

Special Interest Division on Fluency and Fluency Disorders

These guidelines are an official statement of the American Speech-Language-Hearing Association (ASHA). They are guidelines for practice in stuttering treatment but are not official standards of the Association. They were developed by members of the Steering Committee of ASHA's Special Interest Division on Fluency and Fluency Disorders (Division 4): C. W. Starkweather, Kenneth St. Louis, Gordon Blood, Theodore Peters, Janice Westbrook, Hugo Gregory, Eugene Cooper, and Charles Healey, under the guidance of Crystal Cooper, vice president for professional practices. Lyn Goldberg provided support from the National Office. The Steering Committee acknowledges the assistance of Diane L. Eger, vice president for professional practices, 1991-1993.

I. Introduction

The document that follows was developed by the Special Interest Division on Fluency and Fluency Disorders (Division 4) of ASHA in response to the affiliates' belief that the field lacked standards for the treatment of stuttering. It was felt too that the parallel move toward specialization made it necessary to define more clearly the role of nonspecialists. At the same time, the ASHA document, "Preferred Practice Patterns for the Professions of Speech-Language Pathology and Audiology" (*Asha* Supplement No. 11, March 1993), was published but addressed only Fluency Assessment and only in the most general terms. The failure of this document to address the treatment of fluency disorders left a gap to be filled.

It should be noted that the Steering Committee felt that the state of knowledge in several key areas—specifically treatment efficacy and the measurement of stuttering—was not developed well enough to al-

low the promulgation of "standards." It was decided to provide less prescriptive "guidelines."

Another issue concerned the base of knowledge used to determine whether a goal is desirable or a practice appropriate to achieve a goal. The Steering Committee felt that a set of criteria for determining guidelines that was based entirely on empirical evidence would be too restrictive. Some treatment practices may be quite useful even though their efficacy has not yet been determined empirically. The committee felt that both common practice and published data should be considered.

Finally, the document does not take a position on stuttering theory or advocate a specific philosophy of treatment. Instead, it puts forward what is hoped to be an agreed upon set of goals and the procedures that are used to achieve them.

II. General Guidelines for Practice

Timing and Duration of Sessions

There is considerable variation in the timing and duration of treatment sessions and in the total duration of treatment. Some residential programs treat clients very intensively, 6 or more hours each day for a number of weeks. Private clinicians may see clients one, two, or three times a week for a longer period of time. In the schools and hospitals, the timing and duration of sessions is restrained by overriding schedules. Intensive treatment may be expected to achieve more rapid change, but the intensive treatment alters the client's daily activity more extensively, creating a barrier to transfer that the clinician considers in planning treatment activities. Nonintensive treatment, on the other hand, disrupts the client's everyday life far less, but it may achieve change so slowly that the client becomes discouraged. Clinicians who see clients less frequently can sequence treatment activity for early success, or provide for other motivational activities that will keep the client interested in continuing treatment.

Reference this material as: American Speech-Language-Hearing Association. (1995, March). Guidelines for practice in stuttering treatment. *Asha, 37* (Suppl. 14), pp. 26-35.

Index terms: Stuttering, fluency, Special Interest Division, assessment/fluency, treatment, practice guidelines/stuttering, management goals, competencies/fluency

The Setting of Treatment

Clients are seen in a wide variety of settings. Some programs are residential, providing treatment, usually intensive, in a setting removed from the client's everyday life. Others treat clients in the communities where they live. Both residential and nonresidential treatment programs provide activities for effective transfer of new behaviors to the ordinary social situations of everyday life. Transfer can be achieved through carefully sequenced, monitored practice in real-life social situations. Programs that treat the client only in a limited setting and do not provide for monitored practice of newly learned behaviors in natural settings fall outside the guidelines of good practice. There are a number of ways to monitor a client's practice: (1) direct observation, in which the clinician is present during the practice session, (2) interviews with the client after practice sessions, and (3) listening, with the client, to audiotape recordings of practice sessions. In each case, monitoring should include opportunities for the clinician to discuss the practice session with the client so as to increase understanding, and opportunities to provide immediate feedback on the client's performance. Listening to audiotape recordings that are submitted by mail and responded to with written comments from the clinician falls outside the guidelines of good practice, if it is the only method of transfer. It should be recognized, however, that there are circumstances— when a client lives in a remote area, for example— where it may be impossible to provide service that is within the guidelines. The best practice, in these circumstances, is to make sure that both client and clinician are aware of any necessary limitations on treatment.

There is also variation in the duration of individual sessions. In general, clinicians plan sessions so that they are long enough to accomplish some stated objective, but not so long as to lose clients' attention through fatigue or boredom. The client's age and ability to attend are taken into consideration in determining the duration of sessions.

Duration of Treatment

The total duration of treatment is an important variable of practice. Clinicians want to be sure that treatment lasts long enough for effective change, but they do not want to continue to provide treatment when there is no longer any further benefit. Our field is in the process of researching the variables that affect treatment duration, but we cannot yet say with certainty what these variables are. It seems clear that more intensive treatment produces more rapid change than nonintensive treatment (Prins, 1970). It also seems likely, but not yet demonstrated, that the complexity of a client's problem may influence the duration of treatment. People who stutter in a way that is unusually complex behaviorally, or who have other coexisting problems or disorders are likely to require considerable time in treatment. Those who are cognitively impaired, or who cannot attend easily, for example, would be expected to take longer in treatment. Also, the presence of a coexisting language or articulation disorder, or a psychoemotional disturbance, can lengthen treatment.

A client's personal level of motivation and commitment to the treatment process will also influence the duration of treatment. School-age, adolescent, and adult stutterers require longer durations of treatment than preschool children. In spite of the uncertainty that remains in this area, clinicians try to provide to clients and their families some sense of how long treatment may take, including the processes of maintenance and follow-up.

Complexity of Treatment

Stuttering is typically a complex problem. It may begin simply, but it usually, and sometimes quickly, becomes complex because of the reactions, defensive behaviors, and coping strategies of the person who stutters and the reactions of significant others in the listening environment. Furthermore, in older children and adults, the communicative difficulties that stuttering creates present barriers to social, educational, and vocational life that can greatly complicate the problem. In some cases, there can be serious emotional disturbance, such as depression or sociopathic behavior. These complexities create issues that clinicians help their clients deal with through treatment and referral. Stuttering treatments that do not address the complete problem in whatever complexity it presents are not within the guidelines of good practice.

The Cost of Treatment

As independent professionals, clinicians working with stutterers have the responsibility of setting their own fees. In doing so, they consider a number of factors. People who stutter sometimes seek help with an intense longing for relief, and in some cases feel quite desperate. Clinicians, in setting their fees, do not exploit these feelings. In addition, the client's desire for help can be increased through statements by the clinician implying that the treatment is highly effective. The prohibition in the Code of Ethics of ASHA against misrepresentation in public statements has particular relevance for stuttering treatment. When clinicians make public statements about their own treatment programs, they are appropriately cautious about its effectiveness. It would seem well outside the guidelines of good practice for a clinician to make a public statement that a new technique could solve every stutterer's problem, and then charge far more than is the usual practice.

Typically, the amount of time the clinician spends in face-to-face contact with the client is the main yardstick by which the value of treatment is determined. Telephone contact, tape recordings, paper and electronic mail contact also have value, although not many clinicians charge for these services. The value of treatment for people who stutter lies in the supportive nature of the client-clinician relationship and in the clinician's ability to hear and see the stutterer's behavior and respond to it in a way that helps the client learn to talk more effectively.

III. Attributes of Clinicians Who Work With People Who Stutter

It is desirable for clinicians to have certain personal attitudes and qualities and a fund of certain information. The following list is an expanded version of the Texas Speech and Hearing Association Fluency Task Force's list of "Personal Clinician Competencies":

Personal Attributes

1. Is interested in and committed to the treatment of people with fluency disorders.

2. Is willing to develop as much knowledge and skill as possible related to diagnosis and treatment of stuttering and keeps abreast of current developments.

3. Is willing to refer clients when the need for more assistance is necessary.

4. Is willing to take an active role in the profession to know about specific services that are available both locally and nationally to clients who stutter.

5. Has good problem-solving skills and uses them when things do not go according to plan in evaluation and treatment.

6. Is flexible in thinking and planning.

Learned Attributes

7. Has a general understanding of the literature relative to the etiology and development of stuttering.

8. Has an adequate level of knowledge of the phenomenology of stuttering, particularly with regard to those phenomena that influence therapeutic practice, such as, episodic variation, clustering, paradoxical intention, adaptation and consistency, spontaneous recovery, fluency enhancement, arousal effects.

9. Has a general understanding of the literature on

normal and language-based (dis)fluency, rate, prosody, rhythm, and effort, and the development of these speech characteristics and has the skill to gain new information from the literature as new findings are incorporated into it.

10. Has a view of stuttering that is focused enough to provide guidance in the planning of treatment but broad and adjustable enough to accommodate new research findings and theoretical perspectives.

11. Has an understanding and appreciation of the possible relations between a person's normal and abnormal speech behavior on the one hand, and their beliefs, upbringing, and cultural background on the other.

12. Has an understanding and appreciation of the basic processes of dynamic clinical interaction, such as transference, denial, grief, victimization.

13. Can communicate relevant ideas about stuttering to clients and their families.

14. Has a general working knowledge of psychopathology.

15. Has a general working knowledge of cognitive and behavioral learning theory.

In addition, the specialist in fluency should meet the guidelines listed below:

IV. Specific Guidelines for Practice–Goals, Processes, and Competencies

This section contains three parts. First, a list of goals, appropriate to the treatment of fluency disorders, is described. The criterion for including goals is that they be acceptable and desirable for speech-language pathologists to try to reach with clients with fluency disorders. These goals follow from the nature of fluency disorders, and it is expected that few will disagree with the choice of goals. Indeed, peer review of the guidelines revealed a broad consensus on the goals.

The philosophy of treatment that a clinician believes in will, of course, strongly determine which goals are considered most important. This list is intended to include all goals that are considered appropriate by all philosophies of treatment currently held by speech-language pathologists who treat people who stutter. The order of goals presented in this document does not reflect their order of importance.

It is recognized that certain goals may be desirable for (some) clients to reach but are nevertheless outside the scope of practice for most speech-language pathologists, e.g., psychotherapeutic goals unrelated to fluency, or parenting issues unrelated to a child's fluency.

The second part lists processes that are useful for achieving specific goals. The inclusion of processes in this list in no way mandates their use by clinicians. Some clinicians will rely exclusively on a few processes; others will combine many different processes. The list is an attempt to set down processes that are in widespread use by speech-language pathologists who treat stuttering.

The criteria for selecting processes combine empirical knowledge, theory, and common practice. For example, one goal is a reduction in the frequency of stuttering behaviors. Processes that have been shown empirically to reduce stuttering behaviors in a lasting way, for example, slowed parental speech rate for young stuttering children, have consequently been included. Another process, for example, instrumental extinction, might be included for more theoretical reasons. In some cases, either the empirical or the theoretical support is weak, and this weakness is pointed out in the document.

The third part identifies competencies—skills and knowledge—that clinicians can use to engage in the processes identified in part two. The criteria for inclusion in this list of competencies are simply logical. If the modification of cognitive structures that make it difficult for clients to think about their speech in a productive manner is a desirable goal, then cognitive restructuring is a useful process, and a competency in that technique is useful for clinicians to have. It is understood that not all clinicians will have all competencies, although it is expected that clinicians will continue to augment their current competencies through continuing education.

A. Assessment

Desirable goals in the assessment of fluency disorders:

Assessment Goal 1

Obtain a speech sample that is as representative as possible of the client's speech in everyday use.

Assessment Goal 2

Obtain a sample of the client's speech under circumstances that are constant from one client to the next.

Assessment Goal 3

Generate, from obtained speech samples and incidental observations, quantitative and qualitative descriptions of the client's fluent and disfluent speech behaviors that can be related where applicable to vocal tract physiology, and that are communicable to other interested professionals.

Assessment Goal 4

Obtain information about variables that affect the client's fluency level and apply this to treatment planning.

Assessment Goal 5

Obtain information about a client's early social, physical, behavioral, and speech development, including information about variables that might be related to the origin of the disorder or its course of development, and apply this information to treatment planning.

Assessment Goal 6

Obtain information about variables that might influence clinical outcome and/or the prognosis for treatment and apply this to treatment planning.

Assessment Goal 7

Obtain information about other communicative problems or disorders that may or may not be related to fluency.

Assessment Goal 8

Generate descriptions of the results of assessment that are communicable to other professional and lay persons.

Processes for achieving the goals of assessment

Processes for achieving Assessment Goal 1 — achieving a representative sample

1. Observation and recording of the client's speech during an interview with the clinician about the client's stuttering disorder.

2. Observation and recording of the client talking to a relative or friend prior to meeting with the clinician.

3. Observation and recording of a child playing with parents after instructions to the parents to play with the child as they normally would at home (Family Play Session).

4. Tape recordings made by the client of conversations during daily activities at work, home, or anywhere.

Processes for achieving Assessment Goal 2 — a speech sample from a constant setting

1. Observation and recording of the client's speech in response to being asked to describe a standard stimulus picture.

2. Observation and recording of the client's speech while reading a standard passage aloud.

3. Observation and recording of the client's speech while the client plays a "barrier game"[1] with the clinician, or, preferably, with a third party.

4. Observation and recording of the client's speech during a structured interview, in which the clinician asks the same question of each client by referring to an interview form.

5. Observation and recording of the client's speech while performing a specific speech task, such as describing a job or a favorite activity or a school subject.

Processes for achieving Assessment Goal 3 — quantitative and qualitative description of the client's fluency level

1. Administering any of a variety of published tests of fluency, stuttering severity, attitudes toward stuttering and speech, self-efficacy as a speaker, situational fears, and avoidance behavior.

2. Administering any of a variety of systematic protocols for coding speech sample(s) so as to reflect the categories of disfluency, and the extent of fluency or nonfluency, and the presence and type of secondary behaviors.

3. Transcribing a speech sample verbatim in such a way as to accurately reflect all fluent and nonfluent speech behavior.

4. Identifying and counting the frequency of primary and secondary stuttering behaviors.

5. Measuring the duration of discontinuous and continuous speech elements.

6. Measuring speech rate (syllables per second with pauses included) and articulatory rate (syllables per second with pauses excluded).

7. Observing and recording behavioral and/or physiological measurements of oral, laryngeal, and respiratory behavior so as to relate specifically identified stuttering behaviors to possible vocal tract events and to assess the capacity for fluent speech production.

8. Describing qualitatively any of the nonmeasurable aspects of fluency, such as apparent level of muscular tension, emotional reactivity to speech or stuttering behaviors, coping behaviors, nonverbal aspects of stuttering behavior, or anomalies of social interaction such as poor eye contact, generalized low muscle tonus, poor body posture.

---

[1] In the barrier game, the client and another person sit opposite each other at a table. A barrier is erected across the table so that the two cannot see each other. The client has to direct the other person in the assembly of, for instance, a puzzle, piece of equipment, or toy.

Processes for achieving Assessment Goal 4 — assessing variables that affect fluency

1. Developing and systematically testing hypotheses about variables that might affect fluency level, for example, talking slowly to a stuttering child to see if a measurable improvement in fluency can be obtained.

2. Interviewing the client or the client's family about social circumstances, words, listeners, sentence types, speech sounds, that improve or exacerbate fluency.

3. Playing videotapes or audiotapes of parent-child interactions to the parents of a child who presents with a potential or actual fluency disorder.

4. Conducting a variety of brief trial treatment procedures, such as delayed auditory feedback, whispering, rate modification.

Processes for achieving Assessment Goal 5 — getting and using a developmental history

1. Developing questionnaires or other written materials (e.g., fluency autobiography) designed to obtain potentially relevant background information.

2. Interviewing the client, the client's family, or others about developmental milestones of motor control, social-emotional behavior, speech and language, and cognitive level.

Processes for achieving Assessment Goal 6 — getting and using prognostic information and information that will optimize treatment planning

1. Administering tests or reading reports of others who have administered formal tests of intelligence, attitudes, motivation, comprehension, ability to take direction, or other prognostic indicators.

2. Making informal tests and observations related to intelligence, attitudes, motivation, comprehension, ability to take direction, or other prognostic indicators.

Processes for achieving Assessment Goal 7 — getting and using information about coexisting problems

1. Administering tests or reading reports of others who have administered formal tests of language, voice, articulation, psychoemotional function, learning disability, cognitive level, or auditory or visual deficits and using this information to plan for treatment and to provide prognostic information.

2. Making informal observations of language, voice, articulation, psychoemotional function, learning disability, cognitive level, or auditory or visual deficits, and using this information to plan for treatment and to provide prognostic information.

Processes for achieving Assessment Goal 8 — communicating the results of assessment

1. Writing reports of assessment processes designed to be read by physicians, psychologists, and other nonspeech-language pathology professionals.

2. Writing comprehensive reports of assessment processes designed to be read by the current or subsequent clinicians.

3. Reporting the results of assessment processes, formally or informally, to the client and/or the client's family/significant others.

Clinician competencies related to assessment [2]

1. Can differentiate between a child's normally disfluent speech, language-based disfluency, the speech of a child at risk for stuttering, and the speech of a child who has already begun to stutter.

2. Can distinguish cluttered from stuttered speech and understands the potential relationship between these two disorders.

3. Can relate the findings of language, articulation, voice, and hearing tests to the development of stuttering.

4. Can obtain a thorough case history from an adult client or the family of a child client.

5. Can obtain a useful speech sample and evaluate it for stuttering severity both informally by subjective impression and formally by calculating relevant measures such as the frequency of disfluency, duration of disfluency, speaking rate.

6. Is familiar with the available diagnostic tests for stuttering that serve to objectify aspects of the client's communication pattern (secondary features, avoidance patterns, attitudes, etc.) that may not be readily observed.

7. Is able to identify, and measure where feasible, environmental variables (i.e., aspects, such as time pressure, emotional reactions, interruptions, nonverbal behavior, demand speech, or the speech of significant others) that may be related to the onset, development, and maintenance of stuttering and to fluctuations in the severity of stuttering.

8. Can identify disfluencies by type (prolongation, repetition, etc.) and, in addition, can describe qualitatively the fluency of a person's speech.

9. Can relate, to the extent possible, what stuttered speech sounds like to the vocal tract behavior

that is producing it (for example, recognizing the subtle acoustic cues that signal vocal straining).

10. Can, in appropriate consultation with the client or parents, construct a treatment program, based on the results of comprehensive testing, on the client's personal emotional and attitudinal development, and on past treatment history, that fits the unique needs of each client's disorder(s).

11. Can administer predetermined programs in a diagnostic way so that decisions with regard to branching and repeating of parts of the program reflect the unique needs of each client's disorder(s).

12. Can explain clearly to clients or their families/ significant others what treatment options, including the various types of speech treatment, medication, devices, self-help groups, and other forms of treatment are available, why they may or may not be appropriate to a specific case, and what outcomes can be expected from each, based on knowledge of the available literature.

B. Management

Desirable goals in the management of fluency disorders:

Management Goal 1

Reduce the frequency with which stuttering behaviors occur without increasing the use of other behaviors that are not a part of normal speech production.

Management Goal 2

Reduce the severity, duration, and abnormality of stuttering behaviors until they are or resemble normal speech discontinuities.

Management Goal 3

Reduce the use of defensive behaviors.[3]

Note that when clients use avoidance behaviors that are successful (in that they avoid stuttering behavior) they will appear to have made progress toward Management Goal 1, but in fact will have done so by including some additional, and abnormal, behavior. For example, clients who are able to change

---

[2] This list of competencies is an expanded and revised version of a list prepared originally by the Texas Speech and Hearing Association Fluency Task Force.

[3] Defensive behaviors are behaviors performed so as to prevent, avoid, escape from, or minimize aversive events, real or imagined (Bandura, 1969). A somewhat broader category than avoidance behaviors, defensive behaviors include also struggled stuttering behavior, trying to force a word or sound out, rushing through a phrase so as to "get past" the stuttering.

words so as to avoid saying a word that they will stutter on will have a reduced frequency of stuttering behavior, but they will also have an increased frequency of cognitive behaviors involved in the search for and retrieval of substitute words.

Management Goal 4

Remove or reduce processes serving to create, exacerbate, or maintain stuttering behaviors.

In children, this might entail modification of the child's parents' behavior so as to reduce maladaptive reactions to the child's stuttering behavior. In adults it might include teaching the client how to change his or her listeners' behavior. In some cases, there may be reinforcement for stuttering, such as excuses for failure, or getting attention that is otherwise not forthcoming. In other cases, denial may prevent an adult from perceiving the extent to which stuttering affects his or her life.

Management Goal 5

Help the person who stutters make treatment (e.g., adaptive) decisions about how to handle speech and social situations in everyday living.

This includes such things as helping the client learn how to respond to people who try to talk for him or her, or helping the client learn not to use behaviors that avoid, rather than confront, specific social situations such as using the telephone, ordering in a restaurant, or helping the client learn that changing words costs something in personal self-esteem. This also includes teaching the client how to politely influence listeners' behavior so that the client's fluency can be improved.

Management Goal 6

Increase the frequency of social activity and speaking.

Clients who have adopted reticence as a strategy to deal with stuttering will need help in regaining a normal amount of social speech.

Management Goal 7

Reduce attitudes, beliefs, and thought processes that interfere with fluent speech production or that hinder the achievement of other treatment goals.

In some adults this might involve modifying their attitude toward very brief stuttering behaviors so as to prevent stuttering from returning at a later date. Similarly, certain attitudes toward fluency and disfluency, or beliefs about these attitudes, can maintain stuttering behaviors, for example, perfectionist fluency, abhorrence of normal disfluency, rigidity in speech behavior. Some clients may have attitudes

toward themselves that serve to exacerbate or maintain stuttering behaviors, for example, low self-esteem, lack of confidence, or feelings of worthlessness.

Management Goal 8

Reduce emotional reactions to specific stimuli when these have a negative impact on stuttering behavior or on attempts to modify stuttering behavior.

For example, fear of specific social situations, word fears, a sense of intimidation by specific categories of listeners, a sense of helplessness or fear of specific speech tasks, such as answering the telephone or asking questions in class, or a fear of the embarrassment of stuttering in public. This should not be confused with the reduction of defensive behavior, which is one kind of reaction to these fears. Both fear reduction and defensive behavior reduction can be appropriate.

Management Goal 9

Where necessary, seek helpful combinations and sequences of treatments, including referral, for problems other than stuttering that may accompany the fluency disorder, such as, cluttering, learning disability, language/phonological disorder, voice disorder, psychoemotional disturbance.

Management Goal 10

Provide information and guidance to clients, families, and other significant persons about the nature of stuttering, normal fluency and disfluency, and the course of treatment and prognosis for recovery.

In addition, help clients and families/significant others understand the nature of past treatment and the availability and possible utility of other options, including other forms of treatment, devices, and self-help groups.

Processes for achieving the goals of management

It is not the intention of this document to assert that all processes should be used with all clients. A process for reducing excitement is useful only with a client whose fluency is adversely influenced by excitement. For each client, clinicians choose a set of appropriate goals, based on a careful evaluation of the client. Having established what are appropriate goals for a client, a selection of processes to achieve these goals is made. At times during treatment, both goals and processes should be re-evaluated, and after treatment, it is likewise appropriate to review the selection of goals and processes and evaluate them with regard to the outcome of treatment.

Note that processes are not exactly the same as techniques. There might be several techniques for engaging in a particular process. For example, one process mentioned below is "Identify reinforcers for stuttering." A clinician could engage in this process by interviewing clients and asking what happens after they stutter, or spend some time with clients, observing them in real speaking situations, or interview people who know the clients well, such as parents, siblings, or partners. Each of these techniques would or could result in the identification of reinforcers that are contingent on stuttering behavior.

Note that referral and consultation are processes that may be used to achieve goals.

Processes for achieving Management Goal 1–Reducing the frequency of stuttering behaviors

1. Fluency-shaping approach:

    a. Slowed rate of speech movements.

       • typically taught in stages of speed (e.g., Rate I, Rate II, and Slow-Normal Rate)

    b. Easy onset of voicing.

       • slow inhalation

       • soft but true voice changing to full voice before vowel initiation

       • practice in order to shorten the time taken up by the onset of voicing period

    c. Blending, or continuous voicing.

    d. Light articulatory contacts.

    e. Smooth, slow speech movements.

    f. Use of computer-assisted feedback to train clients in fluency — producing coordinated speech production movements.

2. Vocal control treatment approach.

    a. Better vocal tone, breath support, full resonance, efficient and relaxed voice, adequate loudness.

    b. Typically accompanied by systematic desensitization.

3. Contingency management:

    a. Combined reinforcement for fluent speech and mild, nonaversive punishment for stuttering behaviors.

    b. Successive approximation (shaping) toward fluent speech.

    c. Practice in a systematically sequenced series of steps from where fluent speech is easiest to achieve toward where fluency is more difficult to achieve, for example, through gradually increasing the length and complexity of an utterance, or through a hierarchy of feared social situations.

    d. Use of fluency-enhancement, in the clinic, or via a wearable device, may be a useful way to establish the behavior in the first place.

    e. Use of computer-assisted devices to ensure rapid and consistent feedback.

    f. Systematically administered reinforcement for more natural-sounding speech.

4. Reduction of speech-associated anxiety:

    a. Systematic desensitization to social situations.

    b. Desensitization to the experience of stuttering (confrontation).

    c. Pseudostuttering (voluntary stuttering, or faking).

    d. With children, through counseling parents, reduction or removal of as many anxiety-producing events as possible.

5. Reduction of speech-associated excitement:

    a. With children, through counseling parents, reduction of as many exciting events as practical and reasonable.

6. In prevention, training parents to speak more slowly but with normal intonation, timing, and stress patterns.

7. In prevention, training parents to talk less often, and with simpler language, to interrupt less often, and to ask fewer questions requiring long complex answers.

Processes for achieving Management Goal 2–reducing the abnormality, severity, or duration of stuttering behaviors

1. Disfluency shaping:

    a. Help the client learn ways to be disfluent in a more normal way.

    b. Remove, through modeling and practice, one behavior at a time until disfluencies are normal in type.

2. Muscle tension reduction:

    a. Reduction of oral and vocal muscular tension during speech.

       • slowed rate and rate control

       • direct suggestion to reduce muscle tension in specific parts of the vocal tract

       • referrals for the possible use of medication to achieve muscle relaxation

       • attitude modification via techniques described below

3. Repair treatment:

a. Teach client the various types of speech sounds and how they are fluently produced.

b. Teach client the types of stuttering behaviors used by client.

c. Teach client types of repairs — ways of changing from the stuttered to the nonstuttered type of production.

d. Practice repairs in different environments.

e. Work on one or two specific sounds or sound category at a time.

4. Stuttering modification sequence:

a. Post-block modification, or cancellation.

b. In-block modification, or pull-out.

c. Pre-block modification, or prep-aratory set.

5. Counterconditioning techniques:

a. Associating stuttering with pleasant events, for example, "reinforcement" for stuttering, or tag game.

b. Voluntary stuttering.

6. Confrontational (nonavoidance) techniques:

a. Discussion with the client of specific behaviors, the circumstances under which they occurred, and the variables that may have influenced them.

b. Listening to or watching with clients audio or videotapes of themselves while speaking and discussing specific behaviors and reactions with them.

Processes for achieving Management Goal 3–reducing defensive behaviors

1. Extinction of defensive behavior:

a. For secondary (avoidance) behavior:

• direct instructions to stop performing the secondary behavior, accompanied by an alternative to stuttering behavior, for example, in-block modification (pull-outs), or slowed speech, or monitored vocalization

• punishment (time-out, response cost or other nonaversive punishment only) accompanied by an alternative to stuttering behavior

b. For primary (escape) behavior, that is, struggled disfluency:

• stuttering modification sequence of post-block, in-block, pre-block modification

• modeling stuttering that is easy and free of struggle, then reinforcing the client for disfluency that is less struggled

• direct suggestions, accompanied by cuing and reminders

• discussions about the client's stuttering pattern, approaching feared situations, to toughen attitudes toward stuttering

2. In prevention, training parents in the relaxed production of occasional disfluencies that are normal for their child's age.

Processes for achieving Management Goal 4–removing processes that may be maintaining stuttering behaviors

1. Instrumental (operant) conditioning:

a. Identify reinforcers for stuttering.

b. Remove conditions in the environment, including in the client's "internal environment" that are reinforcing stuttering or defensive behavior.

2. Defensive counterconditioning:

a. Identify aversive consequences for stuttering.

b. Identify stimuli, or constellations of stimuli (situations) associated with or predictive of aversive consequences, as in a hierarchy of speech situations.

c. Identify behaviors that terminate or avoid the aversive consequences.

d. Provide experiences for the client in which the conditioned stimuli occur, but the avoidance behaviors are NOT performed and no aversive consequences follow.

e. Help client learn how to handle pressure situations while still using newly learned fluency skills.

3. Vicarious conditioning:

a. Identify speech models who are reinforced for stuttering, or who avoid stuttering or try to avoid stuttering (i.e., use defensive behavior), or who demonstrate negative emotional reactions to disfluency.

b. Counsel, train, or modify the behavior of these models so as to remove or reduce the occurrence of vicarious conditioning.

4. Environmental manipulation:

a. Alter the client's environment, external or internal, so as to remove any conditioning process that is exacerbating or maintaining stuttering behavior:

• by counseling significant others

• by counseling the client

• by providing for experiences that will alter attitudes or beliefs that result in deleterious conditioning processes.

Processes for achieving Management Goal 5–helping clients learn how to make decisions about everyday speaking situations

1. Identification of specific decisions about social behavior that may affect fluency, for example, deciding to let a colleague answer the phone even though the client is closer to it.

2. Counseling, including sensitive explanations about how decisions based on defensive reactions serve to increase fear and decrease self-confidence.

3. Identify, with the client's help, attainable behavioral goals for more effective decision-making.

4. Plan activities that will provide opportunities for the client to make better decisions.

5. Reinforce client for making decisions that are more conducive to speaking fluently and with confidence.

6. Help clients foresee the natural consequences of their decisions to use or not use learned treatment techniques in day-to-day activities.

7. Attendance in a support group with other people who stutter.

Processes for achieving Management Goal 6–increasing social activity and speaking behavior

1. Provide reinforcement for entering speech situations previously feared.

2. Encouragement and reinforcement for talking more often and in a wider variety of situations, structured hierarchically from least to most stressful or intimidating.

3. Encourage client to participate in a self-help group.

4. Use of a fluency-enhancing device to make possible social activity that would otherwise be too intimidating for the client.

Processes for achieving Management Goal 7–improving self esteem or revising a perfectionist attitude toward speech

1. Counsel the client so as to provide for successful experiences of any kind.

2. Counsel the client so as to provide for successful speech experiences.

3. Validation of the client as a person and speaker:

a. Listen to the client and demonstrate appreciation of the client as a person.

b. Listen to the client and validate aspects of speech that are unrelated to fluency, through expressed appreciation for aspects of the client's speech that are normal or superior, e.g., voice quality, expressiveness, word choice, articulation.

c. Listen to the client and validate fluency, where appropriate, by expressed appreciation for stuttering behaviors that are less struggled or less abnormal.

d. Transfer similar listening skills to client (self-listening).

4. Provide for increased attention from significant others.

5. Help client attain better identification of self through support group or other activities.

6. Provide for increased tolerance of failings through counseling, modeling.

7. Positive self-talk and affirmation training.

Processes for achieving Management Goal 8–reducing negative reactions to stuttering and social situations that have included stuttering in the past

1. Confrontational desensitization to stuttering events:

a. Talk about stuttering with the client in an objective way.

b. Have clients learn, through self-demonstration, that speech improves when they "give permission to stutter" or stutter on purpose.

c. Stuttering on purpose in the clinical setting.

d. Stuttering on purpose in real situations.

e. Keep a record of situations in which clients have stuttered on purpose or allowed themselves to stutter.

2. Desensitization to anxiety-provoking speech situations:

a. Traditional systematic desensitization:

• constructing a hierarchy of feared words, listeners, and situations

• inducing a physically and emotionally relaxed state

• imagining feared situations while in a relaxed state

• imagining oneself talking to feared listeners while in a relaxed state

• imagining oneself producing feared words while in a relaxed state

• imagining oneself stuttering while in a relaxed state

• testing the effects of these experiences in real situations

b. in vivo systematic desensitization:

• ...feared words, listeners, and situations

• systematically talking in real life situations, starting with the easiest elements in the hierarchy, and gradually increasing the level of difficulty. A fluency-enhancing device may provide a place to begin this process, although it will be important to wean the client from the device so as not to create a dependency on it.

Processes for achieving Management Goal 9–dealing with coexisting problems:

1. Referral to other professionals with regard to psychoemotional or learning disability problems.

2. Team treatment with other speech-language pathologists so as to work simultaneously on language, phonological, or voice problems.

3. Sequencing treatment so as to deal with one problem at a time. Usually this means postponing work on language, voice, or articulation until fluency is under control, but sometimes it means postponing work on fluency until some progress is made on the other disorder, for example, improved intelligibility.

4. Designing treatment plans that deal simultaneously with stuttering and coexisting problems.

Processes for achieving Management Goal 10–providing information to significant others:

1. Direct counseling of parents, spouses, siblings, and others.

2. Bibliotherapy for parents, spouses, physicians, psychologists, and others.

3. Use of audio and videotape to present to clients and the parents of clients examples of specific behaviors and reactions.

4. Provide information about other treatment approaches, treatment devices, self-help and consumer advocate groups.

5. Provide information about third-party payment options.

Clinic competencies related to management

1. Is familiar with the appropriate goals of treatment and the processes for achieving them and can engage these processes, choosing techniques that are best for the client, and administer them with an attitude that balances the goal of normal speech with a tolerance for abnormal speech.

2. Has flexibility in choosing and changing the level of difficulty of tasks based on fluency level of the client.

3. Can teach clients to produce vocal tract behaviors that result in normal sounding speech production.

4. Has sufficient counseling skills so as to interact with clients of all ages and develop a reasonable set of expectations in the client.

5. Has a thorough understanding of, and knows how to put into practice, the principles of conditioning and learning so as to achieve a successful and appropriate modification of speech behavior.

6. Understands the relations between stuttering and other related disorders of fluency, such as cluttering, neurogenic and psychogenic stuttering, as well as disorders of language, articulation, learning, and so on, and can with flexibility identify sequences and combinations of treatment options that are helpful to the client.

7. Understands the dimensions of normal fluency and the relation of normal fluency to speech situations and is able to work toward normal speech, with an awareness of the compromises among effort, fluency, and natural-sounding communication.

8. Understands that some stuttering behaviors may be reactions to other stuttering behaviors and knows how to plan treatment to account for this.

9. Can evaluate available treatment programs with regard to treatment application for a wide variety of clients.

10. Is able to decide, based on objective progress, motivational level, and cost in time and money when it is appropriate to terminate treatment.

11. Is aware of the continuous nature of fluency and can identify subtle changes in speech or other behaviors related to treatment change and explain their importance to the client.

12. Can explain stuttering and treatment for stuttering to lay persons, such as day care workers, teachers, baby sitters, grandparents, and others who may influence the life of children who stutter.

13. Knows how to develop a plan for assessing objectively the efficacy of treatment in an ongoing way.

14. Can recognize problems that are treated by professionals other than speech-language pathologists and can guide a client to acceptance of an appropriate referral.

C. Transfer and Maintenance

Desirable goals in the transfer and maintenance of acquired fluency behaviors

Transfer and Maintenance Goal 1

Generalization of the behavioral changes learned in the treatment setting to speech situations in the client's everyday life.

Transfer and Maintenance Goal 2

A sense of committed interest and self-reliance on the part of clients in managing their own speech behavior, balanced against an awareness of the need for occasional help (professional or otherwise) as needed.

Transfer and Maintenance Goal 3

Ability on the client's part at recognizing the earliest signs of returning emotional reactions and/or stuttering behaviors and knowledge and skill for dealing with these occurrences.

Transfer and Maintenance Goal 4

In parents, knowledge and skills needed to facilitate their child's further development of fluency.

Processes for achieving transfer and maintenance goals

Processes for achieving Transfer and Maintenance Goal 1 — generalization of behavior to external settings.

1. Variation of speech use within the treatment setting.

2. Role-playing of social interactions while using new behaviors.

3. Hierarchically structured practice in the client's everyday life, monitored by the clinician via tape recordings and/or interviews.

4. Continued practice in the treatment setting.

5. Use of self-help and support groups.

Process for achieving Transfer and Maintenance Goal 2 — self-reliance and commitment.

1. Counseling clients to assist themselves in taking over the process of decision making in treatment.

2. Providing exercises for the client designed to increase skills at self-evaluation and self-treatment planning.

3. Gradually reducing the clinician's input in making decisions about treatment.

4. Gradually decreasing the frequency of contact between clinician and client.

5. Use of self-help and support groups.

Processes for achieving Transfer and Maintenance Goal 3 — self-monitored maintenance.

1. Practice at self-listening and identification of stuttering behaviors, even brief or barely noticeable ones.

2. Counseling and training in the modification of brief and barely noticeable stuttering behaviors.

3. Counseling and training at recognizing changes in client's attitude, specifically increasing tendency to avoid speech situations and/or stuttering.

4. Use of self-help and support groups.

Processes for achieving Transfer and Maintenance Goal 4 — parent facilitation of child's fluency development

1. Counseling and training families in recognition of subtle signs of returning struggle.

2. Desensitization and empowerment of parents so as to reduce anxious reactions to signs of returning struggle behavior.

3. Training parents and other family members in skills useful in providing a fluency-enhancing atmosphere.

4. Use of family support groups.

Clinician competencies related to transfer and maintenance

1. Is aware of the principles of stimulus generalization and response transfer.

2. Has knowledge of, and can implement a variety of procedures to achieve transfer and maintenance of behavior changes achieved in the clinical setting.

3. Can, through guidance and counseling, help clients develop an attitude toward maintenance that includes an understanding of their own responsibility for their speech yet permits occasional booster session (e.g., the dental model) and that tolerates failure yet appreciates success.

4. Can help the client develop an awareness of the subtler forms of (returning) abnormality and know how to deal with them in a variety of ways, such as the use of home practice, graded hierarchical practice in social situations, and support groups.

5. Knows how to counsel parents regarding changes they can make at home that will facilitate their child's fluency development or encourage the generalization of gains made in treatment.

Reference

Prins, D. (1970). Improvement and regression in stutterers following short-term intensive therapy. *Journal of Speech and Hearing Disorders, 35,* 123-135.

SUBJECT INDEX